PRETERM BIRTH
CAUSES, CONSEQUENCES, AND PREVENTION

Committee on Understanding Premature Birth and
Assuring Healthy Outcomes
Board on Health Sciences Policy

Richard E. Behrman and Adrienne Stith Butler, *Editors*

INSTITUTE OF MEDICINE
OF THE NATIONAL ACADEMIES

THE NATIONAL ACADEMIES PRESS
Washington, D.C.
www.nap.edu

THE NATIONAL ACADEMIES PRESS   500 Fifth Street, N.W.   Washington, DC 20001

NOTICE: The project that is the subject of this report was approved by the Governing Board of the National Research Council, whose members are drawn from the councils of the National Academy of Sciences, the National Academy of Engineering, and the Institute of Medicine. The members of the committee responsible for the report were chosen for their special competences and with regard for appropriate balance.

This study was supported by Contract No. N01-OD-4-2139, Task Order No. 145 between the National Academy of Sciences and the National Institute for Child Health and Human Development, Centers for Disease Control and Prevention, Health Resources and Services Administration, Environmental Protection Agency, and NIH Office of Research on Women's Health; and contracts with the March of Dimes, Burroughs Wellcome Fund, American College of Obstetricians and Gynecologists, American Society for Reproductive Medicine, and the Society for Maternal-Fetal Medicine. Any opinions, findings, conclusions, or recommendations expressed in this publication are those of the authors and do not necessarily reflect the view of the organizations or agencies that provided support for this project.

Library of Congress Cataloging-in-Publication Data

Preterm birth : causes, consequences, and prevention / Committee on
Understanding Premature Birth and Assuring Healthy Outcomes,
Board on Health Sciences Policy ; Richard E. Behrman, Adrienne
Stith Butler, editors.
p. ; cm.
Includes bibliographical references and index.
ISBN-13: 978-0-309-10159-2 (hardback)
ISBN-10: 0-309-10159-X (hardback)
1. Labor, Premature. I. Behrman, Richard E., 1931- . II. Butler,
Adrienne Stith. III. Institute of Medicine (U.S.). Committee on
Understanding Premature Birth and Assuring Healthy Outcomes.
[DNLM: 1. Premature Birth—diagnosis—United States. 2. Premature
Birth—economics—United States. 3. Premature Birth—prevention &
control—United States. 4. Public Policy—United States.
WQ 330 P9413 2006]
RG649.P744 2006
618.3'97—dc22
2006028538

Additional copies of this report are available from the National Academies Press, 500 Fifth Street, N.W., Lockbox 285, Washington, DC 20055; (800) 624-6242 or (202) 334-3313 (in the Washington metropolitan area); Internet, http://www.nap.edu.

For more information about the Institute of Medicine, visit the IOM home page at: www.iom.edu.

The serpent has been a symbol of long life, healing, and knowledge among almost all cultures and religions since the beginning of recorded history. The serpent adopted as a logotype by the Institute of Medicine is a relief carving from ancient Greece, now held by the Staatliche Museen in Berlin.

"Knowing is not enough; we must apply.
Willing is not enough; we must do."
—Goethe

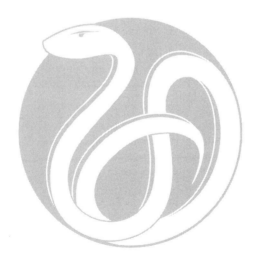

INSTITUTE OF MEDICINE
OF THE NATIONAL ACADEMIES

Advising the Nation. Improving Health.

THE NATIONAL ACADEMIES
Advisers to the Nation on Science, Engineering, and Medicine

The **National Academy of Sciences** is a private, nonprofit, self-perpetuating society of distinguished scholars engaged in scientific and engineering research, dedicated to the furtherance of science and technology and to their use for the general welfare. Upon the authority of the charter granted to it by the Congress in 1863, the Academy has a mandate that requires it to advise the federal government on scientific and technical matters. Dr. Ralph J. Cicerone is president of the National Academy of Sciences.

The **National Academy of Engineering** was established in 1964, under the charter of the National Academy of Sciences, as a parallel organization of outstanding engineers. It is autonomous in its administration and in the selection of its members, sharing with the National Academy of Sciences the responsibility for advising the federal government. The National Academy of Engineering also sponsors engineering programs aimed at meeting national needs, encourages education and research, and recognizes the superior achievements of engineers. Dr. Wm. A. Wulf is president of the National Academy of Engineering.

The **Institute of Medicine** was established in 1970 by the National Academy of Sciences to secure the services of eminent members of appropriate professions in the examination of policy matters pertaining to the health of the public. The Institute acts under the responsibility given to the National Academy of Sciences by its congressional charter to be an adviser to the federal government and, upon its own initiative, to identify issues of medical care, research, and education. Dr. Harvey V. Fineberg is president of the Institute of Medicine.

The **National Research Council** was organized by the National Academy of Sciences in 1916 to associate the broad community of science and technology with the Academy's purposes of furthering knowledge and advising the federal government. Functioning in accordance with general policies determined by the Academy, the Council has become the principal operating agency of both the National Academy of Sciences and the National Academy of Engineering in providing services to the government, the public, and the scientific and engineering communities. The Council is administered jointly by both Academies and the Institute of Medicine. Dr. Ralph J. Cicerone and Dr. Wm. A. Wulf are chair and vice chair, respectively, of the National Research Council.

www.national-academies.org

NORMAN J. WAITZMAN, Associate Professor, Deparment of Economics, University of Utah, Salt Lake City

XIAOBIN WANG, Director and Mary Ann and J. Milburn Smith Research Professor, Children's Memorial Hospital and Children's Memorial Research Center, Chicago, IL

Health Sciences Policy Board Liaison

GAIL H. CASSELL, Vice President, Scientific Affairs, Distinguished Lilly Research Scholar for Infectious Diseases, Eli Lilly and Company, Indianapolis, IN

IOM Project Staff

ADRIENNE STITH BUTLER, Study Director
EILEEN J. SANTA, Research Associate
THELMA L. COX, Senior Program Assistant

Copy Editor

MICHAEL HAYES

Reviewers

This report has been reviewed in draft form by individuals chosen for their diverse perspectives and technical expertise, in accordance with procedures approved by the NRC's Report Review Committee. The purpose of this independent review is to provide candid and critical comments that will assist the institution in making its published report as sound as possible and to ensure that the report meets institutional standards for objectivity, evidence, and responsiveness to the study charge. The review comments and draft manuscript remain confidential to protect the integrity of the deliberative process. We wish to thank the following individuals for their review of this report:

GLEN AYLWARD, Southern Illinois University School of Medicine
PAULA A. BRAVEMAN, University of California, San Francisco School of Medicine
CHRISTOS COUTIFARIS, University of Pennsylvania Medical Center
JANET CURRIE, Columbia University
M. SEAN ESPLIN, University of Utah Health Sciences Center
NEIL FINER, University of California, San Diego
THOMAS J. GARITE, Professor Emeritus, University of California, Irvine
LAURA GLYNN, University of California, Irvine
JOHN GODDEERIS, Michigan State University
MAUREEN HACK, Case Western Reserve University
HOWARD HU, Harvard School of Public Health

KATHY S. KATZ, Georgetown University Hospital
CHARLES LOCKWOOD, Yale University School of Medicine
JEROME F. STRAUSS, Virginia Commonwealth University School of Medicine
MICHELLE A. WILLIAMS, University of Washington School of Public Health and Community Medicine

Although the reviewers listed above have provided many constructive comments and suggestions, they were not asked to endorse the conclusions or recommendations nor did they see the final draft of the report before its release. The review of this report was overseen by NANCY E. ADLER. Appointed by the National Research Council, she was responsible for making certain that an independent examination of this report was carried out in accordance with institutional procedures and that all review comments were carefully considered. Responsibility for the final content of this report rests entirely with the authoring committee and the institution.

Preface

Preterm birth and its consequences constitute a major health problem in the United States and worldwide. However, there has been relatively little attention from the public and research community despite the significant impact preterm birth and prematurity have on infant mortality and subsequent disabilities of many survivors, and on societal and economic costs to the nation. This health problem is associated with multiple complex and poorly understood, but interrelated, biologic, psychologic, and social factors that appear to be expressed in the common pathway of preterm birth. Low socioeconomic status alone does not explain the increase in preterm births among African Americans compared to the white non-Hispanic population.

Prenatal care is currently primarily directed at identifying and managing preeclampsia; maternal infections, diabetes, and other major illnesses; birth defects; and intrauterine fetal growth failure. As our knowledge and understanding of preterm birth increase, prenatal care will provide a health infrastructure for women from which it is possible to prevent, diagnose, and treat preterm births.

The nature of this health problem and the charge to the committee required a comprehensive assessment as well as an in depth analysis resulting in a large-volume report. The Committee suggests that readers first review the executive summary for essential ideas and recommendations, then turn to the abstracts of each chapter before reading each of the individual chapters.

Richard E. Behrman, M.D.
Chair
Committee on Understanding Premature Birth
and Assuring Healthy Outcomes

Acknowledgments

Several individuals and organizations made important contributions to the study committee's process and to this report. The committee wishes to thank these individuals, but recognizes that attempts to identify all and acknowledge their contributions would require more space than is available in this brief section.

To begin, the committee would like to thank the sponsors of this report. Funds for the committee's work were provided by the National Institute for Child Health and Human Development, the Centers for Disease Control and Prevention, the Health Resources and Services Administration, March of Dimes, Burroughs Wellcome Fund, American College of Obstetricians and Gynecologists, Environmental Protection Agency, National Institutes of Health Office of Research on Women's Health, American Society for Reproductive Medicine, and the Society for Maternal-Fetal Medicine. The committee thanks Capt. Donald Mattison, Scott Grosse, and Samuel Posner, who served as project officers and who were instrumental in the initiation of this activity. The committee thanks Ann Koontz, Marina Weiss, Nancy Green, Lisa Potetz, Enriqueta Bond, Nancy Sung, Ralph Hale, Nicole Owens, Lanelle Bembenek Wiggins, Vivian Pinn, Loretta Finnegan, Robert Rebar, and Richard Depp for their support and guidance on the committee's task. Special recognition is also given to Eli Adashi and Gloria Sarto for the fundamental roles they played in the initiation of this activity.

The committee found the perspectives of many individuals and organizations to be valuable in understanding the causes and consequences of preterm birth. The committee thanks the numerous individuals and organizations who generously provided information and assistance during deliberations. Appendix A of this report contains the names of those who participated in the committee's meetings by providing important information at its open workshops.

The committee also gratefully acknowledges the contributions of the many individuals who assisted the committee in its work, either by providing data and research support or by assisting in the preparation of draft material. The committee would like to thank Brent James and Intermountain Healthcare (IHC) for data used to generate the cost estimates provided in the chapter, "Societal Costs of Preterm Birth." In particular, Pascal Briot, Russell Staheli, and Erick Henry performed much of the data generation used for the medical care estimates. C. Jason Wang of the RAND Corporation served as an appointed consultant and assisted the committee in preparation of the chapter, "Public Policies Affected by Preterm Birth." James Perrin of Massachusetts General Hospital, and Wendy Chavkin and Blair Johnson of Columbia University's Mailman School of Public Health also served as appointed consultants and provided information on policies related to preterm birth. Stavros Petrou of the University of Oxford, an appointed consultant, provided information and assistance on the economic consequences of preterm birth. Ciaran Phibbs of Stanford University; Wanda Barfield of the Massachusetts Department of Public Health; Charles Mercier of the University of Vermont; Joyce Martin of the Centers for Disease Control and Prevention; Mona Rowe of the National Institutes of Health; Ralph Hale, Albert Strunk, Bernice Rose, Nonda Wilson, Donna Kovacheva of the American College of Obstetricians and Gynecologists; Mario Merialdi of the World Health Organization; and Vipul Mankad of the University of Kentucky provided information, reports, and data. The committee thanks each of these individuals.

Finally, the committee would also like to thank the authors whose paper contributions added to the evidence base that the committee examined. These include John A.F. Zupancic, Harvard Medical School; Gerri R. Baer and Robert M. Nelson, The Children's Hospital of Philadelphia and the University of Pennsylvania School of Medicine; and Greg R. Alexander, University of South Florida.

Contents

Summary		1
1	Introduction	31
Section I Measurement		53
2	Measurement of Fetal and Infant Maturity	55
	Section I Recommendations	84
Section II Causes of Preterm Birth		87
3	Behavioral and Psychosocial Contributors to Preterm Birth	89
4	Sociodemographic and Community Factors Contributing to Preterm Birth	124
5	Medical and Pregnancy Conditions Associated with Preterm Birth	148
6	Biological Pathways Leading to Preterm Birth	169
7	Role of Gene-Environment Interactions in Preterm Birth	207
8	The Role of Environmental Toxicants in Preterm Birth	229
	Section II Recommendations	255
Section III Diagnosis and Treatment of Preterm Labor		259
9	Diagnosis and Treatment of Conditions Leading to Spontaneous Preterm Birth	261
	Section III Recommendations	308

Section IV Consequences of Preterm Birth   311
10   Mortality and Acute Complications in Preterm Infants   313
11   Neurodevelopmental, Health, and Family Outcomes for
     Infants Born Preterm   346
12   Societal Costs of Preterm Birth   398

     Section IV Recommendations   430

Section V Research and Policy   433
13   Barriers to Clinical Research on Preterm Birth and Outcomes
     for Preterm Infants   435
14   Public Policies Affected by Preterm Birth   455

     Section V Recommendations   473

15   A Research Agenda to Investigate Preterm Birth   477

REFERENCES   493

APPENDIXES
A   Data Sources and Methods   591
B   Prematurity at Birth: Determinants, Consequences, and
     Geographic Variation   604
C   A Review of Ethical Issues Involved in Premature Birth   644
D   A Systematic Review of Costs Associated with Preterm Birth   688
E   Selected Programs Funding Preterm Birth Research   725
F   Committee and Staff Biographies   732

INDEX   741

PRETERM BIRTH

Summary

ABSTRACT

In 2004, 12.5 percent of births in the United States were preterm; that is, born at less than 37 completed weeks of gestation. This rate has increased steadily in the past decade. There are significant, persistent, and very troubling racial, ethnic, and socioeconomic disparities in the rates of preterm birth. The highest rates are for non-Hispanic African Americans, and the lowest are for Asians or Pacific Islanders. In 2003, the rate for African-American women was 17.8 percent, whereas the rates were 10.5 percent for Asian and Pacific Islander women and 11.5 percent for white women. The most notable increases from 2001 to 2003 were for white non-Hispanic, American Indian, and Hispanic groups.

Infants born preterm are at greater risk than infants born at term for mortality and a variety of health and developmental problems. Complications include acute respiratory, gastrointestinal, immunologic, central nervous system, hearing, and vision problems, as well as longer-term motor, cognitive, visual, hearing, behavioral, social-emotional, health, and growth problems. The birth of a preterm infant can also bring considerable emotional and economic costs to families and have implications for public-sector services, such as health insurance, educational, and other social support systems. The annual societal economic burden associated with preterm birth in the United States was at least $26.2 billion in 2005. The greatest risk of mortality and morbidity is for those infants born at *the earliest gestational ages. However, those infants born nearer to term represent the greatest number of infants born preterm and also experience more complications than infants born at term. Preterm birth is a complex cluster of problems with a set of overlapping factors of influence. Its causes may include individual-level behavioral and psychosocial factors, neighborhood characteristics, environmental exposures, medical conditions, infertility treatments, biological factors, and genetics. Many of these factors occur in combination, particularly in those who are socioeconomically disadvantaged or who are members of racial and ethnic minority groups.*

The current methods for the diagnosis and treatment of preterm labor are currently based on an inadequate literature, and little is know about how preterm birth can be prevented. Treatment has been focused on inhibiting contractions. This has not reduced the incidence of preterm birth but has delayed delivery long enough to allow the administration of antenatal steroids and transfer of the mother and fetus to a hospital where they may receive appropriate care. These interventions have reduced the rates of perinatal mortality and morbidity. Although improvements in perinatal and neonatal care have significantly improved the rates of survival for infants born preterm, these infants remain at risk for a host of acute and chronic health problems. Therapies and interventions for the prediction and the prevention of preterm birth are thus needed.

Upon review of the literature assessing the causes and consequences of preterm birth, the diagnosis and treatment of women at risk for preterm labor, and treatments for infants born preterm, the committee proposes a research agenda for investigating the problem of preterm birth that is intended to help focus and direct research efforts. Priority areas are: (1) the establishment of multidisciplinary research centers; (2) improved research in three areas including better definition of the problem of preterm birth with improved data, clinical and health services research investigations, and etiologic and epidemiologic investigations; and (3) the study and informing of public policy. The committee hopes that its efforts will help provide a framework for working toward improved outcomes for children born preterm and their families.

The prevalence of preterm birth in the United States constitutes a public health problem, but unlike many health problems, the rate of preterm birth has increased in the last decade. In 2004, 12.5 percent of births were preterm, or in which the infants were born at less than 37 weeks of gestation (CDC, 2005a). Since 1981, the rate has increased more than 30 percent (from 9.4 percent) (CDC, 2005a). The birth of a preterm infant results in significant health consequences to the infant and emotional and economic costs for families and communities. Although advances in perinatal and neonatal care have improved the survival for preterm infants, those infants who do survive have a greater risk of developmental disabilities, health, and growth problems than infants born at full term. Whereas the group of infants with the greatest risk of morbidity and mortality comprises those born at less than 32 weeks of gestation, infants born between 32 and 36 weeks represent the greatest number of infants born preterm. The latter group of infants also experiences a greater risk for health and developmental problems compared with the risk for infants born at term. To date, no single test or sequence of assessment measures that may accurately predict preterm birth are available, and efforts at the prevention of preterm birth have primarily focused on the treatment of women with symptomatic preterm labor.

STUDY CHARGE

The persistent and troubling problem of preterm birth prompted the Institute of Medicine (IOM) to convene a committee, the Committee on Understanding Premature Birth and Assuring Healthy Outcomes, to assess the current state of the science on the causes and broad consequences of preterm birth. Specifically, the charge to the committee was as follows:

An IOM committee will define and address the health related and economic consequences of premature birth. The broad goals are to (1) describe the current state of the science and clinical research with respect to the causes of premature birth; (2) address the broad costs—economic, medical, social, psychological, and educational—for children and their families; and (3) establish a framework for action in addressing the range of priority issues, including a research and policy agenda for the future. In support of these broad goals, the study will:

- Review and assess the various factors contributing to the growing incidence of premature birth, which may include the trend to delay childbearing and racial and ethnic disparities;
- Assess the economic costs and other societal burdens associated with premature births;
- Address research gaps/needs and priorities for defining the mechanisms by which biological and environmental factors influence premature birth; and
- Explore possible changes in public health policy and other policies that may benefit from more research.

In order to assess research gaps and needs, the committee will plan an additional meeting that will address barriers to clinical research in the area of preterm birth. A workshop hosted by the committee will seek to

• Identify major obstacles to conducting clinical research, which may include the declining number of residents interested in entering the field of obstetrics and gynecology and the resulting effect on the pipeline of clinical researchers; the impact of rising medical malpractice premiums on the ability of academic programs to provide protected time for physicians to pursue research; and ethical and legal issues in conducting research on pregnant women (for example, the consideration of safety issues and informed consent); and
• Provide strategies for removing barriers—including those targeting resident career choices, departments of obstetrics and gynecology, agencies and organizations that fund research, and professional organizations.

Through this process the committee learned four key lessons. The first is that preterm birth is a complex expression of many conditions. Second, little is known about how preterm birth can be prevented. Great strides have been made in treating infants born preterm and improving survival. However, any significant gains to be made in the study of preterm birth will be in the area of preventing its occurrence. Third, racial-ethnic and socioeconomic disparities are striking and largely unexplained. Fourth, infants who are born near term or late preterm (at 32 to 36 weeks of gestation) are at increased risk for adverse health and developmental outcomes that should not be ignored.

This summary presents an overview of the committee's recommendations. Below, these recommendations are preceded by text summarizing the evidence base from which they are drawn. For full findings and justification of each recommendation, the reader is referred to the full committee report.

APPROACH TO THE PROBLEM

Three themes repeatedly emerged at the start of the committee's deliberations that helped to organize the committee's thinking and approach to this problem. The first was a need for clarity of terminology. In the literature, terms characterizing the duration of gestation, fetal growth, and maturation have been applied inconsistently and have been used interchangeably. This has made it difficult to interpret the data on the causes and consequences of preterm birth and to evaluate treatments. The committee uses the term *preterm birth,* which is based on the period of gestation, to assess this population. The evidence contained in this report draws first on the literature that uses gestational age, preterm birth, and small for gestational age as outcomes. In the absence of this information, low birth weight and other related outcomes are cited, as needed. The committee recognizes that the weight of the evidence in this field has used low birth weight to assess this population.

The second theme that guided the committee's approach to its task was the troubling evidence of long-standing disparities in the rates of preterm birth among different groups in the U.S. population. Certain subpopulations categorized by their racial, ethnic, or socioeconomic status have a greater risk and a higher proportion of preterm births. The most striking rates are for African-American women. In 2003, the proportions of preterm births for specific racial and ethnic groups were 10.5 percent for Asian Pacific Islander women, 11.5 percent for non-Hispanic white women, 11.9 percent for Hispanic women, 13.5 percent for American Indian/Alaska Native women, and 17.8 percent for non-Hispanic African American women (CDC, 2005i). Although the rate for African American women has decreased in the last decade, overall these women continue to experience a much higher proportion of preterm births. The most notable increase in the percentages of preterm birth from 2001 to 2003 was for white non-Hispanic, American Indian, and Hispanic groups. Although the rates for Hispanic and Asian Pacific Islander women are the lowest among the ethnic and racial minority groups in the United States, these are not homogeneous populations, and considerable variation in the rates of preterm birth exist among subpopulations.

The third theme that guided the committee's framing of this problem and formulation of recommendations is the complexity of the problem that it was charged with assessing. Preterm birth is not one disease for which there is likely to be one solution or cure. Rather, the committee considers preterm birth a cluster of problems with a set of overlapping factors of influence that are interrelated. This complexity makes the detection of solutions to the problem difficult. There will be no silver bullet. The complex nature of this problem led the committee to consider its causes in an integrated manner. These causes are multiple and may vary for different populations. Individual-level behavioral and psychosocial factors, neighborhood social characteristics, environmental exposures, medical conditions, infertility treatments, biological factors, and genetics may play roles to various degrees. Many of these factors are present together, particularly among women of low socioeconomic or minority status.

After reviewing the evidence, the committee proposes a research agenda for investigating the problem of preterm birth. The agenda is presented to help focus and direct research efforts. The recommendations are grouped and prioritized and therefore presented in a different sequence than they appear in the full report; however, their numeric designation remains the same.

Priority areas are grouped as follows:

I.   Establish Multidisciplinary Research Centers

II.   Priority Areas for Research

- *Better define the problem of preterm birth with improved data*
  Recommendations included in this category pertain to the need for
  improved collection of surveillance and descriptive data in order to
  better define the nature and scope of the problem of preterm birth.
  1. Improve national data
  2. Study the economic outcomes for infants born preterm

- *Conduct clinical and health services research investigations*
  Recommendations in this category pertain to the need to examine
  and improve the clinical treatment of women who deliver preterm
  and infants born preterm and the health care systems that care for
  them.
  1. Improve the methods of identifying and treating women at risk
  for preterm labor
  2. Study the acute and the long-term outcomes for infants born
  preterm
  3. Study infertility treatments and institute guidelines to reduce
  the number of multiple gestations
  4. Improve the quality of care for women at risk for preterm labor and infants born preterm
  5. Investigate the impact of the health care delivery system on
  preterm birth

- *Conduct etiologic and epidemiologic investigations*
  Recommendations in this category pertain to the need to examine
  the potential causes of preterm birth and its distribution in the population.
  1. Investigate the etiologies of preterm birth
  2. Study the multiple psychosocial, behavioral, and environmental risk factors associated with preterm birth simultaneously
  3. Investigate racial-ethnic and socioeconomic disparities in the
  rates of preterm birth

III. **Study and Inform Public Policy**
      Recommendations in this final group pertain to the need to under-
      stand the impact of preterm birth on various public programs and
      how policies can be used to reduce rates of preterm birth.

Categories under group II are not prioritized because the committee believes that they are actions that should occur simultaneously. However, recommendations within the categories are prioritized. The policy recommendations are listed last, as information resulting from previous recommendations will be needed in order to analyze and improve policies pertaining to preterm birth.

AN AGENDA TO INVESTIGATE PRETERM BIRTH

I. Establish Multidisciplinary Research Centers

The complexity of interrelated biological, psychological, social, and environmental factors that are involved in preterm birth necessitates a multidisciplinary approach to research directed at understanding its etiologies, pathophysiology, diagnosis, and treatment. In addition to the scientific and clinical challenges, other important barriers must be addressed. Although some of these barriers are common to physician scientists in all clinical disciplines, others are unique to physician scientists trained in obstetrics and gynecology. Of primary importance are the recruitment and participation of scientists in the types of investigations that must be pursued to address preterm birth. In general, there has been a chronic lack of the resources needed to train clinical investigators and support clinical research (IOM, 1994; Nathan and Wilson, 2003; NIH, 1997; NRC, 2000, 2004). A major roadblock to advancing research on preterm birth and its consequences is thus the lack of experienced clinician scientists to conduct research and serve as mentors in obstetrics and gynecology. Other barriers include problems related to the career choices and training of new physicians (Gariti et al., 2005); the difficulties with conducting clinical investigations, particularly drug studies, during pregnancy; the relatively low levels of research funding, given the size of the problem; ethical and liability issues (A. Strunk, personal communication, January 10 and January 12, 2006); and the need for coordinated scientific leadership in the field (see Chapter 13).

Recommendation V-1: *The National Institutes of Health and private foundations should establish integrated multidisciplinary research centers. The objective of these centers will be to focus on understanding the causes of preterm birth and the health outcomes for women and their infants who were born preterm.*

Consistent with the Roadmap initiative of the National Institutes of Health, these activities should include the following:

• Basic, translational, and clinical research involving the clinical, basic, and behavioral and social science disciplines is needed. This research should include but not be limited to investigations covered by recommendations pertaining to the etiologies of preterm birth; the psychosocial, behavioral, sociodemographic, and environmental toxicant exposure-related risk factors associated with preterm birth; the disparities in the rates of preterm birth by race and ethnicity; the identification and treatment of women at risk of preterm labor; quality of health care provided to infants born preterm; and health services research.

• Sustained intellectual leadership of these research activities is essential to make progress in understanding and improving the outcomes for women and their infants who have been born preterm.

• Mentored research training programs should be integral parts of these centers. Fostering the development of basic and clinical researchers, including facilitating opportunities for funding and promotion, is critical.

• Funding agencies should provide ample and sustained funds to allow these centers to investigate the complex syndrome of preterm birth, analogous to programs developed to study cancer and cardiovascular disease.

II.   Priority Areas for Research

Better Define the Problem of Preterm Birth with Improved Data

1. Improve National Data

The concept of prematurity involves biological immaturity for extrauterine life. Maturation is the process of achieving full development or growth. Infants born preterm have immature organ systems that often need additional support to survive. The degree of maturity, therefore, is the major determinant of mortality and morbidity (the short- and long-term complications) of preterm birth.

Accurate definitions of preterm birth are essential for comparing and interpreting the various studies that evaluate the etiologies and mechanisms of preterm birth; the efficacies of treatments for the prevention of preterm birth; the health and neurodevelopmental outcomes of infants born preterm; and efficacies of the strategies used to treat infants born preterm. Early efforts at defining prematurity relied on birth weight. The primary problem with the use of birth weight as a proxy for prematurity is that it identifies infants who are heterogeneous for fetal development and may miss some preterm infants. At any given gestational age, there is a distribution of birth weights such that some infants appear to be within the norm for their gestational age, some appear to be relatively light, and others appear to be quite heavy (Battaglia and Lubchenco, 1967). These categorizations of growth for gestational age have implications for mortality and morbidity. Thus, many preterm infants who are large for gestational age have normal birth weights but have rates of mortality and morbidity different from those of full-term infants with normal birth weights. Few studies report outcomes by gestational age category.

The inaccuracy of data on gestational age is a major problem for research on preterm birth. Several methods are used to determine gestational age. Early prenatal ultrasounds (before 20 weeks of gestation) are more accurate than any other prenatal or postnatal estimate of pregnancy duration (Alexander et al., 1992; Chervenak et al., 1998; Nyberg et al., 2004). Despite its accuracy in estimating gestational age, the routine use of prenatal ultrasounds to estimate the duration of pregnancy is limited by several factors. Access to prenatal care is an issue for many of the women who are at the highest risk of preterm delivery (i.e., young, poor, and immigrant women); and there are racial disparities in prenatal care. In addition, the United States has no national standard for the routine use of prenatal ultrasound. Although more pregnant women in the United States are receiving ultrasounds than in the past (68 percent in 2002 versus 48 percent in 1989), many may be performed too late in pregnancy or the quality of the ultrasound may not be sufficient for the accurate and reliable estimation of the duration of pregnancy (Martin et al., 2003). Although early prenatal ultrasound is a good recommendation for obstetric practice, for research an earlier ultrasound (well within the first trimester) would be better, as it would allow investigation of potential factors that affect the growth trajectory earlier in pregnancy.

Although much attention has been paid to obtaining accurate obstetric estimates of gestational age, there is a similar need for more methods of assessing fetal and infant maturity. Maturity assessment is even more important when gestational age is unknown or uncertain. In lieu of functional measures of fetal or infant maturity, accurate measures of gestational age are essential for clinical care as well as research on the causes, mechanisms, and outcomes of preterm birth.

The National Center for Health Statistics develops standards for uniform reporting of live births and fetal, neonatal, and infant deaths to national public health databases. Although birth certificates are intended to establish the date of birth, citizenship, and nationality, they contain valuable public health information and are the only national source of birth weight and gestational age data. Large state and national population databases with birth and death certificate data have been used to plot gestational age distributions, birth weight for gestational age, and gestational age- and birth weight-specific rates of neonatal mortality. Gestational age is used to calculate a variety of statistical indicators used to monitor the health of mothers and their children in a population. These indicators can be used to target public health interventions and monitor their effects.

Recommendation I-1: *Promote the collection of improved perinatal data. The National Center for Health Statistics of the Centers for Disease Control and Prevention should promote and use a national mechanism to collect, record, and report perinatal data.*

The following key elements should be included:

• The quality of gestational age measurements in vital records should be evaluated. Vital records should indicate the accuracy of the gestational age determined by ultrasound early in pregnancy (less than 20 weeks of gestation).
• Birth weight for gestational age should be considered one measure of the adequacy of fetal growth.
• Perinatal mortality and morbidity should be reported by gestational age, birth weight, and birth weight for gestational age.
• A categorization or coding scheme that reflects the heterogeneous etiologies of preterm birth should be developed and implemented.
• Vital records should also state whether fertility treatments (including in vitro fertilization and ovulation promotion) were used. The committee recognizes that the nature of these data is private and sensitive.

Recommendation I-2: *Encourage the use of ultrasound early in pregnancy to establish gestational age. Because it is recognized that more precise measures of gestational age are needed to move the field forward, professional societies should encourage the use of ultrasound early in pregnancy (less than 20 weeks of gestation) to establish gestational age and should establish standards of practice and recommendations for the training of personnel to improve the reliability and the quality of ultrasound data.*

Recommendation I-3: *Develop indicators of maturational age. Funding agencies should support and investigators should develop reliable and precise perinatal (prenatal and postnatal) standards as indicators of maturational age.*

2. Study the Economic Outcomes for Infants Born Preterm

To date, research on the medical cost of prematurity has focused nearly exclusively on inpatient care and has primarily focused on the cost for the initial hospitalization of the infant (see the review by John Zupancic in

Appendix D). Several of these studies have provided estimates of the hospitalization cost exclusively by low birth weight (Rogowski, 1999), others have provided estimates exclusively by gestational age (Phibbs and Schmitt, 2006), whereas still others have provided estimates by both gestational age and low birth weight (Gilbert et al., 2003; Schmitt et al., 2006). This literature has drawn specific attention to the high costs associated with neonatal intensive care for preterm infants. Little is known, however, about the medical care costs of preterm birth beyond early hospitalization or about the costs associated with early intervention services, special education, or indirect costs, such as lost productivity. Lifetime estimates of cost, however, have been made for certain critical conditions and developmental disabilities associated with preterm birth and low birth weight, such as specific birth defects (Waitzman et al., 1996), cerebral palsy (CDC, 2004c; Honeycutt et al., 2003; Waitzman et al., 1996), mental retardation, and hearing loss and vision impairment (CDC, 2004c; Honeycutt et al., 2003).

On the basis of new estimates provided by the committee, the annual societal economic burden associated with preterm birth in the United States was at least $26.2 billion in 2005, or $51,600 per infant born preterm. Nearly two-thirds of the societal cost was accounted for by medical care. The share that medical care services contributed to the total cost was $16.9 billion ($33,200 per preterm infant), with more than 85 percent of those medical care services delivered in infancy. Maternal delivery costs contributed another $1.9 billion ($3,800 per preterm infant). Early intervention services cost an estimated $611 million ($1,200 per infant), whereas special education services associated with a higher prevalence of four disabling conditions, including cerebral palsy, mental retardation, vision impairment, and hearing loss among premature infants added $1.1 billion ($2,200 per preterm infant). Lost household and labor market productivity associated with those disabling conditions contributed $5.7 billion ($11,200 per preterm infant).

Recommendation IV-2: *Investigate the economic consequences of preterm birth. Researchers should investigate the gaps in understanding of the economic consequences of preterm birth to establish the foundation for accurate economic evaluation of the relative value of policies directed at prevention and guidelines for treatment.*

This research should:

• Assess the long-term educational, social, productivity, and medical costs associated with preterm birth, as well as the distributions of such costs;

• Undertake multivariate modeling to refine the understanding of what drives the large variance of the economic burden, even by gestational age at birth;

• Be ongoing to provide the basis for ongoing assessments; and

• Establish the basis for refined economic assessment of policies and interventions that would reduce the economic burden.

Conduct Clinical and Health Services Research Investigations

1. Improve the Methods of Identifying and Treating Women at Risk for Preterm Labor

In the past 30 years, important strides in obstetric and neonatal tertiary care have been made to reduce the rates of infant morbidity and mortality as a result of preterm birth. However, the primary and secondary interventions implemented to date have not reduced the rate of preterm birth. Current prenatal care is focused on risks other than preterm birth. Birth defects, adequate fetal growth, preeclampsia, gestational diabetes, selected infections, and the complications of postdate pregnancy are emphasized in the prenatal record (see Chapter 9). Preterm birth has historically not been emphasized in prenatal care, in the belief that the majority of preterm births are due to social rather than medical or obstetrical causes (Main et al., 1985; Taylor, 1985) or are the appropriate result of pathological processes that would benefit the mother or infant.

African-American women deliver their infants before 37 weeks of gestation twice as often as women of other races and deliver their infants before 32 weeks of gestation three times as often as white women. The strongest risk factors in all ethnic groups are multiple gestations, a history of preterm birth, and vaginal bleeding.

The prevention of preterm birth by the use of interventions targeting a variety of risk factors has been attempted, but these interventions have largely been without success. The diagnosis and treatment of preterm labor are currently based on an inadequate literature and are compromised by an incomplete understanding of the sequence and timing of events that precede clinical evidence of preterm labor. The accurate diagnosis of early preterm labor is difficult because the symptoms (Iams et al., 1994) and signs (Moore et al., 1994) of preterm labor occur commonly in normal women who do not deliver preterm and because manual examination of the cervix in early labor is not highly reproducible (Berghella et al., 1997; Jackson et al., 1992). Treatment efforts are primarily focused on inhibiting contractions in women with preterm labor. This approach has not decreased the incidence of preterm birth but can delay delivery long enough to allow administration of antenatal steroids and to transfer the mother and fetus to the appropriate hospital, two interventions that have consistently been shown to reduce perinatal mortality and morbidity (Towers et al., 2000; Yeast et al., 1998). The goal of the prevention of preterm birth is subordinate to the goal of improved perinatal morbidity and mortality. This goal is important, because the continuation of pregnancy in women with preterm parturition in some instances may increase the health risks for the mother or the fetus, or both.

Recommendation III-1: *Improve methods for the identification and treatment of women at increased risk of preterm labor. Researchers should investigate ways to improve methods to identify and treat women with an increased risk of preterm labor.*

Specifically:

• The content and structure of prenatal care should include an assessment of the risk of preterm labor.
• Improved methods for the identification of women at increased risk of preterm labor both before pregnancy and in the first and second trimesters are needed.
• Combinations of known markers of preterm labor (e.g., a prior preterm birth, ethnicity, a short cervix, and biochemical and biophysical markers) and potential new markers (e.g., genetic markers) should be studied to allow the creation of an individualized composite assessment of risk.
• More accurate methods are needed to
    • diagnose preterm labor,
    • assess fetal health to identify women and fetuses that are and that are not candidates for the arrest of labor, and
    • arrest labor.
• The success of perinatal care during preterm birth should be based primarily on perinatal morbidity and mortality rates as well as the rate of preterm birth, the numbers of infants born with low birth weights, or neonatal morbidity and mortality.

2. Study Acute and Long-Term Outcomes for Infants Born Preterm

Although the mortality rate for preterm infants and the gestational age-specific mortality rate have improved dramatically over the last three to four decades, preterm infants remain vulnerable to many complications. These complications often arise from still immature organ systems that are not yet prepared to support extrauterine life. There is a progressive increase in the risk for complications of prematurity and acute neonatal illness with decreasing gestational age, reflecting the fragility and immaturity of the brain, lungs, immune system, kidneys, skin, eyes, and gastrointestinal system. In general, the more immature the preterm infant is, the greater the degree of life support required. The outcomes for preterm infants are also influenced by the extrauterine environment, which includes the neonatal intensive care unit (NICU), the home, and the community.

Among the earliest concerns about the health of premature infants is the increased risk for neurodevelopmental disabilities. The spectrum of neurodevelopmental disabilities includes cerebral palsy, mental retardation, visual impairment, and hearing impairment. The more subtle disorders of central nervous system function include language disorders, learning disabilities, attention deficit hyperactivity disorder, minor neuromotor dysfunction or developmental coordination disorders, behavioral problems, and social-emotional difficulties. The literature demonstrates wide variations in the prevalence of neurodevelopmental disabilities (Allen, 2002; Aylward, 2005). Many of these variations are due to methodological problems; for example, a lack of uniformity in sample selection criteria, the method and the length of follow-up, follow-up rates, the outcome measures used, and diagnostic criteria. The variabilities in the outcome frequencies reported also reflect differences in the population base and in clinical practice. The mortality and neurodevelopmental disability rates for moderately preterm infants with gestational ages of 33 to 36 weeks are higher than those for full-term infants (although they are lower than those for more-preterm infants). Children born near term have also been reported to have greater delays in achieving infant developmental milestones (and more difficulty with hyperactivity, fine motor skills, mathematics, speaking, reading, and writing) (Hediger et al., 2002; Huddy et al., 2001).

The most frequently cited evidence of a higher risk for adverse health status among preterm infants is an increased risk of rehospitalization during the first few years of life (Hack et al., 1993; McCormick et al., 1980) and a disproportionate duration of stay for those hospitalizations (Cavalier et al., 1996; McCormick et al., 1980). Among the conditions leading to poorer health are reactive airway disease or asthma, recurrent ear infections, and the possible sequelae of problems encountered as a neonate, like strabismus (McGauhey et al., 1991).

Families caring for a child born preterm also face long-term and multilayered challenges. The limited research on this topic suggests that the impact is largely negative (Macey et al., 1987; McCormick et al., 1986; Taylor et al., 2001; Veddovi et al., 2001), such as maternal depression and psychological distress, although some studies have found positive outcomes (Macey et al., 1987; Saigal et al., 2000a; Singer et al., 1999), such as positive interactions with friends and within the family. Furthermore, the impact varies according to sociodemographic factors as well as the severity of the child's health condition (Eisengart et al., 2003; McCormick et al., 1986; Rivers et al., 1987; Saigal et al., 2000a).

Early intervention programs have been demonstrated to be effective, at least in the short term, in improving some cognitive outcomes for individual children born preterm. They also have the potential to lead to important improvements in family function (Berlin et al., 1998; Majnemer and Snider, 2005; McCormick et al., 1998; Ramey and Ramey, 1999; Ramey et al., 1992). Although evidence on the long-term effects of early intervention programs is inconclusive, some longitudinal follow-up studies have noted that they have continued beneficial effects (McCormick et al., 2006).

Recommendation IV-1: *Develop guidelines for the reporting of infant outcomes. The National Institutes of Health, the U.S. Department of Education, other funding agencies, and investigators should develop guidelines for determining and reporting outcomes for infants born preterm that better reflect their health, neurodevelopmental, educational, social, and emotional outcomes across the life span and conduct research to determine methods that can be used to optimize these outcomes.*

Specifically,

• Outcomes should be reported by gestational age categories, in addition to birth weight categories; and better methods of measuring fetal and infant maturity should be devised.

• Obstetrics-perinatology departments and pediatrics-neonatology departments should work together to establish guidelines to achieve a more uniform approach to evaluating and reporting outcomes, including ages of evaluation, measurement tools, and the minimum duration of follow-up. The measurement tools should cover a broad range of outcomes and should include quality of life and the elicitation of outcome preferences from adolescents and adults born preterm and their families.

• Long-term outcome studies should be conducted into adolescence and adulthood to determine the extent of recovery, if any, and to monitor individuals who were born preterm for the onset of disease during adulthood as a result of being born preterm.

• Research should identify better neonatal predictors of neurodevelopmental disabilities, functional outcomes, and other long-term outcomes. These will allow improved counseling of the parents, enhance the safety of trials of interventions for mothers and their infants by providing more immediate feedback on infant development, and facilitate planning for the use of comprehensive follow-up and early intervention services.

• Follow-up and outcome evaluations for infants involved in maternal trials of prenatal means of prevention or treatment of threatened preterm delivery and infant trials of means of prevention and treatment of organ injury not only should report the infant's gestational age at delivery and any neonatal morbidity but also should include neurological and cognitive outcomes. Specific outcomes should be tailored to answer the study questions.

• Research should identify and evaluate the efficacies of postnatal interventions that improve outcomes.

3. Study Infertility Treatments and Institute Guidelines to Reduce the Number of Multiple Gestations

The use of infertility treatments has risen dramatically in the past 20 years and has been associated with the trend to delay childbearing. In 2002, 33,000 American women delivered babies as a result of assisted reproductive technology (ART) procedures, more than twice the number who had done so in 1996 (Meis et al., 1998). More than 50 percent of these women were 35 years of age or older. In recent years, an unintended consequence of these technologies, multiple gestations and the increased risk for preterm delivery, has become a focus of attention. There is also evidence of an association between the underlying causes of infertility and subfecundity (long time to becoming pregnant) and preterm birth (Henriksen et al., 1997; Joffe and Li, 1994). Preterm birth in relation to ART may be different in its pathogenesis than most other cases.

ART involves procedures in which the egg and sperm are handled in the laboratory, including in vitro fertilization (IVF) procedures. Since 1996, the federal government has mandated that all clinics performing ART procedures report their outcomes to the CDC (Meis et al., 1998). Even though ART use must be reported, other reproductive technologies not classified as ART are not. The CDC definition of ART does not include treatments in which only sperm are handled (for example, for intrauterine or artificial insemination) or procedures in which a woman takes medication to stimulate egg production without the intention of having eggs retrieved. The frequency of use and the number of births attributable to this technique are unknown. This is an important gap in current knowledge.

Multiple gestations are more common in assisted reproduction than in natural conception. The major cause underlying the increased risk of multiples with ART is the number of embryos transferred. National data indicate that in the United States, the majority of ART cycles involve the transfer of more than one embryo, with more embryos transferred as maternal age increases (CDC, 2001). There is a direct relationship between the rise in assisted reproduction use and the increase in multiple gestations. Fifty-three percent of 45,751 infants born through the use of ART in the United States in 2002 were multiples. Much of the focus on the causes of multiple gestations has been placed on the role of ART, particularly IVF. Much less attention has been paid to the role of ovulation promotion (superovulation-intrauterine insemination and conventional ovulation induction), which is equally important in terms of the contribution to multiple gestations. The risk of multiple gestations secondary to these treatments is less well documented, as reporting data are not mandated.

The primary concern regarding ART and ovulation promotion is the risk of preterm delivery in association with multiple gestations. Among the infants conceived through ART specifically, 14.5 percent of singletons, 61.7 percent of twins, and 97.2 percent of higher-order multiples were born at gestational ages of less than 37 weeks (CDC, 2005a). The results of a recent meta-analysis revealed that singletons conceived by IVF are twice as likely to be born preterm and die within 1 week of birth compared with the risk for those not conceived through IVF (McGovern et al., 2004). The etiology of this type of preterm birth remains unknown. This is an important area for future research.

In 1999, the American Society for Reproductive Medicine issued guidelines that recommended limiting the number of embryos transferred. The guidelines were further refined in 2004. A demonstrable drop in the rate of triplet gestations from 7 to 3.8 percent from 1996 to 2002 has been cited as evidence of the success of these practice guidelines (Barbieri, 2005). Despite success in reducing rates of higher-order multiples, the United States does not fare as well as European countries in minimizing the risk of multiple gestations (Anderson et al., 2005).

> **Recommendation II-4:** *Investigate the causes of and consequences for preterm births that occur because of fertility treatments. The National Institutes of Health and other agencies, such as the Centers for Disease Control and Prevention and the Agency for Healthcare Research and Quality, should provide support for researchers to conduct investigations to obtain an understanding of the mechanisms by which fertility treatments, such as assisted reproductive technologies and ovulation promotion, may increase the risk for preterm birth. Studies should also be conducted to investigate the outcomes for mothers who have received fertility treatments and who deliver preterm and the outcomes for their infants.*

Specifically, those conducting work in this area should attempt to achieve the following:

- Develop comprehensive registries for clinical research, with particular emphasis on obtaining data on gestational age and birth weight, whether the preterm birth was indicated or spontaneous, the outcomes for the newborns, and perinatal mortality and morbidity. These registries must distinguish multiple gestations from singleton gestations and link multiple infants from a single pregnancy.

• Conduct basic biological research to identify the mechanisms of preterm birth relevant to fertility treatments and the underlying causes of infertility or subfertility that may contribute to preterm delivery.

• Investigate the outcomes for preterm infants as well as all infants whose mothers received fertility treatments.

• Understand the impact of changing demographics on the use and outcomes of fertility treatments.

• Assess the short- and long-term economic costs of various fertility treatments.

• Investigate ways to improve the outcomes of fertility treatments, including ways to identify high-quality gametes and embryos to optimize success through the use of single embryos and improve ovarian stimulation protocols that lead to monofollicular development.

Recommendation II-5: *Institute guidelines to reduce the number of multiple gestations. The American College of Obstetricians and Gynecologists, the American Society for Reproductive Medicine, and state and federal public health agencies should institute guidelines that will reduce the number of multiple gestations. Particular attention should be paid to the transfer of a single embryo and the restricted use of superovulation drugs and other nonassisted reproductive technologies for infertility treatments. In addition to mandatory reporting to the Centers for Disease Control and Prevention by centers and individual physicians who use assisted reproductive technologies, the use of superovulation therapies should be similarly reported.*

4. Improve the Quality of Care for Women at Risk for Preterm Labor and Infants Born Preterm

Beyond the content of prenatal care, little is known about the quality of care throughout the reproductive spectrum. For infants born preterm, there are also few indicators of high-quality NICU care. Knowledge of the quality of care received during pregnancy and delivery has the potential to reduce the rates of preterm birth. However, few quality measures related to the perinatal period have been developed. Reporting systems such as the National Center on Quality Assurance's HEDIS (Health Plan Employer Data and Information Set; www.ncqa.org/Programs/HEDIS) measures contain only a few basic indicators related to the timing and content of prenatal care and the birth outcome.

In general, large variations in outcomes exist across NICUs that cannot be explained by patient mix or other readily observable hospital characteristics, such as patient volume and level of care. Recent research has suggested a role for the organizational and management structures of NICUs in ensuring good patient outcomes (Pollack et al., 1993). More research on the determinants of high-quality care will be needed to be able to send patients to the best hospitals.

Recommendation V-2: *Establish a quality agenda. Investigators, professional societies, state agencies, payors, and funding agencies should establish a quality agenda with the intent of maximizing outcomes with current technology for infants born preterm.*

This agenda should:

• Define quality across the full spectrum of providers who treat women delivering preterm and infants born preterm;
• Identify efficacious interventions for preterm infants and identify the quality improvement efforts that are needed to incorporate these interventions into practice; and
• Analyze variations in outcomes for preterm infants among institutions.

5. Investigate the Impact of the Health Care Delivery System on Preterm Birth

Policy makers have focused on expansion of access to prenatal care since the 1980s in an effort to improve birth outcomes in general, including a reduction in preterm birth rates. These efforts have primarily been achieved through the expansion of Medicaid eligibility for pregnant women at the state level. A direct link between the availability of increased insurance and the receipt of early prenatal care was demonstrated in a study of Medicaid expansion in Florida (Long and Marquis, 1998).

Alternately, states can increase access to prenatal care outside of the confines of Medicaid by expanding programs that target uninsured pregnant women to provide them with access to prenatal care through Maternal and Child Health block grants (Schlesinger and Kornesbusch, 1990). Coverage for prenatal care services has also been extended through expansion of the State Children's Health Insurance Program (SCHIP) [Title XXI, Social Security Act, Pub. I, No. 74-271 (49 Stat 620) (1935)].

Evaluations of the Medicaid expansions have not found reduced rates of preterm birth or improvements in maternal outcomes in association with these increases in the levels of insurance coverage for pregnant women (Piper et al., 1990). One reason that the expansions may not have been effective in reducing the rates of preterm birth may be that current prenatal care is focused on risks other than preterm birth (see Chapter 9). Nonetheless, prenatal care provides the framework though which interventions can be implemented and thus plays an important role in the potential to reduce preterm birth rates in the future.

The organization of the health care delivery system has long been viewed as a key determinant of birth outcomes. In the 1970s, the March of Dimes developed practice guidelines advocating for the regionalization of perinatal care in the United States (Committee on Perinatal Health, 1976), based on research linking the regionalization of neonatal care with improved neonatal survival and overall outcomes. As initially envisioned, regionalized perinatal care involved the designation of three levels of care on the basis of the clinical conditions of the patients—both the mother and the infant. Level I centers were able to provide basic or routine obstetrical and newborn care, whereas Level II centers had the capability to care for patients of moderate risk, with Level III centers being reserved for those with the ability to tend to the most specialized high-risk cases. In addition to the designation of levels, regionalized perinatal care was to include the coordination of care among the region's hospitals.

Research demonstrated an increase in regionalization with a concomitant marked improvement in the rates of survival of the neonates (McCormick et al., 1985). By the latter half of the decade, however, the emphasis on the regionalization of perinatal care was being replaced by an interhospital competition driven by the reimbursement policies of an increasingly managed care environment. To compete for managed care contracts and to maintain and attract obstetric patients, smaller community hospitals were hiring neonatalogists and building new NICUs, even in the absence of increased obstetric volume or the ability to provide comprehensive neonatal services.

Follow-up studies revealed a reversal in regionalization, increased competition between hospitals, and blurred distinctions between levels of care (Cooke et al., 1988). Between 1990 and 1994 an increase in the number of self-designated Level II facilities occurred compared with the number between 1982 and 1986, with a concomitant decrease in the number of Level I institutions (Yeast et al., 1998). However, the relative risk of neonatal mortality for infants born with very low birth weights was twofold higher in Level II centers than in Level III centers.

More recently, the private sector has begun a trend toward moving patients to high-quality hospitals through evidence-based selective referral.

Evidence-based hospital referral in its broadest sense means making sure that patients with high-risk conditions are treated in hospitals with the best outcomes. Evidence-based hospital referral standards for infants with very low birth weights required that infants with expected birth weights of less than 1,500 grams, a gestational age of less than 32 weeks, or correctable major birth defects should be delivered at a regional NICU with an average daily census of 15 patients or more. Evidence suggests that although patient volume and NICU level of care are statistically significant determinants of outcomes, they explain little of the variation in the rates of mortality among very-low-birth-weight infants among hospitals (Rogowski et al., 2004a). In general, large variations in outcomes exist among NICUs that cannot be explained by patient mix or other readily observable hospital characteristics, such as volume and level of care. More research will be needed on the determinants of high-quality care so that patients may be sent to the best hospitals.

Recommendation V-3: *Conduct research to understand the impact of the health care delivery system on preterm birth. The National Institutes of Health, the Agency for Healthcare Quality and Research, and private foundations should conduct and support research to understand the consequences of the organization and financing of the health care delivery system on access, quality, cost, and the outcomes of care as they relate to preterm birth throughout the full reproductive and childhood spectrum.*

Conduct Etiologic and Epidemiologic Investigations

1. Investigate the Etiologies of Preterm Birth

It is clear that the causes of preterm labor are multifactorial and vary according to gestational age. Biological pathways include systemic and intrauterine infections (which are responsible for the majority of extremely preterm births), maternal stress, uteroplacental thrombosis and intrauterine vascular lesions associated with fetal stress or decidual hemorrhage, uterine overdistension, and cervical insufficiency. Each of these pathways may be influenced by gene-environment interactions. In the past, obstetricians and epidemiologists have tended to combine, for statistical purposes, all preterm births occurring between 20 and 37 weeks of gestation. This has obscured the opportunity to study preterm birth as a final common end point and has led to uniform, largely empirical, and unsuccessful treatment strategies. Each pathway to preterm labor can be characterized by its own unique upstream initiators of preterm parturition. Nonetheless, all share common downstream effectors of preterm contractions.

There is much interest in using relevant animal models to help understand the mechanisms of preterm birth and the sequelae of preterm birth for the neonate and to develop rational and effective treatment and prevention strategies. The most compelling data from animal models are derived from the role of infection and inflammation in preterm birth (Gravett et al., 1994; Vadillo-Ortega et al., 2002; see Elovitz and Mrinalini [2004] for a review) and the positive effects of treatment with antibiotics and immunomodulators (Gravett et al., 2003).

Until recently, the roles of genetic susceptibility and gene-environment interactions in preterm birth have largely been unexplored. There is some evidence of a genetic predisposition to preterm birth and the existence of gene-environment interactions. To date, however, only limited studies on the role of gene-environment interactions in preterm birth have been published (Genc et al., 2004; Macones et al., 2004; Nukui et al., 2004; Wang et al., 2000, 2002). Nevertheless, the available literature has provided some evidence of a familial or intergenerational influence on low birth weight and preterm birth (Bakketeig et al., 1979; Carr-Hill and Hall, 1985; Khoury and Cohen, 1987; Porter et al., 1997; Varner and Esplin, 2005). With recent advances in human genetics and molecular biology, assessment of the genetic contributions to human diseases has progressed from indirect measurements based on family history to direct measures of an individual's genotype at particular loci. Nevertheless, the family history and a woman's past medical history remain valuable tools in assessment of the risk for preterm birth. Understanding these factors and their interactions could lead to improvements in the diagnosis, prevention, and treatment of women at risk for preterm birth. This quickly expanding field will require new paradigms for interdisciplinary collaborations, as reflected in Recommendation V-1.

The potential risk of preterm birth as a result of exposures to environmental pollutants is poorly understood. Few environmental pollutants have been investigated for their potential to increase the risk for preterm birth, and even among those pollutants that have been studied, the information available for most of them is limited. This lack of knowledge presents a potentially significant shortcoming for the design of public health preventive strategies. The most robust support for the relationship between exposures and preterm birth are for lead (see Andrews et al. [1994] for a review) and environmental tobacco smoke (Ahlborg and Bodin, 1991; Ahluwalia et al., 1997; Jaakkola et al., 2001), for which the weight of evidence suggests that maternal exposure to these pollutants increases the risk for preterm birth. In addition, a number of epidemiological studies have found significant relationships between exposures to air pollution and preterm birth, particularly for sulfur dioxide and particulates, suggesting that exposure to these air pollutants may increase a woman's risk for preterm birth (Liu et al., 2003; Mohorovic, 2004; Xu et al., 1995).

Recommendation II-1: *Support research on the etiologies of preterm birth. Funding agencies should be committed to sustained and vigorous support for research on the etiologies of preterm birth to fill critical knowledge gaps.*

Areas to be supported should include the following:

• The physiological and pathologic mechanisms of parturition across the entire gestational period as well as the pregestational period should be studied.
• The role of inflammation and its regulation during implantation and parturition should be studied. Specifically, perturbations to the immunologic and inflammatory pathways caused by bacterial and viral infections, along with the specific host responses to these pathogens, should be addressed.
• Preterm birth should be defined as a syndrome of multiple pathophysiological pathways, with refinement of the phenotypes of preterm birth that recognizes and accurately reflects the heterogeneity of the underlying etiology.
• Animal models, in vitro systems, and computer models of human implantation, placentation, parturition, and preterm birth should be studied.
• Simple genetic and more complex epigenetic causes of preterm birth should be studied.
• Gene-environment interactions and environmental factors should be considered broadly to include the physical and social environments.
• Biological targets and the mechanisms and biological markers of exposure to environmental pollutants should be studied.

2. Study Multiple Psychosocial, Behavioral, Sociodemographic, and Environmental Risk Factors Associated with Preterm Birth Simultaneously

Behavioral determinants of preterm birth have been of interest, given the fact that they are subject to change and could reduce the frequency of preterm birth directly. A large number of observational studies on a variety of behaviors have been conducted, including tobacco, alcohol, and illicit drug use; nutrition; physical and sexual activity; employment; and douching. Although each of these behaviors poses specific challenges in discerning cause-and-effect relationships, two key, generic concerns crosscut them all.

First, it is a challenge to measure many of these behaviors with accuracy because of their inherent complexity, the inability of individuals to completely recall past behaviors, or the stigma associated with the behavior. The challenge is especially heightened for women who are pregnant. Behavioral factors are highly susceptible to confounding, so that any true causal effects of the behavior of interest on preterm birth are distorted by the association of that behavior with antecedent factors like socioeconomic conditions or with other behaviors. However, when considered in conjunction with other lines of research involving mechanistic studies and randomized trials, observational studies of behavioral influences on preterm birth, when it is feasible to conduct such studies, have been highly informative.

Cocaine use is associated with an increased risk for preterm birth (Holzman and Paneth, 1994), and leisure time physical activity has been associated with a reduced risk of preterm birth (Evenson et al., 2002). Dietary constituents have been examined to a limited degree, with mixed evidence on the potential benefits of increased levels of iron (Villar et al., 1998), long-chain fatty acids (Olsen et al., 2000), folate (Rolschau et al., 1999; Savitz and Pastore, 1999), and vitamin C (Siega-Riz et al., 2003) being found. Although none of these dietary constituents is well established as having effects that prevent preterm birth, all warrant further evaluation.

The findings of research on psychosocial factors and preterm birth have accumulated rapidly in recent years. Psychosocial factors such as stress, life events (for example, divorce, illness, injury, or job loss), anxiety, depression, and racism are distinct factors. Consistent evidence indicates that some factors, such as major life events (Dole et al., 2003, Zambrana et al., 1999), chronic and catastrophic stress (Lederman et al., 2004; Misra et al., 2001; Stein et al., 2000), maternal anxiety (Rini et al., 1999), racism (Collins et al., 2004), and intendedness of pregnancy (Orr et al., 2000), are associated with an increase in preterm birth. A small but growing body of work suggests that women who experience domestic or personal violence during pregnancy are at risk for adverse birth outcomes (Amaro et al., 1990; Coker et al., 2004; Parker et al., 1994a; Rich-Edwards et al., 2001; Shumway et al., 1999). The extent to which this is the result of stress processes rather than other mediating processes is unclear, however.

Neighborhood conditions that are hypothesized to either directly or indirectly influence health are features of the neighborhood's social environment (e.g., neighborhood cohesion, crime, socioeconomic composition, and residential stability), service environment (e.g., access to quality health care, grocery stores, recreational facilities), and physical characteristics (e.g., exposure to toxicants, noise and air pollution, and housing quality). A number of studies have documented a significant association between neighborhood-level socioeconomic disadvantage and birth outcomes (Collins and David, 1990, 1997; Elo et al., 2001; O'Campo et al., 1997; Roberts, 1997).

These studies have used birth weight rather than gestational age, which is a major limitation of this work. Differences in the rates of low birth weight according to race and ethnicity remain, with African-American mothers bearing a substantially higher risk than white mothers, even after individual and community-level factors are taken into account (Roberts, 1997). Some specific neighborhood-level characteristics that have been associated with birth weight and the risk of low birth weight include indicators of neighborhood economic deprivation and crime (Elo et al., 2001). Adverse neighborhood conditions have also been found to lessen the effects of protective factors, such as prenatal care (O'Campo et al., 1997).

Recommendation II-2: *Study multiple risk factors to facilitate the modeling of the complex interactions associated with preterm birth. Public and private funding agencies should promote and researchers should conduct investigations of multiple risk factors for preterm birth simultaneously rather than investigations of the individual risk factors in isolation. These studies will facilitate the modeling of these complex interactions and aid with the development and evaluation of more refined interventions tailored to specific risk profiles.*

Specifically, these studies should achieve the following:

• Develop strong theoretical models of the pathways from psychosocial factors, including stress, social support, and other resilience factors, to preterm delivery as a basis for ongoing observational research. These frameworks should include plausible biological mechanisms. Comprehensive studies should include psychosocial, behavioral, medical, and biological data.
• Incorporate understudied exposures, such as the characteristics of employment and work contexts, including work-related stress; the effects of domestic or personal violence during pregnancy; racism; and personal resources, such as optimism, mastery and control, and pregnancy intendedness. These studies should also investigate the potential interactions of these exposures with exposure to environmental toxicants.
• Emphasize culturally valid measures in studies of stress and preterm delivery to consider the unique forms of stress that individuals in different racial and ethnic groups experience. Measurement of stress should also include specific constructs such as anxiety.
• Expand the study of neighborhood-level effects on the risk of preterm birth by including novel data in multilevel models. Data that address this information should be made more available to researchers for such activities. Interagency agreements for the sharing of data should be reached to support the development of cartographic modeling of neighborhoods.

• Work toward the development of primary strategies for the prevention of preterm birth. When there is evidence of modest effects of multiple causes, interventions that address all of these factors should be considered.

• Have designs that are common enough to allow for pooling of data and samples, and consider studying high-risk populations to increase the power of the study.

3. Investigate Racial-Ethnic and Socioeconomic Disparities in the Rates of Preterm Birth

As discussed above, preterm birth rates vary substantially by race and ethnicity. The greatest differences in the rates of preterm birth are between African-American and Asian women. Knowledge can be gained by obtaining an understanding of the differences between groups as well as differences among Asian subgroups. Preterm birth rates also vary by nativity and the duration of residence. In 2003, the preterm birth rate was 13.9 percent for foreign-born African Americans but 18.2 percent for U.S.-born African Americans (CDC, 2005i). It is not known, however, why foreign-born and U.S.-born women of the same racial descent have such disparate rates of preterm birth, given their supposedly common genetic ancestry. Even the duration of residence seems to have an effect on preterm birth rates. A study in California found that long-term Mexican immigrants who had lived in the United States for more than 5 years were more likely to deliver their infants preterm than newcomers who had lived in the United States for 5 years or less (Guendelman and English, 1995).

A number of explanations have been studied, including differences in socioeconomic status (SES), maternal risk behaviors, prenatal care, maternal infection, maternal stress, and genetics. Findings related to SES suggest that the disparities in the rates of preterm birth between African American and white women persist after attempts to adjust for socioeconomic differences (Collins and David, 1997; McGrady et al., 1992; Schoendorf et al., 1992; Shiono et al., 1997). Disparities in preterm birth rates by SES have been well documented not only in the United States (Parker et al., 1994a) but also in other countries, such as Canada (Wilkins et al., 1991), Sweden (Koupilova et al., 1998), Finland (Olsen et al., 1995b), Scotland (Sanjose et al., 1991), and Spain (Rodriguez et al., 1995), where the levels of poverty are lower and where the population has universal access to high-quality prenatal and other medical care. Furthermore, socioeconomic disparities are associated with other factors, such as maternal nutrition (Hendler et al., 2005), maternal drug use (Kramer et al., 2000), maternal employment (Mozuekewich et al., 2000), prenatal care (CDC, 2005i), and maternal infection. Given the serious doubt about the effects of prenatal care on reducing the risk of preterm birth (Alexander and Kotelchuck, 2001; Lu and Halfon, 2003), it too seems an unlikely mediator of socioeconomic disparities in preterm birth. Bacterial vaginosis is more common among women of low SES (Hillier et al., 1995; Meis et al., 1995); however, clinical trials of screening and treatment have yielded conflicting results (Carey et al., 2000; McDonald et al., 2005). Finally, women of low SES women experience more stressful life events and more chronic stress (Lu et al., 2005; Peacock et al., 1995), which are linked to preterm birth.

Other behavioral and social differences between African American and white women have been evaluated as potential causes of the disparity in preterm birth rates. Proportionately fewer African American women smoke cigarettes (Beck et al., 2002; Lu et al., 2005) and their rate of use of drugs and alcohol is no higher than white women's (Serdula et al., 1991). The effectiveness of prenatal care for preventing prematurity has yet to be conclusively demonstrated (Alexander and Kotelchuck, 2001; Lu and Halfon, 2003; CDC, 2005i). African American women are more likely than white women to experience infections, including bacterial vaginosis and sexually transmitted infections (Fiscella, 1995; Meis et al., 2000). However, the cause of this increased susceptibility to infections among pregnant African American women largely remains unknown, and treatment has yielded modest or no benefits (Carey et al., 2000; King, 2002; McDonald et al., 2005). Insofar as African American women may experience more stress in their daily lives than white women, it has been suggested that maternal stress may contribute to the disparities in the rates of preterm birth between African American and white women (James, 1993; Krieger, 2002; Lu and Chen, 2004). Although a woman's genetic makeup undoubtedly plays a role in the pathogenesis of preterm birth, the potential genetic contribution to racial disparities in preterm birth is unknown (Cox et al., 2001; Hassan et al., 2003; Hoffman et al., 2002; Varner and Esplin, 2005).

Recommendation II-3: *Expand research into the causes and methods for the prevention of the racial-ethnic and socioeconomic disparities in the rates of preterm birth. The National Institutes of Health and other funding agencies should expand current efforts in and expand support for research into the causes and methods for the prevention of the racial-ethnic and socioeconomic disparities in the rates of preterm birth. This research agenda should continue to prioritize efforts to understand factors contributing to the high rates of preterm birth among African American infants and should also encourage investigation into the disparities among other racial-ethnic subgroups.*

III. Study and Inform Public Policy

Because preterm birth is concentrated in populations of low socioeconomic status, the cost of preterm birth generates a considerable burden on public programs, many of which target low-income and other vulnerable populations. As noted above, pregnant women who have received ART may not be representative of all pregnant women (among other things, evidence suggests that they are from socioeconomically advantaged backgrounds). Thus, this fact should be taken into account when generalizations are made from the findings for births that result from ART.

The costs of preterm birth extend beyond the medical costs associated with the actual birth of the infant. There are significant lifetime consequences of preterm birth for many infants. Therefore, the consequences of preterm birth span a broad range of services and social supports. These may include early intervention programs; special education; income supports, including those provided by the Supplemental Security Income program and Temporary Assistance to Needy Families; Title V Maternal and Child Health Programs; foster care; and the juvenile justice system. Little is known about the magnitude of the public burden, aside from the costs associated with the medical care provided through Medicaid. It is not possible to assign dollar costs associated with preterm birth to other services and programs because of a lack of data.

A second aspect of public policy is that it can be used to potentially reduce preterm birth rates and improve health outcomes for infants. Public policies have the potential to reduce the rates of preterm birth and improve outcomes for children and families through the financing of health care, the organization of care and improvements in the quality of care, and other social policies. Better measures of the quality of health care need to be developed to enable quality improvement efforts and guide public policy. However, effective public policies will require a better understanding of the determinants of preterm birth.

Recommendation V-4: *Study the effects of public programs and policies on preterm birth. The National Institutes of Health, the Centers for Medicare and Medicaid Services, and private foundations should conduct and/or support research on the role of social programs and policies on the occurrence of preterm birth and the health of children born preterm.*

Recommendation V-5: *Conduct research that will inform public policy. In order to formulate effective public policies to reduce preterm birth and assure healthy outcomes for infants, public and private funding agencies and organizations, state agencies, payors, professional societies, and researchers will need to work to implement all of the previous recommendations. Research in the areas of better defining the problem of preterm birth, clinical investigations, and etiologic and epidemiologic investigations is critical to conduct before policy makers can create policies that will successfully address this problem.*

CONCLUDING REMARKS

Although significant improvements in treating infants born preterm and improving survival have been made, little success has been attained in understanding and preventing preterm birth. The challenge remains to identify interventions that prevent preterm birth, reduce the rates of morbidity and mortality of the mother or the infant once a preterm birth occurs, and reduce the incidence of long-term disability among children who were born preterm in the most comprehensive and cost-effective manner possible. The recommendations of this report are intended to assist policy makers, academic researchers, funding agencies and organizations, third-party payers, and health care professionals with the prioritization of research activities and to inform the public about the problem of preterm birth. The ultimate goal of the committee's efforts is to work toward improved outcomes for children and their families.

1

Introduction

The period of gestation is one of the most important predictors of an infant's subsequent health and survival. In 2004, more than 500,000 infants, or 12.5 percent of all infants, were born preterm, which is considered birth at less than 37 completed weeks of gestation (CDC, 2005a). On the basis of new estimates provided in this report, the annual societal economic burden associated with preterm birth in the United States was in excess of $26.2 billion in 2005 (this estimate represents a lower boundary).

The percentage of preterm deliveries has risen steadily over the last 2 decades. Most of this increase has been among children born at 32 to 36 weeks gestation. In the past, low birth weight has been used as an indicator for preterm birth; however, the present Institute of Medicine (IOM) committee considers low birth weight to be a poor surrogate and has specifically focused its analysis on preterm birth.

Compared with infants born at term (37 to 41 weeks of gestation), preterm infants have a much greater risk of death and disability. Approximately 75 percent of perinatal deaths occur among preterm infants (Slattery and Morrison, 2002). Almost one-fifth of all infants born at less than 32 weeks gestation do not survive the first year of life, whereas about 1 percent of infants born at between 32 and 36 weeks of gestation and 0.3 percent of infants born at 37 to 41 weeks of gestation do not survive the first year of life. The infant mortality rate (IMR) per 1,000 live births for infants born at less than 32 weeks of gestation was 180.9, nearly 70 times the rate for infants born at between 37 and 41 weeks of gestation (Mathews et al., 2002).

Advances in medical technologies and therapeutic perinatal and neonatal care have led to improved rates of survival among preterm infants, including those born when they are as young as a gestational age of 23 weeks. However, surviving infants have a higher risk of morbidity. Neurodevelopmental disabilities can range from major disabilities such as cerebral palsy, mental retardation, and sensory impairments to more subtle disorders, including language and learning problems, attention deficit hyperactivity disorder, and behavioral and social-emotional difficulties. Preterm infants are also at increased risk for growth and health problems, such as asthma or reactive airway disease (see Chapter 11 for review).

Although significant improvements in treating preterm infants and improving survival have been made, little success in understanding and preventing preterm birth has been attained. The complexity of factors that are involved in preterm birth will require a multidisciplinary approach to research directed at understanding its etiologies, pathophysiology, diagnosis, and treatments. However, there are barriers to the recruitment and participation of scientists in these investigations. A critical barrier to research is the demand on clinical researchers in academic centers to provide clinical income and other duties that take them away from research. This necessitates the development of new ways to provide support to allow the time to conduct this important research.

The challenge for researchers and clinicians remains to identify interventions that prevent preterm birth; reduce the morbidity and mortality of the mother or the infant, or both, once preterm birth occurs; and reduce the incidence of long-term disability in children in the most comprehensive and cost-effective manner possible.

CONTEXT AND CHARGE TO THE COMMITTEE

The persistent and troubling problem of preterm birth prompted IOM to convene a committee to assess the current state of the science on the causes and broad consequences of preterm birth. This interest was generated by the IOM Roundtable on Environmental Health Sciences, Research, and Medicine, which convened a workshop in October 2001 focused on the role of the environment in preterm birth. In 2003, the Roundtable published a factual summary of this workshop in *The Role of Environmental Hazards in Premature Birth* (IOM, 2003). The Roundtable members, concerned that research into understanding preterm birth was not progressing as fast as was hoped, believed that progress could be made if researchers had an agenda to follow, an agenda that would help focus and direct research efforts for the variety of disciplines needed to address this problem.

With assistance from the study sponsors, the Committee on Understanding Premature Birth and Assuring Healthy Outcomes was established. The sponsors include the National Institute of Child Health and Human

Development, the Centers for Disease Control and Prevention, the National Institutes of Health Office of Research on Women's Health, the Health Resources and Services Administration, the Environmental Protection Agency, the March of Dimes, the Burroughs Wellcome Fund, the American College of Obstetricians and Gynecologists, the American Society for Reproductive Medicine, and the Society for Maternal-Fetal Medicine. Specifically, the charge presented to the committee of 17 members was as follows:

> An IOM committee will define and address the health related and economic consequences of premature birth. The broad goals are to (1) describe the current state of the science and clinical research with respect to the causes of premature birth; (2) address the broad costs—economic, medical, social, psychological, and educational—for children and their families; and (3) establish a framework for action in addressing the range of priority issues, including a research and policy agenda for the future. In support of these broad goals, the study will:
>
> • Review and assess the various factors contributing to the growing incidence of premature birth, which may include the trend to delay childbearing and racial and ethnic disparities;
> • Assess the economic costs and other societal burdens associated with premature births;
> • Address research gaps/needs and priorities for defining the mechanisms by which biological and environmental factors influence premature birth; and
> • Explore possible changes in public health policy and other policies that may benefit from more research.
>
> In order to assess research gaps and needs, the committee will plan an additional meeting that will address barriers to clinical research in the area of preterm birth. A workshop hosted by the committee will seek to
>
> • Identify major obstacles to conducting clinical research, which may include the declining number of residents interested in entering the field of obstetrics and gynecology and the resulting effect on the pipeline of clinical researchers; the impact of rising medical malpractice premiums on the ability of academic programs to provide protected time for physicians to pursue research; and ethical and legal issues in conducting research on pregnant women (for example, the consideration of safety issues and informed consent); and
> • Provide strategies for removing barriers—including those targeting resident career choices, departments of obstetrics and gynecology, agencies and organizations that fund research, and professional organizations.

During the 21-month study, the committee convened for six meetings and hosted three public workshops (see Appendix A for the study methods).

PREVIOUS REPORTS ADDRESSING PRETERM BIRTH AND LOW BIRTH WEIGHT INFANTS

Several reports on the problem of preterm birth, low birth weight, and other infant outcomes have been published by the Institute of Medicine, in addition to the workshop summary on *The Role of Environmental Hazards in Premature Birth*. *Preventing Low Birthweight* (IOM, 1985) defined the significance of the problem of low birth weight, reviewed data on risk factors and etiology, and examined state and national trends in the incidence of low birth weight among various groups. This report also described approaches to prevent low birth weight and their economic costs and identified research needs. *Prenatal Care: Reaching Mothers, Reaching Infants* (IOM, 1988) examined 30 prenatal care programs, analyzed surveys of mothers who did not seek prenatal care, and made recommendations for improving the nation's maternity system and increasing the use of prenatal care programs. Two recent reports: *Reducing Birth Defects: Meeting the Challenges in the Developing World* (IOM, 2003) and *Improving Birth Outcomes: Meeting the Challenges in the Developing World* (IOM, 2003) address issues specific to developing countries.

Two IOM reports are specifically related to the committee's charge to address research barriers; *Medical Professional Liability and the Delivery of Obstetrical Care* (IOM, 1989) and *Strengthening Research in Academic OB/GYN Departments* (IOM, 1992). The first report addressed medical liability and its effect on access to and delivery of obstetrical care; and civil justice and insurance systems, medical liability issues, and their combined effect on health care for mothers and children. The second report examined the ability of departments of obstetrics and gynecology to conduct research within academic departments in order to improve women's health and the outcomes of pregnancy.

Research and other activities addressing preterm birth are also being conducted and supported by a variety of federal agencies and private foundations (see Chapter 13 for review). A major effort has been undertaken by the March of Dimes to address the problem of preterm birth. In January 2003, the Foundation launched its Prematurity Campaign to raise awareness of the problem of prematurity and reduce the rate of premature births. Components of the campaign include funding research, providing support to families affected by prematurity, working for access to insurance and health care coverage, helping providers learn ways to help reduce the risk for preterm delivery, and educating women about how to reduce their risk and recognize symptoms of preterm labor. The March of Dimes recently published a research agenda for preterm birth (Green et al., 2005). Major recommendations outlined six primary research topics including epidemiologic studies, genes and gene-environment interactions, racial-ethnic disparities, role of inflammatory responses, stress responses and preterm birth, and clinical trials.

Other reports have also highlighted knowledge gaps and identified research priorities. The National Institute of Child Health and Human Development and American Academy of Pediatrics Section on Perinatal Pediatrics convened a workshop in 2004 focusing on research in neonatology. The published summary of this workshop (Raju et al., 2005) identifies research opportunities in neuroscience, cardiopulmonary research, fetal and neonatal nutrition, gastrointestinal research, perinatal epidemiology, and neonatal pharmacology. Similarly, a workshop sponsored by the National Institute of Child Health and Human Development, National Institute of Neurologic Disorders and Stroke, and Centers for Disease Control and Prevention focused on follow-up care of high risk infants. The publication from this workshop (Vohr, 2004) provided suggestions to improve the long-term follow-up of this population. Suggestions included measuring the long-term impact of interventions for populations enrolled in randomized-controlled trials. Challenges were identified for multicenter networks, including standardizing study materials, achieving adequate follow-up rates, defining the study population and the timing of enrollment, and engaging a cost-effective and appropriate control population.

The current report makes a novel contribution by recommending directions for action and an organizational structure that will help focus research and policy directives on a variety of dimensions of preterm birth, based on a comprehensive assessment of the status of knowledge and scientific research regarding the causes and the broad short- and long-term consequences of preterm birth. In completing its task, the committee does not, however, provide an exhaustive review of the literature examining the various etiologies of preterm birth or its consequences for infants and children. Rather, the goal of this report is to summarize and synthesize this literature and to evaluate it to identify the gaps in knowledge and recommend a research agenda to address these gaps. The committee's recommendations are based on scientific evidence and expert judgment.

The findings and recommendations of this report are intended to assist policy makers, academic researchers, funding agencies and organizations, third party payors, and health care professionals in prioritizing research and to inform the public about the problem of preterm birth. The ultimate goal of the committee's efforts is to work toward improved outcomes for children who have been born preterm and their families.

RECURRING THEMES

At the beginning of its deliberations, the committee noticed three topics that repeatedly emerged. These topics became themes that helped to organize the committee's thinking and approach to the issue of preterm birth. The first was a need for clarity in terms. The population of preterm infants is diverse, with preterm births having various etiologies and infants born preterm having various complications and outcomes. A variety of terms have been used to characterize the duration of gestation, fetal growth, and maturation. These terms have been inconsistently applied and used interchangeably in the literature. The inconsistent use of terms has made it difficult to interpret the data on the causes and consequences of preterm birth and to evaluate the appropriate treatments for children who are born preterm. Early on in its deliberations, the committee decided to use the term *preterm birth*, which is based on the period of gestation, to assess this population of infants (Chapter 2 provides a discussion of terminology used in the literature and various methods of determining gestational age). Although low birth weight is more often used as an outcome than preterm birth, the committee considers low birth weight to be a poor proxy. However, it recognizes that the preponderance of the evidence in this field has used low birth weight to identify the infants under study. The committee also recognizes the limitations of the various methods used to estimate gestational age (Chapter 2). The evidence contained in this report therefore draws first on the literature that uses gestational age, preterm birth, and small for gestational age as outcomes. In the absence of these outcomes, low birth weight and other related outcomes are cited as needed.

The committee also discussed the need to distinguish *spontaneous preterm birth* (which occurs naturally as a result of preterm labor or preterm premature rupture of fetal membranes) and *indicated preterm birth* (in which labor is initiated by medical intervention because of dangerous pregnancy complications). There has been a tendency to group births that occur as a result of these complications together, although the etiologies and the initiators of these types of birth may be quite distinct. When the data allow, the committee distinguishes spontaneous and indicated preterm births in its review of the evidence.

The second theme that guided the committee's approach to its task was the troubling evidence of long-standing disparities in the rates of preterm birth among different subpopulations of the overall U.S. population. There is a greater risk and a higher proportion of preterm births among certain racial-ethnic, and socioeconomically disadvantaged subpopulations. Several explanations for this long-standing trend have been cited, including racial differences in genetics, cigarette smoking, substance use or abuse, work and physical activity, maternal behaviors, stress, institutional racism, access to and the use of prenatal care, and infections. The committee reviews these proposed explanations and discusses the need for a more integrative approach to understanding racial-ethnic and socioeconomic disparities in preterm birth. Research needs in the area of the disparities are also discussed.

Third, the committee highlights the complexity of the problem that it was charged to assess. Preterm birth is not one disease for which there is likely to be one solution or cure. Rather, the committee considers preterm birth to be a cluster of problems that comprise a set of overlapping factors of influence that are interrelated. Its causes are multiple and may vary for different populations. Individual psychosocial and behavioral factors, neighborhood social characteristics, environmental exposures, medical conditions, assisted reproductive technology (ART), biological factors, and genetics may play roles to various degrees. Many of these factors co-occur, particularly in those who are socioeconomically disadvantaged or members of minority populations. It is difficult to assess the extent to which each potential factor accounts for the proportion of preterm births. This complexity makes the detection of solutions to the problem difficult. There will be no silver bullet.

The complex nature of preterm birth led the committee to consider its multiple causes in an integrated manner. Several perspectives provided background for the committee's framing of this problem. *New Horizons in Health: An Integrative Approach* called for a need to focus on "multiple pathways to diverse health outcomes" (NRC, 2001, p. 2). It emphasized that for a more complete understanding of disease etiology, these pathways should incorporate information from the molecular and cellular levels into information from the psychosocial and community levels. Furthermore, the report states that "mechanisms underlying racial, ethnic, and social inequalities in health . . . cannot be fully understood without integrated pathway characterizations" (p. 2).

Understanding that multiple determinants across the life span need to be considered in the examination of perinatal health outcomes, Misra and colleagues (2003) proposed a framework, adapted from the Evans and Stoddart (1990) health field model, that incorporates distal factors (such as the genetic, physical, and social environments) that affect an individual's predisposition or exposure and proximal factors (including biomedical and behavioral responses) that have a direct impact on an individual's health. These risk factors are connected to a woman's life course through the transition from preconception and interconception to the pregnancy. Lu and Halfon (2003) also called for a reexamination of the racial and ethnic disparities from a similar integrated life-course perspective. These views guided the committee's approach to examining the causes of preterm birth, which include not only individual demographic, psychosocial, and behavioral factors but also broader social factors, medical and pregnancy conditions, biological pathways, gene-environment interactions, and environmental toxicants.

THE PROBLEM OF PRETERM BIRTH

With the proportion of preterm births reaching 12.5 percent of all births in the United States in 2004, the prevalence of preterm birth constitutes a public health problem. There are three primary reasons for this concern (Mattison et al., 2001). First, unlike many health problems, there has been a troubling increase in the rates of preterm birth in the past decade. Second, the birth of a preterm infant brings significant emotional and economic costs to families and communities. Third, there are notable disparities in the rates of preterm births across populations in the United States, and this disparity is particularly striking between African American women and Asian women. It is clear that the prevention of preterm birth is crucial to improving pregnancy outcomes.

This introduction provides an overview of these issues. First, major trends in preterm birth; that is, the rates or proportions of preterm births by gestational age at birth, geographic location, and maternal age and preterm births resulting from ARTs, are reviewed. Second, the broad costs of preterm birth are briefly described. Outcomes—including the health of the infant born preterm, the consequences of preterm birth on daily functioning, its impact on families, and the economic costs—are discussed in detail in later sections of the report. Last, evidence regarding the presence of disparities in the rates of preterm birth is introduced. As discussed above, this issue served as a broad theme that guided the committee's approach to its task. Potential explanations for these disparities are discussed throughout the report.

Trends in Preterm Birth

As many reports have indicated, the proportion of preterm births has risen fairly steadily since 1990 (Figure 1-1). Note, however, that some of the change in the rate of preterm birth is likely reflective of changes in the way in which gestational age is measured (see Chapter 2 for a discussion). In the early to mid-1990s the percentage of preterm births remained stable at about 11 percent. There was a slight decline from 11.8 percent in 1999 to 11.6 percent in 2000. In 2004, the percentage rose to its highest level since 1990, from 10.6 to 12.5 percent. Since 1981 (when the percentage was 9.4 percent), the proportion has increased more than 30 percent (CDC, 2005a).

Gestational Age

Changes in the distribution of preterm births by degree of prematurity have occurred over time. Although the group of infants with the greatest morbidity and mortality are those who are born at less than 32 weeks, infants born at between 32 and 36 weeks represent the greatest number of preterm births. Figure 1-2 illustrates that between 1990 and 2000, the per-

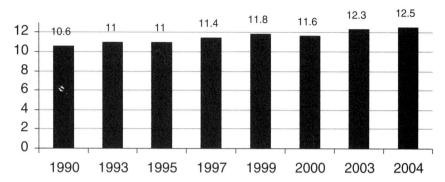

FIGURE 1-1 Preterm births as a percentage of live births in the United States, 1990 to 2004.
SOURCES: CDC (2001, 2002a, 2004a, 2005a).

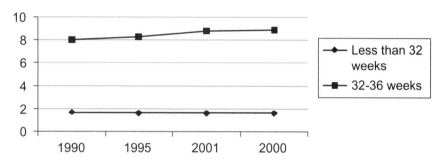

FIGURE 1-2 Preterm births as a percentage of live births by gestational age.
SOURCE: CDC (2002a).

centage of preterm birth was the highest for infants born at between 32 and 36 weeks of gestation. Among singleton births, the 7 percent rise in preterm births between 1990 and 2002 was attributable to the birth of infants of these gestational ages (CDC, 2005a). In contrast, during the same time period the proportions of preterm births occurring at less than 32 weeks of gestation declined from 1.69 to 1.57 percent. (See Appendix B for further discussion of gestational age distribution and trends by race and ethnicity.)

Mortality Associated with Preterm Birth

The overall Infant Mortality Rate (IMR) decreased from 9.1 deaths per 1,000 live births in 1990 to 6.9 in 2000. An interruption in this steady

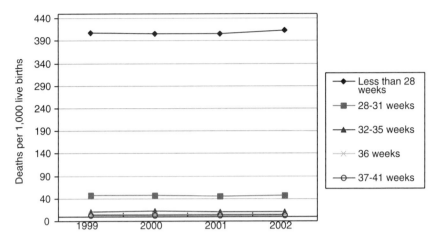

FIGURE 1-3 IMRs by gestational age, United States, 1999 to 2002.
SOURCE: CDC (2005c).

decline was evidenced in 2002, with an increase in the IMR to 7.0 deaths
from 6.8 deaths per 1,000 live births in 2001, the first rise since 1958 (CDC,
2003a, 2005e). Analyses assessing the relative contribution of the change in
the distribution of births by gestational age and in gestational age-specific
IMRs to the change in the IMR revealed that 61 percent of the rise in the
IMR from 2001 to 2002 was due to changes in the distribution of births by
gestational age. Thirty-nine percent of the increase was due to changes in
gestational age-specific mortality rates (CDC, 2005c,d).

In 2002, the IMR for infants born at less than 37 completed weeks of
gestation was 37.9 deaths per 1,000 live births, whereas the IMR was 2.5
deaths per 1,000 live births for infants born at between 37 and 41 weeks of
gestation (full term). Figure 1-3 displays IMRs by gestational age from 1999
to 2002. In 2002, approximately 64 percent of all infant deaths were for the
12.1 percent of infants who were born at less than 37 weeks of gestation
and 53.7 percent of all infant deaths were for the 2 percent of infants born
at less than 32 weeks of gestation. (Also see Appendix B for data reflecting
gestational age-specific IMRs and geographic variations in mortality rates.)

Geographic Differences

The proportion of preterm births varies considerably across different
regions of the country (Figure 1-4). This variation may be related to state
demographics, such as the distribution of maternal ages, multiple births,
and race and ethnicity (CDC, 2005b). In 2003, the lowest percentages were

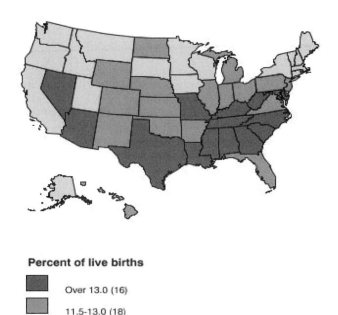

Percent of live births

■ Over 13.0 (16)

■ 11.5-13.0 (18)

□ Under 11.5 (17)

FIGURE 1-4 Percentage of preterm births by U.S. state, 2003.
SOURCE: MOD (2005d).

in the Northeast states (particularly New England), followed by the West, the Midwest, and the South. It is notable that within the western region of the country, where many states have proportions of preterm birth below the national average, Nevada's was 13 percent. Among southern states, Georgia and Virginia had the lowest percentages of preterm birth: 12.6 and 11.8 percent, respectively.

The trends within the four major geographic regions show that the proportion of preterm births in the Northeast increased throughout the 1990s, with a small decline from 1999 to 2000 (MOD, 2005a,b,c,d). From 1996 to 2002, the proportion remained below the national percentage (12.1 percent). The percentage of preterm births in the Midwest during this time period was roughly equivalent to the national percentage. Western states had the lowest proportion of preterm births from 1996 to 2002 compared with the percentages in other parts of the country. Southern states had the highest percentage of preterm births in the United States from 1996 to 2002. This percentage steadily increased and remained above the national average during this period. (See Appendix B for further discussion of the geographic and sociodemographic variations in the rates of preterm births.)

International Comparisons

It is widely reported that the rates of preterm birth in the United States are anomalously high compared with those in other developed countries. However, there is a paucity of published international reports providing unbiased comparisons of the rates of preterm birth among countries. Many of the data that are available have compared countries by the rates of low birth weight. For example, the United Nations Children's Fund (UNICEF) and the World Health Organization (WHO) (UNICEF and WHO, 2004) reported estimates of the incidence of low birth weight. Nevertheless, such reports emphasize that international comparisons and trends must be interpreted cautiously and typically do not allow conjectures on the range of determinants that may underlie the observed differences in the rates of preterm birth to be made. Table 1-1 displays the incidence of low birth weight in selected developed and developing countries.

TABLE 1-1 UNICEF and WHO Estimates of the Incidence of Low Birth Weight

Country	Year	% Low-Birth-Weight Infants	No. of Low Birth Weight (1,000s)	% of Births Not Weighed
Australia	2000	7	16	NA
Canada	2000	6	19	NA
China	1998-1999	6	1,146	NA
Cuba	2001	6	8	NA
Denmark	2001	5	3	NA
Finland	2001	4	3	NA
France	1998	7	51	NA
Germany	1999	7	49	NA
Guatemala	1999	13	53	22
India	1999	30		NA
Ireland	1999	6	7,8373	71
Japan	2000	8	93	NA
Malaysia	1998	10	53	NA
Mexico	1999	9	212	NA
Norway	2000	5	3	NA
Russian Federation	2001	6	79	NA
South Africa	1998	15	155	32
Spain	1997	6	23	NA
Sudan	1999	31	335	NA
Sweden	1999	4	4	NA
Switzerland	1999	6	4	NA
United Kingdom	2000	8	52	NA
United States	2002	8	323	NA

NOTE: NA = Not available.
SOURCE: UNICEF and WHO (2004).

Several cautions are noted in comparing these data across countries (UNICEF and WHO, 2004). First data from industrialized countries are obtained mostly from service-based data and national birth registration systems, while data from developing countries are derived from national household surveys and other routine reporting systems. In addition, the majority of infants in developing countries are not weighted at birth, although an attempt is made to adequately adjust the data. Among developed countries, there are differences in definitions used reporting births (for example, cutoffs for registering births and birth weight). These data are also not corrected for variables such as maternal age, race, social and economic disadvantage, and health care factors.

A report by the Canadian Perinatal Surveillance System cited a rate of 7.1 preterm births per 100 live births in 1996; in comparison, the rate in Australia was 6.9 and that in the United States was 11.0 (McLaughlin et al., 1999). Reporting of data on preterm birth rates at the international level is problematic, however, because substantial differences in the definitions of live births and fetal deaths exist in different countries, which affects the rates of preterm birth. These differences stem from variations in vital record reporting, laws, and procedures. Among the different countries, the impact of different standards of practice related to the measurement of gestational age is often unclear (see Chapter 2 for discussion of measurement issues). It may not be known what measure is typically used to estimate gestational age; for example, ultrasound or the first day of the mother's last menstrual period. Some nations rely on periodic surveys rather than vital records to establish preterm birth rate trends. In addition to measurement issues, there are variations in demographic and health variables, as described above. Therefore, observations of marked differences in preterm rates between European countries and the United States are fraught with the potential for error. Currently, the twofold and greater differences in very preterm rates among U.S. states are largely unexplained. Establishing which factors underlie similar or greater variations among countries is an even larger task.

Method of Delivery

There has been a shift toward earlier delivery for infants of all gestational ages, which may reflect the increase in use of practices such as induction of labor and cesarean delivery (CDC, 2005i; MacDorman et al., 2005). In 2003, the rate of cesarean delivery was 27.5 percent of all births. The rate was 20.7 percent of all births in 1996 and 26.1 percent of all births in 2002. While the total rate of cesarean births increased for all gestational ages between 1996 and 2003, the highest increase was for preterm infants born at 32 to 36 weeks and those born full term (37 to 41 weeks gestation). In 2003, 49.5 percent of infants born at less than 32 weeks gestation and

37.3 percent of infants born at 32 to 36 weeks gestation were delivered by cesarean.

The rise in cesarean rates corresponds to a rise in maternal age. In 2003, the cesarean delivery rate for women 25 to 29 was 26.4 percent. For 35-39 year old women, the rate was 36.8 percent. This may be related to increased multiple births for older women, biological factors, or patient-practitioner concerns (Ecker et al., 2001; CDC, 2005i). Some findings suggest relatively low risks for maternal morbidity (for example, anesthesia-related complications, infection) (Bloom et al., 2005; Lynch et al., 2003), while others suggest that there are increased risks such as readmission in the postpartum, infection, and complications related to anesthesia, among others (Koroukian, 2004; Hager et al., 2004; Liu et al., 2005; Lumley, 2003).

Maternal Age

Dramatic demographic changes in the late 20th century have resulted in increased levels of education and rates of employment among women, including the employment of married women and mothers of young children. The U.S. Department of Labor (DOL, 2005) reported that in 2003 more than half of married American women and more than half of mothers of young children were employed, with the most highly educated women being the most likely to be working. The current proportion of women in the civilian workforce (56 percent) presents a 54 percent change from the proportion in 1980 (DOL, 2004). There has been an increasing trend for women to delay childbearing into their 30s. In 2003, women ages 30 to 34 experienced the highest birth rate for women in this age group since the mid-1970s and women ages 40 to 44 had the highest birth rate for women in this age group since the late 1960s (CDC, 2005a). For women ages 35 to 39, the birth rate increased 47 percent between 1990 and 2003, although the increase in the population of women aged 35 to 39 was only 7 percent (CDC, 2004a, 2005a) (Figure 1-5). A slight increase in the birth rate among women between the ages of 25 and 29 was observed in 2003. In contrast, over the past decade, the birth rates among adolescents (ages 15 to 19) and women ages 20 to 24 have decreased. The current birth rate among adolescents is the lowest rate recorded for this age group in the United States (CDC, 2005a).

Women age 35 and older have increased rates of preterm birth (see Figure 4-1 for discussion and also see Appendix B). Although adolescents also have increased rates of preterm delivery, the numbers of births among women in this age group, as noted above, have decreased in the last decade. Older mothers are more likely to have underlying medical conditions, such as diabetes and hypertension. The rates of these diagnoses reported in birth certificate data have risen since the early 1990s, in tandem with the rise in

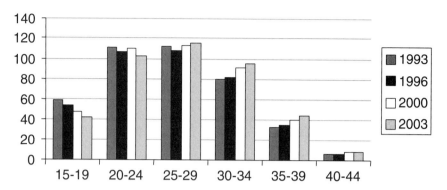

FIGURE 1-5 Birth rates by age of mother, 1993 to 2003. The rates represent the number of live births per 1,000 women in each group.
SOURCE: CDC (2005a).

the mean maternal age (CDC, 2003c). These chronic health problems are associated with adverse birth outcomes, such as growth restriction, preeclampsia, and abruption, leading, in turn, to increases in the rates of indicated preterm deliveries.

ARTs, Multiple Births, and Preterm Birth

The incidence of multiple births has risen steadily in the past 20 years (Figure 1-6). Between 1980 and 2003 the rates of twin births climbed from 18.9 to 31.5 per 1,000 live births. The rates of triplets or higher-order multiple births increased from 37 to 187.4 per 100,000 live births. Multiple births are much more likely than singletons to be born preterm. The rise in multiple births is largely due to the use of ART (in vitro fertilization and other procedures in which the egg and the sperm are handled in the laboratory) (NCCDPHP, 2005), which is more frequently used by older women (see Chapter 5 for a discussion). In 2002, approximately 1 percent of infants born were conceived through the use of ART (NCCDPHP, 2005). Although the use of ARTs must be reported to the Centers for Disease Control and Prevention, this is not the case with other fertility treatments not classified as ARTs. These other treatments include those in which only sperm are handled (i.e., intrauterine insemination, which is also known as artificial insemination) or procedures in which a woman takes medication to stimulate egg production without the intention of having the eggs retrieved. The latter procedure is used to improve fertility, but the frequency of use of this technique and the number of births attributable to the use of this technique are not precisely known.

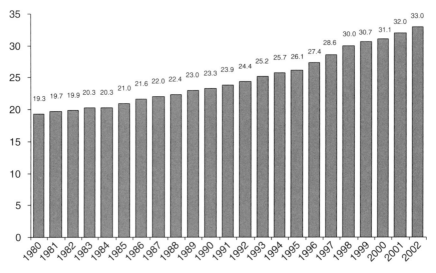

FIGURE 1-6 Multiple births as the number per 1,000 live births, 1980 to 2002.
SOURCE: CDC (2003c).

Women in their mid- to late 30s had the highest percentages of births
conceived through the use of ART (Figure 1-7). Low birth weight infants
are also a result of ART treatments, separate from their increased risk of
preterm birth. Interestingly, singletons conceived through the use of ART
have an increased risk of preterm birth than naturally conceived singletons.
The incidence of multiple births is also related to the trend to delay child-

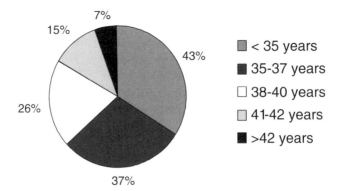

FIGURE 1-7 Percentage of live births from ART by maternal age, 2002.
SOURCE: NCCDPHP (2005).

bearing. The reasons for this are unknown. Older mothers also are more likely than younger mothers to naturally conceive multiple fetuses.

Costs of Preterm Birth

In addition to the health problems associated with preterm birth described at the outset of this chapter, preterm birth is accompanied by broad emotional and financial costs and lost opportunities for families. The birth and hospitalization of preterm infants are associated with maternal distress (Eisengart et al., 2003; Singer et al., 2003) and maternal depressive symptoms (Davis et al., 2003). Longer-term outcomes are also apparent. Evidence suggests greater stress in families of school-age children who were born with very low birth weights; including perceptions of less parenting competence and more difficulty in parental attachment to the child (Taylor et al., 2001). The family as a unit is affected by the greater likelihood of not having additional children (Cronin et al., 1995; Saigal et al., 2000a), the financial burden (Cronin et al., 1995; Macey et al., 1987; McCormick et al., 1986; Rivers et al., 1987), limits on family social life (Cronin et al., 1995; McCormick et al., 1986), high levels of adverse family outcomes (family stress and dysfunction) (Beckman and Pokorni, 1988; Singer et al., 1999; Taylor et al., 2001), and parents' difficulty maintaining employment (Macey et al., 1987; Saigal et al., 2000a). The impact of caring for a child born preterm may also contribute to the strength of the family. There is evidence that parents may perceive positive interactions with friends and within the family stemming from their efforts to care for their child born with birth weight less than 1,000 grams. These parents also reported enhanced personal feelings and improved marital closeness (Saigal et al., 2000a).

On the basis of estimates prepared by the committee (see Chapter 12), the annual societal economic burden associated with preterm birth in the United States was in excess of $26.2 billion in 2005, or $51,600 per infant born preterm. The share that medical care services contributed to the total cost was $16.9 billion ($33,200 per preterm infant), or about two-thirds of the total cost, with more than 85 percent of that medical care delivered during infancy. Maternal delivery costs contributed another $1.9 billion ($3,800 per preterm infant). Special education services associated with a higher prevalence of four disabling conditions (cerebral palsy, mental retardation, hearing loss, and visual impairment) among preterm infants added $1.1 billion ($2,200 per preterm infant), whereas lost household and labor market productivity associated with such disabling conditions contributed $5.7 billion ($11,200 per preterm infant).

Racial and Ethnic Disparities in Preterm Birth

The large disparities in the proportion of preterm births and other birth outcomes between racial and ethnic groups in the United States have been persistent and troubling. The categorization of racial and ethnic groups is difficult and controversial because there is no simple method for defining these groups or subgroups. However, it is important to collect data on race and ethnicity to document and assess health status and health outcomes for various groups of the U.S. population. The U.S. Office of Management and Budget provides a classification system of race and ethnicity to study the social, demographic, health, and economic characteristics of various groups in the United States (EOP, 1995). That system comprises five racial group categories (American Indian or Alaska Native, Asian, black or African American, Native Hawaiian or other Pacific Islander, and white) and two categories for ethnic groups (Hispanic or Latino and not Hispanic or Latino) (EOP, 1995). Newborn infants and fetal deaths are categorized on the basis of the self-reported race of the mother (CDC, 2005d). The data presented in this section were obtained from the National Center for Health Statistics, and the discussion in this section uses this classification system.

Explaining and trying to remedy the significant racial disparities in the proportion of preterm births should be a priority for the research and the health care communities. The most striking disparities are between non-Hispanic white and black women and between Asian or Pacific Islander women and black women (Figure 1-8). Although the highest percentages of

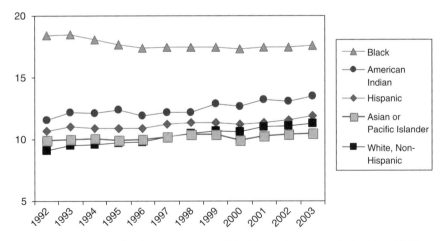

FIGURE 1-8 Preterm births as a percent of live births, by race and ethnicity, 1992 to 2003.
SOURCE: CDC (2004a).

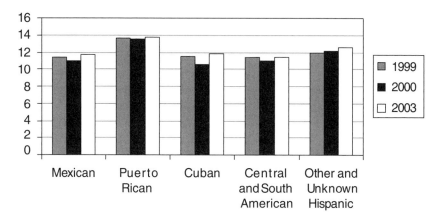

FIGURE 1-9 Preterm births as a percent of live births, by Hispanic subgroups, 1999, 2000, and 2003.
SOURCES: CDC (2001, 2002a).

preterm births occur among non-Hispanic blacks and the lowest percentages occur among Asians and Pacific Islanders, the most notable increases in the percentages of preterm births from 2001 to 2003 were for the white non-Hispanic, American Indian, and Hispanic groups. Overall, the rise in the proportion of preterm births in the United States was due mostly to the increase among the non-Hispanic white population.

The proportion of preterm births among white non-Hispanic women increased from 8.5 percent in 1990 to 11.3 percent in 2003. The proportion has remained fairly stable among Asian and Pacific Islander women (at about 10 percent). Among black women, although the proportion decreased from 18.9 percent in 1990 to 17.8 percent in 2003, overall, these women continue to experience much higher proportions of preterm births.

Although the proportion of preterm births among Hispanic and Asian-Pacific Islander women are the lowest of those among the ethnic and racial minority groups, these are not homogeneous populations. Considerable variation in preterm birth percentages exists among subpopulations of these populations. Although the percentage of preterm births for Hispanics in the United States was 11.9 in 2003, the percentages within subgroups of the Hispanic population ranged from 11.4 to 13.8 percent (Figure 1-9). Compared with other Hispanic subgroups, Puerto Rican women had the highest percentages and Central and South American women had the lowest.

In 2002, the Asian and Pacific Islander subgroups of American women had preterm birth percentages that ranged from 8.3 to 12.2 (Figure 1-10). The Hawaiian (11.7 percent) and Filipino (12.2 percent) subgroups of

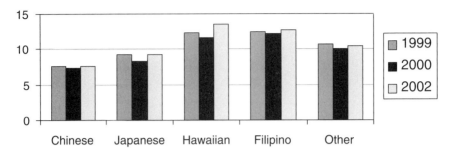

FIGURE 1-10 Preterm births as a percent of live births by Asian and Pacific Islander subgroups, United States, 1999, 2000, and 2002.
SOURCES: CDC (2001, 2002a).

American women had the highest percentages, which were also above the overall percentage among Asians and Pacific Islanders (10.6 percent). Women of Chinese descent had the lowest percentages from 1999 to 2002.

Significant disparities in the mortality rates among infants born preterm also exist (Figure 1-11) (see also Appendix B for an additional discussion of the gestational age-specific IMRs among black and white infants). The mortality rates are significantly higher for non-Hispanic black infants than for

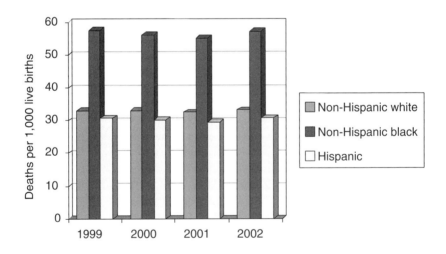

FIGURE 1-11 Mortality rates for preterm infants (less than 37 weeks of gestation) by race or ethnicity, 2002.
SOURCE: CDC (2005c).

non-Hispanic white and Hispanic infants. In 2002, there were 57.3 deaths per 1,000 live births for black infants born at less than 37 weeks of gestation. In contrast, the mortality rates were 33.2 deaths per 1,000 live births for white infants and 30.7 deaths per 1,000 live births for Hispanic infants. Many believe that differences in family socioeconomic conditions explain the differences in the risk for preterm birth by race, particularly between African American and white, non-Hispanic women. However, evidence suggests that the differences in the rates of preterm birth between African American women and white women, as well as the differences in the birth weights and the rates of infant mortality, remain after attempting to adjustment for the family's socioeconomic condition (Collins and Hawkes, 1997; McGrady et al., 1992; Schoendorf et al., 1992; Shiono et al., 1997). Investigators have noted that even after attempting to adjust for socioeconomic condition, substantial differences in income and other related variables remain (Schoendorf et al., 1992). (see Chapter 4 for a full discussion of the sociodemographic factors associated with preterm birth).

CONTENT AND STRUCTURE OF THE REPORT

The purpose of this report is to assess the state of the science on the causes of preterm birth, address the health and economic costs of preterm birth for children born before term and their families, and establish a framework for action in addressing the range of priority issues, including a research and policy agenda for the future. The report is divided into five sections (Table 1-2). Section I reviews and discusses the definitions and terms used to describe the population of preterm infants (Chapter 2). Section II reviews the major categories of research investigating the causes of preterm birth: behavioral and psychosocial factors, sociodemographic and community factors, medical and pregnancy conditions, biological pathways, gene-environment interactions, and environmental toxicants (Chapters 3 to 8). Section III assesses the current understanding of the diagnosis and treat-

TABLE 1-2 Report Organization

Section	Chapter(s)
I. Measurement	2
II. Causes	3 to 8
III. Diagnosis and Treatment	9
IV. Consequences	10 to 12
V. Research and Policy	13 to 15

ment of spontaneous preterm labor (Chapter 9). Section IV explores the consequences of preterm birth including health, developmental, social, psychological, educational, and economic outcomes (Chapters 10 to 12). The final section explores research and policy considerations and concludes with the committee's proposed research agenda for the investigation of preterm birth (Chapters 13 to 15). Recommendations are provided at the end of each section. Table 1-3 describes the points of the committee's charge and the corresponding chapters in which they are addressed.

TABLE 1-3 Committee Charge Points and Report Location Where Addressed

Committee Charge	Chapter(s)
Review and assess the various factors contributing to the growing incidence of premature birth	3 to 8
Assess the economic costs and other societal burdens associated with premature births	10, 12
Address research gaps/needs and priorities for defining the mechanisms by which biological and environmental factors influence premature birth	15
Explore possible changes in public health policy and other policies that may benefit from more research	14
Identify major obstacles to conducting clinical research, which may include • the declining number of residents interested in entering the field of obstetrics and gynecology and the resulting effect on the pipeline of clinical researchers • the impact of rising medical malpractice premiums on the ability of academic programs to provide protected time for physicians to pursue research • the ethical and legal issues involved with conducting research with pregnant women	13
Provide strategies for removing barriers, including those targeting resident career choices, departments of obstetrics and gynecology, agencies and organizations that fund research, and professional organizations	13

SECTION I

MEASUREMENT

2

Measurement of Fetal and Infant Maturity

ABSTRACT

The heterogeneity of the population born preterm is striking. Although pregnancy duration, fetal growth, and fetal or infant physical and neurological maturity are all interrelated and associated with neonatal mortality and morbidity, they are conceptually distinct entities that are differentially influenced by internal and external conditions. Progress in understanding the etiologies and mechanisms of preterm birth and its consequences requires the use of precise definitions, recognition of the limitations of the measures used, and an understanding of the relationships among them. This field requires a better classification of preterm infants into subgroups on the basis of pathogenic pathways, placental findings, genomic markers, and environmental exposures, as well as the recognition that any given individual infant has unique combinations of risk factors and exposures. Outcomes should be reported by gestational age categories, but birth weight for gestational age is an important indicator of the adequacy of fetal growth. Research on methods of quantifying fetal and infant maturity should be encouraged. Pre- and postnatal markers of organ system maturity and predictors of morbidity and functional outcomes that are more effective than birth weight or gestational age should be identified and developed.

Precise definitions of preterm birth are essential for comparing and interpreting the various studies that address the complex problems of preterm birth. These include: (1) studies of the etiologies and mechanisms of preterm birth, (2) trials of the safety and efficacy of strategies for prevention of preterm birth, (3) health and neurodevelopmental outcome studies of preterm infants, (4) trials of the safety and efficacy of medication and treatment strategies for preterm infants, and (5) regional and international comparisons of preterm birth rates.

The concept of prematurity involves biological immaturity for extrauterine life. Maturation is the process of achieving full development or growth. The embryo and fetus matures in utero until organ systems are capable of supporting extrauterine life. Although full-term newborns (neonate) have basic needs (warmth, milk), they are generally capable of sustained breathing, crying when hungry, sucking from a nipple, digesting milk, and complex physiological functions, including gas exchange, blood pressure control, glucose metabolism, and regulation of body fluids. Infants born preterm have immature organ systems that often need additional support to survive. Neonatal intensive care has developed to attend to those needs. Degree of maturity, therefore, is the major determinant of mortality and morbidity (the short- and long-term complications) of preterm birth. Born too soon, preterm infants are more vulnerable to organ injury, death, chronic illness, and neurodevelopmental disability than fullterm newborns (see Chapters 10 and 11). Because there are not good direct measures of degree of maturity, gestational age denotes duration of the pregnancy and is used as a proxy measure of degree of maturity.

Prematurity is not a defined disease or syndrome, and there is no one specific cause or fixed set of outcomes. Moreover, proximal antecedents of prematurity, such as preterm labor or preterm rupture of membranes, may be the cumulative effect of many environmental and genetic factors. Indeed, delivery before term may be required because of threats to the health of mother or fetus from complications of pregnancy. Some causes originate at or even before conception. In addition, as described in Chapter 11, the outcomes for preterm infants are influenced by factors that lead to preterm birth, organ immaturity, neonatal management, and the postnatal environment. Preterm birth is therefore a common, complex condition that results from multiple interactions between the maternal and the fetal genomes and conditions in the intrauterine environment, the mother's body, and her external environment.

While immaturity is the primary characteristic of preterm infants, degree of immaturity varies, even when controlling for duration of pregnancy. As with older children, there is a biologic continuum, and similar gestational ages and fetal sizes may not indicate similar levels of maturity. Just as a 10-year-old may be tall or short and mature or immature for his or her age, an infant born 4 months early may be large or small and more or less mature for an infant born at 24 weeks gestation. This biologic individual variation in size and maturity is the result of different genotypes and different intrauterine and extrauterine environments and experiences. Thus, the complexity of preterm birth and its causes and complications makes it impossible at this time to predict the outcome for an individual preterm infant at delivery with any degree of certainty.

Careful attention to definitions that distinguish between different methods of determining gestational age and recognition of the limitations of measurement methods are necessary to achieve an understanding of the complexities of preterm birth. In lieu of functional measures of fetal or infant maturity, accurate measures of gestational age are essential for clinical care as well as research on the causes, mechanisms, and outcomes of preterm birth. This chapter is devoted to clarifying definitions, describing methods of determining gestational age and their limitations, and demonstrating the implications of the use of precise definitions of the terms used. The reader is referred to Appendix B for further discussions of the definitions of preterm birth and the measurement of gestational age.

DEFINITION OF PRETERM BIRTH

The World Health Organization (WHO) has defined *preterm birth* as delivery before 37 completed weeks of gestation. By convention, gestational age is reported in terms of completed weeks (i.e., one never rounds gestational age up, so 36 weeks and 6 days of gestation is 36 weeks and not 37 weeks of gestation). This definition makes the distinction between being born early and being born too small. Determining when natural conception takes place is difficult (see below), so birth weight (not gestational age) was initially used as a proxy measure for maturity. Although some infants are both too small and born too early, small infants can be either fullterm or preterm (Figure 2-1).

Although it has long been recognized that pregnancy lasts 9 months and that infants who were born before 9 months gestation or who were born small were at risk for death or disability, it was not until the end of the 19th century that systematic attention to the care of preterm infants began. Early efforts at defining prematurity relied on birth weight, with a birth weight less than 2,300 or 2,500 grams considered low birth weight (LBW). LBW was first used as a standard by Nikolaus T. Miller, physician-in-chief of the Moscow Foundling Hospital, and also in 1888 by Pierre Budin, an obstetrician who was a leader in the care of premature infants. The American Academy of Pediatrics adopted this standard in 1935 (Cone, 1985). In 1948, the WHO defined prematurity as a birth weight of 2,500 grams (5 pounds, 8 ounces) or less.

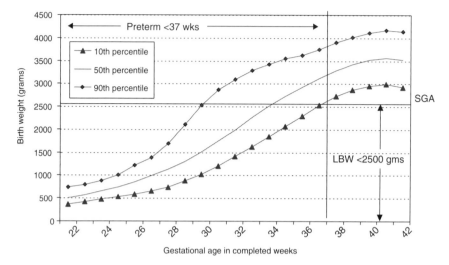

FIGURE 2-1 Fetal growth curves (birth weight percentiles by gestational age), United States, 1999 to 2000. Percentile based on gestational age calculated from LMP (first day of the mother's last menstrual period); SGA = small for gestational age.
SOURCE: Provided by Greg Alexander, 2006.

    The primary problem with the use of birth weight as a proxy for prematurity is that it identifies a group of infants heterogeneous for fetal development and may miss many preterm infants. In the 1960s, Battaglia and Lubchenco (1967) used measurements from a large population of infants to develop norms for fetal growth. At any given gestational age, the distribution of birth weights was such that some infants appeared to be within the norm for their gestational age (defined as "appropriate for gestational age"), some were relatively light (less than the 10th percentile for gestational age, or "small for gestational age"), and others were quite heavy (greater than the 10th percentile for gestational age, or "large for gestational age"). Battaglia and Lubchenco (1967) demonstrated that these categorizations of growth for gestational age had implications for mortality and morbidity. Thus, many preterm infants are large for gestational age but have a normal birth weight, and the rates of mortality and morbidity for these infants differ from those for term infants of normal birth weight. Moreover, at any gestational age, infants who had grown less well (small for gestational age) had poorer outcomes than heavier infants at that gestational age (Lubchenco and Butterfield, 1983). Since then, a number of neonatal growth curves have been published, with the standard diagnosis of small for gestational age based on a birth weight less than 10 percent of the birth weight norm (Alexander et al., 1996, 1999; Kramer et al., 2001a; Usher and McLean, 1969) (Figure 2-1).

Because of the higher accuracy of measures of birth weight, until recently, most researchers have continued to use birth weight cutoffs to designate infant risk. These included very low birth weight (VLBW) infants, whose birth weights are less than 1,500 grams (3 pounds, 5 ounces), and extremely low birthweight (ELBW) infants, whose birth weights are less than 1,000 grams (2 pounds, 3 ounces). The metric system is preferred because an ounce is not small enough to denote significant differences in weights. Moreover, not all researchers used the same birth weight categories, with some using birth weight categories of birth weight less than 2,000, 1,700, 1,250, 800, 750 grams, or, most recently, 600 or 500 grams (Chapter 11). Some researchers who subdivided their study cohort of infants with birth weight less than 1,500 g into two more categories used the term VLBW to describe infants with birth weights of 1,000 to 1,499 grams. The lack of commonly used birth weight categories makes this literature difficult to summarize. Unfortunately, few studies report outcomes by gestational age category. It has only been in the last several decades that gestational age estimates have become more accurate, primarily because of the increase in use of prenatal ultrasounds.

Finding 2-1: Birth weight is an incomplete surrogate for gestational age for determination of the risk of perinatal morbidity and mortality.

MEASUREMENT OF GESTATIONAL AGE

To operationalize the current definition of prematurity, accurate measures of the duration of pregnancy (i.e., gestational age) are needed. Several methods are used to determine gestational age, but many are based on prenatal ultrasounds, which have provided a window onto the fetus and allowed observation of fetal growth and development (Goldstein et al., 1988; Neilson, 2000; Nyberg et al., 2004; Timor-Tritsch et al., 1988; Warren et al., 1989). Most often, prenatal ultrasounds determine pregnancy duration with early measures of fetal size, when there is little individual variation in fetal growth. Individual variations in fetal growth increase with the duration of the pregnancy and become quite prominent by the third trimester. It is ironic that gestational age, which reflects time (duration of pregnancy), is in fact often operationally determined by measures by fetal growth. A number of fetal growth curves have been generated and used to monitor fetal growth during pregnancy.

Use of Date of Last Menstrual Period

Except for women who have used assisted reproductive technologies (ARTs; e.g., in vitro fertilization), the timing of the initiation of a pregnancy is imputed from the first day of the mother's last menstrual period (LMP). Obstetricians have traditionally confirmed pregnancy dating by combining information regarding the mother's LMP, periodic measurements of the mother's abdomen, and when fetal heart sounds and movement (i.e., quickening) are detected (Rawlings and Moore, 1970). If a mother's menstrual cycle is regular (i.e., it is 28 to 29 days long) and she receives good prenatal care with no problems with the pregnancy, LMP can be used to estimate the duration of a pregnancy (Rossavik and Fishburne, 1989). However, wide biologic individual variations in the interval between the onset of LMP and conception (from 7 to more than 25 days) can be due to variations in the timing of menstrual cycles, ovulation, and implantation of the blastocyst. Changes in age, levels of physical activity, body mass index (BMI), nutrition, breast-feeding, interpregnancy interval, smoking, alcohol consumption, and stressful life events can influence the length of an individual woman's menstrual cycle and can therefore influence accuracy of LMP in estimating the duration of a pregnancy (Kato et al., 1999; Liu et al., 2004; Munster et al., 1992; Rowland et al., 2002).

In addition to biological variations in menstrual cycles, ovulation, and implantation, many other factors contribute to difficulties with the use of LMP for pregnancy dating. Irregular menses, first-trimester vaginal bleeding, unrecognized spontaneous abortions, oral contraceptive use, and recall errors contribute to errors in calculating the duration of a pregnancy from LMP. Mothers who are socioeconomically disadvantaged are more likely to receive late or no prenatal care and to have a poor recall of LMP (Campbell et al., 1985; Dubowitz and Goldberg, 1981; Buekens et al., 1984). As many as 25 to 50 percent of the women in some samples have had difficulty recalling LMP (Campbell et al., 1985). Determination of gestational age by the use of LMP or by the use of clinical estimates thus causes significant differences in the gestational age distributions and in the preterm and postterm birth rates for large populations (Alexander et al., 1995; Mustafa and David, 2001). LMP data are missing or incomplete on approximately 20 percent of certificates of live births in the United States, especially for women who are socioeconomically disadvantaged, who are most at risk for preterm birth and intrauterine growth restriction (IUGR). Uncertainty about actual dates contributes to the recording of a digit preference for LMP (e.g., the most common day for LMP is the 15th of the month) (Savitz et al., 2002a; Waller et al., 2000).

When LMP is used to determine gestational age, 40 weeks is added to the LMP to calculate the estimated date of confinement (EDC; which is also referred to as the estimated due date); that is, the day when the infant is due

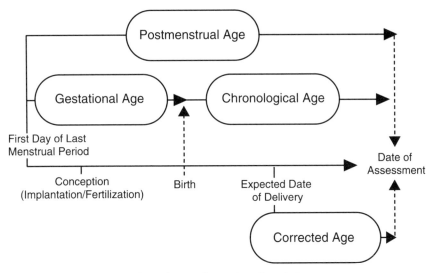

FIGURE 2-2 Age terminology during the perinatal period.
SOURCE: CFN (2004, p. 1363). (Reprinted with permission from *Pediatrics*, Vol. 114, pg. 1363, © 2004 by the AAP.)

to be born (Figure 2-2). This convention of defining gestational age in terms of LMP has been incorporated into the definition of gestational age and used for many years. For women who have used ARTs, EDC is determined from the date of egg retrieval (which is equivalent to the day of ovulation to give a true conceptional age), but gestational age is expressed by use of the conventional definition (thereby adding 2 weeks to the conceptional age, which is approximately the timing of ovulation in a natural cycle). Although it is confusing, gestational age as arbitrarily defined includes an estimated 2 weeks before the embryo is fertilized for the sake of convention and based on the historical use of the term *gestational age.*

Neonatologists and pediatricians have also adopted this arbitrary historical convention from obstetricians regarding gestational age. Neonatologists anticipate the amount of resuscitation and support a preterm infant may need both in the delivery room and in the NICU. Chronological age is the age from the time of birth of an infant, whether the infant was born preterm or fullterm. Postmenstrual age, which suggests (but does not guarantee) a specific degree of maturity/immaturity, is the infant's chronological age (from birth) plus the infant's gestational age at birth (Table 2-1). For office visits following discharge from the NICU, the pediatrician calculates the infant's chronological age (from birth) and the infant's age corrected for degree of prematurity (corrected age, calculated from the infant's due date or EDC.

TABLE 2-1 Methods for Determining Gestational Age

Category	Timing	Measure	Type
Prenatal	First to third trimesters	Last menstrual period	Maternal recall
Prenatal	First to third trimesters	Obstetric clinical estimate*	Maternal exam
Obstetric ultrasound	First trimester	Detection of gestational sac, crown-rump length	Fetal size
Obstetric ultrasound	Second to third trimester	Biparietal diameter, femur length, abdominal and chest circumference	Fetal size
Postnatal	Birth (within first day)	Anthropometric measurements: birthweight, length, head circumference, foot length	Infant size
Postnatal	Birth to 7 days Three to four days after birth to 40 weeks	External physical characteristics	Infant exam
Postnatal	PMA	Neurological assessment: Amiel-Tison	Infant exam
Postnatal	Birth to 4 or 5 days	Combination: Dubowitz, Ballard, New Ballard Score and others**	Infant exam
Postnatal	Any time after birth	Disappearance of pupillary membrane (Anterior Vascular Capsule of Lens)	Infant eye exam

NOTE: PMA = Postmenstrual age.

*Includes onset of pregnancy symptoms, fundal height, time when fetal heartbeat first detected, time of quickening (maternal detection of fetal movement).

**Other combinations have been proposed but are less well known and are used less frequently (See Allen, 2005a for references). The new Ballard Score is most accurate in infants with less than 26 weeks if performed before 12 h after birth (See Allen, 2005a for references).

SOURCE: Allen (2005a). Reprinted with permission from *Mental Retardation and Developmental Disabilities*, Vol. 11, p. 23, © 2005 by Wiley-Liss, Inc.

Use of Ultrasound to Measure Gestational Age

Prenatal gestational age estimates, especially those obtained by early fetal ultrasound, have proven to be more reliable than postnatal estimates of gestational age (Alexander and Allen, 1996; Allen, 2005a; Wariyar et al.,

1997). The accuracy of prenatal ultrasound estimates of gestational age has been confirmed in a number of studies with women who had used ARTs or whose ovulation was confirmed on the basis of basal temperature records (Kalish et al., 2004; Nyberg et al., 2004; Persson and Weldner, 1986; Rossavik and Fishburne, 1989; Saltvedt et al., 2004).

The earlier the ultrasound in the pregnancy, the more accurate the dating of the pregnancy (Drey et al., 2005; Johnsen et al., 2005; Kalish et al., 2004; Neilson, 1998; Nyberg et al., 2004). Measurements of fetal length from head to buttocks (i.e., the crown-rump length) can be used during the first trimester, and it is accurate within 2 to 5 days (Hadlock et al., 1992; Kalish et al., 2004; Wisser et al., 2003). By 14 weeks gestation, a fetus flexes and other measurements are used (e.g., biparietal diameter of the fetal head; head, abdominal and chest circumference; and femur and foot lengths) (Hadlock et al., 1987; Nyberg et al., 2004). Between 14 and 18 weeks gestation, measurement of the biparietal diameter of the fetus's head estimates gestational age to within 9 days (Wariyar et al., 1997), and head circumference estimates gestational age to within 4 days (Chervenak et al., 1998). The use of multiple fetal measurements on a second-trimester ultrasound improves the accuracy of estimation of the gestational age (Chervenak et al., 1998; Hadlock et al., 1987; Johnsen et al., 2005).

Because of increasing individual and pathological variations in fetal growth, gestational age estimates based on fetal measurements from a third-trimester ultrasound are less accurate, especially as the fetus approaches term (Alexander et al., 1999; Altman and Chitty, 1994; Lubchenco et al., 1963; Nyberg et al., 2004). By the third trimester, fetal growth can be adversely influenced by many environmental factors, including uteroplacental insufficiency, maternal drugs or toxins, and congenital infections. Racial, ethnic, and gender variations in birth weight by gestational age are the most prominent during the third trimester (Alexander et al., 1999). In multiple gestations, intrauterine crowding and competition for resources often results in IUGR. Intrauterine growth in twin pregnancies begins to diverge from that in singleton pregnancies at as early as 28 to 30 weeks gestation, with significant differences detected by 35 weeks gestation (Alexander et al., 1998; Min et al., 2000). Intrauterine growth variation is further compromised with higher-order multiples (e.g., triplets and quadruplets) (Alexander et al., 1998; Luke, 1996).

Early prenatal ultrasounds before 20 weeks gestation are more accurate (95 percent confidence interval = ± 3 to 5 days) than any other prenatal or postnatal estimate of pregnancy duration (Alexander et al., 1992; Chervenak et al., 1998; Nyberg et al., 2004; Wisser and Dirscheld, 1994). Studies that have compared ultrasound with LMP have found that more infants were born within 1 to 2 weeks of their due date if the due date was calculated by ultrasound rather than by LMP (Mongelli and Gardosi, 1996;

Savitz et al., 2002b; Yang et al., 2002c). These studies have also noted that the population mean gestational age at birth, as estimated from prenatal ultrasound, was approximately 1 week lower than the mean estimated from LMP. The use of ultrasound to estimate gestational age resulted in the birth of many fewer infants at what was considered postterm and a small increase in the numbers of infants delivered at what was considered preterm.

Despite its accuracy in estimating gestational age, the routine use of prenatal ultrasounds to estimate duration of pregnancy is limited by access to health care issues. Early prenatal ultrasounds require early prenatal care. In the United States, only 84 percent of pregnant women receive prenatal care during the first trimester, and 3.5 percent did not access prenatal care until the third trimester or had no prenatal care (CDC, 2004d). Access to prenatal care is a more serious issue for many women who have the highest risks of preterm delivery (i.e., young, poor, and immigrant women) and there are racial disparities in prenatal care (6.0 percent of non Hispanic black mothers and 5.3 percent of Hispanic mothers had no or late prenatal care, as compared with 2.1 percent of non-Hispanic white mothers (Goldenberg et al., 1992; CDC, 2004d). The United States has no national standard for the routine use of prenatal ultrasound. Although more pregnant women in the United States are receiving ultrasounds than in the past (68 percent in 2002 versus 48 percent in 1989), many may be performed too late in pregnancy or the quality of the ultrasound may not be sufficient for the accurate and reliable estimation of duration of pregnancy (CDC, 2004d).

In the absence of a known date of conception, the more liberal use of early prenatal ultrasounds enhances the best obstetric dating of a pregnancy (Neilson, 1998). Although an ultrasound in the first trimester is most accurate, as mentioned above (Kalish et al., 2004; Salvedt et al., 2004), unless an ultrasound is clinically indicated earlier in the pregnancy, the American College of Obstetricians and Gynecologists practice guidelines note that a single ultrasound at 16 to 20 weeks of gestation can also screen for fetal anomalies (ACOG, 2004). In a meta-analysis of nine trials of routine vs selective use of prenatal ultrasound examinations, routine ultrasounds were associated with earlier detection of multiple pregnancies, reduced rates of induction of labor for post-term pregnancies and increased terminations of pregnancy for fetal congenital anomalies (Neilson, 1998). There were no differences in perinatal mortality, but the studies would have to have had much larger sample sizes to be able to detect a difference.

Although it may be difficult to demonstrate other benefits, there is no doubt that better obstetric dating has clinical benefits for both the mother and the child. Better obstetric dating assists the clinician with making many important decisions, including those related to the timing and the mode of delivery, intrauterine treatments, the inhibition of labor, or the administration of steroids in anticipation of a preterm delivery. Accurate dating is most important at the extremes of prematurity. For example, decisions on whether attempts should be made to try to postpone the delivery of infants who may be born at the lower gestational age for viability (i.e., 22 to 24 weeks of gestation) hinge on accurate estimates of gestational age. Inadvertent elective delivery of the late preterm (or near term) infant could be avoided (and complications of prematurity reduced with more accurate estimates of gestational age) with elective delivery once the fetus is fullterm (see Chapters 10 and 11).

A large increase in health care costs (estimated at one billion dollars a year in the United States) from instituting routine prenatal ultrasounds before the third trimester (there appear to be no benefits of routine late prenatal ultrasounds) can be considered against the benefits of better assessments of gestational age, earlier detection of multiple pregnancies and detection of unsuspected fetal malformations before the third trimester (Neilson, 1998; Bricker and Neilson, 2000). There is no evidence that prenatal ultrasounds have any harmful effects on the mother or fetus. Research regarding preterm birth would benefit, however, from more accurate population data on gestational age, and by including information on how gestational age was estimated in research and national databases, including birth certificate data.

Finding 2-2: The establishment of reliable gestational age estimates by ultrasound early in pregnancy facilitates both research and practice on the identification of multiple gestations; the diagnosis of preterm labor; the need for tocolysis, the administration of steroids, the elective induction of labor; determination of the mode of delivery, the hospital where the birth will take place, whether resuscitation will be needed in the delivery room; and the adequacy of fetal growth.

MEASUREMENT OF FETAL AND INFANT MATURATION

Although much attention has been paid to accurate obstetric estimates of gestational age, there is a similar need for more methods of assessment of fetal and infant maturity. The assessment of maturity is even more important when the gestational age of the fetus is unknown or uncertain. For most preterm infants, the most important determinant of their survival, the development of complications, health sequelae, and neurodevelopmental outcome is the infant's degree of maturation at birth (although the infant's genotype and subsequent environment are also important). The number and frequency of acute complications and the long-term health and neurodevelopmental consequences of preterm delivery have made other measures of fetal immaturity imperative.

Finding 2-3: Neither gestational age nor birth weight is a sufficient or complete indicator of the level of immaturity of a newborn.

Biophysical Profile

Obstetricians need accurate estimates of fetal maturity to make decisions about the optimal time for delivery of the preterm fetus in an adverse intrauterine environment. Fetal heart rate, movement, and responses to stimuli can be monitored to determine fetal well-being. A single measure that combines many of these measures, the biophysical profile, is often used to monitor high-risk pregnancies (Manning, 1995). The likelihood of mortality and morbidity with an immediate preterm birth is weighed against the risks of worsening intrauterine conditions (which at some point could lead to fetal demise) and, on occasion, worsening maternal status. Accurate estimates of fetal maturity would thus facilitate planning for delivery and postnatal management.

Measures of Fetal Lung Maturity

In the 1970s, obstetricians began to analyze chemically the amniotic fluid surrounding the fetus to measure fetal lung maturity (Gluck and Kulovich, 1973a; Gluck, 1971; Gluck et al., 1974; Philip and Spellacy, 2004; Spellacy and Buhi, 1972). The respiratory distress syndrome associated with immature lungs is due in part to the deficient production of surfactant, which stabilizes the alveoli (air sacs) (Chapter 10). With fetal breathing, surfactant is dispersed into the amniotic fluid. Gluck (1971) and Gluck and Kulovich (1973a) measured increasing concentrations of lecithin in comparison with the concentrations of sphingomyelin (i.e., the L/S ratio) in amniotic fluid obtained by amniocentesis (i.e., insertion of a needle into the amniotic sac to obtain amniotic fluid) with gestational age. A low L/S ratio (less than 2) signals fetal lung immaturity and a high probability of respiratory distress syndrome (RDS) if the fetus is delivered (whereas post-term fetuses had L/S ratios as high as 7). Other amniotic fluid tests for fetal lung maturity include the shake test; lamellar body count; and measurement of the phosphatidylglycerol, saturated phosphatidylcholine, fluorescent polarization, or lung phospholipid profile (Torday and Rehan, 2003; Wijnberger et al., 2001).

Physiological Severity Measures

The number, type, and severity of complications of prematurity are directly proportional to neonatal immaturity and physiological instability. Early markers of immaturity or physiological instability would alert health care providers to anticipate other complications and take actions to prevent or treat them as early as possible. Several measures of severity of acute illness (e.g., Scoring for Neonatal Acute Physiology and Clinical Risk Index for Babies) have been developed and are associated with mortality and morbidity rates in preterm infants, although these are not methods for the estimation of gestational age (Gagliardi et al., 2004; Richardson et al., 1993, 1999b). These systems of scoring for the severity of acute illness can be used to compare neonatal intensive care units (NICUs) for quality improvement initiatives and for insight into why complications and outcomes differ among NICUs (Richardson et al., 1999a).

Postnatal Estimates of Maturity

In the 1960s to 1970s, missing or inaccurate gestational age data for many newborns led to a search for postnatal methods of determining gestational age. These methods invariably focused on the degree of infant maturation (Allen, 2005a; Philip et al., 2003). Farr et al. (1966) described the maturation of a number of external physical characteristics in preterm and term infants. Hittner et al. (1977, 1981) proposed a systematic method of grading the disappearance of the pupillary membrane (i.e., the anterior vascular capsule of the lens of a preterm infant's eye) at 2-week intervals from 27 to 34 weeks of gestation. French investigators developed a method of measuring neurological maturity from observations of the changes in neck, trunk, and extremity flexor tone and posture with gestational age (Amiel-Tison, 1968; Amiel-Tison et al., 2002; Philip et al., 2003; Saint-Anne Dargassies, 1977). A number of postnatal clinical measures of the degree of maturation of external physical characteristics or neurological muscle tone, or both, were developed to estimate gestational age of preterm and fullterm infants (Allen, 2005a; Ballard et al., 1979, 1991; Dubowitz et al., 1970; Parkin et al., 1976).

These clinical postnatal measures are less predictive of gestational age (i.e., pregnancy duration at birth) at the extremes of gestation (i.e., in preterm and postterm infants) and in very sick infants (Alexander et al., 1990; Sanders et al., 1991; Shukla et al., 1987; Spinnato et al., 1984). The most widely used postnatal measures, the New Ballard Score (Ballard et al., 1991) and the Dubowitz gestational age assessment (Dubowitz et al., 1970), overestimate gestational age by 2 or more weeks in 45 to 75 percent of preterm infants with birth weights less than 1,500 grams (Sanders et al., 1991; Shukla et al., 1987; Spinnato et al., 1984). The accuracies of these measures decrease with an increase in gestational age (Alexander et al., 1990; Sanders et al., 1991). Gestational age is more often overestimated in African-American preterm infants than in white preterm infants, even when

LMP, sociodemographic variables, pregnancy complications, and delivery characteristics are controlled for (Alexander et al., 1992).

Although some of these postnatal gestational age measures are extensively used to estimate gestational age at birth, first- and second-trimester ultrasounds are far more accurate at estimating gestational age (Alexander et al., 1990, 1992; Mitchell, 1979; Wariyar et al., 1997). In a comparison study, Wariyar et al. (1997) found that ultrasound before 20 weeks of gestation was the most accurate (95% confidence interval = ±9 days, whereas the 95% confidence interval = ±17 days for postnatal methods). For preterm infants with gestational ages of less than 30 weeks, an ultrasound performed before 20 weeks of gestation was more accurate than an ultrasound performed at or after 20 weeks of gestation for determination of gestational age at birth (95% confidence intervals = ±9 days and ±15 days, respectively), the New Ballard Score (95% confidence interval = ±24 days), and the Dubowitz gestational age assessment (95% confidence interval = ±34 days).

The difficulty of using postnatal measures of degree of maturation of external physical characteristics and neurological muscle tone to estimate gestational age at birth highlights the difference between pregnancy duration and degree of maturation (Allen, 2005a). Although conceptually the use of the words "gestational age" implies a time interval, duration of pregnancy, the measurement of gestational age has historically involved either measures of fetal or infant size, or measures of degree of infant maturation. Since degree of fetal maturation plays an important role in infant mortality and morbidity rates, and may play a role in the signaling mechanisms for the normal initiation of labor at term, clarity in how gestational age is defined and determined is essential for understanding the mechanisms leading to preterm birth.

Measures of Functional Maturity

Neuromaturational changes in brain structural and functional development have been noted in preterm infants. These changes can be detected by detailed neurological examination, neuroimaging (especially cranial ultrasound), electroencephalography (EEG), amplitude-integrated EEG (a-EEG), electroretinography and neurophysiological measures of conduction time after auditory, visual, or tactile stimulation (Allen, 2005a; Amiel-Tison and Gosselin, 2001; Burdjalov et al., 2003; Finnstrom, 1972; Henderson-Smart et al., 1985; Kesson et al., 1985; Klimach and Cooke, 1988; Leaf et al., 1995; Miller et al., 1983; Olischar et al., 2004a,b). Prenatal ultrasounds have detected sonographic landmarks of normal fetal cortical development, which is important to know for the prenatal detection of fetal brain malformations (Perri et al., 2005).

Wide variations in responses at each gestational age or postmenstrual age, and the need for special equipment and expertise for the most part limits their use for estimating gestational age at birth. However, current research focuses on using clinical and neurophysiological measures of neuromaturation (e.g., amplitude-integrated EEG and comprehensive neurodevelopmental examinations) to assess ongoing development and integrity of the central nervous system (CNS) in high-risk preterm infants in an NICU (Allen, 2005a; Amiel-Tison and Grenier, 1986; Burdjalov et al., 2003; Olischar et al., 2004a,b). Better measures of fetal and infant neuromaturation have the potential to detect abnormalities; predict neurodevelopmental outcomes for more effective counseling of the parents and the more effective use of limited community resources; evaluate the effects of various prenatal and NICU interventions on CNS development; and provide insight into the various causes of CNS injury, neuroprotective factors, and mechanisms of CNS recovery after injury.

HETEROGENEITY OF THE PRETERM INFANT POPULATION

Intrauterine Growth Restriction, Small for Gestational Age, and Fetal Maturation

Intrauterine growth restriction (IUGR, also known as fetal growth restriction) is as complex and multifactorial a condition as preterm delivery, and many of its etiologies and mechanisms are just as poorly understood. The fetus may be small for familial reasons (i.e., the parents are small) or because of a chromosomal disorder, dysmorphic syndrome, or congenital infection. When other causes of IUGR have been ruled out, *uteroplacental insufficiency* and *fetal deprivation of supply* are catchall terms used to identify fetuses whose poor growth is assumed to be due to an inadequate placental supply of nutrition, inadequate gas exchange, or the lack of other resources. Fetuses with a declining growth rate (i.e., IUGR) may be delivered before they have actually achieved a weight that would make them small for gestational age (birth weight less than the 10th percentile for gestational age). Declining body growth in response to inadequate intrauterine supply but with a relative preservation of brain growth has been viewed as an adaptive response that protects fetal brain development (Warshaw, 1985).

Some controversy exists as to how the appropriateness of growth for gestational age should be diagnosed and what growth standards should be used. The standard has been any one of a number of published curves that plot the birth weight of live-born infants against their gestational age at delivery, in which small for gestational age is defined as birth weight less than the 10th percentile for gestational age (Alexander et al., 1999; Kramer et al., 2001b; Lubchenco et al., 1963; Usher and McLean, 1969). The more rigorous small-for-gestational-age definition of a birth weight that is 2 or more standard deviations below the mean is seldom used. Because of geographical or population differences, birth weights for gestational age curves vary (for example, birth weights are lower in Colorado because of the higher altitude (Alexander et al., 1999; Kramer et al., 2001b; Lubchenco et al., 1963). Because of significant differences in the distributions of birth weights, Kramer et al. (2001b) reported birth weight percentiles by gender and Alexander et al. (1999) reported birth weight percentiles for gestational age by race, Hispanic origin, and gender. There is no agreement whether a diagnosis of small for gestational age should be based on racial, ethnic, or gender norms. The focus has been on identifying small for gestational age infants on the basis of their birthweight for gestational age, but identifying fetal growth restriction by comparing weight for length or head circumference growth has also been suggested.

Weight for gestational age distribution curves are very different when fetal weights are imputed from prenatal ultrasound data and are compared to birthweight for gestational age distribution curves for infants born in a similar population (Bernstein et al., 1994). Ultrasound estimates of fetal weights are valid, in that the 95 percent confidence intervals for individual estimates are ±15 percent, errors are not systematic, and estimates of the mean population fetal weight in a large sample are accurate (Hadlock et al., 1984). Comparison of these curves demonstrates that at the lower gestational ages, infants delivered preterm as a group are much smaller than fetuses that remained in utero and delivered closer to fullterm. A change from the use of data generated from infants born at a given gestational age less than 36 weeks to the use of weight data estimated from prenatal ultrasounds at that gestational age increases the proportion of infants diagnosed at birth as being small for gestational age from 10 to 25 percent. This approach has not been widely adopted, but these data raise a convincing argument for the use of the ultrasound estimates of fetal weight data to define small for gestational age (Bernstein, 2003). Furthermore, these data suggest an overlap between preterm birth and IUGR.

In addition to a relative preservation of brain growth, some data suggest that fetuses make other adaptations to adverse intrauterine conditions, such as the acceleration of lung and brain maturation (Amiel-Tison et al., 2004a,b). Several studies of chemical amniotic fluid analyses have noted that some preterm fetuses that had IUGR or that were from pregnancies complicated by chronic placental abruption, prolonged rupture of membranes, placental infarction, severe preeclampsia, chronic hypertension, or amnionitis had L/S ratios that were higher than expected for their gestational age, indicating that the fetuses had more mature lungs (Gluck and Kulovich, 1973b; Gould et al., 1977). Amiel-Tison (1980) and Amiel-Tison et al. (2004a,b) have noted accelerated neuromaturation in some infants with IUGR, infants born to mothers with hypertension, and infants of multiple gestations. Others have noted higher than expected Ballard or Dubowitz scores (they were more mature) among infants of known gestational age who are small for gestational age and who have been born to hypertensive mothers; and a few have noted lower than expected scores (they were less mature) for the infants of diabetic mothers (Ballard et al., 1979; Dubowitz and Dubowitz, 1985; Spinnato et al., 1984). When preterm IUGR infants and infants of multiple gestations are born after 33 to 34 weeks gestation, they may have fewer complications of prematurity than expected for their gestational age (Allen, 2005b; Ley et al., 1997). Infants born with IUGR before 34 weeks gestation have greater mortality and morbidity than preterm appropriate for gestational age infants of the same gestational age (Garite et al., 2004; Tyson et al., 1995).

Accelerated neuromaturation, as measured by electrophysiological measures of auditory and visual neuromaturation, has also been observed among fetuses growing under adverse intrauterine conditions. Conduction times decrease as the CNS matures and becomes more efficient at conducting impulses. Investigators have noted shorter than expected conduction times in preterm infants who are small for gestational age, preterm infants who are born to hypertensive mothers or after stressed pregnancies, and preterm infants with Doppler flow evidence of fetal brain sparing (Henderson-Smart et al., 1985; Pettigrew et al., 1985; Scherjon et al., 1992, 1993). Amiel-Tison and Pettigrew (1991) and Amiel-Tison et al. (2004a) have reviewed this evidence and concluded that accelerated neuromaturation is not an all-or-nothing phenomenon but is "a progressive response by variable degree" (Amiel-Tison et al., 2004a, p. 20).

There is a physiological cost to fetal development for accelerated fetal maturation in the face of adverse intrauterine circumstances. Scherjon et al. (2000) found a lower mean intelligence quotient score (87 versus 90) and a higher incidence of cognitive impairment (54 versus 20 percent) in 5-year-old children who had had Doppler flow evidence of fetal brain sparing and accelerated neuromaturation than in those without accelerated neuromaturation. These data from a longitudinal study of adaptive mechanisms in infants who encountered IUGR is a reminder that survival under adverse intrauterine circumstances has many costs over the life span.

The long-term effects of IUGR and its adaptive mechanisms on fetal brain development and health and functioning as an adult are not well understood and need to be studied further. Adverse intrauterine circumstances can overwhelm adaptive mechanisms and lead to organ injury and death. Obstetricians face the challenge of recognizing and delivering these infants before decompensation and organ injury occur, and must weigh the consequences of earlier preterm birth against increasing IUGR.

Perinatal Mortality of Infants Born at the Limit of Viability

Although WHO has defined the upper limit of prematurity as a gestational age of 36 weeks and 6 days, the lower limit is determined by fetal organ development and advances in high-risk obstetric and neonatal intensive care. Dramatic decreases in neonatal mortality rates and gestational age-specific neonatal mortality rates have been associated with a concomitant lowering of the limit of viability (Alexander et al., 1999; Allen et al., 2000; Appendix B). A current concern is that a biological limit has been reached and that major new technological advances will be required for any further lowering of the limit of viability (Hack and Fanaroff, 1999).

A limiting factor in interpreting all studies of survival and complications at the lower limit of viability is the accuracy of gestational age determination. In these studies, various proportions of each population sample studied did not have ultrasound confirmation of the dates of conception. At the limit of viability, each week of gestation makes a difference in the rate of survival of an infant born preterm and the complications that the infant may encounter (Allen et al., 1993; Wood et al., 2000). However, how much information is lost in these studies because of incorrect gestational age data? Could some of the infants who were born at 22 or 23 weeks of gestation and who survived have been misclassified and have actually been born at 24 or 25 weeks of gestation? Improvements in the accuracy of gestational age data will provide more reliable data on survival and outcomes at the limit of viability and enhance clinicians' ability to counsel the parents.

For infants born at the lower limit of viability, the aggressiveness of resuscitation at delivery varies considerably from region to region, as does the degree to which parents participate in the medical decision making (Hakansson et al., 2004; Haumont, 2005; Ho and Saigal, 2005; Lorenz and Paneth, 2000; Partridge et al., 2005; Appendix C). Infants born at 22 to 25 weeks gestation die if they are not resuscitated at birth and provided with neonatal intensive care. Many studies do not report the proportion of live births who were resuscitated. Concerns about the ultimate survival of infants born at the limit of viability to adulthood and the likelihood of significant disability or chronic illness, pain, and suffering cause parents and health providers to question how these infants should be managed. Although most very immature infants die during the first day after birth, another concern is that further advances in neonatal intensive care may merely prolong their dying for days to weeks. Although there are sporadic reports of survival at the lowest gestational ages (21 or 22 weeks gestation) or birth weights (400 grams), some have defined the lower limit of viability as that gestational age or birth weight at which 50% survive (Alexander et al., 1999; Allen et al., 2000).

Discussion of the management and survival of infants born at the lower limit of viability requires extreme precision and attention to how mortality and outcome rates are calculated. For example, data should be provided as to what proportion of infants were resuscitated at delivery and provided with neonatal intensive care. The proportion of infants with congenital anomalies, especially anomalies that contribute to the infant's death, should be reported. Care should also be taken to describe the chronological age at which survival is ascertained. The conventional definition of the neonatal mortality rate excludes infants who survive past 28 days but who die before they leave the NICU. Likewise, studies that report survival to the time of NICU discharge may miss deaths later in the first year of life that would be captured by infant mortality rates.

When reviewing mortality rates for infants born at the limit of viability, attention to the denominator used to calculate mortality rates at the limit of viability is important (Allen et al., 1993; Evans and Levene, 2001). Many tertiary-care NICUs report birth weight- and gestational age-specific mortality rates that use the number of infants admitted to the NICU as the denominator. However, many infants born at 22 to 25 weeks gestation die shortly after delivery, and are never admitted to an NICU. In addition, a large proportion of infants born at a gestational age of less than 23 weeks or with a birth weight of less than 500 grams are stillborn (60 to 89 percent and 68 to 77 percent, respectively) (Sauve et al., 1998; Wood et al., 2000).

Although there are guidelines for distinguishing between a fetal death and live birth (Table 2-2), the clinical distinction is not as clear as one might think. A fetal death occurs before the fetus is completely delivered and excludes induced terminations. The clinician must distinguish between evidence of life (e.g., beating heart, pulsation of the umbilical cord, or the movement of voluntary muscles) from transient or fleeting cardiac contractions, gasps, or jerks of the limbs. This is most difficult in fetuses born at 21 to 24 weeks of gestation. How many of these infants have been categorized in the past as live births instead of fetal deaths is unknown, as is how this categorization varies from region to region and even among health care providers at the same institution. A willingness to resuscitate a very immature infant who has a transient heart beat or gasp at delivery changes the classification of that infant from a fetal death to an infant death. This type of change in how an infant is classified has only a small impact on the preterm birth rate (because so many more infants are born after 26 weeks gestation), but could contribute substantially to rising U.S. Infant Mortality Rates. The use of perinatal mortality rates (the number of deaths of infants with gestational ages greater than 20 weeks/1,000 total births) may be a more useful measure of the outcomes of very preterm infants, since it includes infants who are stillborn and infants who die immediately after birth.

TABLE 2-2 Definitions of Spontaneous Abortion, Fetal Death, Stillbirth and Live Birth

Spontaneous abortion	Abortion occurring without medical or mechanical means to empty the uterus.
Fetal death or stillbirth	Death before the complete expulsion or extraction from its mother of a product of conception, irrespective of the duration of pregnancy. The death is indicated by the fact that after such separation, the fetus does not breathe or show any other evidence of life, such as beating of the heart, pulsation of the umbilical cord, or definite movement of voluntary muscles. A death that occurs at 20 or more weeks of gestation constitutes a fetal death and after 28 weeks it is considered a late fetal death.
Live birth	The term used to record a birth whenever the newborn at or sometime after birth breathes spontaneously, or shows any other sign of life such as a heartbeat or definite spontaneous movement of voluntary muscles. Heartbeats are to be distinguished from transient cardiac contractions, and respirations are to be distinguished from fleeting respiratory efforts or gasps.

SOURCES: CDC (2004e), Cunningham et al. (2005).

Marked regional variations in the management and the rates of survival of infants born at the lower limit of viability and variations in the methods used to estimate gestational age make it difficult to evaluate trends over time with respect to live birth rates by gestational age and fetal death rates (Costeloe et al., 2000; Lorenz et al., 2001; Sanders et al., 1998; Tyson et al., 1996). For infants born at the lower limit of viability, an accurate estimate of gestational age is essential for guiding discussions about the many decisions to be made during and after delivery, including the timing and mode of delivery and whether antenatal steroids and aggressive resuscitation should be used at the time of delivery. Discussions of management and outcomes should focus not on when survival is possible but on a working definition of the limit of viability, when chances of survival, or of survival without major disability, are substantial (for example, 50 percent). Furthermore, better measures of fetal and infant maturity have the potential to improve the clinical care that is provided, improve the ability to predict short- and long-term outcomes, and assist families and health care providers in making difficult care management decisions.

Late-Term or Near-Term Infants Born at the Upper Border of Prematurity

At all times during a pregnancy, accurate dating of the pregnancy and accurate estimates of fetal maturity provide better information for decision making by the health care provider and the family. Although this is especially true for the high-risk pregnancies noted above, the information also assists the health care provider and the family with making decisions on how a threatened preterm delivery is managed and the optimal timing and mode of delivery as a pregnancy approaches fullterm. Accurate gestational age and maturity information facilitates better prenatal counseling about the anticipated chance of survival, complications, and the long-term health and neurodevelopmental outcomes of the preterm infant born near to fullterm.

There is not a standard accepted definition of this category of infants. Studies have varied as to whether they included infants with gestational ages from 32, 33, or 34 completed weeks gestation to 36 completed weeks gestation (Amiel-Tison et al., 2002). These infants have been called near-term infants, late-term infants, and macropremies, but "late-term infants" serves as a reminder that they are not yet fullterm.

The majority of preterm infants are born at 33 to 36 weeks of gestation (Table 2-3) (Appendix B). From 1995 to 2000, 8.9 percent of all U.S. births were infants born at 33 to 36 weeks gestation, whereas only 3 percent were born at gestational ages of less than 33 weeks. As many as 34 percent of twins are born at 32 to 35 weeks gestation, 31 percent are born at 36 to 37 weeks of gestation, and only 24 percent are born after 37 weeks gestation (Min et al., 2000). Many near-term preterm infants have normal birth weights, and most receive routine care in well-baby nurseries (Amiel-Tison et al., 2004a; Wang ML et al., 2004).

TABLE 2-3 Proportion of Births for Various Gestational Age Categories, United States,1985 to 1988 and 1995 to 2000

Gestational Age (weeks)	Gestational Age Categories	1985–1988	1995–2000
≤28	Extremely preterm	0.66	0.82
≤32	Very preterm	1.9	2.2
33-36	Moderately preterm	7.7	8.9
<37	Preterm	9.7	11.2
42+	Postterm	11.9	7.0

SOURCE: Alexander (2006 [Appendix B]).

Although their outcomes are better than outcomes of preterm infants with gestational ages of less than 32 or 33 weeks, late preterm infants remain vulnerable to the complications of prematurity. They are more likely than fullterm infants to experience cold stress, hypoglycemia, respiratory distress syndrome, jaundice, and sepsis, yet there are wide variations among hospitals in treatments and resource use for late preterm infants (Amiel-Tison et al., 2002; Laptook and Jackson, 2006; Lewis et al., 1996; McCormick et al., 2006; Wang ML et al., 2004). Despite a relative lack of information regarding long-term outcomes, retrospective studies of children with cerebral palsy report that 16 percent to 20 percent were born between 32 and 36 weeks gestation (Hagberg et al., 1996; MacGillivray and Campbell, 1995).

Accurate estimates of gestational age and better measures of fetal and infant maturity would provide important information for clinical decision making. Recognizing the higher mortality and morbidity rates for late preterm infants than fullterm infants, health care providers and families need to weigh carefully the advantages of earlier delivery against the health, financial, and economic costs of preterm delivery.

IMPLICATIONS FOR PUBLIC HEALTH AND RESEARCH

Although the complex interplay between the duration of pregnancy, fetal and infant size and maturity, and how they are measured are sources of some confusion, evaluation of the interrelationships among these factors provides an opportunity to gain some insight into the factors contributing to preterm birth. For example, racial disparities in all aspects of health have long been recognized, and the causes of these disparities are poorly understood. Public health databases with data on births, health problems, and deaths for large populations are available for exploration; but it must be recognized that the definitions of these variables may have changed over time.

Racial and Ethnic Disparities

Although controversy exists over inclusion criteria for racial and ethnic subgroups, racial and ethnic disparities in preterm birth rates, birth weight distributions for gestational age, neonatal and infant mortality rates, and gestational age- and birth weight-specific neonatal mortality rates have been consistently reported (see Appendix B). In the United States in 2003, preterm birth rates were 10.5 for Asian and Pacific Islanders, 11.3 percent for whites, and 17.8 percent for African Americans (Chapter 1). In 1997, the birth rates for white, Hispanic, and African American infants with gestational ages less than 28 weeks were 0.35, 0.45, and 1.39 percent, respectively

(Alexander et al., 2003). Racial, ethnic, and gender differences in birth weight for gestational age become increasingly prominent as pregnancies approach term (Alexander et al., 1999). At 40 weeks of gestation, birth weight for African American infants tends to be lower than those for white, Hispanic, and Native American infants.

Furthermore, despite overall dramatic reductions over the decades, racial and ethnic disparities in neonatal and infant mortality rates in the United States persist (Alexander et al., 2003). Although mortality rates are higher for full-term African American infants than for full-term white infants, the smaller and more preterm the infant is, the more of a survival advantage that preterm African American infants have over preterm white and preterm Hispanic infants (Alexander et al., 1999, 2003; Allen et al., 2000; Demissie et al., 2001). As gestational age-specific neonatal mortality has decreased over the last several decades, this gap has narrowed but still exists for the more immature or smaller preterm infants (Allen et al., 2000; Hamvas et al., 1996, Appendix B). Borrowing the pharmacologists' concept of the 50 percent lethal dose (LD50), which is the point at which 50 percent of a population dies and 50 percent survives, that 50 percent point decreased from 26.8 weeks gestation in 1975–1979 to 24.5 weeks in 1990–1994 for white infants born in South Carolina (Allen et al., 2000). For African American infants, the gestational age at which 50 percent survive decreased from 25.2 to 23.9 weeks. The gap in survival between white and African American infants decreased during those two time periods, from a difference of 1.6 weeks to 0.5 week of gestation, respectively.

Although racial disparities in preterm birth rates and mortality rates have been noted for many years, the reasons for these differences are complex and not well understood. Some have suggested that many of the obstetric and neonatal intensive care advances (e.g., surfactant and antenatal steroid use) disproportionately improved the rates of survival for white preterm infants (who had higher incidences of RDS within each gestational age category) (Hamvas et al., 1996). Gender disparities, with higher mortality and pulmonary morbidity rates in preterm male infants are presumed to be based on not yet elucidated biological mechanisms (Stevenson et al., 2005). Others are concerned that neonatal mortality rates are higher in hospitals that serve predominantly minority populations (Morales et al., 2005). The reported racial and ethnic differences in risk factors for and presentations of preterm birth suggest that the etiologies of preterm birth may play a role (Ananth et al., 2005; Reagan and Salsberry, 2005). From 1989 to 2000, the rate of preterm birth following preterm labor increased by 3 percent for whites but decreased by 27 percent for African Americans (Ananth et al., 2005). Medically indicated preterm birth increased for both groups, but at different rates: 55 and 32 percent for whites and African Americans, respectively. Preterm births following ruptured membranes decreased for both groups: 23 and 37 percent, respectively. Declines in neonatal mortality were associated with increases in medically indicated preterm births in white preterm infants but with declines in preterm birth following labor or ruptured membranes in black preterm infants. An important question is how racial disparities in preterm birth are influenced by the broad social context (see Chapter 4).

An important consideration for all of these issues is that the method used to estimate gestational age may play a complex (and interfering) role. Postnatal estimates of gestational age, especially the Ballard and Dubowitz gestational age assessments, tend to overestimate gestational age in preterm infants, but the magnitude of the overestimation varies with race and ethnicity. Even when a variety of maternal sociodemographic variables, pregnancy complications, and the type of delivery are controlled for, African American infants had significantly higher mean postnatal gestational age estimates for each gestational age interval (Alexander et al., 1992). The Ballard gestational age estimate was higher for African Americans for each gestational age interval, whether gestational age was determined by LMP or prenatal ultrasound (for a subset of infants for whom these data were available). In this study, the proportion of preterm births changed, depending on whether gestational age was estimated from LMP or Ballard score, and the amount of change varied by race. Since the Ballard estimates gestational age from physical and neurological infant characteristics, these and other similar data raise the question as to whether African-American infants mature more rapidly than white infants.

In response to missing data for gestational age as determined by LMP on many U.S. birth certificates, a location for insertion of the clinical estimate of the infant's gestational age was added to U.S. birth certificates in 1989 and was intended to be a cross-check of the gestational age determined by LMP. It is likely that postnatal estimates factored into the clinical gestational age estimates recorded on the birth certificate, although the magnitude of this tendency is unknown. Any data obtained by using these clinical gestational age estimates are therefore difficult to interpret, especially when one is trying to discern true racial and ethnic differences from artifacts of data reporting (i.e., the use of postnatal gestational age estimates). This problem has implications for the use of the clinical gestational age estimates to evaluate differences in gestational age distributions, birth weights for gestational age, and gestational age-specific mortality data. Rather than reverting to a reliance only on birth weight data, this problem argues for moving toward the adoption of early ultrasound to establish or confirm the gestational age or EDC for all pregnancies. The earlier in gestation that the prenatal ultrasound is performed, the greater the validity that the gestational age estimates for all racial and ethnic groups becomes.

Public Health Databases

Developed countries have set up complex public health systems to collect data on births, deaths, and other indicators of health for their populations. In the United States, the recording of vital events is the responsibility of each of the states and not the federal government. The National Vital Statistics System is a collaborative effort between state and territory agencies and, as federal representatives, the Centers for Disease Control and Prevention and the National Center for Health Statistics (NCHS) (Martin and Hoyert, 2002). NCHS develops standards for the uniform reporting of live births and fetal, neonatal, and infant deaths to national public health databases through cooperative agreements. Although birth certificates are intended to establish the date of birth, the citizenship, and the nationality of a newborn infant, they contain valuable public health information and are the only national source of birth weight and gestational age data. Large state and national population databases with birth and death certificate data have been used to plot gestational age distributions, birth weights for gestational age, and gestational age- and birth weight-specific neonatal mortality rates.

The systematic and random misclassification of birth weight, gestational age, and other birth and death certificate data is a continuing problem with all population databases, although procedures have been established to clean the data to eliminate those that are implausible. A consistent finding in many sets of perinatal data is a bimodal distribution of birth weight for gestational age, which is often attributed to the occasional miscoding of gestational age in fullterm infants with normal birth weights (David, 1980; Platt, 2002). One study noted frequent errors when obstetrics estimates of gestational age were transferred to infants' medical records: in 15 percent of the cases, the gestational age was wrong by at least a week (Wariyar et al., 1997). Some were systematic errors, such as recording of the gestational age at the time of maternal hospital admission and not the gestational age at birth and the lack of attention to high-quality antenatal data. Similar errors may be made on original birth and death certificates, depending on the recorder's training, experience, and level of attention to detail.

Gestational age is used to calculate a variety of statistical indicators used to monitor the health of the mothers and children in a population. These indicators include the proportion of infants born preterm (before 37 weeks gestation), very preterm (before 32 weeks gestation), with an LBW (birth weight less than 2,500 grams) or a VLBW (birth weight less than 1,500 grams), and small for gestational age. The gestational age of a fetus at the time of initiation of prenatal care is one factor included when the prenatal care index is computed. All of this information can be used to target public health interventions and monitor their effects.

Changes in how gestational age is estimated and recorded have implications for all fetal and neonatal health indicators and for time and regional comparisons of fetal and neonatal health. Although birth certificates have recorded the duration of pregnancy since 1939 (initially in months), LMP has been recorded only since 1968. Although the addition of a clinical estimate of gestational age was recommended in 1989, the method used to determine that estimate was not specified on the birth certificate. The proportion of clinicians who base the clinical gestational age estimate on postnatal assessments is unknown. The magnitude by which postnatal assessments overestimate gestational age varies with both gestational age and race or ethnicity (Alexander et al., 1990, 1992; Sanders et al., 1991; Shukla et al., 1987; Spinnato et al., 1984). As discussed earlier in this chapter, an additional problem with postnatal assessments of gestational age is that they are generally based on signs of maturity, and infants with IUGR and from complicated pregnancies can demonstrate accelerated maturation after 30 weeks of gestation (Amiel-Tison et al., 2004a,b).

As a remedy, in 2003 NCHS recommended that the clinical estimate of gestational age be replaced with the best obstetric estimate of gestational age, which "should be determined by all perinatal factors and assessments such as ultrasound, but *not* the neonatal exam" (CDC, 2004b, p. 172). States will be gradually making this change over the next several years. Agencies and researchers will need to consider these changes when they analyze the trends and state-to-state comparisons using gestational age.

Fortunately, the change in gestational age determination from the use of LMP to ultrasound-based data has less of an effect on the preterm birth rate than it does on the birth rate for postterm infants born after 41 weeks gestation. Studies agree that this shift decreases the postterm birth rates, but the increase in the preterm birth rate is less (Goldenberg et al., 1989; Kramer et al., 1988; Savitz et al., 2005; Yang et al., 2002c). The timing of the ultrasound assessment is important: ultrasounds early in pregnancy increase the number of births determined to be fullterm by LMP but reclassified as preterm by ultrasound assessment more than ultrasounds late in the pregnancy. Multiparous mothers and mothers with small stature, diabetes, and high prepregnancy BMIs and fetuses with chromosomal anomalies were more likely to have large ($\geq$7-day) discrepancies between LMP- and early ultrasound-based gestational ages (Morin et al., 2005). Thus, a gradual shift toward the use of prenatal ultrasound to determine or confirm gestational age may be contributing to the rising preterm birth rates.

Administrators and researchers working with data from these large databases need to recognize and specifically state how gestational age variables were calculated, used, and imputed, especially when the data are interpreted and used. Differences in gestational age variables interfere with and complicate comparisons among states and countries and over time. For example, one study defined gestational age in completed weeks as estimated from LMP when it was available, imputed gestational age if the month and the year were recorded, but had to rely on clinical estimates in 4 to 5 percent of the cases and had to eliminate from the calculations birth certificates with missing data (2 percent of white infants, 2.7 percent of African American infants, and 3.6 percent of Hispanic infants) (Alexander et al., 2003). These proportions will change in the coming years as more states begin to record best obstetric estimates and the rate of clinical use of early ultrasound to date pregnancies increases.

Clarifying Mortality Rates

The decentralized system for the reporting of vital statistics in the United States has made it difficult to compare state-to-state variations in preterm birth, fetal death, and infant mortality rates (Martin and Hoyert, 2002). In addition to variations in the reporting of gestational age on birth certificates, state requirements for the reporting of fetal deaths vary. There are also regional differences in the rates of underreporting of fetal deaths and missing data on fetal deaths. As attention has shifted toward survival at the lower limits of viability, the definitions of a fetal death and a live birth require attention. How life and death are defined and how very immature and critically ill fetuses are managed at delivery may have important effects on a number of recent trends, including rising preterm birth, neonatal and infant mortality rates, and decreasing fetal death rates.

Less attention has generally been paid to fetal deaths than to neonatal and infant deaths. Approximately 16 percent of all pregnancies end in the death of the fetus (Martin and Hoyert, 2002; Ventura et al., 2001). Fetal death generally includes spontaneous abortions, miscarriages, and stillbirths. The majority (more than 90 percent) of fetal deaths occur in the first 20 weeks pregnancy; 5 percent occur at 20 to 27 weeks gestation; and 2 percent occur late in pregnancy; that is, after 27 weeks gestation. The greatest decrease has been in fetal deaths after 27 weeks gestation. States have different requirements on the data on fetal deaths that must be reported; some require gestational age (gestational age at or beyond 16 weeks, 20 weeks, or 5 months), some require birth weight (birth weight at or above 350, 400, or 500 grams), and some require both gestational age and birth weight criteria. Missing data regarding initiation of prenatal care vary from 17 percent of the records of fetal deaths at 20 to 27 weeks of gestation to 11 percent of fetal deaths beyond 27 weeks of gestation and 2.8 percent of live births.

The possibility exists that changing practices in the categorization and reporting of live births and fetal deaths have contributed to falling fetal death rates and rising preterm birth and infant mortality rates in the United

States (Martin and Hoyert, 2002). Earlier obstetric intervention when the fetus is not doing well, prompt aggressive resuscitation in the delivery room, and the initiation of neonatal intensive care may save the lives of a few fetuses that formerly died in utero. However, many die within a few days (or weeks) of birth. Such efforts may have a significant impact on infant mortality rates (CDC, 2004f; MacDorman et al., 2005).

If more infants are born alive at the limit of viability but die within days of delivery, thereby contributing to infant deaths, then a small rise in the infant mortality rate should not be viewed with alarm. It might generate a discussion of relative costs (emotional as well as financial) and how limited health care resources should be used, but it is not an indicator of worsening child health. Similarly, intensive prenatal care of high-risk mothers facilitates the detection of fetuses whose adaptive systems become overwhelmed by adverse intrauterine circumstances. An indicated preterm delivery that prevents a fetal death is not an indicator of worsening infant health, even if it does contribute to a higher preterm birth rate

Consideration should be given to using perinatal mortality rates as another child health indicator. Perinatal mortality rates include fetal death rates as well as neonatal mortality rates and would not be expected to change in the two scenarios presented above. However, calculating perinatal mortality rates as an indicator of child health requires that attention be given to how perinatal data are collected and reported, especially regarding fetal deaths.

Attention to the quality of data regarding causes of death could provide insight into the mechanisms of preterm birth as well as the causes of fetal and early neonatal deaths. This approach would require clinicians to vigorously search for causes of death whenever a fetal or early neonatal death occurs. Petersson et al. (2004) found that 11.5 percent of fetal deaths that would have been characterized as unexplained were due to infections with parvovirus, cytomegalovirus, or enterovirus. Other possible causes that should be explored include thrombophilias (e.g., Factor V Leiden), fetomaternal hemorrhage, chorioamnionitis (which would include pathologic examination of the placenta and the umbilical cord), uterine anomalies, umbilical cord or placental anomalies, toxin or drug exposures, and maternal illness (e.g., diabetes, hypertension with or without preeclampsia, thyroid disease, and autoimmune diseases) (Gardosi et al., 2005). Because the most common condition associated with fetal deaths is IUGR (43 percent), research into the mechanisms of IUGR, how to better detect IUGR, and the effect of IUGR on fetal organ systems should be encouraged.

Every avenue that might lead to a better understanding of the causes and mechanisms of preterm birth, fetal and infant mortality, complications of prematurity, health sequelae, and neurodevelopmental disabilities should be explored. The costs to infants, their families, and society as a whole are too high to continue to ignore this lack of knowledge.

CONCLUSIONS

The use of caution with the terms used and attention to their definitions is essential in efforts to understand the causes and consequences of preterm birth. It is important to recognize the limitations and variations in the data collected and entered into large administrative and research public health databases. Every effort should be made to improve the quality of national vital records, especially data on the gestational ages of newborns and the rates of preterm births. Uniform data collection and reporting procedures facilitate comparisons among states, over time, and with data from other countries.

The impact of early dating of gestational age by ultrasound on clinical factors such as labor, tocolysis, administration of steroids, timing of elective induction of labor, determination of the mode of delivery, in utero transport, delivery room resuscitation, and determination of adequacy of fetal growth should be evaluated. Professional societies should encourage the routine use of early (before 20 weeks gestation) ultrasound for the establishment of gestational age. Standards of practice and recommendations for training of personnel to improve the reliability and the quality of ultrasound data should be established.

Section I

Measurement

Recommendation I-1: *Promote the collection of improved perinatal data.* *The National Center for Health Statistics of the Centers for Disease Control and Prevention should promote and use a national mechanism to collect, record, and report perinatal data.*

The following key elements should be included:

• The quality of gestational age measurements in vital records should be evaluated. Vital records should indicate the accuracy of the gestational age determined by ultrasound early in pregnancy (less than 20 weeks of gestation).

• Birth weight for gestational age should be considered one measure of the adequacy of fetal growth.

• Perinatal mortality and morbidity should be reported by gestational age, birth weight, and birth weight for gestational age.

• A categorization or coding scheme that reflects the heterogeneous etiologies of preterm birth should be developed and implemented.

• Vital records should also state whether fertility treatments (including in vitro fertilization and ovulation promotion) were used. The committee recognizes that the nature of these data is private and sensitive.

Recommendation I-2: *Encourage the use of ultrasound early in pregnancy to establish gestational age.* Because it is recognized that more precise measures of gestational age are needed to move the field forward, professional societies should encourage the use of ultrasound early in pregnancy (less than 20 weeks of gestation) to establish gestational age and should establish standards of practice and recommendations for the training of personnel to improve the reliability and the quality of ultrasound data.

Recommendation I-3: *Develop indicators of maturational age.* Funding agencies should support and investigators should develop reliable and precise perinatal (prenatal and postnatal) standards as indicators of maturational age.

SECTION II

CAUSES OF PRETERM BIRTH

3

Behavioral and Psychosocial Contributors to Preterm Birth

ABSTRACT

Although individual behaviors have not been proven to have a strong influence on the risk of preterm birth, consistent evidence suggests that a constellation of favorable lifestyle factors are associated with more favorable pregnancy outcomes. These include a reduced risk of preterm birth among women who engage in leisure time physical activity, women who do not use cocaine, and those who have a favorable diet. There is clear evidence that a favorable lifestyle and a greater degree of health consciousness are associated with a reduced risk of preterm birth above and beyond what can be measured effectively and controlled in observational studies. Despite the lack of success in pinpointing behaviors that affect the occurrence of preterm birth, continued efforts are needed to better understand and ultimately pinpoint the aspects of a favorable lifestyle that are associated with a reduced risk of preterm birth. The results of research on psychosocial factors and preterm birth have accumulated rapidly in recent years. What is most clear from this large body of evidence is that psychosocial factors should not be grouped together as if they were one risk factor. Rather, they must be studied as the distinct theoretical risk factors that they are. Evidence indicates that some psychosocial factors in the etiology of preterm birth include major life events, chronic and catastrophic stress, maternal anxiety, personal racism, and lack of support.

This chapter reviews a number of individual-level factors that have been thought to contribute to preterm birth (birth at less than 37 weeks of gestation), including the available evidence for each factor, with an emphasis on the data and findings from recent and more definitive studies. The section on behavioral factors covers tobacco use, alcohol use, illicit drug use, nutrition (prepregnancy weight, weight gain in pregnancy, dietary composition, and fish and fish oil consumption), sexual activity, physical activity, employment, and douching. The section on psychosocial factors includes findings on stress (life events and chronic and catastrophic stress), emotional responses and affective states (anxiety and depression), racism, social support, personal resources, and intendedness of pregnancy. Suggestions for the understanding and prevention of preterm delivery on the basis of the review of the effects of these individual-level factors appear at the end of the chapter.

BEHAVIORAL INFLUENCES ON PRETERM BIRTH

A special interest in behavioral influences on preterm birth is well justified, given that these are subject to change and could reduce the frequency of preterm birth directly. As previously reviewed in some detail (Berkowitz and Papiernik, 1993; Savitz and Pastore, 1999), a large number of observational studies of a range of health behaviors, including tobacco and alcohol use, nutrition, and physical activity, have been conducted. Although each of these behaviors poses specific challenges in discerning cause-and-effect relationships, two key, generic concerns crosscut them all. First, it is a challenge to measure many of these behaviors with accuracy because of their inherent complexity, the inability of individuals to completely recall past behaviors (e.g., diet and physical activity), or the stigma associated with the behavior (e.g., alcohol and illicit drug use). The challenge is especially heightened for women who are pregnant. This inaccurate recall ability is accompanied by the potential for a distorted recall of the facts when these behaviors are assessed after pregnancy outcomes have occurred, as well as by a likely dilution of measures of association because of random error. Second, the decisions about these behaviors that women make render them highly susceptible to confounding, in which any true causal effects of the behavior of interest on preterm birth are distorted by the association of that behavior with antecedent factors like socioeconomic conditions or with other behaviors. For example, smoking during pregnancy has become increasingly strongly linked to lower socioeconomic condition, much more so than smoking by other segments of the population (Cnattingius, 2004), so that isolation of the effect of smoking per se from the socioeconomic context is challenging. In addition, unfavorable health behaviors tend to cluster, so that women with poor diets often also exhibit other potentially detrimental behaviors, such as a lack of physical activity, and vice versa.

For a number of these behaviors, observational studies are inherently limited, no matter how carefully conducted and how attentive investigators are to controlling for other exposures (which are themselves difficult to measure accurately and to thus fully control). Nonetheless, when considered in conjunction with other lines of research involving mechanistic studies and randomized trials, observational studies of behavioral influences on preterm birth, when it is feasible to conduct such studies, have been highly informative. The subsections that follow review tobacco use, alcohol use, illicit drug use, nutrition, employment, physical activity, sexual activity, and douching.

Tobacco Use

Cigarette smoking is recognized to be among the most prevalent, preventable causes of adverse pregnancy outcomes. Smoking is strongly related to placental abruption, reduced birth weight, and infant mortality (Cnattingius, 2004); but the relationship of cigarette smoking to preterm birth is rather modest and not entirely consistent. The influence of smoking on pregnancy outcome is dependent on whether it occurs in the later part of pregnancy, and no increased risk has been detected for former smokers who quit before the onset of pregnancy or early in pregnancy.

Many studies have examined the association between smoking and preterm birth, as reviewed previously (Berkowitz and Papiernik, 1993; Savitz and Pastore, 1999), and they generally find modest associations. Recent studies continue to show such a pattern (Cnattingius et al., 1999; Hellerstedt et al., 1997; Lang et al., 1996; Savitz et al., 2001; Wen et al., 1990; Wisborg et al., 1996). However, some reports suggest a stronger association (Nordentoft et al., 1996) and others suggest no association at all (Goldenberg et al., 1998). The variability in results is limited, and evidence of relative risks (RRs) of about 1.2 to 1.5 for smoking 10 to 20 cigarettes per day and an RR of 1.5 to 2.0 for smoking 20 or more cigarettes per day is fairly consistent throughout the literature.

Some studies have suggested more pronounced effects for subsets of preterm birth or for subgroups of women. For example, a few studies (Berkowitz et al., 1998; Harger et al., 1990) have found stronger effects of smoking on preterm birth presenting as premature rupture of membranes than on preterm births due to the spontaneous onset of labor or for medical indications. Given that a primary cause of medically indicated preterm birth is pregnancy-induced hypertension, which is less frequent among smokers (England et al., 2002; Newman MG et al., 2001), different patterns of smoking effects across preterm birth subtypes might be expected. Some studies suggest greater or lesser effects of smoking among African American women than among white women in the United States (Lubs, 1973; McDonald et al., 1992), suggesting a race-smoking interaction, and among older mothers (Cnattingius et al., 1993; Savitz and Pastore, 1999; Wen et al., 1990).

Alcohol Use

High levels of alcohol use during pregnancy have obvious adverse effects on fetal development (AAP, 1993; Spohr et al., 1993). There is consistent support of an adverse effect for heavier users of alcohol; for example, women who have more than one drink per day, on average, have an increased risk of preterm birth (Albertsen et al., 2003; Kesmodel et al., 2000; Larroque, 1992; Lundsberg et al., 1997; Parazzini et al., 2003). Subject to the question of the accuracy of self-reported information on alcohol consumption and some variation across studies in the definition of "heavier alcohol use," recent data provide evidence of an association between moderate alcohol use and preterm birth (Savitz and Pastore, 1999). However, some studies reported modest inverse associations between the consumption of small amounts of alcohol and preterm birth, but this may be a result of a higher prevalence of small alcohol use among women who are more socioeconomically advantaged (Albertsen et al., 2004; Kesmodel et al., 2000). A report from the Preterm Prediction Study, a recent large project to evaluate predictors of preterm birth, suggested a substantial reduction in the risk of medically indicated preterm birth in association with alcohol use (Meis et al., 1998). Research on alcohol use is limited by the quality of the self-report and the absence of biological markers that are well suited to epidemiological studies. Given that challenge, plus evidence that different effects may be observed at different dose levels and the suggestion that the effect differs by subtype of preterm birth, the issue of whether a relationship exists between alcohol use and preterm birth remains unresolved.

Illicit Drug Use

Marijuana and cocaine are the drugs that have been most commonly studied for their potential effects on preterm births. There is little indication that marijuana use influences preterm birth (Shiono et al., 1995). Either the psychoactive agents or the combustion products derived from the act of smoking could be harmful, but given that cigarette smoking produces only modest effects, it is unlikely that marijuana smoking would cause a discernible increase in risk through the inhalation of combustion products alone.

Cocaine has been much more intensively studied, and there is a sizable literature demonstrating an association between cocaine use and preterm birth (Holzman and Paneth, 1994). Cocaine users experience an approximately twofold increased risk of preterm birth compared with that for nonusers. Although plausible preterm birth-related mechanisms of action of cocaine involving vasoconstriction have been detected and the association is found with reasonable consistency, there are real uncertainties regarding whether the association is causal. First, women who use cocaine during pregnancy often have other strongly associated lifestyle factors that could well constitute the underlying cause of preterm birth, such as infection or poor nutrition. Second, the ways in which cocaine use is detected may make identified cocaine users a particular subset of all cocaine users. That is, when screening is done on the basis of a suspicion or a known history of drug abuse, the women who are found to be positive for cocaine use may well be at higher risk of preterm birth on the basis of the factors that marked them as potential cocaine users rather than on the basis of the use of cocaine per se. Some studies suggest that more systematic assessments by the use of sensitive methods for the detection of cocaine use results in a smaller association or, in some cases, the absence of any association at all (Kline et al., 1997; Savitz and Pastore, 1999; Savitz et al., 2002a). Although there are many good reasons to discourage the use of cocaine during pregnancy, it is not at all clear that this is a major contributor to the etiology of preterm birth.

Nutrition

Prepregnancy Weight

Prepregnancy weight is not a behavior per se but is somewhat associated with patterns of diet and nutrition and thus is covered here. Evidence suggests that a low prepregnancy weight is associated with an increased risk of preterm birth (Kramer et al., 1995; Savitz and Pastore, 1999; Siega-Riz et al., 1996), although in the aggregate, the data in the literature are not consistent (Berkowitz and Papiernik, 1993). In general, the studies that do report on the association between low prepregnancy weight and preterm birth find modest associations, with RRs on the order of 1.5. In the Preterm Prediction Study, a low prepregnancy body mass index (BMI) was strongly associated with an increased risk of preterm birth, with the RRs being greater than 2.5 (Goldenberg et al., 1998), and obese women were at a markedly decreased risk of spontaneous preterm birth (Hendler et al., 2005). A recent meta-analysis of this topic found that prepregnancy BMI had little or no relationship with the risk of preterm birth overall (Honest et al., 2005), counter to the conventional wisdom regarding this association.

Weight Gain During Pregnancy

A low level of weight gain during pregnancy is associated with an increased risk of preterm birth (Berkowitz and Papiernik, 1993; Carmichael and Abrams, 1997), particularly for women who are not overweight or obese (Savitz and Pastore, 1999), with RRs for low weight gain and preterm birth being on the order of 1.5 to 2.5. Studies that adjust for infant weight by subtracting it from the total weight gain of the mother sometimes find that this adjustment eliminates the association (Berkowitz and Papiernik, 1993; Kramer et al., 1995). What is less certain is the extent to which the association reflects a causal effect of the weight gain on the risk of preterm birth compared with the extent to which the low weight gain and preterm birth are manifestations of some shared etiology. Weight gain during pregnancy reflects in part the duration of gestation (longer pregnancies allow more weight gain), which must be considered by calculating week-specific weight gain. Furthermore, weight gain in pregnancy is due not only to increased caloric intake and fat deposition but also to fluid retention.

Dietary Composition

A series of studies dating to the 1970s indicate that calorie supplementation during pregnancy does not reduce the risk of preterm birth. The challenges to addressing the hypothesized protective effects of micronutrient intake are profound. First, diet reflects individual choice and lifestyle, making it difficult to isolate the impact of individual micronutrients from one another or from the overall dietary patterns. Second, socioeconomic and behavioral correlates of diet can introduce confounding. Finally, accurate measurement of diet is extremely challenging, and with the rapid changes that occur over the course of pregnancy, it is particularly difficult to assess the composition of the diet and its relation to preterm birth. Randomized studies in both developed and developing countries have noted an absence of benefit from dietary supplementation in preventing preterm birth (Berkowitz and Papiernik, 1993). Furthermore, protein supplementation specifically has not been found to reduce the risk of preterm birth and possibly increases the risk (Berkowitz and Papiernik, 1993; Rush et al., 1980), as does multivitamin supplementation (Villar et al., 1998).

Relatively limited research has addressed the possibility that specific micronutrients, with the exception of long-chain fatty acids (discussed below), affect the risk of preterm birth. Limited iron levels in the bodies of pregnant women, which manifest as anemia, have been examined in a number of studies, but it is unclear the extent to which the results reflect actual iron intake. Iron deficiency anemia, which has been found to be correlated with an increased risk of preterm birth in a number of studies, is unlikely to be an actual cause of preterm birth after the timing of measurement of iron levels (Berkowitz and Papiernik, 1993; Klebanoff et al., 1989) and the extent to which iron deficiency simply reflects maternal blood volume expansion rather than the influence of iron intake are taken into account. Serum ferritin reflects a response to inflammation and infection, not necessarily an influence of iron intake, and it is thus difficult to interpret serum ferritin levels as a marker of diet. Despite the reasons to question whether anemia is part of a causal pathway that leads to preterm birth, there is some consistency in the evidence from randomized trials that iron supplementation may reduce the rates of preterm birth (Villar et al., 1998).

Folate has been studied mostly in relation to birth defects, but several studies have related increased folate levels to the risk of preterm birth. There are plausible biological pathways by which folate levels could influence preterm birth (Scholl and Johnson, 2000). The empirical assessment of that relationship has generated mixed findings, with some evidence indicating that higher levels of folate reduce the risk of preterm birth (Savitz and Pastore, 1999; Scholl et al., 1996; Siega-Riz et al., 2004) and some evidence indicating that such an association does not exist (Czeizel et al., 1994; Savitz and Pastore, 1999; Shaw et al., 2004). A large randomized study reported that increased folate levels have a marginally positive effect in reducing the rate of preterm labor (Rolschau et al., 1999).

Isolated observational studies have addressed vitamin C levels and the risk of preterm birth, with some indication that low vitamin C levels are associated with an increased risk of premature rupture of membranes, leading to preterm birth (Siega-Riz et al., 2003). Increased levels of calcium have also been possibly associated with a reduced risk of preterm birth (Siega-Riz et al., 2003).

Zinc

The impact of zinc supplementation on fetal growth has also been studied. In a U.S. study of a low income population, Goldenberg and colleagues (1995) found an effect of supplementation on birth weight, such that mothers with a lower body mass index (BMI) who received supplementation had babies with greater birth weight than women with low BMI who did not receive supplementation. There was no difference among supplemented women with a higher BMI. With respect to studies examining preterm birth, evidence is conflicting (Castillo-Durán and Weisstaub, 2003; Caulfield et al., 1998; Merialdi et al., 2003; Villar et al., 2003a,b). Methodological limitations have hindered progress in this area and should be addressed by future research.

Fish and Fish Oil

A series of studies have addressed the hypothesis that the intake of larger amounts of the long-chain fatty acids found in certain fish might increase the duration of gestation and fetal growth (Olsen, 1993). Those studies were motivated by the relationship between prostaglandin levels and the timing of parturition and fetal growth. Investigators have compared aggregate populations who live in the Faroe Islands and Denmark, with one key difference between the two populations being the very high levels of intake of fish and whale by the population in the Faroe Islands. On average, the longer gestation times in the Faroe Islands contribute to the birth of infants born 100 grams heavier than infants in Denmark, and higher fetal growth rates contribute to infants who are 100 grams heavier. The n-3 fatty acids in erythrocytes were associated with an increased duration of gestation among Danish women but not among Faroese women (Olsen et al., 1986). One study of fish consumption and fetal growth (Olsen et al., 1990) found no overall relation between the frequency with which the mother ate fish and the duration of her pregnancy, but a positive association was found when the population was restricted to nonsmokers. A study with 965 pregnant Danish women for whom information on their levels of intake of n-3 fatty acids was available found no indication that the level of intake of n-3 fatty acids was associated with gestational duration, birth weight, or birth length (Olsen et al., 1995a). In an observational study conducted in the Faroe Islands, the levels of fatty acids in blood were examined as predictors of gestational age and birth weight (Grandjean et al., 2001). The levels of eicosapentanoic acid in serum were also found to be associated with an increased duration of gestation but a decreased birth weight for gestational length, which is a measure of the fetal growth rate. The report of seafood intake and pregnancy outcome in Denmark (Olsen and Secher, 2002) reported a rather strong but imprecise association between low levels of seafood consumption and the risk of preterm birth (odds ratio [OR] = 3.6; 95% confidence interval [CI] = 1.2–11.2).

Additional evidence of an association between fish oil consumption and an increased duration of gestation comes from randomized trials (Olsen et al., 1992). The investigators evaluated 533 pregnant Danish women who were divided into three groups: one group received fish oil, one group received olive oil, and one group received capsules with no oil. The gestational age distributions among these three groups of women varied at the time of delivery, with a shift toward prolonged gestation among the fish oil consumers; the group receiving no oil had gestation lengths that were intermediate among those of the three groups, and the group receiving olive oil had the shortest gestations. Comparison of the group receiving fish oil and the group receiving olive oil showed that gestations were 4 days longer and the birth weight was 107 grams greater in the group receiving fish oil, with the apparent benefit derived from prolonged gestation and not from an increased rate of growth.

A multicenter trial involving 19 centers throughout Europe enrolled women with high-risk pregnancies (defined as a history of certain complications or adverse outcomes) or twin pregnancies (Olsen et al., 2000). Fish oil and olive oil were given to equal numbers of women in each arm of the trial. A notable protective effect against the recurrence of preterm birth was found, with an OR of 0.54 (95% CI 0.30–0.98), and fish oil was found to delay delivery across all centers involved in the trial.

Although randomized trials suggest a possible benefit of fish oil consumption on pregnancy duration, the information in the literature as a whole is not consistent in supporting a beneficial effect of seafood consumption and includes some indications of reduced growth rates, despite the prolonged gestation or the positive effects, which were limited to subgroups in the populations studied. This remains an active area of research, and both observational studies and randomized trials continue.

Employment

Employment during pregnancy has been of interest as a possible cause of increased risk of preterm birth for some time (Saurel-Cubizolles and Kaminski, 1986). The challenge of studying paid employment as an "exposure" is the many implications of work and the variability in the character of paid employment across geographic settings, time periods, and socioeconomic groups. Work has been conceptualized as a source of physical work demand, which is relatively rare in developed countries but which is common in many other parts of the world, or as a source of psychological stress because of its demands on the pregnant woman. In contrast, work is also a source and indicator of favorable socioeconomic circumstances; that is, the ability to have and maintain a job, the insurance benefits that employed women receive, and the psychological satisfaction resulting from certain types of jobs.

Recent studies have generally found no increased risk of preterm birth in association with employment per se but have provided suggestions that long work hours, physically demanding work, or other stressful conditions may be associated with an increased risk (see section below on Physical Activity). A large study across 16 European countries (Saurel-Cubizolles et al., 2004) found no association overall; but RRs for preterm birth on the order of 1.3 were found for women who work more than 42 hours per week, women who stand for more than 6 hours per day, and women with low levels of job satisfaction. However, a study of Thai women found that increased risks of small-for-gestational-age births but not preterm births were associated with physically demanding work conditions (Tuntiseranee et al., 1998).

A more specific entity, premature rupture of membranes, was studied as a possible consequence of occupational fatigue, which was defined on a five-item scale that considered posture, work with industrial machines, physical exertion, mental stress, and environmental stress (Newman RB et al., 2001). Although these realms are diverse, each can be considered a work-related challenge, and in fact, a linear relationship between the number of sources of fatigue reported and the risk of premature rupture of membranes was observed, with an RR about 2.0 found among women reporting four or five sources of fatigue.

Given these and other findings, the continued study of employment-related physical activity and psychosocial stress offers an opportunity to study potential modifiable causes of preterm birth, but the consideration of paid employment in the aggregate in relation to preterm birth is unlikely to be helpful in identifying modifiable causes or improving the understanding of the causes of preterm birth more generally. The impact of employment is highly dependent on the socioeconomic conditions in the geographic location of the study, the implications of employment for economic resources and medical care access, and the particular character of the work. Given that heterogeneity, drawing inferences across studies of the impact of paid work is not possible.

Physical Activity

Evidence has found a clear pattern of a reduced risk of preterm birth in association with being employed generally compared with the risk in association with being unemployed (Saurel-Cubizolles and Kaminski, 1986; Savitz and Pastore, 1999; Savitz et al., 1990). However, among employed women, a number of reports suggest that jobs that require physical exertion may be associated with an increased risk of preterm birth (Mamelle et al., 1984; see the reviews of Berkowitz and Papiernik [1993] and Saurel-Cubizolles et al. [1991]). It is difficult to isolate the impact of physical exertion in the workplace from other aspects of employment, however. The key question is whether, among working women, physical activity on the job is associated with an increased risk of preterm birth, and here the evidence is distinctly mixed (Berkowitz and Papiernik, 1993; Savitz and Pastore, 1999; Shaw, 2003). Standing, lifting, and other measures of exertion, such as long work hours and the challenges of shift work, have been examined in a large number of studies, with modest and inconsistent associations with preterm birth detected (Ahlborg et al., 1990; Fortier et al., 1995; Xu et al., 1994). Among the candidate markers of physical work demands, none has emerged as the most important or the most promising as having a causal influence on preterm birth on the basis of consistent empirical support for an association. The limited qualities of the assessments, the use of inconsistent definitions, and susceptibility to confounding may have blurred the findings for the association of interest. Nevertheless, despite the sizable number of studies that have evaluated whether such an association exists, there is as yet little basis for asserting that physical work is associated with an increased risk of preterm birth.

Leisure activities and their association with preterm birth have been of increasing interest in recent years. Historically, the primary concern was with an adverse effect of physical activity on fetal growth and the duration of gestation (Dye and Oldenettel, 1996). In more recent times, the focus has shifted toward the potential for a protective effect of being physically active on preterm birth (Sternfeld, 1997). Evidence suggests that the longer in pregnancy that exercise continues, the greater the reduction in the risk of preterm birth is (Evenson et al., 2002). Although intense activity has physiologic effects that raise concern over an increased risk of preterm birth, relevant mechanisms involving glucose metabolism and vascular effects would be consistent with a reduction in the risk of preterm birth.

Sexual Activity

The potential for adverse effects of sexual activity, particularly intercourse, during pregnancy has been of concern for some time due to the potential for direct effects of semen on initiating preterm labor, alteration of vaginal microflora, or other hypothesized pathways leading to preterm birth. Much of the interest and research on this question appeared in the 1980s, with consistent evidence that remaining sexually active during pregnancy was not associated with preterm birth (Klebanoff et al., 1984; Mills et al., 1981; Rayburn and Wilson, 1980). There was some suggestion that intercourse in the presence of certain infections; namely, *Trichomonas vaginalis* and *Mycoplasma hominis*, might increase risk for preterm birth (Read and Klebanoff, 1993), but more recent studies have continued to report not just an absence of increased risk associated with sexual activity but a notably diminished risk of preterm birth (Sayle et al., 2003). This may well be a reflection of selection for remaining sexually active, i.e., having a partner who may provide social support, having an absence of contraindications to remaining active, and the subjective sense of well-being that motivates continued activity.

Douching Before and During Pregnancy

A number of indirect lines of evidence suggest that the practice of vaginal douching might increase the risk of preterm birth. Douching is a common behavior and is more common among African American women than white women, consistent with the increased prevalence of bacterial vaginosis (BV) and preterm birth among African American women (Bruce et al., 2000). Furthermore, douching alters the vaginal microflora and may well facilitate the passage of vaginal pathogens to the upper reproductive tract, which contributes to inflammation and, possibly, to preterm birth. Few empirical evaluations of this hypothesis have been conducted thus far.

Women rarely douche during pregnancy, so the analyses have focused on douching during the period before pregnancy begins. Bruce et al. (2002) reported no association, after adjustment for confounders, between douching at any time before pregnancy and preterm birth, with ORs ranging from 0.7 to 1.1. However, among the small proportion of women who did report that they douched during pregnancy, the OR for preterm birth was 1.9 (95% CI 1.0–3.7). In another study (Fiscella et al., 2002), frequent and long durations of douching before pregnancy were found to be associated with an increased risk of preterm birth. Given the racial disparity in douching practices and the high degree of plausibility that douching influences pathways linked to preterm delivery, continued evaluations of the effects of this behavior are warranted.

PSYCHOSOCIAL FACTORS AND PRETERM BIRTH

In 1985 the Institute of Medicine (IOM) issued a report on low birth weight that concluded that stress was one promising avenue for future research (IOM, 1985). Since then, the findings of many more investigations have been published, as have numerous reviews, partial reviews, and commentaries on this area of research (Istvan, 1986; Kramer et al., 2001a; Lederman, 1986; Lobel, 1994; Paarlberg et al., 1995; Savitz and Pastore, 1999). However, existing reviews are outdated because of the burgeoning papers that have been published since the year 2000. This reflects the high level of scientific interest and public health attention to the topic of psychosocial factors and preterm delivery, especially research on stress and preterm delivery. This section summarizes the scientific findings on stress (including racism as a stressor), social support, and the intendedness of a pregnancy and their relation to the occurrence of preterm delivery.

Stress

Stress is defined as demands that tax or exceed the adaptive capacity of an organism and that result in psychological and biological changes (Cohen and Syme, 1985). This definition includes both environmental demands and the responses to them at multiple levels of analysis (cognitive, affective, immune, endocrine, cardiovascular, and so on). The breadth of this construct has led to confusion among health care researchers and has muddled conceptual and measurement issues in the literature on stress and preterm delivery. Reframing stress as an umbrella concept (Lazarus and Folkman, 1984) that contains these distinguishable components has opened the way for stronger theory and research on stress and health in general (Cohen, 1995) and on birth outcomes more specifically (Lobel, 1994). Thus, this body of research can be divided by specific subtopics; namely, the effects of environmental demands, the effects of emotional and cognitive responses to those demands, and the role of biological stress responses such as hypothalamic pituitary axis (HPA) and cardiovascular and immune responses. Moreover, theoretical analyses have linked these distinct areas of empirical inquiry together into proposed pathways from the existence of stressors to the occurrence of preterm delivery (Hogue and Bremner, 2005; Holzman et al., 2001; Livingston et al., 2003; Lockwood, 1999; Rich-Edwards et al., 2005; Schulkin, 1999; Wadhwa, 2001).

The empirical research on stress and preterm delivery has become increasingly sophisticated in the past decade in several ways. First, the designs of observational studies have shifted from predominantly retrospective to predominantly prospective, measuring stress before rather than after delivery. Second, sample sizes are larger, in general, affording better power to test the effect(s) of interest. Third, the means of both the conceptualization and the measurement of stress have been strengthened. Fourth, most researchers now analyze data with attention to separating preterm labor and delivery from infant birth weight rather than studying only one of these outcomes without controlling for the other or lumping together several outcomes into what was sometimes termed "complications." Finally, studies have involved greater control for potential confounders of the stress-preterm birth relationship. Thus, the methodological problems that have plagued past research on stress and preterm delivery (Hoffman and Hatch, 1996; Lobel, 1994) are being ameliorated by trends in current research. Nonetheless, the findings of experimental studies that can provide firmer evidence for causality than observational studies are not yet available. Interventions in pregnancy that are aimed at reducing stress have generally used multifaceted treatment packages, including smoking cessation, support provision, prenatal education, and other ingredients, which prevents any conclusions of the effects of stress on preterm birth independent of the effects of other factors from being made (IOM, 2000). To date, prenatal intervention trials have not used state-of-the-art methodologies to isolate the effects of stress reduction from other psychosocial components; and none have examined the mediating processes involved to determine which components successfully reduced stress, which did not, or why (West and Aiken, 1997).

Although intervention trials on stress per se and preterm birth are absent or their findings are inconclusive, a handful of more rigorous observational studies on stressors (environmental demands) and preterm birth now exist. A second group of acceptable studies that have evaluated emotional, affective, or cognitive stress-related states and preterm birth exist. In addition, a number of notable animal and human studies on specific linkages between stress or emotion and various hypothesized mediators of preterm birth have been published. These mediators include BV (Culhane et al., 2001), cytokines (Coussons-Read et al., 2005), corticotropin-releasing hormone (Hobel et al., 1998; Lockwood, 1999; Mancuso et al., 2004), cortisol (Obel et al., 2005), blood pressure (McCubbin et al., 1996; Stancil et al., 2000), uterine artery resistance (Teixeira et al., 1999), and pregnancy-induced hypertension (Landsbergis and Hatch, 1996). This literature is discussed elsewhere in this report (Chapter 6). Finally, a small group of more recent studies has linked prenatal stress or emotion to a wide range of developmental outcomes, and both animal and human research in this area has been reviewed (Huizink et al., 2004; Schneider et al., 2002). The results have linked prenatal stress to outcomes ranging from fetal neurobehavioral indices (DiPietro et al., 2002; Wadhwa et al., 1996; also see the review by DiPietro [2005]) and fetal brain development (Graham et al., 1999; Hansen et al., 2000; Lou et al., 1994) to infant temperament and related infant outcomes (Huizink et al., 2002, 2003) and even some outcomes in toddlers (Laplante et al., 2004) and school age children (Rodriguez and Bohlin, 2005; Van Den Bergh and Marcoen, 2004; Van Den Bergh et al., 2005). Extensions of this work to the role of fetal stress programming in adult health outcomes are also capturing great interest (Barker, 1998; Huizink, 2005; Nathanielz, 1999).

Altogether these research developments strengthen the theoretical premises that causal pathways link maternal and fetal environmental stress exposures and maternal emotional states through biological mediators to preterm delivery or low birth weight and, furthermore, to developmental outcomes across the life span. However, the evidence to date is not sufficient or strong enough to draw firm conclusions on the many pieces of the complex and diverse pathways linking psychosocial factors to maternal and fetal outcomes. Nonetheless, it is possible to draw some tentative conclusions from recent research on the narrower topic of stressors or emotions as risk factors for preterm delivery. Much more intensive and rigorous scientific inquiry is needed before it will be known where, when, and how stress operates in pregnancy to influence developmental outcomes at any point in the life course (also see Chapter 6). Given the high levels of enthusiasm for research in this area, equal doses of objectivity, rigorous study, and the cautious drawing of conclusions on the effects of prenatal stress on distal outcomes are called for at this time.

This review begins where Savitz and Pastore (1999) ended their review of 20 methodologically acceptable studies. As they stated, the conclusions that one can draw from that group of studies are hampered by method-ological limitations, including retrospective study designs, sampling of spe-cial populations, small samples sizes, the use of various definitions of stress, the use of weak measures, and study enrollment often late in pregnancy. Nonetheless, the pattern of findings is informative. Of the 20 psychosocial studies reviewed, 11 studies assessed life events and tested the associations of those life events with preterm birth or gestational age. Of those 11 stud-ies, 5 reported significant effects (Berkowitz and Kasl, 1983; Hedegaard et al., 1996; Mutale et al., 1991; Newton and Hunt, 1984; Newton et al., 1979), whereas 6 did not (Honnor et al., 1994; Lobel et al., 1992; MacDonald et al., 1992; Pagel et al., 1990; Stein et al., 1987; Wadhwa et al., 1993). Eleven studies assessed the associations of preterm birth and gestational age with anxiety, depression, or emotional distress. Of those 11 studies, 6 found significant effects (Copper et al., 1996; Hedegaard et al., 1993; Lobel et al., 1992; Orr and Miller, 1995; Steer et al., 1992; Wadhwa et al., 1993), whereas 5 did not (MacDonald et al., 1992; Molfese et al., 1987; Pagel et al., 1990; Perkin et al., 1993; Stein et al., 2000). In short, approximately half of the tests of stress measures and their association with preterm birth or gestational age outcomes were statistically significant.

Two notable early studies stand out because of their prospective de-signs and large sample sizes. In a sample of 5,873 Danish women, Hedegaard et al. (1996) found that experiencing one or more highly stress-ful life events at between 16 and 30 weeks of pregnancy was associated with a risk of preterm delivery (OR = 1.76). In an investigation of nearly 2,600 pregnant women in a large multisite U.S. study, Copper et al. (1996) reported that a two-item stress measure that assessed the extent to which women felt nervous, tense, and strained in general at 26 weeks of gestation predicted preterm birth, after controlling for race, age, marital status, insur-ance coverage, education, and substance use. Savitz and Pastore (1999) con-clude that "psychosocial stress is among the more promising targets for [preterm birth] prevention strategies" (p. 93). This conclusion rests partly on the results of these stronger observational studies and also on specific criteria for interventions contained in the review, such as the modifiability of stress.

Studies published after the 1999 review continued to be somewhat methodologically uneven, but in general, research on stress and preterm birth has improved substantially since 1996 or 1997 in terms of the hypoth-eses and conceptualizations used, the measures used, sample sizes, and data analyses. Some of the newer studies are methodologically quite innovative. The IOM committee review of electronic databases yielded more than two dozen newly published reports on stress and its effects on preterm birth or birth weight. Databases containing data on low birth weight are viewed as potentially different, in terms of the mechanisms underlying the causes of low birth weight, from those containing data on preterm births; but they are noted because of the substantial overlap of the two outcomes. Of 27 published reports, 21 were deemed of acceptable methodological quality for review and represent data from approximately 19 independent databases.[1] Many of the studies assessed multiple aspects of stress, such as major life events, anxiety, and depression. Of the 17 investigations (which evaluated data from 16 independent databases) that assessed any stress variables and that had preterm birth or gestational age as the outcome, only 2 obtained no significant findings. All four investigations on low birth weight that measured stress also found significant associations.[2] In sum, the overall pattern of findings since they were last reviewed suggests that more rigorous approaches are yielding more definitive results regarding the effects of stress on preterm delivery and gestational age, although the exact nature and strength of these effects are not yet clear. This led the committee to turn to examining the specific forms of stress involved, especially in more definitive studies, to obtain clues on the patterns of exposures.

Life Events

Life events are major events that individuals experience, such as divorce, a death in the family, illness, injury, or the loss of a job (Cohen et al., 1995). Eight studies assessed life events and tested whether a count of the number of events occurring during pregnancy or the severity or the impact of those events predicted preterm birth. Three obtained nonsignificant results, including one large prospective study (Goldenberg et al., 1996a), one prospective study with a small sample size (Lobel et al., 2000), and one analysis of a very large data set with data collected retrospectively (Lu and Chen, 2004). The other five studies all reported significant associations of some aspects of life events with preterm birth. In a large prospective study (in which maternal age, cohabitation, and education were controlled), Nordentoft et al. (1996) assessed life events at 20 weeks of gestation in a cohort of 2,432 Danish women and found that severe life events predicted preterm birth (adjusted OR = 1.14) but did not predict intrauterine growth restriction. Similarly, Dole and colleagues (2003) found an increased risk of preterm birth in women with negative-impact life events (RR = 1.8) in 1,962 pregnant women in North Carolina. Whitehead and colleagues (2002) analyzed two cohorts of women from a large study of 70,840 women in the

---

[1] In some cases, publications have addressed different issues within subgroups of the same database.

[2] Of the 6 studies deemed methodologically weaker than the original 21, 3 reported that stress had significant effects on preterm birth, gestational age, or birth weight.

United States (the Pregnancy Risk Assessment Monitoring System) by assessing life events 2 to 6 months after delivery (retrospectively). Experiencing more than two life events predicted preterm birth in primiparous pregnancies in one cohort (1994 and 1995), and more than five life events predicted preterm birth in multiparous pregnancies in the other cohort (1990 to 1993). Why these results did not cross replicate across cohorts is unclear (also see the findings of Lu and Chen [2004], based on a third cohort from the same study).

However, the results presented above are consistent with those of two additional studies restricted to African-American women. In one study, the number of prenatal major life events, as assessed prospectively, was associated with gestational age in a sample of 179 pregnant women selected from a larger data set (Parker Dominguez et al., 2005). The other study of African-American women (Collins et al., 1998), which had a case-control design, indicated that three or more life events in pregnancy were significantly associated (OR = 3.1) with very low birth weight (all cases were also preterm births; see also Sable and Wilkenson [2000]). Zambrana et al. (1999) also found a bivariate association between life events and gestational age in a large sample of women of Mexican origin or descent and African-American women studied in the second trimester. However, the strongest effect in that study was detected when life events were combined with other stress measures into a latent factor in a multivariate model.

Thus, there is some consistent evidence that major life events are associated with preterm birth, although the evidence is by no means uniform. High numbers of life events and severe life events or life events with the greatest impact have been more consistently predictive of preterm birth across studies.[3] On the whole, the focus in the future should be on approaches to the study of life events that delineate events by their severity and emphasize those with the highest negative impacts.

Chronic and Catastrophic Stress Exposures

A second set of studies involved a common chronic stressor, such as being imprisoned (Hollander, 2005) or homeless (Stein et al., 2000) during pregnancy or experiencing a catastrophic event occurring during pregnancy (Glynn et al., 2001; Lederman et al., 2004). For example, Lederman and colleagues (2004) assessed the impact of the time of gestation at the time of the World Trade Center terrorist attack on September 11, 2001, among

---

[3]One exception is the finding of Goldenberg et al. (1996a) that a low frequency of positive life events during pregnancy was weakly associated with preterm birth.

300 nonsmoking women in New York City who were pregnant at the time. Women who were in the first trimester at the time of the attack delivered infants of significantly shorter gestations, and women whose place of employment was within 2 miles of the World Trade Center had marginally shorter gestations. Strikingly similar effects were found by Glynn and colleagues (2001), who examined gestational age at delivery of 40 women who experienced a major earthquake in the first, second, or third trimester or postpartum. They found a significant effect of the timing of the earthquake during pregnancy on gestational age, such that the later in pregnancy that an earthquake occurred, the longer the gestation was. The longest gestational age in that study was among women who had already delivered at the time of the event (and who were effectively unexposed), and the shortest gestation was among women who experienced the earthquake in the first trimester. Although the sample size was small and some alternative explanations cannot be ruled out, these results are intriguing, especially because of their similarity to those of Lederman et al. (2004), as they indicate that the timing of sudden traumatic environmental stressors during pregnancy may affect the timing of delivery. Although the methodological strengths of these studies vary, they avoid some of the pitfalls encountered in life events approaches because all the participants in the studies experienced the same stressor.[4]

Turning to more chronic forms of exposure, Stein et al. (2000) studied 237 homeless women interviewed at 78 shelters or meal programs. The severity of homelessness, especially the variable of the percentage of the woman's lifetime that she had been homeless, predicted both preterm birth and low birth weight (each of which controlled for the other). The analyses controlled for many other variables, such as substance use, trauma and distress, prior birth complications, race-ethnicity, income, and various medical risk factors. The severity of homelessness is a fairly objective measure of chronic stress or strain and not merely a measure of perceived stress or distress; but it may have been confounded nonetheless by inadequate nutrition or general health neglect, as the authors point out, which could account in part for these effects. Nonetheless, these are unique findings on the possible role of chronic stress in preterm birth and low birth weight.

Misra and colleagues (2001) also retrospectively studied chronic stress during pregnancy in 739 low-income African-American non-Hispanic women interviewed after delivery. Multivariate analyses indicated that chronic stress predicted preterm delivery (adjusted OR = 1.86) when several

---

[4]See also earlier studies by Kuvacic et al. (1996) on the effects of expatriation on preterm birth and Levi et al. (1989) on the effects of the Chernobyl nuclear disaster on preterm birth.

biomedical and other psychosocial factors were controlled for. The chronic stress measures contained 12 items that assessed financial, family, work, health, and other forms of ongoing stress.

In sum, studies of chronic and catastrophic stress exposures are suggestive of an association between stress and preterm birth, although the findings are not yet definitive. Such studies offer an opportunity to use quasiexperimental designs instead of correlational designs, and these quasiexperimental studies may add to the ability to draw inferences (Cook and Campbell, 1979; Shaddish et al., 2002), and also have the potential to test competing theories about acute versus chronic stress exposures and their effects on preterm birth.

Emotional Responses and Affective States

Anxiety

The early research on psychosocial risk factors for preterm delivery and low birth weight focused on maternal anxiety (Gorsuch and Key, 1974). Other studies over the years have focused on the role of general distress. Determination of whether either depression or anxiety is a risk factor for preterm delivery has, however, been difficult for many reasons. Among these is the fact that the two emotional states are often comorbid, although they are distinguishable clinically. However, the questionnaire measures used in obstetric research to assess anxiety and depression are not well suited to their differentiation. Thus, many studies have investigated general distress by using the General Health Questionnaire (Hedegaard et al., 1993, 1996; Perkin et al., 1993) or the Hopkins Symptom Checklist (Paarlberg et al., 1996). General emotional distress may not be as clear-cut a risk factor as the potentially separable effects of either anxiety or depression.

Recent studies suggest that anxiety may be a potentially important risk factor for preterm delivery. The IOM committee found 12 studies in total that tested the emotional components of stress as predictors of preterm birth. Eleven studies had prospective designs; of these, nine tested the association of anxiety with gestational age or preterm birth. Two found no significant effects for state anxiety (Lobel et al., 2000; Peacock et al., 1995); one study found that general anxiety was associated with intrauterine growth restriction (but not with preterm birth), but only in white patients (Goldenberg et al., 1996a); and one study found that general anxiety was associated with preterm labor in women who had a history of preterm labor (Dayan et al., 2002).

Four more investigations were very consistent in finding that anxiety concerning the pregnancy itself was associated with gestational age or preterm birth. For example, Rini et al. (1999) reported that prenatal anxiety (a combination of state anxiety and pregnancy anxiety), assessed by interviews with women at 28 to 30 weeks of gestation, was associated with gestational age in 230 Hispanic and white women when other sociodemographic, medical, and behavioral risk factors were controlled for (estimated OR for preterm birth = 1.59). In a larger prospective study, Dole et al. (2003) replicated these findings; pregnancy-related anxiety at 24 to 29 weeks of gestation predicted preterm birth in a sample of 1,962 women (RR = 2.1) when the data were adjusted for alcohol and tobacco use. This effect was robust for women with spontaneous preterm labor rather than the medical induction of labor, with medical comorbidities controlled for, and was a stronger effect than that of the life events noted above.

Mancuso and colleagues (2004) also replicated these findings with a sample of 282 women assessed twice during their pregnancies (Behavior in Pregnancy Study [BIPS]). Pregnancy-specific anxiety at 28 to 30 weeks of gestation (but not at 18 to 24 weeks of gestation) significantly predicted gestational age. In addition, Mancuso et al. (2004) reported that corticotropin-releasing hormone levels mediated the effects of pregnancy anxiety on gestational age (see also Hobel et al. [1999]). Further multivariate analyses of this sample reported by Roesch et al. (2004) sought to determine which of three stress indicators (state anxiety, pregnancy anxiety, and perceived stress) was most predictive of gestational age in the women participating in BIPS. They determined that pregnancy anxiety was the only significant predictor of gestational age when all three indicators were included in the model. Other studies of perceived stress that used the standard scale in BIPS (PSS) have had mixed results for this component (Lobel et al., 1992, 2000; Sable and Wilkenson, 2000; Zambrana et al., 1999).

When considered together, these results are quite consistent in pointing to anxiety as a possible risk factor. Although results of studies on general anxiety are somewhat mixed, studies on anxiety regarding the pregnancy itself are more consistent in predicting gestational age at birth or preterm birth. The most vulnerable times in pregnancy for emotions to have effects on physiology are not yet clear, but some research points to weeks 24 and 30 of gestation (Rini et al., 1999). The possibility of the confounding of anxiety over existing medical risk conditions was considered and controlled to some extent in some of these investigations, suggesting that anxiety over existing medical risk conditions does not fully account for the effects. That is, high-risk pregnancies may elicit anxiety, but this does not appear to account for these findings; in short, anxiety resulting from knowledge of one's medical risk conditions is not implicated as a risk factor per se. Follow-up research on anxiety and its timing and mechanisms of effects on preterm labor and delivery is recommended.

Depression

Ten studies on depression and preterm birth or low birth weight were reviewed. All studies had prospective designs. Of these, four reported non-significant effects (Dole et al., 2003; Goldenberg et al., 1996a; Lobel et al., 2000; Misra et al., 2001; Peacock et al., 1995). Three found that prenatal depression in the mother affected fetal growth (Hoffman and Hatch, 2000) and birth weight percentiles (Paarlberg et al., 1999). Two studies reported associations of depression and preterm delivery (Dayan et al., 2002; Jesse et al., 2003; Orr et al., 2002). One found significant effects only among women who were underweight (BMI < 19) before the pregnancy (Dayan et al., 2002). Another was a large study of African American women only (Orr et al., 2002) reporting adjusted OR of 1.96 for spontaneous preterm birth among women in the top 10 percent on a standard depression measure.

Overall, recent prospective studies on depression do not suggest a strong pattern for depression as a general risk for preterm delivery consistent with the results of earlier studies (Copper et al., 1996; Perkin et al., 1993) with some exceptions. For example, depression in African American women seems to be an area worthy of further investigation. Effects of depression on birth weight or fetal growth is also inconsistent but there are some indications that depression may be a risk factor for fetal growth or low birth weight. Further research is needed to clarify this topic of research. Pathways from emotion to low birth weight through health behaviors such as diet and nutrition, substance use, sleep, and inactivity are important to elucidate. Women who are depressed or anxious during pregnancy are unlikely to take care of themselves as adequately as those who are not. Anxiety may be linked to different behavioral implications than depression. Studies of these states also must address their frequent confounding as well. This is a potential topic for follow-up research.

Other Forms of Stress Exposure

A relatively small number of studies have assessed the effects of daily stressors on preterm birth but have shown nonsignificant results (Paarlberg et al., 1996; Wadhwa et al., 1993). It is possible that these measures do not capture levels of stress exposure high enough to influence pathways to prematurity. Although daily stressors may operate in combination with other stress exposures, such as major life events, and interact with responses such as anxiety or depression to contribute to the risk of preterm birth, they do not seem promising overall for predictive purposes.

Two other bodies of research are relevant to the role of stress and preterm delivery. One is on the effects of occupational or work stress on preterm delivery (Woo, 1997). This area is related to but distinct from the topics of physical activity and employment discussed earlier in this chapter. Whether or not a woman is employed, she may engage in various degrees of daily physical activity or strain, but only women who are employed would potentially experience occupational stress. Savitz and Pastore (1999) highlighted previous studies on occupational stress and preterm birth that were consistent in showing significant associations of either occupational stress or physical strain with preterm labor or delivery (Brandt and Nielsen, 1992; Brett et al., 1997; Henriksen et al., 1994; Homer et al., 1990). In a related study, Pritchard and Teo (1994) found that assessments of household strain were significant predictors of preterm birth in 393 Swedish women.

This area is complex because it has sometimes been framed as an issue of whether employment during pregnancy is itself risky or whether the characteristics of a woman's employment are the preterm birth risk-associated factor. Key issues include the type of work activities, the number of hours of work each day or week, the time during pregnancy when a woman works, the work environment, and the psychological strain (cognitive and emotional) that may be associated with work. When these factors are quantified, it may be found that some employed women are at risk and others are not. This is another topic worthy of future investigation.

A second area relevant to stress is that on exposure to personal violence. A small but growing body of work suggests that women who experience domestic or personal violence during pregnancy are at risk for adverse birth outcomes (Amaro et al., 1990; Coker et al., 2004; Parker et al., 1994a; Rich-Edwards et al., 2001; Shumway et al., 1999). The extent to which this is the result of stress processes rather than other mediating processes is unclear, however. In addition, most studies appear to view domestic or personal violence as a chronic stressor and have observed that violence affects birth weight but not preterm birth.

Mechanisms Linking Stress and Emotions to Preterm Birth

Maternal stress can cause the release of increased levels of catecholamines and cortisol, which could prematurely activate placental corticotropin-releasing hormone, thereby precipitating the biological cascade leading to the onset of preterm labor (see Chapter 6). Stress can also alter immune function, leading to increased susceptibility to intra-amniotic infection or inflammation (Wadhwa et al., 2001). Additionally, stress may induce high-risk behaviors as a means of coping with stress (Whitehead et al., 2003). Evidence is also accumulating that infections may play a key role in the pathogenesis of preterm birth, particularly very preterm delivery (see Chapter 6). Although researchers have recently focused on bacterial vaginosis (BV), several other infections, including asymptomatic bacteriuria, sexually transmitted infections, and periodontal infections, have all been implicated.

There is a need for investigation of the specific pathways whereby distinct stress and emotional and affective factors contribute to preterm birth. Past research provides some clues to possible avenues of investigation. For example, maternal anxiety has been implicated more in early labor and delivery via HPA pathways, whereas depression has been associated with poor health behaviors and their consequences for fetal growth. In particular, greater theoretical analysis of the intensity and duration of distinct emotional states such as anxiety and depression and their consequences for pregnancy outcomes, such as spontaneous preterm labor, spontaneous rupture of membranes, and fetal growth restriction, is needed. (See Chapter 6 for a more extensive review and discussion of the pathways from stress to preterm birth.)

More specifically, the role of anxiety in the preterm pathogenesis process has not been adequately evaluated (Kurki et al., 2000; McCool et al., 1994). One notion, built on common anecdotes, is that a single episode of strong emotion, such as anxiety from being in New York City when the World Trade Center was attacked, in New Orleans during Hurricane Katrina, or in Los Angeles during the Northridge Earthquake, can precipitate early labor. A second possibility is that a chronic state of anxiety resulting from a clinically diagnosable anxiety disorder or subclinical set of symptoms places a woman at risk for preterm delivery. A third possibility is that a combination of the first two possibilities, in the form of an anxious disposition combined with a highly stressful acute event or series of events, may interact to cause early labor.

Limiting the inquiry to the role of anxiety and its biological consequences may prove more fruitful than earlier and cruder approaches to studying general distress and its influence on preterm delivery. Earlier, such studies served the field well in identifying potentially new risk factors, but more scientific precision on the emotional experience of pregnancy and its consequences is greatly needed now to obtain a further understanding of the association of stress with preterm delivery. For example, emerging research indicates that physiologic stress reactivity (e.g., endocrine and cardiovascular) decreases across gestation (de Weerth and Buitelaar, 2005; Glynn et al., 2001, 2004; Matthews and Rodin, 1992; Schulte et al., 1990), which has substantive implications for the role of psychosocial factors as both risk factors and targets for intervention.

Culture, Race, Ethnicity, and Stress

A complication of research on stress in general and on emotional states during pregnancy more specifically is that emotional experience and responses to emotion are at least partially culturally grounded (Mesquita and Frijda, 1992). That is, people of different cultures differ in their comprehension of and ability to accept the expression of emotions, such as anxiety and sadness. In some subgroups in the United States, the expression of anxiety may be much more normative and accepted than in others, in which it may be frowned upon, misunderstood, or ignored. Languages may also differ in their abilities to translate the word "stress." The Spanish language, for example, does not have a specific translation for the word "stress." Anxiety, or *nervios*, is understood in Spanish, whereas stress in general is not. Thus, studies of stress as a risk factor by the use of standard scale assessments delivered in Spanish may or may not be assessing the same phenomenon that these scales assess when they are delivered in English. This poses a special challenge to researchers.

Similarly, African American women, whose rates of preterm delivery and infant mortality are the highest in the United States, have unique experiences of stress, yet there is a dearth of studies on African American cultural factors pertaining to stress, emotion, or pregnancy. Parker Dominguez and colleagues (2005) found that neither anxiety nor perceived stress was significantly correlated with gestational age or low birthweight among 179 pregnant African American women. Instead, a newer measure of the extent to which women experienced intrusive thoughts or rumination about their two most severe major life events was associated with lower birth weight when gestational age in linear multiple regression analyses was controlled for. Intrusive thought is a recognized symptom of trauma containing both cognitive and emotional components (and is often symptomatic of post-traumatic stress disorder).

The possibility that low-income African American women experience more symptoms of trauma and that these are more important risk factors for preterm birth than depression or anxiety for this or other groups is intriguing. More generally, researchers must address the possibility that the same aspects of stress may not pose a risk for preterm birth in the same manner for all racial and ethnic groups. In-depth studies of specific racial-ethnic and cultural groups that include culturally specific stress measures may yield answers to whether stress is a risk factor for preterm birth for specific groups. The answers may be more complex than has been imagined. Anxiety may be a stronger risk factor for Latinos and whites, whereas depression, posttraumatic stress disorder, or racial stressors may be more potent individual-level risk factors for African American women. These possibilities might help to explain why research on stress and pregnancy outcomes has yielded equivocal findings and also why the findings from studies in foreign countries with more homogeneous populations, such as Denmark, have been more definitive. Furthermore, these possibilities suggest very different intervention strategies for different racial and ethnic groups (Norbeck and Anderson, 1989).

Racism

The pressing need to reduce the racial disparities in infant mortality, low birth weight, and preterm birth in the United States has led to new theories and new research directions on the pregnancies of African-American women (Hogue and Vasquez, 2002; Rich-Edwards et al., 2001; Rowley, 1994, 2001; Rowley et al., 1993). In particular, attention is being directed to the role of racism and discrimination in health outcomes in general (Krieger, 2000) and in pregnancy outcomes specifically (Collins et al., 2000, 2004). Racism is defined as racially motivated interpersonal and institutional discrimination (Krieger, 2000). Several research teams have developed self-report measures of racism, and these measures have been used in a handful of case-control and prospective studies of pregnancy. Collins and colleagues (2000) published the first study on this issue with a sample of low-income African American women in Chicago who delivered very low birth weight infants (n = 25), all of which were preterm, or matched controls with infants of normal birth weight (n = 60). They used Krieger's measures developed for the CARDIA study (Krieger, 1990; Krieger and Sidney, 1996). These measures query participants about their experiences of racism at work, at school, when getting medical care, when receiving service at stores or restaurants, and when finding housing. Mothers with infants with very low birth weights were twice as likely to report experiences of racial discrimination during pregnancy as women who delivered infants of normal birth weight. After adjustment for socioeconomic condition, levels of social support, cigarette smoking, alcohol intake, and illegal drug use, the adjusted OR was 3.2.

Four subsequent studies have been published since publication of the first one by Collins et al. (2000), two of which had case-control designs (Collins et al., 2004; Rosenberg, 1965) and two of which had prospective designs (Dole et al., 2003; Mustillo et al., 2004). Mustillo and colleagues (2004) examined racial discrimination using the CARDIA data set, which included data from a 10-year prospective study of a large cohort of African American and white men and women. Their sample comprised the 352 African American and white women who gave birth to live infants at 20 weeks gestation or longer. Racism was measured by use of the Krieger measure at year 7 of the study, and low birth weight for an intervening pregnancy was assessed by self-report at year 10. Several findings are of interest. First, race was a risk factor for preterm birth, as expected (OR = 2.54); but the risk estimate was reduced after adjustment for lifetime experiences of racism, suggesting that racism may mediate the racial-ethnic difference in preterm birth rates. Smoking, alcohol intake, depression, and the amount of weight gained during pregnancy did not have such effects. Second, women who had experienced lifetime discrimination were nearly five times more likely to deliver a low birth weight infant than those who had not experienced racism. This relationship was reduced by including preterm birth in the model, suggesting that the effect of discrimination on birth weight was as a result of the effects of racism on the likelihood of an earlier delivery. Thus, lifetime experiences of racism explained the racial and ethnic disparities in the rates of both preterm birth and low birth weight.

Collins and colleagues (2004) also considered lifetime exposure to racism as well as pregnancy exposure in a case-control study of 104 African American women in Chicago who delivered very low birth weight preterm infants and 208 matched controls who delivered normal birth weight infants. Lifetime exposure to racial discrimination in three or more domains of life was associated with very low birth weight (OR = 3.2; OR = 2.6 adjusted for age, education, and cigarette smoking). The outcomes were not associated with perceived prenatal racial discrimination. The authors conducted post hoc tests, whose results suggested that the effects detected were not attributable to recall bias because of infant illness among the low birth weight infants. In addition, the strongest risk was for college-educated African American women. Collins and colleagues (2004) conclude that "lifelong accumulated experiences of racial discrimination by African American women constitute an independent risk factor for preterm delivery" (p. 2132). One apparent pathway whereby racism appears to influence health and possibly prenatal processes is by cardiovascular functioning (Krieger, 1990; Krieger and Sidney, 1996). (For a complete review of the literature on racial and ethnic disparities in pregnancy outcomes, definitions and measures of racism, the conceptualization of racism as stress, and findings, see the work of Giscombe and Lobel [2005]).

The following are key questions to be resolved in future research: Is racism a risk factor for preterm birth or fetal growth restriction or both, and, if so, by what pathways? Does racism act in association with other factors, such as social class, age, medical risk factors, or other stress or emotional factors to pose a risk? If racism is a potent risk factor, are there effective, practical, and cost-effective ways to mitigate its effects on maternal and infant outcomes?

In general, the emerging literature on racism and preterm delivery suggests that racism may be a potent stressor throughout the lifetimes of African American women that contributes to an explanation of the racial and ethnic disparities in the rates of both preterm birth and low birth weight. However, further study is needed to replicate and extend the existing studies. One challenge researchers face is the difficulty of assessing experiences of racism. Many factors contribute to underreporting of the experience. This challenge requires further precise work by investigators in future.

Social Support

The term *social support* incorporates research on social integration, social networks, and social support (House et al., 1988). The last element (social support per se) has been studied mainly as a perception that others will provide the mother with specific resources during pregnancy if she should need them (Sarason et al., 1987). Alternatively, social support refers to a set of interactions or exchanges with others in which emotional concern, instrumental aid, or information about the environment or one's self are provided (House, 1981). *Instrumental aid* includes task assistance and material aid. *Emotional concern* includes affection, opportunities to express feelings, and empathy and understanding. *Information* includes constructive feedback, validation, advice, and guidance. For the purposes of this report, all of these conceptualizations (social integration, network characteristics, perceived available support, and actual receipt of support) and their associated measures are relevant.

In the small body of observational research on preterm delivery, many different ways of defining and measuring social support have been adopted, with, for the most part, no consensus or overlap across studies. Not surprisingly, intervention research has focused on the actual provision of support during pregnancy. Support may be provided by professionals, paraprofessionals, other pregnant women, family members, friends, or a woman's partner. The majority of past intervention research has been on the professional or paraprofessional support provided by telephone calls, by home visits, or in prenatal care settings. In contrast, observational research has been slanted toward family or partner support. Notably, the specific sources of support that women of different subgroups use differ by their racial-ethnic, cultural, and sociodemographic backgrounds (Dunkel-Schetter, 1998). For some groups, the baby's father may be the most important source, whereas for other groups, the pregnant woman's mother or family may be her most likely source of support (Sagrestano et al., 1999).

Observational Studies

Early observational studies drew attention to the possibility that prenatal social support might reduce the incidence of adverse outcomes either directly or as a result of their ability to buffer the effects of stress (see the reviews by Brooks-Gunn [1991], Dunkel-Schetter [1998], and Oakley [1988]). However, early research on psychosocial factors and birth outcomes tended to lump together distinct factors such as stress and social support (Nuckolls et al., 1972) and to combine distinct outcomes such as preterm birth and low birth weight into one category of complications (Boyce et al., 1985, 1986; Norbeck and Tilden, 1983).

The next set of observational studies corrected for some of these problems but did not confirm the direct link between social support and gestational age or preterm birth (Molfese et al., 1987; Pagel et al., 1990; Reeb et al., 1987), although associations were detected in some specific racial-ethnic groups (Berkowitz and Kasl, 1983; Norbeck and Anderson, 1989). These studies were followed by another generation of studies (after 1990) involving larger sample sizes, improved study designs (prospective), better measures, and more carefully controlled analyses. The results of these studies were highly consistent: virtually every study found significant associations between social support variables and birth weight or fetal growth (Buka et al., 2003; Collins et al., 1993; Feldman et al., 2000; Mutale et al., 1991; Pryor et al., 2003; Turner et al., 1990). However, those that tested for an association between social support variables and preterm labor or delivery specifically found no evidence that such a relationship exists (Dole et al., 2003; Feldman et al., 2000; Misra et al., 2001).

Thus, the results of observational studies over two decades do not confirm the hypothesized correlation between social support and preterm delivery, but they do provide fairly consistent evidence for a direct association between prenatal maternal social support and infant birth weight. The magnitude of this effect is difficult to determine from existing research.

Intervention Research

Enthusiasm for the theoretical premise that the provision of social support to pregnant women could reduce adverse pregnancy outcomes fueled a handful of controlled intervention studies published in the late 1980s and 1990s (Heins et al., 1990; Oakley et al., 1990; Olds et al., 1986; Rothberg and Lits, 1991; Spencer et al., 1989). Some of these combined social support with other programmatic elements, such as nutrition or smoking cessation interventions. Many aimed to reduce adverse pregnancy outcomes overall, including both low birth weight and preterm birth, in a composite outcome variable. These intervention studies have been extensively reviewed elsewhere (Blondel, 1998; Elbourne and Oakley, 1991; Elbourne et al., 1989; Olds and Kitzman, 1993). In 1999, Goldenberg and Rouse concluded their review as follows: "there is little evidence to support the belief that a significant reduction in preterm birth can be achieved through the systematic provision of psychosocial support" (Goldenberg and Rouse, 1999, p. 114).

A recent Cochrane review that used meta-analytic techniques systematically evaluated 16 trials involving 13,651 women in total (Hodnett and Fredericks, 2003). The study design used randomization to the treatment and the control groups, and additional support was provided to women in the treatment group in the first or second trimester if they were at risk of preterm delivery or fetal growth restriction. The interventions included standardized or individualized programs that were provided on several occasions in home visits by midwives, nurses, or social workers; during regular antenatal clinic visits; or by telephone. Meta-analyses revealed that overall these interventions were not associated with reductions in the rates of preterm birth (11 trials) or low birth weight (13 trials). The authors concluded that the provision of additional support did not reduce the likelihood of giving birth too early or of delivering an infant who was smaller than expected (Hodnett and Fredericks, 2003). These conclusions are consistent with those of another recent review (Lu et al., 2005), in which it was found that only 1 of 12 randomized controlled trials of the provision of psychosocial resources to reduce low birth weight was effective (Norbeck et al., 1996). However, some of the randomized controlled trials showed that the provision of psychosocial resources affected a range of other outcomes, such as anxiety, satisfaction with care, awareness and knowledge of risk conditions, perceived mastery, and engagement of the mother in health-promoting behaviors (Klerman et al., 2001).

The inability of intervention trials to demonstrate the effects of social support on either preterm birth or low birth weight is puzzling to experts and is in some ways a source of controversy. Although study designs can always be improved, the high degree of consistency of the results across numerous trials, combined with the fact that at least some of the studies were quite rigorous, tends to refute the possibility that the studies had general design flaws or methodological explanations as the sole reason for the lack of demonstration of an effect of social support. A more specific possibility raised by Hodnett and Fredericks (2003), however, is that the ability to identify women at high risk of delivering infants preterm or of low birth weight is so imprecise that many women in these trials were not actually at higher risk.

The identification of women at high risk of preterm birth might be improved; and with greater understanding of the etiology of preterm birth and with the availability of better indicators of risk, greater precision in targeting the subset(s) of pregnant women who could benefit from supportive interventions of specific kinds may be achieved. Lu et al. (2005) echo this sentiment, pointing out that most trials do not have effective risk screening procedures; only 2 of the 12 trials that they reviewed even evaluated the effectiveness of their risk screening procedures for the untreated group. Moreover, in some studies, the risk factors did not predict outcomes for the untreated study participants, as would be expected. If investigators are not successfully targeting selected risk groups, then the trials are not likely to have expected effects.

In addition, it has been pointed out that the treatments must be much better matched to the risk factors (Lu et al., 2005; Olds and Kitzman, 1993).

Norbeck et al. (1996), for example, selected pregnant women for intervention partly on the basis of inadequate social support, and then provided social support to those in the treatment group, which produced a reduction in the numbers of infants born with low birth weights. Thus, because of limitations in risk screening and intervention matching, the matter of whether supportive interventions of some kinds might reduce the rates of preterm birth for at least a subset of women has probably not yet been adequately tested.

A further concern is the absence of a strong theoretical basis for support intervention trials. For example, only 5 of 12 of the studies reviewed by Lu et al. (2005) had a predictive model on which the intervention was based. Contributing to this concern is the fact that, despite the large number of experimental trials, the causal mechanisms that might underlie a relationship between low levels of social support and early labor or delivery have not been specified. Research indicating that social support is associated with various demographic factors, better health behaviors, more optimal prenatal care, and greater wantedness of the pregnancy may be informative about the pathways linking social support to fetal growth.

Interestingly, considerable theoretical findings on the association of social support and health more broadly are available, but these have not been applied in a significant way to the study of pregnancy (Cohen, 1988; Cohen and Syme, 1985; Taylor, 2006). Furthermore, little has been culled from the available rigorous research and theory on social support interventions for other medical conditions (Cohen, 2000), such as cancer (Helgeson and Cohen, 1996). Drawing from what is known about how to conceptualize, assess, administer, and evaluate support resources in other populations requiring health care may provide new perspectives on how to do so for pregnant women.

A final possibility raised by Hodnett and Fredericks (2003) is that no matter how much or how effective social support is, it may not be sufficiently powerful to improve substantially the outcomes of pregnancy, especially given the long-standing conditions of social deprivation endured by the women at the highest risk. This possibility must be considered in the case of preterm birth, for which neither observational research nor randomized controlled trials have offered any empirical basis for further research and plausible theoretical mechanisms are lacking.

Personal Resources

The emerging literature on personal resources warrants attention in multilevel research attempts to understand preterm birth better. The term *personal resources* refers to individual differences in views about one's self and the world, such as self-esteem, mastery, perceived control, and optimism. These are conceptualized as relatively stable characteristics of individuals that are generally protective of the individual's health and that function as coping resources (Lachman and Weaver, 1998; Thoits, 1995). They can be more broadly conceptualized as resilience resources, along with social support and other values, beliefs, and personality traits, which function similarly. Studies to date on personal resources and preterm birth have shown some interesting results. In a prospective study of 553 nulliparous African American pregnant women at less than 26 weeks of gestation, Edwards et al. (1994) found that two specific questions from a standard self-esteem measure predicted gestational age and preterm birth, and one item predicted infant head circumference. Jesse et al. (2003) found that the same standard self-esteem measure predicted a lower risk of preterm birth (RR = 0.865) in 120 pregnant women studied at 16 to 28 weeks of gestation, but that the effect became marginally significant when other variables were controlled for in the analyses. Rini et al. (1999), using the same standard measure used by Jesse et al. (2003), combined with standard scales of mastery and optimism into a broader personal resources factor, reported that self-esteem again predicted birth weight but not gestational age in more than 200 pregnant women assessed in midpregnancy. The findings of these studies are contradictory as to whether self-esteem influences preterm birth independently of birth weight. In addition, there is little discussion in the literature of the mechanisms by which such an effect would occur. It is possible that women with higher levels of self-esteem take better care of themselves during pregnancy, which has plausible pathways to fetal growth and to the use of health care for the management of risk factors for preterm birth and intrauterine growth restriction. However, these pathways remain to be fully explicated and tested.

Other pertinent studies have evaluated mastery, which is a sense of efficacy over one's environment (Copper et al., 1996), and dispositional optimism, which refers to expectations for positive life outcomes in future (Lobel et al., 2000). In general, however, those studies did not find an association of these factors with preterm birth (see also the work by Rini et al. [1999]). However, Misra et al. (2001) report that locus of control was an independent predictor of preterm birth (unadjusted OR = 2.22; adjusted OR = 1.75 after controlling for biomedical factors). Women who perceived that they could influence the health of their children at birth had lower rates of preterm birth.

In sum, the few available studies on self-esteem, mastery, optimism, and perceived control in women expecting infants do not consistently predict preterm birth. It may be that these factors are more related to fetal growth and low birth weight or that these factors are more relevant to particular subgroups of pregnant women, such as populations of women who are socioeconomically disadvantaged. There is a need for the development of hypothesized pathways to preterm birth as a basis for any future study of these factors. In addition, the study of these factors in combination with social factors, such as race and ethnicity, social class, and neighborhood factors (see Chapter 4), is recommended.

Intendedness of Pregnancy and Preterm Delivery

The term *unintended* refers to those pregnancies that are unwanted or mistimed (i.e., they occur earlier than desired by the parents). Intentions are measured by self-report by using standard survey questions that can distinguish between whether the woman wanted a child now, not now but at some point (mistimed), or not at all (unwanted). These questions are answered after conception and in many studies are answered after delivery, which may introduce retrospective bias.

It is estimated that approximately 60 percent of all pregnancies are unintended, and of these, about half end in a live birth (IOM, 1995). Women with unintended pregnancies are less likely to seek early prenatal care (Bitto et al., 1997; IOM, 1995; Kost et al., 1998; Pagnini and Reichman, 2000) and are more likely to use alcohol or tobacco (IOM, 1995). They also appear to be more likely to experience high levels of exposure to psychosocial stress and depressive symptoms (Orr and Miller, 1997). Although unintended pregnancies occur among women across the sociodemographic spectrum, they are disproportionately likely among mothers who are adolescent, unmarried, or over age 40 (Bitto et al., 1997; IOM, 1995). The child of an unwanted pregnancy (as opposed to the child of a wanted or a mistimed pregnancy) is at greater risk of low birth weight, death in the first year of life, abuse, and receiving insufficient resources for optimal early child development (IOM, 1995). Additional consequences occur for the parents of unwanted pregnancies. For example, a study that used data from the Pregnancy Risk Assessment Monitoring System database of 39,348 women in 14 states who delivered a live-born infant (Goodwin et al., 2000) found that women with unintended pregnancies had a 2.5 times greater risk of physical abuse.

Having an unintended pregnancy is estimated to increase the odds of delivering an infant of low birth weight by about 1.2 to 1.8 (IOM, 1995). However, only three studies on intentions and preterm birth were available as of 1995, and of those three studies, two were unpublished. On the basis of the findings from these preliminary studies, IOM (1995) indicated that the increased risk of low birth weight because of an unintended pregnancy appeared to be related to preterm delivery rather than intrauterine growth restriction. Subsequently, at least one further study has been conducted with a sample of 922 African American, low-income pregnant women recruited in four hospital-based prenatal clinics in Baltimore, Maryland (Orr et al.,

2000). Women with unintended pregnancies were 1.82 times more likely to deliver their infants preterm, after adjustment for clinical and behavioral factors associated with preterm delivery.

Thus, although the research available on the association of the intendedness of pregnancy and preterm delivery is limited, that which is available suggests that women with unintended pregnancies are more likely to deliver preterm, and as a consequence, their infants are at higher risk of being of low birth weight. Understanding the pathways from unintended conception to preterm labor and delivery by the use of multilevel approaches would be useful in elucidating the etiology of preterm birth for at least some subgroups of women. Unmeasured socioeconomic factors that may be confounded with unintended pregnancies must be carefully controlled in future studies. In addition, it is critical to refine measures of intendedness to be sure they are valid and reliable if this arena of research is to be pursued. Reducing unintended pregnancies through family planning and other mechanisms could indirectly reduce the rates of preterm delivery and related adversities (IOM, 1995). Disparities in pregnancy outcomes, including preterm birth, could also be reduced by paying attention to the intendedness of a pregnancy (Hogue and Vasquez, 2002).

SUMMARY AND FUTURE DIRECTIONS FOR RESEARCH

Among the behavioral and psychosocial factors considered, the one that shows the most consistent evidence of having an adverse impact on the risk of preterm birth is cocaine use. Dietary constituents have been examined to a limited degree, with mixed evidence on the potential benefits of increased levels of iron, long-chain fatty acids, folate, and vitamin C being found. Although none of these dietary constituents is well established as having effects that prevent preterm birth, all warrant further evaluation. Leisure time physical activity has been associated with a reduced risk of preterm birth, but the implications for causality are unclear. Employment alone is nonspecific as a factor related to preterm birth, and meaningful etiologic research of this association is likely not possible. Although vaginal douching is of interest as a cause of preterm birth, given the concern with reproductive tract infections and the different prevalences of such infections between African American and white women, evidence of an influence on preterm birth is lacking thus far.

The evidence is fairly consistent that the occurrence of large numbers of major life events and the experiencing of severe life events during pregnancy are associated with preterm birth. Studies of chronic and catastrophic stress exposures are fewer in number, but such exposures also appear to contribute to preterm delivery, although more research in this area is needed. Past research findings are also consistent in pointing to maternal anxiety, especially anxiety over the pregnancy itself, as a risk factor for preterm delivery. In contrast, recent prospective studies on depression do not suggest a strong pattern for depression as a risk factor for preterm delivery; rather, these studies indicate that prenatal maternal depression may predict birth weight and fetal growth. The emerging literature on racism and preterm delivery suggests that racism, a possible stressor throughout the lifetimes of African American women, contributes to the explanation for racial-ethnic disparities in the rates of both preterm birth and low birth weight.

The results of more than two decades of observational studies on naturally occurring social support do not confirm a hypothesized link between maternal social support and preterm delivery; however, the studies do provide fairly consistent evidence for a direct association between social support and infant birth weight. Similarly, the provision of additional support to pregnant women during controlled intervention studies has not reduced the likelihood that the mother will give birth too early, although it does appear to have other benefits for women's health care and psychosocial adjustment. The few available studies on maternal self-esteem, mastery, and optimism provide little evidence for associations with preterm birth specifically, although the concept of perceived control may be a risk factor. Finally, preliminary research on the association of the intendedness of the pregnancy and preterm delivery suggests that women with unintended pregnancies are more likely to deliver their infants preterm.

The foregoing reviews and discussion of behavioral and psychosocial factors involved in the etiology of preterm birth give rise to some suggested future directions for researchers:

• At present, many studies of birth outcomes do not use preterm birth as a study outcome. Instead low birth weight is often used as a proxy. As stated earlier in this report (see Chapter 2), low birth weight can be caused by both preterm birth and fetal growth restriction, two conditions with some overlapping but also divergent determinants and pathways. Future research needs to define preterm birth and small for gestational age as specific and distinct study outcomes and should not use low birth weight as a proxy for preterm birth. In addition, attention should be paid to whether the onset of labor is spontaneous.

• Studies of behavioral risk factors and preterm birth should examine constellations of lifestyle factors rather than individual behaviors in isolation to elucidate possible etiologic pathways for specific subtypes of preterm delivery.

• Studies of stress and preterm birth should focus on specific components or factors, such as anxiety and hypothesized pathways from this condition to preterm birth. There is a pressing need for more theoretical analyses on the intensity and duration of distinguishable emotional states and their consequences for pregnancy outcomes, such as spontaneous preterm labor, spontaneous rupture of membranes, and fetal growth restriction.

• Future studies on the association between stress and preterm birth should consider the unique forms of stress that specific racial and ethnic groups experience by using culturally valid measures in efforts to determine the optimal risk factors for specific subgroups of the population.

• Studies on the association between racism and preterm birth warrant follow-up for replication and further clarification to understand the specific exposures and mechanisms that pose a risk.

• Understudied topics that may be promising avenues for future research are the characteristics of daily activity and employment, as well as activity in the home and work contexts, including physical strain, occupational stress, and the effects of domestic violence during pregnancy.

• Attention to the intendedness of pregnancy is warranted to determine whether it is a risk factor for preterm birth rather than other outcomes, such as intrauterine growth restriction, and the pathways to such outcomes.

• Further research on personal resources, such as self-esteem, mastery, and control, may be warranted if it is conducted with a strong theoretical basis on the pathways to preterm birth. More generally, there is a need for theoretical models of the pathways from the presence of psychosocial conditions, including stress, social support, and other resilience factors, to preterm birth as a basis for ongoing observational research. These models should address the interrelationships of psychosocial conditions with biological and behavioral conditions by use of a multilevel approach.

• A more integrative approach to understanding individual-level factors in prematurity is needed. This will require the use of both a longitudinal integration linking a woman's life history to her vulnerability to preterm delivery and a contextual integration linking a woman's individual biology, psychosocial processes, and behaviors to the multilevel, multiple determinants of preterm birth (Misra et al., 2003).

4

Sociodemographic and Community Factors Contributing to Preterm Birth

ABSTRACT

A number of maternal sociodemographic characteristics are associated with an increased risk for preterm birth. Young maternal age, maternal age over 35, and pregnancy for single mothers and those cohabitating outside of marriage (except in countries where cohabitation is common) are associated with an increased risk. As discussed in preceding chapters, there are significant inter- and intragroup variations in the rates of preterm birth. Proposed explanations include socioeconomic condition, maternal behaviors, stress, and infections, and racial differences in genetics. However, these factors do not fully account for the disparities in the rates of preterm birth. In addition to disparities by race and ethnicity, disparities by socioeconomic condition, independent of race-ethnicity, are well documented. Nutrition, cigarette smoking, substance use or abuse, work and physical activity, prenatal care, infection, psychological factors and multiple gestations have been explored but do not fully explain these differences. Examining the context of neighborhoods may be a promising avenue of exploration for explaining disparities in preterm birth because of clear patterns of residential segregation that result in unequal exposures to adverse neighborhood conditions. Although the evidence suggests that after adjustment for individual-level attributes, neighborhood conditions are independently and significantly associated with a risk of low birth weight, evidence regarding the relationship between neighborhood context and preterm birth specifically is lacking. Further examination of the social contribution to preterm birth may contribute to an understanding of the disparities in the rates of preterm birth among different segments of the U.S. population.

The preceding chapter reviewed the association between individual-level health behaviors and psychosocial characteristics and the risk of preterm birth. In general, studies have not revealed the individual-level risk factors that are strongly and consistently associated with the risk of preterm birth. However, the literature on racial and ethnic disparities in the rates of preterm birth suggests other individual-level characteristics that may be associated with preterm birth and that should be considered. For example, African American women are disproportionately affected by many individual-level conditions that may be associated with preterm birth, such as the higher likelihood of being unmarried, of having lower levels of income and education, and of having poorer prepregnancy health than white women. Thus, it is important to also consider sociodemographic characteristics in relation to preterm birth. These individual-level factors do not occur in isolation. They are embedded in a social context, which also has implications for preterm birth. This chapter addresses both of these issues. The first section addresses sociodemographic characteristics, such as maternal age, marital status and cohabitation, race and ethnicity, and socioeconomic condition. The second section discusses the association between neighborhood conditions and the potential mechanisms through which the neighborhood context may influence reproductive outcomes.

SOCIODEMOGRAPHIC FACTORS

A number of maternal sociodemographic characteristics are associated with an increased risk for preterm birth. This section evaluates the relationships between maternal age, marital status and cohabitation, race and ethnicity, and socioeconomic condition and preterm birth. Possible causes of racial-ethnic and socioeconomic disparities in preterm birth are also explored.

Maternal Age

Several studies have identified young maternal age as an important risk factor for preterm birth (Amini et al., 1996; Branum and Schoendorf, 2005; Fraser et al., 1995; Hediger et al., 1997; Satin et al., 1994; Scholl et al., 1992, 1994). Hediger et al. (1997) found that young adolescents (less than

16 years of age at the time of their last menstrual period), especially those of young gynecological age (within 2 years of menarche), had a twofold greater risk for preterm delivery compared with the risk for older women (ages 18 to 29 years). Using U.S. natality data, Branum and Schoendorf (2005) also found a nearly twofold greater risk of very preterm delivery (less than 33 weeks gestation) among young adolescents (16 years of age or younger) compared with that among young adults (ages 21 to 24 years); the risk decreased with an increase in the age of the adolescent mothers. It is not known at present whether the increased risk of preterm birth among young adolescents is due to their biological immaturity or to an increased preva- lence of other risk factors associated with their generally poor socioeco- nomic condition (Branum and Schoendorf, 2005; Mitchell and Bracken, 1990; Olausson et al., 2001; Scholl et al., 1992).

Women ages 35 and over are also at increased risk for preterm delivery (Astolfi and Zonta, 2002; Cnattingius et al., 1992). Astolfi and Zonta (2002) found in a population sample of Italian women a 64 percent in- creased odds of preterm delivery among mothers 35 years of age or older compared with that among mother less than 35 years of age when educa- tion, birth order, and fetal gender were controlled for. The risk was particu- larly striking among mothers over 35 years of age delivering their first-born child. The reasons for the increased risk for preterm delivery among older women are not known. By using pooled data for the 1998 to 2000 U.S. birth cohorts from the National Center for Health Statistics (NCHS), the committee identified a similar U-shaped curve that characterizes the rela- tionship between maternal age and preterm delivery (Figure 4-1).

As shown in Figure 4-1, the association between maternal age and the risk of preterm birth is not consistent across racial and ethnic groups. It is observed that the preterm birth rate begins to rise at a younger age for non- Hispanic African Americans (ages 27 to 29) than for non-Hispanic whites (ages 33 to 35), and the slope of the rise with increasing age is greater for African Americans than for whites. Geronimus (1996) attributes this differ- ential rise with increasing age to "weathering." According to the "weather- ing" hypothesis, the effects of social inequality on health compound with age, leading to growing gaps in health status between African American and white women through young and middle adulthood that can affect their reproductive outcomes. However, evidence supporting the weathering hypothesis remains inconclusive, as most studies that use cross-sectional data cannot adequately control for potential cohort effects. Further studies on the interaction effects of maternal age and race-ethnicity on preterm birth are needed.

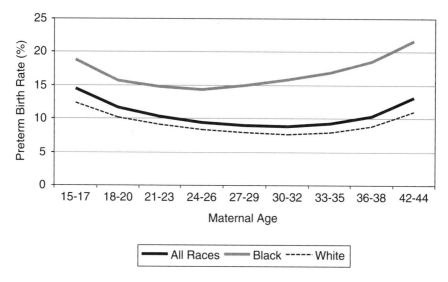

FIGURE 4-1 Relationship between maternal age and preterm birth, by race, 1998 to 2000, U.S. birth cohorts.
SOURCE: NCHS (unpublished data).

MARITAL STATUS AND COHABITATION

Pregnancy in unmarried women has been associated with a higher risk of preterm birth (Blondel and Zuber, 1988; Holt et al., 1997; Luo et al., 2004; Olsen et al., 1995b; Peacock et al., 1995; Raatikainen et al., 2005; Wen et al., 1990; Zeitlin et al., 2002). The rates of preterm birth for unmarried and married women were determined by using NCHS data for the 1998 to 2000 U.S. birth cohorts. As shown in Table 4-1, preterm birth rates are higher for unmarried women than for married women across all racial-ethnic and age groups.

The reasons for the higher rates of preterm birth among unmarried mothers are not known but are commonly attributed to their relative lack of social support and resources (Raatikainen et al., 2005; Waldron et al., 1996). The protective effects of marital status, however, are not uniform across racial-ethnic and age groups; the data in Table 4-1 suggest that marital status appears to offer the greatest protection against preterm birth among older (35 years of age or older) women and non-Hispanic African Americans.

Approximately 40 percent of births that occur outside of marriage now occur to cohabiting couples (CDC, 2000), and the rates of cohabitation have been increasing in the United States within the last few decades. Sev-

TABLE 4-1 Preterm Birth Rates (percent) for Married and Unmarried Women, by Maternal Age and Race-Ethnicity, 1998 to 2000

Age	Non-Hispanic African Americans		Non-Hispanic Whites		Asians-Pacific Islanders		American Indians		Hispanics	
	Married	Unmarried	Married	Unmarried	Married	Unmarried	Married	Unmarried	Married	Unmarried
<20	13.7	17.6	10.4	11.5	12.4	14.3	10.3	12.8	10.6	12.7
20–34	13.7	16.7	7.9	10.8	8.3	11.9	10.2	12.0	9.1	11.0
≥35	16.2	22.9	8.6	14.0	9.9	14.0	13.4	16.0	11.5	14.2

SOURCE: NCHS data for U.S. birth cohorts from 1998 to 2000.

eral studies have examined the relationship between cohabitation outside of marriage and preterm birth (Blondel and Zuber, 1988; Manderbacka et al., 1992). A collaborative case-control study in 16 European countries found that a significantly elevated risk of preterm birth was associated with cohabitation compared with the risk for those who are married (although the odds of preterm birth were substantially lower for women who cohabit with their partners than for single mothers) in countries where less than 20 percent of births occur outside of marriage. In contrast, no excess risk was associated with marital status in countries where out-of-marriage births were more common (Zeitlin et al., 2002). A population-based study in Quebec (where 44 percent of births were to common-law mothers in 1997) found the preterm birth rate among mothers in common-law unions to be higher than that among mothers in traditional marriage relationships but still lower than that among unmarried mothers living alone (Luo et al., 2004). The adjusted odds ratios for preterm birth were 1.14 and 1.41 for common-law and single mothers living alone, respectively, when individual- and community-level characteristics were controlled for. A large hospital cohort study in Finland also found a higher risk of preterm birth among single women than married women (adjusted odds ratio = 1.29), with the risk of cohabiting women being somewhere in between (adjusted odds ratios = 1.15) (Raatikainen et al., 2005).

Race and Ethnicity

Preterm birth rates vary substantially by race and ethnicity in the United States (CDC, 2005i). As discussed in Chapter 1, there are significant inter- and intragroup variations in the risk of premature birth. For example, in 2003 the preterm birth rates among Hispanics ranged from 11.7 percent for Mexicans to 13.8 percent for Puerto Ricans. Preterm birth rates also varied by nativity and duration of residence. In 2003, the preterm birth rate was 13.9 percent for foreign-born blacks but 18.2 percent for U.S.-born African Americans (CDC, 2005i). Even the duration of residence seems to have an effect on preterm birth rates. A study in California found that long-term Mexican immigrants who had lived in the United States for more than 5 years were more likely to deliver preterm infants than newcomers who had lived in the United States for 5 years or less (Guendelman and English, 1995). In general, the literature examining potential causes of racial and ethnic disparities in preterm births is not well developed. Investigations of the effects of nativity are even less developed.

These racial-ethnic disparities have persisted for decades, although the precise reasons are not clear. A number of explanations have been proposed, including racial differences in socioeconomic condition, maternal

TABLE 4-2 Preterm Birth Rates (percent) by Maternal Race-Ethnicity and Educational Attainment, 1998 to 2000

Educational Attainment[a]	Non-Hispanic African Americans	Non-Hispanic Whites	Asians-Pacific Islanders	American Indians	Hispanics
<8	19.6	11.0	11.5	14.8	10.7
8–12	16.8	9.9	10.5	11.8	10.4
13–15	14.5	8.3	9.1	9.9	9.3
≥16	12.8	7.0	7.5	9.4	8.4

[a]Educational attainment indicates the number of years of school completed.

SOURCE: NCHS data for U.S. birth cohorts from 1998 to 2000.

behaviors, stress, infections, and genetics (reviewed by Lu and Halfon [2003]).

Conventional wisdom often regards race as a proxy for socioeconomic condition, and some believe that socioeconomic factors (often measured in terms of educational attainment, household income, or occupational status) explain differences in preterm birth rates by race. African American women, on average, are more socioeconomically disadvantaged than non-Hispanic white women (Oliver and Shapiro, 1995), and a poorer socioeconomic condition is associated with an increased risk for preterm birth. However, in most studies the differences in preterm birth rates (McGrady et al., 1992), birth weights (Collins and Hawkes, 1997; Shiono et al., 1997), and infant mortality rates (Schoendorf et al., 1992) between African American and white women persisted after adjustment for (measured) socioeconomic differences. Furthermore, socioeconomic condition does not confer equal protection across racial-ethnic groups, as shown in Table 4-2.

For example, although within each racial-ethnic group the risk of preterm birth decreases with an increasing level of educational attainment, African American women with more than 16 years of education still have substantially higher preterm birth rates than non-Hispanic white women with less than 9 years of education. Although it is possible that the residual disparities result from misclassification error, measurement error, aggregation bias, or some unmeasured aspect of socioeconomic condition (Kaufman et al., 1997), these studies suggest that differences in socioeconomic conditions cannot fully account for racial disparities in preterm birth rates.

Another popular explanation holds maternal risk behaviors responsible for the racial disparities in preterm birth, such as smoking or drug use. However, several studies have found, albeit by self-report, that proportionately fewer African American women than white women smoke cigarettes during pregnancy (Beck et al., 2002; Lu et al., 2005). Similarly, the reported prevalence of alcohol and drug use among pregnant African American women appears to be no greater than that among pregnant white women (Serdula et al., 1991). Although it is possible that studies may not have considered all risk behaviors (e.g., douching) or interactions between race and behaviors, a few studies have concluded that the contributions of behavioral risk factors during pregnancy to racial disparities in birth outcomes such as preterm birth or low birth weight appear to be modest (Goldenberg et al., 1996a).

Similarly, the delayed and inadequate use of prenatal care among African American women has been identified as an important risk factor for the excess adverse birth outcomes among African American infants, including preterm birth. The expectation that increased access to and use of prenatal care will improve birth outcomes and reduce disparities has shaped national policy for nearly 2 decades (IOM, 1985); however, the effectiveness of prenatal care for the prevention of preterm birth has yet to be demonstrated conclusively (Alexander and Kotelchuck, 2001). A recent review concluded that the standard prenatal care provided today does little that could be expected to reduce preterm birth rates (Lu and Halfon, 2003), and the substantial increased use of early and adequate prenatal care over the past decade has not led to a significant decline in preterm birth rates for either African American or white women (CDC, 2005i). By using NCHS data for the 1998 to 2000 birth cohort, it was found that non-Hispanic African American women who initiated prenatal care in the first trimester or who had adequate prenatal care still experienced higher rates of preterm birth than non-Hispanic white women (Table 4-3).

TABLE 4-3 Preterm Birth Rates (percent) by Maternal Race-Ethnicity and Prenatal Care Use by Trimester of Initiation of Prenatal Care, 1998 to 2000

Trimester	Non-Hispanic African Americans	Non-Hispanic Whites	Asians-Pacific Islanders	American Indians	Hispanics
First	14.7	8.3	8.6	10.4	9.7
Second	17.5	10.2	10.8	12.7	11.0
Third	16.0	10.0	9.5	12.3	10.0
No prenatal care	33.4	21.7	19.4	24.0	19.8

SOURCE: NCHS data for U.S. birth cohorts from 1998 to 2000.

Over the past decade, two risk factors have emerged as promising explanations for the racial disparities in preterm birth rates: stress and infection. As reviewed in Chapter 3, a growing body of research suggests that maternal psychological stress is associated with an increased risk for preterm delivery. Insofar as African American women may experience more stress in their daily lives than white women, it has been suggested that maternal stress may contribute to the disparities in preterm birth rates between African American and white women (James, 1993). For example, Lu and Chen (2004) reported that African American women were significantly more likely to experience stressful life events (e.g., to lose a job or to become separated or divorced) just before or during pregnancy than non-Hispanic white women. As discussed in Chapter 3, African American women are also more likely to experience racism, which can be conceptualized as an additional source of stress (Krieger, 2000).

African American women are more likely than white women to experience a number of infections, including bacterial vaginosis and sexually transmitted infections (Fiscella, 1995; Meis et al., 2000). Insofar as these infections are associated with preterm delivery, they may be responsible for a significant portion of the racial disparities in preterm birth rates (Fiscella, 1995). However, the cause of this increased susceptibility to infections among pregnant African American women remains largely unknown, and to date antibiotic treatment of infections (other than for asymptomatic bacteriuria) during pregnancy has yielded modest or no benefits (Carey et al., 2000; McDonald et al., 2005) (see Chapter 9).

Genetic differences have often been invoked to account for racial disparities in a number of birth outcomes, including preterm birth. Although a woman's genetic makeup undoubtedly plays a role in the pathogenesis of preterm birth, the potential genetic contribution to racial disparities in preterm birth is unknown. First, it is not known which genes contribute to racial disparities in preterm birth rates. For example, interleukin-6 (IL-6), gamma interferon (IFN-γ), and tumor necrosis factor alpha (TNF-α) have all been implicated in the pathogenesis of preterm birth. Although several population-based studies have shown that African Americans are more likely than whites to carry genotypes that induce a high level of expression of IL-6 (Cox et al., 2001; Hassan et al., 2003; Hoffmann et al., 2002), the findings for IFN-γ and TNF-α are less consistent; in some studies the prevalence of individuals with genotypes that induce high levels of expression of these two proinflammatory cytokines was actually lower among African Americans than whites (Cox et al., 2001; Hassan et al., 2003; Hoffman et al., 2002). Second, it is not known how genes interact with the environment to produce racial disparities in preterm birth. Geneticists recognize that the causes of most common, complex diseases and conditions, including preterm birth, consist of a complicated interaction between genes and the environment (Macones et al., 2004; Wang et al., 2002). To date, few studies on preterm birth have untangled this interaction in the context of racial disparities (see Chapter 7). Third, it is not known why foreign-born and U.S.-born women of the same racial descent have such disparate rates of preterm birth, given their supposedly common genetic ancestry. The genetic contributions to racial-ethnic disparities in preterm birth are discussed in greater detail in Chapter 7.

In sum, significant racial-ethnic disparities in preterm birth rates exist in the United States. Racial differences in socioeconomic condition, maternal behaviors (including the use of prenatal care), stress, infection, and genetics cannot fully account for the disparities. More research, perhaps performed by the use of a more integrative approach (Lu and Halfon, 2003; Misra et al., 2003; NRC, 2001), is needed to address this persisting problem. As discussed in the introduction, the greatest difference in rates of preterm birth are between African American and Asian/Pacific Islander women. There could be something learned by understanding those differences as well as differences among Asian subgroups. Although the rates among African American women are strikingly high, they have been decreasing in recent years. In contrast, rates among other racial/ethnic groups have been increasing slightly. Examining these trends or differences may potentially help to shed light on racial and ethnic disparities.

Socioeconomic Condition

Disparities in preterm birth rates by socioeconomic condition have been well documented (Kramer et al., 2000) not only in the United States (Parker et al., 1994a but also in countries such as Canada (Wilkins et al., 1991), Sweden (Koupilova et al., 1998), Finland (Olsen et al., 1995b), Scotland (Sanjose et al., 1991), and Spain (Rodriguez et al., 1995), where the rates of poverty are generally lower than elsewhere in the world and women generally have universal access to high-quality prenatal and other medical care. Although the disparities in preterm birth rates by socioeconomic condition are often closely paralleled (and hence confounded) by disparities by racial and ethnic origin, there are notable exceptions. For example, despite their relative socioeconomic disadvantage, Mexican Americans have preterm birth rates comparable to those of non-Hispanic whites (Table 4-2) (CDC, 2005i).

The reasons for socioeconomic disparities in preterm birth rates are unclear and have been relatively unexplored. A number of factors have been implicated, including maternal nutrition, cigarette smoking, substance use or abuse, work and physical activity, prenatal care, genitourinary tract infection, sexually transmitted diseases, psychological factors, and multiple gestations. A general discussion of these risk factors as they relate to preterm birth is found in Chapters 3 and 5. Kramer and colleagues (2000) reviewed these factors as potential mediators of socioeconomic disparities in preterm birth, and that review is briefly summarized here.

Maternal nutritional status before and during pregnancy may contribute to the risk for preterm birth (WHO, 1995). Women with a low prepregnancy body mass index (BMI) are at increased risk for preterm birth. In the United States, however, BMIs are higher among women who are socioeconomically disadvantaged (Flegal et al., 1988); therefore, the prepregnancy BMI cannot account for socioeconomic disparities in preterm birth rates. Recent evidence suggests that maternal obesity before pregnancy is associated with an increased risk for indicated preterm delivery but with a decreased risk for spontaneous preterm delivery (Hendler et al., 2005); the contribution of maternal obesity to the disparities in preterm birth by socioeconomic condition is not clear. Low gestational weight gain is more common among socioeconomically disadvantaged women (Taffel, 1980); however, because of its modest association with preterm birth, low gestational weight gain is unlikely to be an important mediator of socioeconomic disparities in preterm birth rates (Carmichael and Abrams, 1997). Nutritional intake during pregnancy is generally poorer among socioeconomically disadvantaged women; however, given the weakness of the available evidence linking macro- and micronutrient intakes to preterm birth (Villar et al., 2003a,b), their role in explaining the socioeconomic disparities in preterm birth rates remains unclear.

In the United States, cigarette smoking is more prevalent and heavier among socioeconomically disadvantaged women, and as the adverse effects of smoking during pregnancy have become widely recognized by the general public, the socioeconomic gradient in the rates of cigarette smoking has widened. Cigarette smoking appears to explain some of the socioeconomic disparities in preterm birth, given its higher prevalence among socioeconomically disadvantaged women and its association with preterm birth (Kramer et al., 2000).

Although cocaine use is more common among socioeconomically disadvantaged women and is associated with preterm birth, it has a small etiological effect on preterm birth and thus is unlikely to be an important mediator. In poor, inner-city areas in the United States, however, the prevalence of cocaine use may be high, and in these settings, the mediating role of cocaine use is likely to be more important. Marijuana, alcohol, and narcotic use are also more common among socioeconomically disadvantaged women in the United States, although their independent effects on gestational duration are not clear (Kramer et al., 2000).

Work that is physically demanding, work that requires standing for prolonged periods, shift and night work, or work that creates high levels of cumulative fatigue has been associated with an increased risk for preterm birth (Mozuekewich et al., 2000); and socioeconomically disadvantaged women are more likely to have jobs with these characteristics. However, the etiological effect of these types of work on preterm birth is not known. Even less clear are the contributions of physically demanding work in the home (Pritchard and Teo, 1994) and the stress associated with unemployment or underemployment (Lu et al., 2005).

The rate of use of prenatal care is lower among socioeconomically disadvantaged women (CDC, 2005i); however, given the serious doubt about the effects of prenatal care on reducing the risk of preterm birth (Alexander and Kotelchuck, 2001; Lu and Halfon, 2003), prenatal care also seems to be an unlikely mediator of socioeconomic disparities in preterm birth rates.

Bacterial vaginosis is more common among socioeconomically disadvantaged women (Hillier et al., 1995; Meis et al., 1995). Given its association with preterm birth, it could be an important mediator of socioeconomic disparities in preterm birth rates. However, clinical trials of screening for and treatment of bacterial vaginosis have yielded conflicting results (Carey et al., 2000; McDonald et al., 2005) (see Chapter 9). The potential role of genitourinary *Chlamydia trachomatis* infection in spontaneous preterm birth has remained controversial, and studies of this and other sexually transmitted infections have generated conflicting results (Andrews et al., 2006).

Socioeconomically disadvantaged women experience more stressful life events and more chronic stress (Lu et al., 2005; Peacock et al., 1995). Poverty is associated with poor and crowded housing, living without a partner, unsatisfying marital relationships, violence from an intimate partner, and stressful working conditions. Unintended pregnancies are far more common among socioeconomically disadvantaged women. They also have less social support to limit the impacts of those stressors. Thus, psychosocial factors may prove an important mediator of socioeconomic disparities in preterm birth rates, but their etiologic links with preterm birth require further clarification.

Although socioeconomic differences in multiple gestations have not been well studied, Kramer and colleagues speculate that indirect evidence of increased multiple births attributable to infertility treatment among women in high socioeconomic groups, coupled with the growing contribution of multiple births to the overall incidence of preterm birth, will narrow socioeconomic disparities (Kramer et al., 2000).

Summary of Sociodemographic Factors

A number of maternal sociodemographic characteristics are associated with higher rates of preterm delivery. Specifically, maternal age (less than 16 years of age or 35 years of age or older), marital status (unmarried or cohabiting), race or ethnicity (African American or American Indian), and socioeconomic condition (low income or educational attainment) have been identified as risk factors for prematurity. Most of these sociodemographic factors are closely intertwined with behavioral risk factors, such as smoking and physical activity, and to psychosocial processes, such as stress, discrimination, and social support (see Chapter 3).

Finding 4-1: A particular focus of sociodemographic studies of preterm birth should be on disparities by race-ethnicity and socioeconomic condition, as significant differences in the rates of preterm birth by race-ethnicity and socioeconomic condition continue to exist in the United States. The causes of these persisting disparities remain largely unexplained

COMMUNITY FACTORS

In general, the risks for preterm birth have been individualized; that is, those characteristics of individuals that increase the likelihood of preterm delivery within groups rather than the environmental and social factors that affect the rates of preterm birth among the population as a whole (Goldenberg et al., 1998) are emphasized. However, as discussed in Chapter 3 and the previous section on sociodemographic factors, observational studies do not consistently demonstrate strong associations between the characteristics of the individual and the risk of preterm birth, nor do these individual-level characteristics explain the racial-ethnic differences in the rates of preterm birth.

Some scholars argue that the study of discrete risk factors has led to a rather narrow, static view of perinatal risk assessment (Konte et al., 1988; Main and Gabbe, 1987). In practice, individual risk factors tend to co-occur, resulting in dynamic interactive or synergistic processes that may reflect complex biological mechanisms (Casey and MacDonald, 1988; Challis, 1994; Olson et al., 1995; Petraglia et al., 1996; Romero et al., 1994). Such complex processes may render the contribution of a single risk factor somewhat meaningless. Furthermore, analytic problems arise when individual risk factors have different predictive powers for different populations (Geronimus, 1996; James, 1993; Kleinman and Kessel, 1987), making it difficult to make meaningful adjustments for confounders in studies involving multiple racial groups and resulting in potentially biased estimates of effect (Kaufman et al., 1997).

Several theories exist for the reasons that the identified risk factors do not adequately explain the racial-ethnic and social class disparities in rates of preterm birth. Among these is the idea that adverse social contexts, such as neighborhood conditions, may independently affect health or interact with individual-level characteristics to produce an increased risk of preterm birth. Against this backdrop, some researchers have redirected attention to consideration of the social determinants of reproductive health, calling for new approaches that go far beyond traditional medical risk assessment models and individual-level poverty-driven paradigms to include contextualized research (Holzman et al., 1998; Krieger et al., 1993; Link and Phelan, 1995; Rowley et al., 1993; Susser and Susser, 1996).

Adverse Neighborhood Conditions

The notion that adverse neighborhood conditions influence health outcomes through direct and indirect pathways has recently received increased attention (Robert, 1999). Evidence supporting the contributing role of neighborhood conditions is presented in this section. An important note is that the studies conducted thus far use birth weight as an outcome. A major need in future work is to examine gestational age as well. Neighborhood context may be a fruitful and salient avenue of exploration for explaining differences in preterm birth rates between African American and white women because of clear patterns of residential segregation that result in unequal exposures to adverse neighborhood conditions across racial-ethnic groups. Concentrated poverty and associated neighborhood disadvantages (including a lack of goods and services, health care facilities, and recreational opportunities; poor housing quality; and high crime rates) are more common features of African American neighborhoods than of white neighborhoods (Massey and Denton, 1993; Wilson, 1987). Residents of disadvantaged areas, in turn, not only are at a greater risk of physical injury but also are exposed to higher levels of everyday life stressors.

The social environment, service environment, and physical characteristics of a neighborhood have been hypothesized to affect the health of its residents (Konte et al., 1988). Social environment refers to the level of neighborhood cohesion or disorganization, norms of reciprocity, civic participation, crime, socioeconomic compositions, residential stability, and related attributes. These characteristics are thought to influence health outcomes through pathways such as the availability of social support, the adaptation of coping strategies, and exposure to chronic stress (Casey et al., 1988; Challis, 1994; Geronimus, 1996; Olson et al., 1995; Petraglia et al., 1996; Romero et al., 1994).

The service environment reflects the availability of goods and services, such as access to quality health care, grocery stores, recreational facilities, and police and fire protection. The availability of such services is likely to be affected by the degree of political organization influencing residents' ability to demand public services and recruit private service providers to their neighborhoods. Poor public and private services may have direct and indirect impacts on an individual's health by making residents more susceptible to intentional and unintentional injuries; by limiting access to quality health care, healthy foods, and recreational opportunities; and by increasing crime rates (Holzman et al., 1998; James, 1993; Kleinman and Kessel, 1987; Konte et al., 1988; Mercer et al., 1996). One study of the distribution of food stores found significantly fewer (three to four times) supermarkets in poor and African American communities than in more affluent white communities (Kramer, 1987a).

Finally, the quality of the physical environment and the quality of the housing stock and public space could also have direct effects on health (Main et al., 1987; Olson et al., 1995). Factors that affect the quality of the physical environment include toxicants, noise, and air pollution to which a pregnant woman may be exposed

The concentration of adverse neighborhood conditions along all three dimensions discussed above is often closely tied to the clustering of socioeconomic disadvantage. A number of studies have documented a significant association between neighborhood-level socioeconomic disadvantage and birth outcomes (Cramer, 1995; Kaufman et al., 1997; Krieger et al., 1993). Collins and David (1990) documented variations in the rates of low birth weight in Chicago, Illinois, in 1982 and 1983 among neighborhoods classified by the census-tract median family income. Their results show that in univariate comparisons, the risks of low birth weight for the infants of high-risk African American and white women (whose risk was assessed by measurement of age, level of educational attainment, and marital status) were more similar in poor neighborhoods than in more affluent areas. Low-risk white women had much lower rates of low birth weight than low-risk African American women, no matter where they lived. In a related study of an association between violent crime and low birth weight in Chicago's low-income neighborhoods, defined as census tracts with a median family income of less than $10,000, the same authors found a significant association between the risk of intrauterine growth retardation and the level of violent crime (Collins and David, 1997).

Using 1990 birth record data for Chicago linked to 1990 census data on community-level measures of socioeconomic condition, residential stability, the racial compositions of neighborhoods, and selected housing characteristics, Roberts (1997) modeled the incidence of low birth weight by including individual-level and community-level characteristics in a multivariate logistic regression analysis. The findings indicated that women living in economically disadvantaged communities were more likely to have a low birth weight baby than women living in better off neighborhoods, when individual characteristics available on the birth certificate were controlled for. Several counterintuitive findings were also noted. For example, the percentage of community residents who were African American was inversely associated with low birth weight, as was the rate of crowded housing units, when individual-level determinants and community-level economic status were controlled for. Racial differences in the rates of delivery of low-birth-weight infants remained substantial, however, with African American mothers being about twice as likely to deliver a low-birth-weight infant than white mothers, even after individual- and community-level factors were taken into account (Roberts, 1997, Table 2).

Nested data structures are common meaning that individuals operate within multiple realities such as the household, the neighborhood, the city or town, and the state. Another classic example of nested date derives from the educational world with students, within classrooms, within schools, within neighborhoods, etc. Following the educational example, we can assume that the students within a certain class share common characteristics such as the teacher and the physical surroundings and therefore they are not independent. In other words, students within a specific class are more alike than a random sample of students drawn from the larger population. Given that many statistical techniques require that observations are independent, nested data poses challenges. Until recently nested data would have to be aggregated or disaggregated prior to analyses so that only one level of the data was being assessed (e.g., students, or classrooms or schools but not students, classrooms, and schools). Now, however, nested data can be analyzed using hierarchical linear models or multilevel models. Multilevel models permit the simultaneous assessment of the association between nested data and an outcome of interest.

O'Campo and colleagues (1997) were among the first scientists to use multilevel models to investigate the effects of maternal characteristics and neighborhood conditions on the risk of low birth weight in Baltimore, Maryland, using data recovered from 1985 to 1989 in a multilevel framework. Controlling for individual-level characteristics, which included maternal age, education, prenatal care use, and health insurance coverage, the authors found that women living in census tracts with per-capita incomes of less than $8,000 had a significantly higher risk of delivering an infant of low birth weight than women who lived in higher-income census tracts. They also found a number of significant interactions between neighborhood-level variables and individual-level risk factors for low birth weight. The protective effects of prenatal care, for example, were less strong in neighborhoods with high levels of unemployment, and the elevated risk of low birth weight among women with low levels of schooling was stronger in tracts with higher crime rates. They did not investigate whether these effects varied by race or whether the contextual and individual-level variables explained racial differences in low birth weight.

Pearl and colleagues (2001) conducted a multilevel analysis of the impact of socioeconomic status (SES) on birthweight. SES was measured at the individual level as maternal education, Medi-Cal coverage during pregnancy, and family income. Neighborhood SES was measured by dividing the sample into census tracts and blocks, in which they selected poverty, unemployment, and education as specific SES indicators. Latinas and Asian women were subdivided into U.S. and foreign born. Findings suggest that neighborhood SES was unrelated to the birth weights of children born to white women and U.S.-born Latinas, whereas it was related to a decrease in birth weight among blacks and Asians. Furthermore, foreign-born Latinas living in neighborhoods with high unemployment and poverty delivered infants of higher birth weights and had a lower risk of delivering a low birth weight infant. These findings suggest that both individual and neighborhood level pathways are important, as well as their interactions with ethnicity and nativity.

Elo and colleagues (2001) analyzed linked birth and infant death records in Philadelphia, Pennsylvania, to investigate the effects of individual- and contextual-level variables on birth weight (in grams) and the risk of low birth weight using both fixed-effects and random-effects models. The authors also tested whether their results were sensitive to the level of neighborhood aggregation used; that is, block groups, census tracts, or larger neighborhood aggregations. Using fixed-effects models, the authors found that about a third of the racial difference in birth weight and the risk of low birth weight was explained by the neighborhood context and the characteristics shared by women living in the same neighborhood. The difference was further narrowed when the individual-level characteristics of the women and their births were controlled for. The reduction in the racial difference was greater when neighborhoods were conceptualized as block groups and was somewhat less pronounced when neighborhoods were defined as larger aggregates. The fact that the neighborhood context explained a part of the racial difference in birth weights points to the importance of including neighborhood characteristics in models of birth outcomes. Of the neighborhood-level characteristics examined (income, poverty, education, occupation, health status, household composition, migration, housing, crime, and homelessness), indicators of neighborhood economic deprivation and crime were the most consistently associated with birth weight and the risk of low birth weight.

Research in perinatal health demonstrates modest but consistent effects of neighborhood-level socioeconomic disparities in key pregnancy outcomes (Geronimus, 1996; James, 1993; Kleinman and Kessel, 1987). Low birth weights have been associated with a variety of neighborhood-level socioeconomic variables, including poverty (Cramer, 1995; Geronimus, 1992; Kaufman et al., 1997), unemployment (Geronimus, 1992), education and income (Geronimus, 1992; Kaufman et al., 1997; Krieger et al., 1993), and median rent (Kaufman et al., 1997). In addition to single-variable associations, neighborhood indices representing aspects of economic disadvantage have also been associated with low birth weight. For example, Buka and colleagues (2003) created an index measure of neighborhood economic disadvantage using, among other variables, the percentages of individuals in a neighborhood living below the poverty level according to 1990 census data, receiving public assistance, and being unemployed and found the index to be significantly associated with birth weight. Krieger and colleagues (2003) used multiple indices to assess area-level effects on low birth weight and child lead poisoning, with tract and block group measures of economic deprivation observed to have the strongest effects on low birth weight (odds ratio > 2.0). Although research results have consistently confirmed the effects of neighborhood deprivation on adverse birth outcomes, these findings can be difficult to interpret and compare, owing to the variety of indicators used to measure neighborhood-level deprivation.

Although most studies have documented an association between neighborhood context and health outcomes, whether they are for adults or infants, additional research is needed to more fully specify and test these associations. Future work needs to (1) focus on how best to define context, e.g., whether the context should be administrative or political units or some alternative specifications of neighborhood boundaries; (2) include contextual variables defined at various levels of aggregation on the basis of theoretical considerations, e.g., crime at the block group or smaller levels of aggregation versus service availability at tract or larger levels of aggregation; (3) integrate adequate individual-level information to ensure that neighborhood variables do not reflect individual-level differences; (4) test interactions across levels; and (5) explore various analytical techniques to model the effects of space on health outcomes. In addition, as discussed above, most studies have used birth weight as an outcome, thus confounding with small for gestational age (see Chapter 2). Studies should also use gestational age to investigate prematurity. There are likely different mediators, moderators, and pathways to preterm birth than there are to low birth weight. Using preterm birth as a discrete outcome may not reveal effects. Gestational age should be studied as a continuous variable.

Regardless of how neighborhood-level characteristics are measured, multilevel research has helped to draw attention to the role of social structures in health, particularly with respect to the problem of persistent health disparities. However, as recently reviewed by Oakes (2004), very few such studies have attended to the question of causal inference or recognized that neighborhood effects may not be truly independent effects. Oakes suggests that future multilevel studies make use of social experimental designs to provide a better understanding of the underlying causal processes and to use this understanding to design interventions that more effectively reduce risk and improve public health. Specifically, Oakes suggests that the benefits of studying the independent effect of neighborhood conditions on health are really only realizable through the design, implementation, and rigorous evaluation of randomized clinical trials where a "community-level" treatment is delivered to a randomly selected set of communities. As examples, Oakes suggests community interventions that alter norms with mass media public health messages, change local policies, add green space or clean existing parks, repair sidewalks, or institute community policing strategies. However, Oakes cautions that these types of interventions are very expensive, are hard to evaluate given the long latency between exposure and disease and, most significantly, are hard to design given our limitations in theories linking neighborhoods to health. Given the complex relationships between health and social conditions, this type of methodology might be very productively applied in the field of perinatal epidemiology.

Interaction Between Neighborhood- and Individual-Level Characteristics

Neighborhood-level characteristics may indirectly exert their influence on reproductive outcomes by patterning individual-level economic opportunities and health behaviors. For example, the neighborhood-level opportunity structure may restrict or facilitate access to schooling, training programs, and employment opportunities and thus influence reproductive outcomes through the socioeconomic condition that a woman has attained (Anderson et al., 1996; Konte et al., 1988). Thus, disparities in birth outcomes according to a woman's socioeconomic condition may originate in part from the neighborhood context that shape an individual's life chances.

Furthermore, the social characteristics of neighborhoods, perhaps through shared cultural norms and values, may well influence health behaviors that are linked to reproductive outcomes. For example, individual-level smoking patterns (Cubbin et al., 2000; Diez-Roux et al., 1997), alcohol consumption, and dietary practices (Macintyre et al., 2002; Shepard, 1994; Taylor and Repetti, 1997; Yen and Kaplan, 1999; Yen and Syme, 1999), which seem particularly relevant to this discussion, have been significantly associated with area-level deprivation when individual attributes are controlled for. In addition to health behaviors, adverse conditions such as high crime rates, housing abandonment, and even noise pollution may act as either acute or chronic stressors that exert their influences through stress physiology and are thus potential intervening mechanisms between neighborhood context and reproductive health. Geronimus (1996), for example, has argued that long-term exposure to socioeconomic disadvantage, including residence in socioeconomically disadvantaged neighborhoods, is detrimental to maternal reproductive health and is one of the factors that contributes to more adverse birth outcomes among African American women (O'Campo et al., 1997).

Finally, neighborhood context and individual-level characteristics may interact such that individual-level characteristics may exert a greater influence in certain neighborhoods or such that the effects of the neighborhood context are more pronounced for subgroups of women stratified by socioeconomic condition, race-ethnicity, or other individual attributes. For example, a recent study in Chicago found that high perceived levels of neighborhood support were positively associated with birth weight only for white infants. A significant negative association between birth weight and neighborhood-level economic disadvantage was documented for African American infants (Buka et al., 2003). This association remained significant even after adjustment for maternal characteristics and other neighborhood conditions (Casey and McDonald, 1988). O'Campo and colleagues (1997) found that the early initiation of prenatal care did not have the same beneficial effect for women living in disadvantaged neighborhoods in Baltimore, raising the possibility that prenatal care in deprived settings is unable to address various risks associated with adverse birth outcomes (Holzman et al., 1998; Kaufman et al., 1997). Evidence also suggests that prenatal care has no effect on preterm birth (see Chapter 9 for a discussion).

Effect modification in multilevel models also occurs. This type of effect modification is perhaps most difficult to conceptualize and test because it implies a kind of cross-level effect by which individual-level effects are moderated by community-level conditions. This would mean, for example, that the effect of cigarette smoking on an individual's risk of preterm birth would depend on some attribute of the community in which that individual resides. This effect modification would not be explained by interactions with other individual-level psychological or social exposures. In a study of community characteristics and child maltreatment, The Project on Human Development in Chicago Neighborhoods found that neighborhood social networks interacted with Hispanic ethnicity to affect the amount of physical abuse committed by individual families (Molnar et al., 2003). The authors interpreted this finding to make the point that neighborhood-level interventions may be the most effective way to reduce rates of the child abuse in certain populations. Such findings suggest that studies that examine factors at only one level (either the individual level only or the ecological level only) may underestimate the effects of the social environment and potentially miss an opportunity to use interventions to the reduce risk associated with any particular factor.

Biological Mechanisms

Exposure to acute and chronic stress is one of the hypothesized pathways through which neighborhood context may affect birth outcomes. At the individual level, a growing body of empirical evidence, based on methodologically rigorous studies of pregnant women of different racial-ethnic, socioeconomic, and cultural backgrounds, supports the premise that mothers experiencing high levels of psychological or social stress during pregnancy are at significantly increased risk for preterm birth (relative risk = 1.5 to 2.0), even after adjustment for other biomedical, sociodemographic, and behavioral risk factors (Pearl et al., 2001; Rauh and Culhane, 2001). In addition, adverse neighborhood conditions, such as crime, homelessness, and tax delinquency, were significantly associated with the risk of urogenital tract infection, one of the leading causes of preterm birth (Collins and David, 1997; Roberts, 1997), during pregnancy, even after adjustment for individual-level risk factors (Elo et al., 2001).

Stress both at the individual level and at the neighborhood level may affect preterm birth through physiological pathways (see Chapter 6 for a discussion). The plausibility of the influences of the direct neuroendocrine and the neuroendocrine-immune interaction pathways suggests that stressful exposures may have physiological consequences over and above their possible influences on health-related behaviors. As evidence accumulates that individual-level stressful exposures can become annoying ("get under the skin"), it is not hard to imagine that dangerous and rundown neighborhoods may exert a similar effect. It is therefore possible that neighborhoods can influence health outcomes through direct physiological dysregulation.

Methodological Issues in Modeling Social Context

The inclusion of social conditions in models of cumulative risk depends on the ability to validly measure the various components of social context at appropriate scales of influence. In their simplest form, multilevel studies typically include assessments at the individual and community levels by the use of some standard administrative unit to define community (e.g., health area, zip code, census tract, or block). For example, exposure to poverty or substandard housing may be measured at the individual level (personal income, number of homeless episodes, etc.) and the community level (average income in the census tract, amount of concentrated poverty, proportion of imminently dangerous buildings, etc.).

Advances in statistical analysis techniques that facilitate the modeling of multilevel influences and the growing interest in the use of geographic information systems have made analyses of community- and regional-level variations more feasible (Bellinger, 2004; Diez-Roux, 1999; Kawachi, 2000; Link and Phelan, 1995). A recent review of articles published before 1998 of the effects of local-area social characteristics on various individual health outcomes in developed countries found that all but 2 of the 25 studies reviewed reported a statistically significant association between at least one measure of the social environment and a health outcome, after adjustment for individual-level socioeconomic condition, despite heterogeneity in study designs, substitution of local-area measures for neighborhood-level measures, and probable measurement error (Diez-Roux et al., 2003). Although multilevel studies in environmental health science are still relatively rare compared with individual- or ecological-level investigations, the results of these studies nevertheless point to the potential importance of residential context on health.

Multilevel analysis has the capacity to simultaneously assess the effects of individual- and group-level exposures on individual outcomes (Cassel, 1976). Such studies can address the question of whether local-area characteristics have a measurable effect on outcome over and above individual exposures or whether the apparent associations between aggregate measures and outcomes simply reflect the individual-level characteristics of area residents. For example, does the mean income level in some defined community have an effect on the outcome for an individual beyond the effect of the individual's income, and is the contextual effect independent of a given individual's income (Von Korff et al., 1992)? If individual and contextual factors both influence outcomes, then models that exclude one or the other set of risk factors are likely to be poorly specified and lead to misinterpretation of the effects of both individual- and contextual-level factors.

At the ecological level, the high correlation among various community characteristics poses problems in estimating the effects of distinct community characteristics. One way to get around this problem is to develop indices of related community-level constructs, but such indices may obscure the roles of their distinct components. For example, this approach could underestimate the association between a chemical exposure of interest and a neurobehavioral outcome, if part of the chemical effect is carried by the association between the community quality index and the neurobehavior. Bellinger (2004) suggests the use of more differentiated measures of complex social constructs to control for only those aspects of community quality that do not reflect exposure opportunities.

Despite progress in this area, problems persist with respect to the conceptualization of and the distinctions between micro- and macrolevel social phenomena. Link and Phelan (1995) have proposed the notion of "fundamental social causes" of disease to explain how resources (such as knowledge, power, money, prestige, and social connections) are linked to disease outcomes through multiple (often shifting) risk-factor mechanisms. The notion is that inequalities in health are a function of persistent social inequalities, regardless of the intervening individual-level exposures, many of which can be shown to vary over time. To date, few studies have managed to successfully differentiate macrolevel from microlevel factors, especially with respect to statistical analysis (Diez-Roux, 1999). So-called mixed models and multilevel approaches are now being used in epidemiological studies, but further refinement is needed. In fact, it seems obvious that the classification of "levels" into two or even three categories of influence is somewhat crude, because the definition of the higher-level units and the borders between the various levels are frequently unclear.

CONCLUSION

The overall high rate of preterm birth in the United States and the persistent racial-ethnic gap is one of the most significant public health problems today. Despite many years of observational and clinical research, the exposures that place women at risk are not well understood. The substantial intergroup as well as intragroup variabilities in the risk of preterm birth have been shown to be related related to socioeconomic condition, nativity, acculturation, or other maternal characteristics. Although future research should continue to focus on factors that contribute to the high rates of preterm births among African American infants, much can be learned from examinations of racial-ethnic disparities outside the context of the disparities between African American versus white women, as well as disparities within a particular racial or ethnic group. Common measures of socioeconomic status (e.g., income and education) and other potential mediators may not fully capture the magnitude of group differences. For example, the median income of African American families is about 64 percent of the median income of white families, but the median net worth of African American families is only 12 percent of that of white families (Mishel and Bernstein, 2003).

Similarly, a list of stressful life events cannot adequately measure the multiple dimensions of stress, including acute and chronic stressors, stress appraisal, and the environmental (including social and cultural) contexts of stress. For example, racial discrimination disproportionately affects women of color and is associated with preterm birth, yet it often goes unmeasured in studies linking stress to preterm birth. Thus, better measures (both for "exposures," such as socioeconomic condition and race, and for potential "mediators," such as stress) are needed in research on these disparities.

The paradox of favorable birth outcomes, despite social disadvantages, among some immigrant groups and the increased rates of preterm birth with increasing length of residence in the United States have been attributed, in part, to the loss of resiliency factors with increasing acculturation. This suggests that research on disparities in the rates of preterm birth needs to pay more attention to protective factors (which include such factors as personal resources, social support, and spirituality).

Current research into the causes of the disparities commonly attempts to isolate the effect of a single risk factor, without accounting for the co-occurrence and potential interactions among multiple protective and risk factors (e.g., age and race or education and race) operating at multiple levels and across the life course to produce disparities in the rates of preterm birth. A more integrative approach to understanding racial-ethnic and socioeconomic disparities in the rates of preterm birth is needed (Lu and Halfon, 2003; Misra et al., 2003). Future research on disparities should aim for longitudinal integration linking a woman's life history to her vulnerability for preterm delivery, as well as contextual integration linking individual biology and behaviors to the multilevel, multiple determinants of preterm birth.

Although some individual-level risk factors hold modest associations with a risk of preterm birth, individual-level characteristics do not adequately explain the high rate of preterm birth in the United States or the racial-ethnic differences in the rates of preterm birth. The notion that community-level conditions can produce profound effects on disease susceptibility is long-standing (Cassel, 1976). The questions, however, of whether community-level adversity has a deleterious impact on fetal outcomes, independent of individual-level risk factors, and whether the predictive power of these individual-level factors depends on community-level conditions have only recently been subjected to empirical testing. Numerous reports now show, however, that after adjustment for individual-level attributes, neighborhood conditions are in fact independently and significantly associated with a risk of delivering an infant with a low birth weight. Thus, because exposures to adverse neighborhood conditions are much more common for African American women than for their white counterparts, entire groups of women experience distress. There is also a need to examine the relationship between gestational age and adverse neighborhood conditions.

Exploring the social contribution to this important health outcome may contribute to an understanding of the racial-ethnic differential and provide new avenues for remedial strategies to decreasing the rates of preterm birth that move past the narrow biomedical approach. In addition, it is important to give equal consideration to the concept that social conditions are in fact fundamental causes of diseases and syndromes like preterm birth (Link and Phelen, 1995).

Finding 4-2: Independent of the individual-level attributes that are risk factors for preterm birth, adverse neighborhood conditions such as poverty and crime are risk factors for preterm birth. These data suggest that intervention strategies may need to expand from focusing exclusively on the individual to including the contributions of social structural factors to the risk of preterm birth.

5

Medical and Pregnancy Conditions Associated with Preterm Birth

ABSTRACT

A number of maternal medical conditions are associated with an increased risk of indicated or spontaneous preterm birth, including, for example, chronic hypertension, prepregnancy diabetes mellitus, and systemic lupus erythematosus. Maternal illnesses can alter or limit the placental delivery of oxygen and nutrients to the developing fetus, possibly resulting in fetal growth restriction. In addition, they can increase the risk of preeclampsia and, thus, the risk of indicated preterm birth. Therefore, acute maternal medical conditions might lead to preterm birth. Other risk factors for preterm birth are underweight and obesity. A family history of preterm birth can also be an indicator of higher risk, as can a short interpregnancy interval. Finally, the number of American women using assisted reproductive technologies to achieve pregnancies has increased, and the use of such technologies is associated with multiple gestations and the increased risk for preterm delivery. The existence of any of these risk factors for preterm birth provides a focus for understanding their causative effects and developing interventions.

A number of maternal illnesses, conditions, and medical treatments are associated with indicated or spontaneous preterm birth. Spontaneous preterm birth naturally occurs as a result of preterm labor or preterm premature rupture of fetal membranes. In contrast, indicated preterm occurs when labor is initiated by medical intervention because of dangerous pregnancy complications. This chapter discusses several medical illnesses and conditions, such as low prepregnancy weight, obesity, a family history of spontaneous preterm birth, and short interpregnancy interval, and their relationships to preterm birth. The chapter also provides an overview of infertility treatments and the resulting risk of multiple gestations, which place women at a greater risk for preterm delivery.

MEDICAL ILLNESSES AND CONDITIONS

Indicated preterm birth appears to share a number of risk factors with spontaneous preterm birth. In a cohort of more than 2,900 pregnant women, Meis and colleagues (1998) noted a relation between indicated preterm birth and müllerian duct abnormality (OR 7.02; 95% CI 1.69–29.15, proteinuria at less than 24 weeks of gestation (OR 5.85; 95% CI 2.66–12.89), a history of chronic hypertension (OR 4.06; 95% CI 2.29–7.55), a history of indicated preterm birth (OR 2.79; 95% CI 1.45–5.40), a history of lung disease (OR 2.52; 95% CI 1.32–4.80), previous spontaneous preterm birth (OR 2.45; 95% CI 1.55–3.89), age greater than 30 years (OR 2.42; 95% CI 1.57–3.74), being African American (OR 1.56; 95% CI 1.02–2.40), and working during pregnancy (OR 1.49; 95% CI 1.02–2.19). With the possibility of a significant heterogeneity of risk factors and etiologic overlap, studies of preterm birth should consider indicated and spontaneous preterm births both together and separately as outcomes of interest (Savitz et al., 2005).

A number of maternal medical conditions are associated with an increased risk of indicated preterm birth (Table 5-1). Maternal medical ill-

TABLE 5-1 Examples of Maternal Medical
Problems That May Lead to Indicated Preterm Birth

Chronic hypertension
Systemic lupus erythematosus
Restrictive lung disease
Hyperthyroidism
Pregestational diabetes mellitus
Maternal cardiac disease
Asthma
Gestational diabetes mellitus
Pregestational renal disorders
Hypertensive disorders of pregnancy

nesses such as chronic hypertension, prepregnancy diabetes mellitus, or systemic lupus erythematosus can alter or limit the placental delivery of oxygen and nutrients to the developing fetus, possibly resulting in fetal growth restriction. These same maternal medical illnesses also increase the risk of preeclampsia and, thus, the risk of indicated preterm birth. The mechanism(s) that place a woman at increased risk for preeclampsia are unknown. Acute maternal medical conditions may also result in preterm birth. For example, severe trauma and shock are acute conditions that could create a nonreassuring fetal status or placental abruption and thus lead to indicated preterm birth. The progressive course of some medical illnesses could mandate indicated preterm birth to preserve the health and well-being of the mother. Functional or structural maternal cardiac disease is an example of one such illness. Fetal conditions, such as red cell allo-immunization or a twin-to-twin transfusion sequence, might also progress to require indicated preterm birth in an effort to prevent stillbirth.

There is some evidence for a relationship between birth defects and preterm birth. Rasmussen and colleagues (2001) examined more than 250,000 infants with known gestational ages born between 1989 and 1995 in the Atlanta, Georgia, metropolitan area. Infants born at less than 37 weeks of gestation were more than twice as likely to have a range of birth defects than infants born at term, between 37 and 41 weeks of gestation (RR 2.43; 95% CI 2.30–2.56). The risk of preterm birth in infants with birth defects was 21.5 percent, whereas it was 9.3 percent in infants without birth defects. The relationship between preterm birth and birth defects was also analyzed by smaller gestational age categories (20 to 28 weeks, 29 to 32 weeks, 33 to 34 weeks, and 35 to 36 weeks). Compared to infants born at term, the risk of preterm birth was the highest for those born at between 29 and 32 weeks of gestation (RR 3.37; 95% CI 3.04–3.73). Similar results were found when the analysis was stratified by maternal age, race, and the infant's gender. Data were not specifically provided on the proportion of births that were spontaneous versus indicated. However, the authors note that while some deliveries of babies with birth defects may have been indicated it is unlikely that these deliveries would have performed among infants in the 29 to 32 week gestational age category, unless survival of the fetus was not anticipated. In another study of 2,761 infants born alive with spina bifida between 1995 and 2001 in selected states, approximately 22 percent were born preterm and accounted for more than half of the deaths of infants with spina bifida (Bol, 2006).

In analyses provided to the Committee from the Utah Birth Defects Prevention Network, between 1999 and 2004, about 20 percent of the infants born alive with birth defects in the state of Utah were born preterm. These results are consistent with those reported by Rasmussen et al. (2001) and Bol et al. (2006). It may be that some birth defects increase the risk for preterm birth, that some sociodemographic factors that are associated with preterm birth are also associated with some birth defects, or that the two conditions may share other maternal risk factors or medical conditions (Rasmussen et al., 2001). Further investigation is needed to understand this association.

Underweight and Spontaneous Preterm Birth

Low maternal prepregnancy weight and body mass index (BMI) have consistently been associated with preterm birth. After adjusting for confounders (previous preterm labor, previous low birth weight, standing at work >2 hours, abruptio placentae, urinary tract infection and stress score >5), Moutquin (2003) noted that women with BMIs of less than 20 were nearly four times as likely as heavier women to have a spontaneous preterm birth (OR 3.96; 95% CI 2.61–7.09). Indeed, the relationship between low prepregnancy BMI and spontaneous preterm birth is consistent (OR 1.7–3.9) among North American caucasians (Moutquin, 2003), blacks (Johnson et al., 1994), and urban Latinas (Siega-Riz et al., 1994, 1996).

A low BMI also modifies the contribution of low pregnancy weight gain to the risk of preterm birth (Schieve et al., 2000). Compared with normal-weight women (BMI 19.8–26.0) with adequate weight gain during pregnancy (0.5–1.5 kg/week), the risk of spontaneous preterm birth at less than 37 weeks of gestation is sixfold greater for underweight women (BMI < 19.8) with poor pregnancy weight gain (< 0.5 kg/week) and threefold greater for normal-weight women with poor pregnancy weight gain.

A randomized trial of treatment for bacterial vaginosis (BV) examined the incidence of preterm delivery in at-risk women, including those who were underweight (Hauth et al., 1995). Women who had a previous spontaneous preterm birth or a prepregnancy weight of less than 50 kilograms (N = 624) were randomly assigned to metronidazole and erythromycin antibiotic therapy or placebo. Among the 258 women with BV, a lower rate of preterm delivery in those assigned to the treatment group was observed for women who weighed less than 50 kilograms (N = 81). The incidence of preterm birth was 33 percent in the placebo group and 14 percent in the antibiotic-treated group (p = 0.04). This is in contrast to the findings of several investigators who demonstrated that treatment of BV in a general obstetric population is ineffective (Carey et al., 2000).

Obesity and Spontaneous Preterm Birth

In a cohort of more than 70 percent white women, Sebire and colleagues (2001) noted a decreased frequency of delivery at less than 32 weeks of gestation among women with BMIs greater than or equal to 30 (OR

0.73; 95% CI 0.65–0.82) compared with that among women with BMIs less than 30. Those investigators did not differentiate spontaneous from indicated preterm birth.

In a recent secondary analysis from the National Institute of Child Health and Human Development MFM Units Network Preterm Prediction study, in which 65 percent of the sample was African American, Hendler and colleagues (2005) found a decreased odds of spontaneous preterm birth at less than 37 weeks of gestation among women with prepregnancy BMIs greater than or equal to 30 (OR 0.57; 95% CI 0.39–0.83) compared with that among women with BMIs less than 30.

Even though obesity is detrimental for numerous aspects of human health and disease, high BMIs are associated with better outcomes of both congestive heart failure and atherosclerotic heart disease among people with chronic renal disease (Beddhu, 2004; Kalantar-Zadeh et al., 2004). It has been hypothesized that these epidemiological paradoxes may be the result of obesity-related changes in systemic inflammation (Beddhu, 2004; Kalantar-Zadeh et al., 2004).

Family History and Spontaneous Preterm Birth

Several observations support the hypothesis that spontaneous preterm birth is influenced by a family history of preterm birth. First, evidence from two studies performed with twins suggests a genetic predisposition for preterm birth with estimates of the proportion of preterm births among women with a family history of preterm birth ranging from 20 to 40 percent (Blackmore-Prince et al., 2000; Fuentes-Afflick and Hessol, 2000). Other observations support the idea that genetic factors affect the risk of preterm birth: (1) the leading risk factor for preterm birth is a previous preterm birth (James et al., 1999; Klerman et al., 1998; Shults et al., 1999); (2) an association between race-ethnicity and preterm birth persists in some instances, even if it is corrected for socioeconomic condition (Ekwo and Moawad, 1998); and (3) mothers who were preterm themselves (Basso et al., 1998) or who have a sister who had delivered an infant preterm (Kallan, 1997) have an increased risk of delivering their infants preterm.

Short Interpregnancy Interval and Preterm Birth

Interpregnancy interval is defined as that interval between the termination of one pregnancy and the conception of another. Numerous investigators have found a univariate association between short interpregnancy interval and a number of adverse perinatal outcomes, including preterm birth, low birth weight, and stillbirth (Adams et al., 1997; Al-Jasmi et al., 2002; Basso et al., 1998; Blackmore-Prince et al., 2000; Brody and Bracken, 1987; Conde-Agudelo et al., 2005; Dafopoulos et al., 2002; Ekwo and Moawad,

1998; Erickson and Bjerkedal, 1978; Ferraz et al., 1988; Fuentes-Afflick and Hessol, 2000; Hsieh et al., 2005; Kallan, 1992, 1997; Klebanoff, 1988; Lang et al., 1990; Miller, 1994; Rawlings et al., 1995; Shults et al., 1999; Smith et al., 2003; Zhu and Le, 2003; Zhu et al., 2001). These published reports did not distinguish spontaneous from indicated preterm birth, however. The definition of short interpregnancy interval varies widely across studies; the most common definition is less than or equal to 6 months.

Impacts of Ethnicity and Geography

The relationships between short interpregnancy interval and preterm birth, low birth weight, and small-for-gestational age birth have been noted to be similar in magnitude and significance for African American and white women (James et al., 1999; Kallan, 1992, 1997; Zhu et al., 2001). Most studies have found that the prevalence of short interpregnancy intervals is higher among African American women than white women (James et al., 1999; Kallan, 1992, 1997; Zhu et al., 2001), but others have not found such a higher prevalence (Kallan, 1992; Klerman et al., 1998). International studies have shown that a short interpregnancy interval has been associated with preterm birth in rural Greece, the Philippines, the United Arab Emirates, and Latin America (Blackmore-Prince et al., 2000; Conde-Agudelo et al., 2005; Lang et al., 1990; Zhu et al., 2001).

Magnitude of Effect

The magnitude of the increased risk for preterm birth with an interpregnancy interval of less than 6 months is estimated to be 30 to 60 percent (Kallan, 1997). A single report has suggested that the magnitude and the significance of a short interpregnancy interval are the greatest when the index pregnancy was a preterm birth rather than a term birth (Hsieh et al., 2005).

Role for Intervention

Klebanoff (1988) notes that a short interpregnancy interval is primarily a marker for a woman who is otherwise at high risk of delivering her infant preterm and that modification of that interval alone may be unlikely to have a major impact on low birth weight. Other investigators also support the notion that a short interpregnancy interval may function as a marker of other risk factors rather than exerting an independent effect on preterm birth (Brody and Braken, 1987; Erickson and Bjerkedal, 1978). This concept may be extended to the impact of a short interpregnancy interval on low birth weight. In a Brazilian study, the effect of a short interpregnancy interval on low birth weight was explained by an increased prevalence of underweight among women with short interpregnancy intervals (Ferraz et al., 1988). In the general obstetric population at low risk for adverse pregnancy outcomes, Adams et al. (1997) found that short interpregnancy intervals are rare and are weak risk factors among low-risk women, and thus, efforts to lengthen interpregnancy intervals are unlikely to reduce substantially the rates of adverse pregnancy outcomes among these women. Smith et al. (2003) estimated the attributable risk fractions of a short interpregnancy interval of less than 6 months to preterm birth at 24 to 32 weeks and 33 to 36 weeks of gestation to be 6 and 4 percent, respectively. In a largely African American cohort of women, Blackmore-Prince et al. (2000) found that the median interpregnancy interval was 15 months (range, 1 to 207 months), with 19 (4 percent) of the women having interpregnancy intervals of less than 3 months. After adjustment for parity, gestational age (in weeks), and smoking status, the mean birth weight associated with an interpregnancy interval of 3 or more months was 3,106 grams, 215 grams greater than that for an interpregnancy interval of less than 3 months ($p = 0.06$).

INFERTILITY TREATMENTS AND PRETERM BIRTH

Infertility treatments have allowed thousands of couples who have difficulty conceiving to fulfill their desire to have children. In the United States in 2002, 7.3 million women, or 12 percent of women ages 15 to 44, had physical difficulty becoming pregnant or carrying a baby to term. Approximately 2.1 million of these women, or 7 percent of all women between the ages of 15 and 44, were infertile, defined as not becoming pregnant after 12 months when the couple is not using contraception (CDC, 2002b). Two percent of women had had an infertility-related medical appointment within the previous year, and an additional 10 percent reported that they had received services for infertility at some point in their lives.

The use of infertility treatments has risen dramatically in the past 20 years and has been associated with the trend to delay childbearing (see Chapter 1). In 2002, 33,000 American women delivered babies as a result of the use of infertility procedures; this is more than twice the number who had done so in 1996 (Meis et al., 1998). More than 50 percent of these women were 35 years of age or older. In recent years, an unintended consequence of the use of these technologies, multiple gestations and the increased risk for preterm delivery, has become a focus of attention. There is also evidence that a portion of the reported association between infertility treatments and preterm birth may be attributable to the underlying biological reasons for infertility and subfecundity (long time to becoming pregnant) (Basso and Baird, 2003; Henriksen et al, 1997; Joffe and Li, 1994).

Henriksen and colleagues (1997) examined pregnancy outcomes for two cohorts of approximately 13,000 deliveries in Denmark. The analyses excluded women with chronic illness, multiple fetuses, and unplanned pregnancies. Compared to women who took 6 or less months to conceive before becoming pregnant, women who tried for 7 to 12 months to conceive had a higher adjusted risk (1.3 times) for preterm delivery (95% CI .8–2.1) in both cohorts. Those who tried for 12 months or longer had an adjusted risk of 1.6 (95% CI 1.1–2.2) in the first cohort and 1.7 in the second (95% CI 1.1–2.6). Results held after controlling for infertility treatments.

This section provides an overview of infertility treatments, including Assisted Reproductive Technologies (ARTs) and ovulation promotion procedures, trends in their use and the resulting pregnancies, maternal and child outcomes, and current regulations on the use of these treatments.

Types of ART-Related Treatments and Incidence of Pregnancies Conceived by Use of ART

The Centers for Disease Control and Prevention (CDC) defines ARTs as procedures in which the egg and the sperm are handled in the laboratory, including in vitro fertilization (IVF) as well as related procedures, such as intracytoplasmic sperm injection (ICSI) and gamete intrafallopian transfer (GIFT) or zygote intrafallopian transfer (ZIFT) (Table 5-2). Since 1996, the federal government has mandated that all clinics performing procedures involving ARTs report their outcomes to the CDC (Meis et al., 1998).

TABLE 5-2 Procedures Involving ARTs Defined by the CDC

Treatment	Procedure
In vitro fertilization (IVF)	Extraction of the woman's eggs, fertilization of the eggs in the laboratory, and transfer of the resulting embryos into the woman's uterus; may include intracytoplasmic sperm injection (ICSI), in which a single sperm is injected directly into the egg
Gamete intrafallopian transfer (GIFT)	Use of laparoscope to guide the transfer of unfertilized eggs and sperm into the fallopian tubes through incisions in the abdomen
Zygote intrafallopian transfer (ZIFT)	Fertilization of an egg in the laboratory and use of a laparoscope to guide the transfer of the fertilized eggs into the fallopian tubes

SOURCE: CDC (2003d).

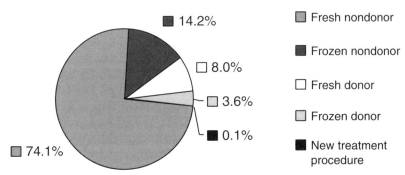

FIGURE 5-1 Types of ART procedures used in the United States, 2003.
SOURCE: CDC (2005f).

ARTs can use a woman's own egg (nondonor egg) or another woman's egg (donor egg). Some eggs are newly fertilized (fresh eggs) or previously fertilized, frozen, and then thawed (frozen eggs). Figure 5-1 depicts the frequency with which procedures involving ARTs were used in the United States in 2003. The majority of the procedures (nearly three-quarters of the cycles of ART) used fresh nondonor eggs. Of those procedures involving fresh nondonor eggs, approximately 44 percent used traditional IVF and another 56 percent used IVF with ICSI. Concern has been raised about the use of ICSI (see section below on Maternal and Child Risks). A small proportion of procedures used GIFT, ZIFT, or a combination of procedures (Figure 5-2).

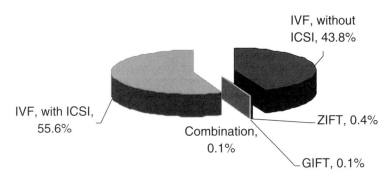

FIGURE 5-2 Types of ART procedures performed with fresh nondonor eggs or embryos, 2003.
SOURCE: CDC (2005f).

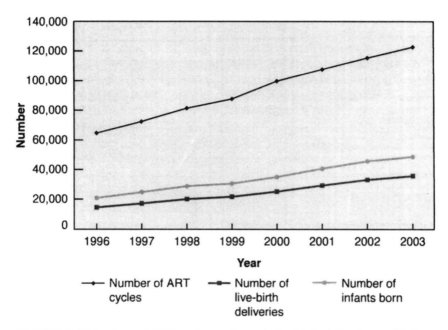

FIGURE 5-3 Numbers of ART cycles performed, live-birth deliveries, and infants born as a result of the use of ARTs, 1996 to 2003.
SOURCE: CDC (2005f).

The rate of use of ARTs has increased significantly in the past several years (Figure 5-3). Between 1996 and 2003, the number of cycles of ART nearly doubled from 64,681 to 122,872. The number of live births resulting from conceptions achieved by the use of ARTs more than doubled from 14,507 to 35,785. Because of the number of multiple births per delivery, the actual number of infants born is greater than the number of deliveries. In 2003, 48,756 infants were born as a result of the use of ARTs, whereas 20,840 were born in 1996.

Although the use of ARTs must be reported, this is not the case with other fertility treatments not classified as ARTs. The CDC definition of an ART does not include treatments in which only sperm are handled (i.e., intrauterine insemination, which is also known as artificial insemination) or procedures in which a woman takes medication to stimulate egg production without the intention of having the eggs retrieved. Superovulation with or without intrauterine insemination is used to improve fertility, but the frequency of use of this technique and the number of births attributable to the use of this technique are unknown. This is an important gap in current knowledge.

Disparities in Infertility Treatment

As discussed in Chapter 4, socioeconomic differences in multiple gestations have not been well studied (Kramer et al., 2000). The literature on infertility, utilization of treatment, and outcomes of treatment has been focused on white and socieconomically advantaged populations. While the extent to which various racial-ethnic minority populations and subpopulations experience fertility problems is not precisely known , a series of recent reports developed from a workshop, *Health Disparities in Infertility,* began to shed light on infertility problems among racial-ethnic minority populations (Berkowitz and Davis, 2006). This workshop was sponsored by the National Institute of Child Health and Human Development, Office of Behavioral and Social Sciences Research, and Office of Research on Women's Health of the National Institutes of Health, and Agency for Healthcare Research and Quality.

In an effort to assess whether racial-ethnic or socioeconomic disparities exist in infertility, impaired fecundity, or infertility treatment, Bitler and Schmidt (2006) analyzed data from the National Survey of Family Growth. The authors reported that infertility was more common for Hispanic, non-Hispanic black, and non-Hispanic women of other races than for non-Hispanic white women. In addition, results suggested disparities by educational attainment. Non-college educated women were more likely to experience problems with infertility and impaired fecundity than women with 4-year college degrees. Despite a higher likelihood of fertility problems for minority and socioeconomically disadvantaged women, these women were less likely to have ever received infertility treatment. Further, state-level infertility insurance mandates (currently in place in 15 states) did not ameliorate these disparities. Within a population of women receiving ART services in the military health care system, clinically significant differences in the live birth rate and statistically significant differences in spontaneous abortions were observed between African American and white women (Feinberg et al., 2006). The authors speculate that this may be due, in part, to higher prevalence of leiomyomas (benign uterine tumors) in the African American women. Other investigations also revealed delayed time to seeking treatment in African American women (Jain, 2006), and economic barriers to care seeking in Arab American (Inhorn and Fakih, 2006) and Latinas women (Becker et al., 2006).

The study by Becker and colleagues also suggests that Latino women raised in the United States may be more likely to seek care, compared with Latino women raised elsewhere. Continued research to understand disparities in infertility, infertility treatment, and outcomes of treatment including multiple gestations and preterm birth is needed.

RISK FOR MULTIPLE GESTATIONS

ARTs

Multiple gestations are more common as a result of assisted reproduction than as a result of natural conception because of the transfer of multiple embryos and a higher incidence of spontaneous twinning with any single embryo. The risk of monozygotic twinning after implantation of a single embryo appears to be increased in pregnancies conceived by IVF compared with the rate during spontaneous conceptions; however, this risk is relatively low, with only a 1 to 2 percent chance of having twins with implantation of a single embryo (Adashi et al., 2004). Therefore, the major cause underlying the increased risk of multiple births as a result of the use of ARTs is the number of embryos transferred. Results from a recent study suggest that IVF with a single blastocyst-stage embryo (at 5 days) versus the typical transfer with an embryo at the cleavage stage (3 days) in women under age 36 results in a higher rate of pregnancy and delivery. Of the two cases of multiple pregnancies, both occurred in the cleavage stage group (Papanikolaou et al., 2006).

National data indicate that in the United States, the majority of ART cycles involve the transfer of more than one embryo, with more embryos transferred as maternal age increases. In 2003, for women under age 35, an average of 2.6 fresh nondonor eggs were transferred per cycle (CDC, 2003d). For women ages 35 to 37, 38 to 40, and 41 to 42, the average numbers of embryos transferred were 2.9, 3.1, and 3.5, respectively. As the techniques involving ARTs have improved, the relationship between the number of embryos transferred and the achievement of a successful live birth is less clear. With the exception of women older than 40 years of age, there appears to be no improvement in the rates of live births when two or more embryos are transferred. Evidence suggests that for women under age 35, the transfer of more than two embryos is not associated with an increased likelihood of conception (Filicori et al., 2005). The transfer of more than two embryos in women over age 40, however, may prove beneficial, as it may result in a successful pregnancy, with fewer risks of multiple gestations (Filicori et al., 2005).

There is a direct relationship between the rise in the use of assisted reproduction and the increase in the numbers of multiple gestations. Fifty-three percent of 45,751 infants born in the United States as a result of the use of ART in 2002 were part of multiple gestations. Although approximately 1 percent of the infants born were conceived through the use of ARTs, these infants represented 0.5 percent of all singleton births and 17 percent of all multiple births. Sixteen percent of twins and 44 percent of higher-order multiple births were conceived by the use of ARTs (CDC, 2005g).

Ovulation Promotion

Much of the focus on the causes of multiple gestations has been placed on the role of ARTs, particularly IVF. Much less attention has been paid to the role of ovulation promotion (superovulation or intrauterine insemination and conventional ovulation induction), which is equally important in terms of its contribution to multiple gestations. The risk of multiple gestations secondary to infertility treatments such as ovulation stimulation with injectable hormones is less well documented, as the collection of data on the frequency of use of these treatments is not mandated. Nonetheless, limited data suggest that these treatments may be associated with an even higher risk of multiple gestations than IVF and ICSI, particularly if the number of developing oocytes is not monitored during the cycle (Adashi et al., 2004).

In 2000, ovulation promotion accounted for 21 percent of twin births, whereas IVF accounted for 12 percent (Figure 5-4) (Reynolds et al., 2003). Ovulation promotion was implicated in 40 percent of higher-order multiple births (Figure 5-5). Forty-two percent of these higher-order multiple births were the result of IVF, whereas 18 percent occurred spontaneously.

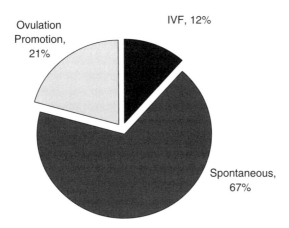

FIGURE 5-4 Contributions (percent) of IVF and ovulation promotion to twin births: 2000.
SOURCE: Reynolds et al. (2003). Reprinted from *American Journal of Obstetrics and Gynecology*, Vol. 190, Pg. 887, © 2004, with permission from Elsevier.

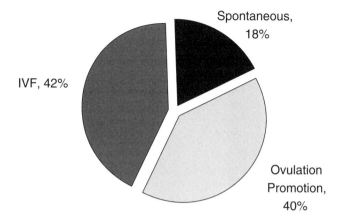

FIGURE 5-5 Contributions (percent) of IVF and ovulation promotion to higher-order multiple births: 2000.
SOURCE: Reynolds et al. (2003). Reprinted from *American Journal of Obstetrics and Gynecology*, Vol. 190, Pg. 887, © 2004, with permission from Elsevier.

Finding 5-1: The prevalence of the use of superovulation with or without artificial insemination is unknown, and no systematic mechanisms are in place to collect these data.

ARTs and Preterm Birth

The primary concern regarding the use of ARTs and ovulation promotion is the risk of preterm delivery that is associated with multiple gestations. For twins, the average gestational age at delivery is approximately 35 weeks, with 58 percent of these deliveries occurring before term (37 weeks of gestation) and with more than 12 percent occurring before 32 weeks of gestation (CDC, 2003d) (Figure 5-6). The risks are even greater for higher-order multiple births. The mean gestational ages of triplets, quadruplets, and quintuplets and higher-order multiples were 32.2, 29.9, and 28.5 weeks, respectively. More than 90 percent of triplets were born at less than 37 weeks of gestation, and approximately 36 percent were born at less than 32 weeks of gestation.

Among the infants conceived through the use of ARTs specifically, 14.5 percent of singleton births, 61.7 percent of twin births, and 97.2 percent of higher-order multiple births were born at gestational ages of less than 37 weeks (CDC, 2005f).

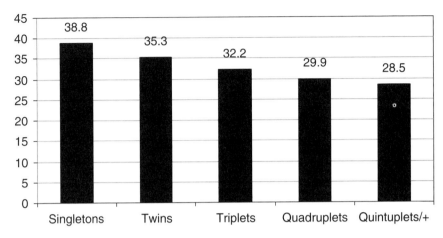

FIGURE 5-6 Mean gestational age (weeks) by number of infants born, United States, 2002.
SOURCE: CDC (2003d).

Singletons Conceived Through ARTs and Preterm Birth

Singletons conceived through the use of IVF are twice as likely to be born preterm and die within 1 week of birth than those not conceived through IVF and 2.7 times more likely to have a low birth weight (Hampton, 2004). A meta-analysis that compiled information from 12,283 singleton births conceived through the use of IVF and 1.9 million spontaneously conceived singleton births noted a twofold increase in the risk of preterm delivery (Jackson et al., 2004). Similarly, the results of a meta-analysis conducted by McGovern and colleagues (2004) found that singleton pregnancies resulting from IVF (embryo transfer) and GIFT were twice as likely as naturally conceived singletons to be delivered preterm. The etiology of this type of preterm birth remains unknown. Recent evidence suggests the possibility of placentation problems in ART pregnancies. A study from the First And Second Trimester Evaluation of Risk trial examined whether the use of ART was associated with an increased risk of chromosomal abnormalities, fetal malformations, or adverse pregnancy outcomes among singleton births (Shevell et al., 2005). Approximately 95 percent of patients did not use any form of ART, 3.4 percent used ovulation induction, and 1.5 percent received IVF treatment. Results indicate that patients who used ovulation induction had an increased risk of placental abruption (OR 2.4; 95% CI 1.3–4.2) and fetal loss after 24 weeks (OR 2.1; 95% CI 1.3–3.6) compared to women who did not receive ART. Patients who used IVF were more likely to develop preeclampsia (OR 2.7; 95% CI 1.7–4.4) have a placental abruption (OR 2.4; 95% CI 1.1–5.2), placenta previa (OR 6.0; 95% CI 3.4–10.7), and undergo a cesarean delivery (OR 2.3; 95% CI 1.8–2.9) compared to women who did not undergo ART. There was no association between ART and fetal growth restriction, aneuploidy, or fetal anomalies after adjusting for a number of sociodemographic and health variables.

Finding 5-2: Fertility treatments are a significant contributor to preterm birth among both multiple and singleton pregnancies.

Finding 5-3: The mechanisms by which conditions of infertility, subfertility, and fertility treatments increase the risk of preterm birth, particularly among singleton pregnancies, are unknown. The mechanisms may be markedly different from the mechanisms suggested when racial and socioeconomic causes of preterm birth are considered.

Maternal and Child Risks

The use of ARTs and ovulation promotion has raised concern about potential risks to the women who undergo these procedures and the children who are conceived as a result. Some investigators have speculated about the effects of fertility drugs on the risk of breast cancer and cancers of the reproductive system. A study by Klip and colleagues (2000), in which a cohort of women in the Netherlands was monitored for 5 to 8 years, found no increase in the risk of breast cancer or ovarian cancer in women who underwent IVF compared with that in subfertile women who had not undergone IVF. The study also found that both women who had undergone IVF and subfertile women did not have an increased risk for endometrial cancer. The authors suggest a potential link between endometrial cancer and subfertility.

Other risks associated with hormonal ovulation stimulation include ovarian hyperstimulation syndrome, in which fluid imbalances and ovary enlargement become problematic; rupture of the ovaries is also a possibility (for a review of the well-being of women during the use of ARTs, see The President's Council on Bioethics [2004]). Multiple pregnancies pose higher risks of mortality and morbidity to the mothers than singleton pregnancies. Mothers with multiple pregnancies are more likely to experience high blood pressure, anemia, preeclampsia, and gestational diabetes and to require delivery by cesarean (Sebire et al., 2001; Wen et al., 2004).

Of central interest in the discussion of the unintended consequences of the use of ARTs is the well-being of the children conceived through the use of these procedures. Although large-scale and long-term follow-up studies of these children are lacking, recent evidence associates some

ART procedures with certain birth defects as a result of defects in DNA methylation, such as Beckwith-Wiedemann syndrome, retinoblastoma, and Angelman syndrome (Jacob and Moley, 2005; Niemitz and Feinberg, 2004). However, the prevalence of these conditions is extremely low. Concern has been raised about the use of intracytoplasmic sperm injection, as this procedure impedes the ovum's natural ability to resist fertilization by a sperm that would otherwise not have the ability to fertilize the egg. However, these risks are considered small, and the greater risk from the use of these procedures results from the consequences of multiple gestations.

Reducing Rates of Multiple Gestation

Nationally, the rate of birth of live twins has continued to increase (Figure 5-7), whereas the rate of birth of live triplets has leveled off since 1998 (Figure 5-8). For births that specifically result from the use of ARTs, the percentage of twin deliveries per ART cycle with fresh nondonor eggs or embryos remained essentially unchanged from 1996 to 2003 (31.4 to 31.0 percent). During this period, the percentage of triplets decreased from 7.0 to 3.2 percent (CDC, 2005f). Despite this trend, the number of multiple deliveries in the United States continues to be a problem and is of concern.

The oversight of ART practices currently occurs at both the governmental (federal and state) and nongovernmental levels, and both govern-

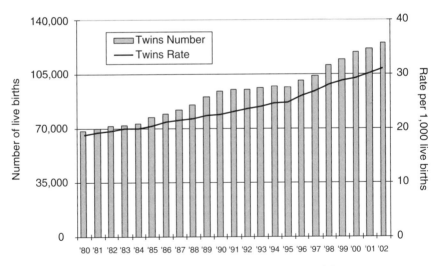

FIGURE 5-7 Trends in live twins births, 1980 to 2002, United States.
SOURCES: CDC (1999a,b, 2002a, 2003b).

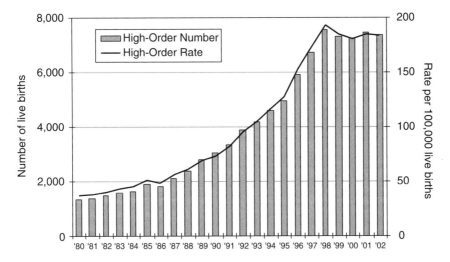

FIGURE 5-8 Trends in live high-order births, 1980 to 2002, United States. SOURCES: CDC (1999a,b, 2002a, 2003b).

mental and nongovernmental entities also provide the public with guidance on such practices. For a more detailed overview of the goals, scope, requirements, mechanisms, and efficacy of ART-related policies, the reader is referred to *Reproduction and Responsibility: The Regulation of New Biotechnologies* (The President's Council on Bioethics, 2004). The Fertility Clinic Success Rate and Certification Act of 1992 was designed to provide consumers with reliable information about the services provided by and the success rates of fertility clinics throughout the United States. Data are reported by the Society for Assisted Reproductive Technology (SART) and are published by the CDC. This act also provides states with a standard process for the accreditation of embryo laboratories. In most states, the states oversee access to services and determine whether and to what extent those services are covered by health insurance. Other states address the prevention of abuse by practitioners and regulate gamete and embryo donations.

Nongovernmental guidance on the practice of ART has come primarily from the American Society for Reproductive Medicine (ASRM) in conjunction with SART. In 1999, ASRM issued guidelines that recommended limiting the number of embryos transferred to no more than two in young women in their first cycle of IVF if sufficient embryos were available for cryopreservation (Barbieri, 2005). A demonstrable drop in the rate of triplet gestations from 7 to 3.8 percent from 1996 to 2002 has been cited as evidence of the success of these practice guidelines (Barbieri, 2005). It is noted that a decrease in the number of triplet live births may be due to factors other than reducing the number of embryos transferred. For example, a distinction should be made between triplet live births and the percent of triplets detected with heart beats since a discordance may exists as a consequence of the use of multifetal reduction. ASRM further refined these guidelines in 2004, recommending the transfer of a single embryo for young women less than 35 years of age with favorable prognoses (PC of SART and ASRM, 2004). The recommendations become less restrictive as maternal age advances and suggest the transfer of no more than two embryos to women with favorable prognoses between the ages of 35 and 37 years and no more than three embryos in women with favorable prognoses between the ages of 38 and 40 years. Transfer of an additional embryo is suggested if an unfavorable prognosis exists. For women over age 40, the recommended limit to the numbers of embryos transferred is no more than five.

Despite the successes in reducing the rates of higher-order multiple births, the United States does not fare as well as European countries in minimizing the risk of multiple gestations (Anderson et al., 2005). The most recent figures released by the European Society of Human Reproduction and Embryology (ESHRE) reported an overall multiple gestation rate of 25.5 percent among pregnancies conceived by the use of ARTs in 2001, when the U.S. ART-related multiple gestation rate was twice that level. Twenty-four percent of European pregnancies conceived by the use of ARTs resulted in twins, and only 1.5 percent resulted in triplets or higher-order multiple births. By 2001, the United States halved its rate of higher-order multiple births to 3.8 percent, but Europe reduced the rate by nearly 60 percent to a low of 1.5 percent. Furthermore, whereas over half of all U.S. ART cycles involve the transfer of three or more embryos, in Europe over 60 percent involve the transfer of only one embryo (12 percent) or two embryos (51.7 percent). A lower number of embryos transferred may result in lower success rate per cycle, especially in women over 40 years. However, continued progress is being made toward addressing the problem of multiple gestations. A recent study examined the results of approximately 200 IVF cycles in which patients had either one or two embryos transferred. Results revealed similar implantation and live birth rates and a significant reduction in the number of twins conceived with single embryo transfer (Criniti et al., 2005).

The international difference in the rates of multiple gestations may reflect the more stringent guidelines regarding the number of embryos transferred. As early as 1993, the Swedish health organizations recommended reductions in the number of embryos transferred from three to two per cycle (Källén et al., 2005). Subsequent voluntary reduction on the part of ART providers virtually eliminated the risk of triplets without lowering the rate of live births (NBHW, 2006). Currently, public funding of ART cycles in Sweden covers only the transfer of single embryos, which has resulted in an even further reduction in multiple gestations. ESHRE guidelines on the recommended number of embryos to be transferred emphasize the elective transfer of a single embryo for women up to 36 years of age if at least one good-quality embryo has been produced. However, there is no scientifically-based definition of what a good quality embryo is and how this can be measured objectively, which affects decisions about which and how many embryos to transfer.

Additional support for single-embryo transfer (SET) comes from a recently published randomized controlled trial comparing two cycles of SET with one cycle of double-embryo transfer (DET) (Lukassen et al., 2005). Two cycles of SET were equally effective in achieving a live birth as a single cycle of DET, with similar costs through 6 weeks postpartum. The investigators estimated that if the lifetime costs of caring for handicapped preterm survivors are included, SET will result in a savings of 7,000 pounds per live birth. The investigators noted that in countries where ART regulation is the strictest, the fee structure supports the use of SET (Ombelet et al., 2005; Papanikolau et al., 2006; Thurin et al., 2004).

The challenge of reducing multiple gestations is also a sensitive and personal issue. The rights and autonomy of patients, the autonomy of providers, and the public good are forces that must be considered (Adashi et al., 2004). Patients may not be rigorously apprised of the risks of multiple gestations or may accept the risks in their desire to conceive. Ovulation enhancement has proceeded without formal guidelines, and advanced training and certification is not required for its practice. With IVF, providers must weigh the goal of a successful singleton pregnancy outcome with the inability to predict the success of implantation of any given embryo. Payers are largely uninvolved in the discussion of the challenge of the risk of multiple gestations. Although some payers underwrite ovulation enhancement, most do not underwrite IVF, the outcome of which is more predictable than that of ovulation enhancement and which results in a lower rate of multiple births. This may be because payers have not been thoroughly informed about the financial consequences of higher-order multiple births.

In an effort to decrease the number of multiple births related to IVF, the Belgian government, in 2003, agreed to reimburse laboratory expenses for the first six IVF trials in women up to age 42. In exchange, restrictions are placed on the number of embryos transferred, depending on the age of the woman (Gordts et al., 2005; Ombelet et al., 2005). For example, in women under 36, single embryo transfer is performed in the first trial and in the second (if high quality embryos are available). Thereafter a maximum of two embryos are transferred. Data reveal that after this policy was instituted, the percentage of singe embryo transfers increased, and overall pregnancy rates did not differ. Twin pregnancies were reduced from 19 percent to 3 percent (Gordts et al., 2005).

Stricter guidelines on the number of embryos transferred should be emphasized by a number of U.S. professional organizations and not just ASRM. Similar best-practice guidelines should be outlined for other infertility treatments that use ARTs, such as ovulation induction. Such guidelines should recommend the use of strict ultrasound guidance and abandonment of a cycle if too many follicles develop. Policy makers should mandate the more systematic collection of data on such procedures and should also consider recommending the use of medication to stimulate egg production. Professional organizations and surveillance activities should redefine success as singleton live births (rather than pregnancy rates). Efforts to reeducate ART consumers on the risks of multiple gestation and preterm birth must transpire simultaneously. Other policies regarding access to assisted reproduction should also be further explored.

Access to reproductive health care and reproductive technology may be a double-edged sword when it comes to ARTs. States with legally mandated coverage for infertility treatment, including ARTs, were the states with the highest rates of ART procedures per million population (Massachusetts, New Jersey, Maryland, the District of Columbia, and Rhode Island) (CDC, 2002b). In Massachusetts, a rise in the state's rate of multiple births can be directly linked to mandated insurance coverage of infertility services (CDC, 1999a). Sweden and Belgium exemplify a contrasting approach, with public funding limited to the coverage of only SET cycles, thus freeing infertile couples from the financial pressure to transfer as many embryos as possible.

6

Biological Pathways Leading to Preterm Birth

ABSTRACT

Preterm birth has usually been treated as a single entity, for epidemiological and statistical purposes. This traditional empiric approach, however, presupposes a single pathologic process for which treatment could be uniform. This approach has met with only limited success in the treatment and prevention of preterm labor. It is now clear that the causes of preterm labor are multifactorial and vary according to gestational age. Important common pathways leading to preterm birth include stress, systemic or maternal genital tract infections, placental ischemia or vascular lesions, and uterine overdistension. These pathways differ in their initiating factors and mediators, but ultimately, they share many common features that result in preterm uterine contractions and birth. Appropriate animal models have been very useful in describing the temporal events leading to preterm birth and the neonatal sequelae of prematurity, particularly in the setting of intrauterine infection. The use of animal models to answer specific questions related to prematurity and to describe the pathophysiological events associated with preterm birth will contribute to the development of rational and efficacious treatment and prevention strategies for preterm birth.

MECHANISMS OF PARTURITION

Parturition

The process of normal spontaneous parturition can be divided into four stages (see the reviews of Challis [2000] and Challis et al. [2000]). During most of pregnancy, the uterus remains relatively quiescent, and this corresponds to Phase 0 (quiescence) of parturition. Phase 1 (activation) involves uterine stretch and fetal hypothalamic-pituitary-adrenal (HPA) activation. Phase 2 (stimulation) refers to stimulation of the activated uterus by various substances, including corticotropin-releasing hormone (CRH), oxytocin, and prostaglandins. These different processes lead to a common pathway to parturition involving increased uterine contractility, cervical ripening, and decidual and fetal membrane activation (Romero et al., 2004a). Phase 3 (involution) corresponds to postpartum involution of the uterus. These unique phases are described below and are summarized in Figure 6-1.

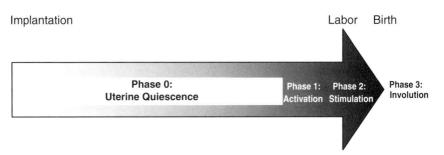

FIGURE 6-1 The stages of parturition. Following implantation, more than 95 percent of gestation is spent in Phase 0, uterine quiescence. During quiescence, myometrial contractility is inhibited by a variety of biological substances, including progesterone. Phase 1, myometrial activation, is characterized by increased expression of contraction-associated proteins, receptors for oxytocin, and prostaglandins, and increased placental estrogen biosynthesis. The signal for myometrial activation is controlled by the fetal HPA axis, which, in turn, is up-regulated by endogenous placental CRH production. Phase 2, myometrial stimulation, involves a progressive cascade of events, beginning with myometrial activation, which results in myometrial contractility, cervical ripening, and decidua and membrane activation. It is likely initiated by the same events of fetal HPA activation that initiate Phase 1. Phase 3, involution, involves placental separation and contraction of the uterus. It is primarily effected by maternal oxytocin.

Phase 0: Quiescence

Throughout most of pregnancy the uterus remains relatively quiescent. Myometrial activity is inhibited during pregnancy by various substances, including progesterone, prostacyclin (PGI2), nitric oxide, relaxin, and parathyroid hormone-related peptide. These substances function by different mechanisms, but in general they increase intracellular levels of cyclic nucleotides (cyclic adenosine monophosphate [cAMP] or cyclic guanosine monophosphate), which in turn inhibit the release of calcium from intracellular stores or reduce the activity of the enzyme myosin light-chain kinase (MLCK). Calcium and MLCK are central to uterine contractility. Calcium is required to activate calmodulin, which in turn induces a conformational change in MLCK, allowing the enzyme to phosphorylate myosin and initiate the coupling of actin and myosin, which leads to myometrial contraction.

Rare uterine contractions that occur during the quiescent phase are of low frequency and amplitude and are poorly coordinated; these are commonly referred to as contractures in animals and Braxton-Hicks contractions in women. The poor coordination of these contractions is primarily due to an absence of gap junctions in the pregnant myometrium (Garfield, 1988). Gap junctions (and their associated proteins, called connexins) allow cell-to-cell coupling. With the onset of labor, there is a massive increase in the numbers of gap junctions, resulting in significantly enhanced electrical coupling and synchronized high-amplitude contractions throughout the myometrium.

Phase 1: Activation

Phase 1 myometrial activation is characterized by increased levels of expression of contraction-associated proteins (CAPs), including connexin-43 (CX-43; the major protein of myometrial gap junctions), and receptors for oxytocin and stimulatory prostaglandins (Lye et al., 1998). Normally, the signals for myometrial activation can come from uterine stretch as a result of fetal growth or from activation of the fetal HPA axis as a result of fetal maturation, or both.

Uterine stretch has been shown in animal models to increase CAP and oxytocin receptor gene expression in the myometrium, but the ability to do so is highly dependent on the endocrine environment. Progesterone blocks stretch-induced increases in the levels of CX-43 expression. However, with progesterone withdrawal at term (see below), uterine stretch is associated with significant increases in the levels of CX-43 expression.

Signals for myometrial activation also come from the fetal HPA axis (Liggins and Thorburn, 1994). It is currently thought that once fetal maturity has been reached (as determined by as yet unknown mechanisms), the fetal hypothalamus and/or the placenta (see below) increase the level of CRH secretion, which in turn stimulates adrenocorticotropic hormone (ACTH) expression by the fetal pituitary and cortisol and androgen production by the fetal adrenals. Fetal androgens are then aromatized into estrogens by the placenta. Ultimately, this initiates a biological cascade that leads to a common pathway of parturition characterized by uterine contractility, cervical ripening and decidual/fetal membrane activation seen in Phase 2 of parturition.

Phase 2: Stimulation

Phase 2 involves a progressive cascade of events that lead to a common pathway of parturition involving uterine contractility, cervical ripening, and decidual and fetal membrane activation. These events are characterized by fetal HPA activation, functional progesterone withdrawal, increasing maternal and fetal estrogens, and rising prostaglandins. The cascade may begin with the placental production of CRH and eventually leads to a functional progesterone withdrawal in the myometrium. The progesterone withdrawal causes increased levels of expression of estrogen receptors and promotes estrogen activity. The increased action of estrogen leads to the formation of many estrogen-dependent CAPs, such as CX-43, oxytocin receptors, and prostaglandins, that promote uterine contractility.

CRH and the "placental clock." Corticotropin-releasing hormone (CRH) is thought to play a central role in fetal maturation and human parturition (McLean et al., 1999; reviewed by Smith R et al. [2002]). CRH, a neuropeptide of predominantly hypothalamic origin, is also expressed in the human placenta and membranes and is released into maternal and fetal compartments in exponentially increasing amounts over the course of gestation. The trajectory of the rise in CRH levels has been associated with the length of gestation (Hobel et al., 1999; Leung et al., 1999; McLean and Smith, 1999). Specifically, women destined to preterm delivery have higher concentrations of maternal CRH in plasma as early as 16 weeks of gestation and a more rapid rise in CRH levels than women who deliver at term. These findings have led some researchers to suggest that placental CRH may act as a "placental clock" that regulates the length of gestation (McLean and Smith, 1999).

Placental CRH synthesis is stimulated by glucocorticoids, in contrast to the inhibitory effect of glucocorticoids on hypothalamic CRH synthesis. Placental CRH, in turn, promotes fetal cortisol and DHEA-S production, and this positive-feedback loop is progressively amplified, thereby driving the process forward from fetal HPA activation to parturition. Placental

CRH, in turn, enhances prostaglandin production by increasing the levels of expression of prostaglandin H2 synthase (PGHS) chorion and amnion cells, creating yet another positive-feedback loop that drives the process of parturition. Paradoxically, during uterine quiescence CRH may act as a myometrial relaxant rather than as a promoter of parturition. Throughout most of pregnancy, the myometrium expresses CRH type 1 receptors that are linked by Gsα regulatory proteins to adenylate cyclase and cAMP, which would promote myometrial relaxation when they are stimulated. At the end of pregnancy, however, an alternative splice variant of the CRH receptor is expressed and the level of expression of Gsα subunits declines, which may promote a contractile phenotype (reviewed by Challis et al. [2000]).

Functional progesterone withdrawal. For most of pregnancy, uterine quiescence is maintained by the action of progesterone. It does so by blocking CAP gene expression and gap junction formation within the myometrium; inhibiting placental CRH secretion; opposing the activity of estrogen (see below); up-regulating systems (e.g., nitric oxide) that promote myometrial relaxation; and suppressing the expression of cytokines and prostaglandins. At the end of pregnancy in most mammals, maternal progesterone levels fall and estrogen levels rise. In women, however, progesterone and estrogen concentrations continue to rise throughout pregnancy until delivery of the placenta. Recent data suggest that functional progesterone withdrawal may occur in women and nonhuman primates by alterations in the levels of progesterone receptor (PR) isoforms (Smith R et al., 2002). In women, the PR-B receptor isoform functions predominantly as an activator of progesterone-responsive genes, whereas the PR-A receptor isoform acts as a repressor of PR-B function and other nuclear receptors. In the term myometrium, the onset of labor is associated with increased levels of PR-A expression relative to the levels of PR-B expression. Because PR-A suppresses the action of progesterone, the increased level of PR-A expression relative to that of PR-B decreases the responsiveness of the myometrium to progesterone, resulting in a functional progesterone withdrawal that enables parturition to proceed.

Estrogens. Unlike the placentas of most other species, the human placenta cannot convert progesterone to estrogen because it is deficient in 17-hydroxylase, which is required for this conversion. Estrogen production in the placenta depends largely on precursor androgens synthesized in the fetal zone of the fetal adrenal; approximately 50 percent of circulating maternal estrone and estradiol are derived from placental aromatization of the fetal androgen, DHEA-S. Placental CRH directly and indirectly (via fetal pituitary secretion of ACTH) stimulates the fetal zone of the fetal adrenals to produce DHEA-S, thereby supplying the precursors needed for estrogen synthesis in the placenta.

Estrogens, in turn, enhance the expression of many estrogen-dependent CAPs, including CX-43 (gap junctions), oxytocin receptor, prostaglandin receptors, cyclooxygenase-2 (COX-2; which results in prostaglandin production), and MLCK (which stimulates myometrial contractility and labor) (Challis, 2000).

Prostaglandins. Extensive evidence supports a central role for prostaglandins in promoting uterine contractiity (Challis et al., 2000). The actions of prostaglandin are effected through specific receptors. PGE2 induces myometrial contractions by binding to EP-1 and EP-3 receptors, which mediate contractions through mechanisms that lead to increased calcium mobilization and reduced levels of production of inhibition of intracellular cAMP. Prostaglandins also enhance the production of matrix metalloproteinases (MMP) in the cervix and decidua to promote cervical ripening and decidual and fetal membrane activation. PGF2α binds to FP receptors to induce myometrial contractions. In contrast, in the lower uterine segment PGE2 induces myometrial relaxation by binding to EP-2 and EP-4 receptors that increase the level of cAMP formation.

Prostaglandins are formed from arachidonic acid by PGHS. In turn, prostaglandins are metabolized to inactive forms by the actions of PGDH. Cortisol, CRH, and estrogens stimulate PGHS activity and cortisone and CRH also inhibit PGDH expression. Thus, increases in fetal steroid hormone production following fetal HPA activation leads to a net increase in prostaglandin levels. Similarly, proinflammatory cytokines such as IL-1 and tumor necrosis factor alpha (TNF-α) up-regulate PGHS expression and down-regulate PGDH expression leading to prostaglandin synthesis associated with preterm delivery in the setting of infection.

In summary, these events initiated by fetal HPA activation and resulting in increased fetal and placental steroid biosynthesis result in a progressive cascade of biological processes lead to a common pathway of parturition involving cervical ripening, uterine contractility and decidual and fetal membrane activation.

Cervical ripening. Cervical changes precede the onset of labor, are gradual, and develop over several weeks. Cervical ripening is characterized by a decrease in the total collagen content, an increase in collagen solubility, and an increase in collagenolytic activity that results in the remodeling of the extracellular matrix of the cervix (Romero et al., 2004a). Prostaglandins, estrogens, progesterones, and inflammatory cytokines (e.g., IL-8) affect the metabolism of the extracellular matrix. PGE2 stimulates collagenolytic activity and the synthesis of subtypes of proteoaminoglycans that are less stabilizing. Estrogen stimulates collagen degradation in vitro, and intravenous administration of 17β-estradiol induces cervical ripening. Progesterone blocks estrogen-induced collagenolysis in vitro and down-regulates IL-8 production by the uterine cervix. In addition to these hormones, nitric oxide may play a role in cervical ripening in some circumstances. Nitric oxide accumulates at sites of inflammation and can act as an inflammatory mediator at high concentrations. Nitric oxide donors (e.g., sodium nitroprusside) have been shown to induce cervical ripening, whereas nitric oxide inhibitors (e.g., L-nitro-arginine methylester) block cervical ripening.

Uterine contractility. Uterine contraction results from the coupling of actin and myosin, which depends on the phosphorylation of myosin by MLCK. MLCK is activated by calcium-calmodulin after an increase in intracellular calcium levels. This increase in generated by the actions of various uterotonins, including oxytocin and prostaglandins. Cell-to-cell coupling, which allows the myometrium to develop synchronous high-amplitude contractions during labor, is facilitated by the formation of gap junctions and their associated proteins (e.g., connexins) (Lye et al., 1998). Their formation is highly dependent on estrogen; estrogen activation, in turn, is induced by a functional progesterone withdrawal at term.

Decidual and fetal membrane activation. Decidual and fetal membrane activation refers to a complex set of anatomical and biochemical events that result in the separation of the lower pole of the membranes from the deciduas of the lower uterine segment and, eventually, in the spontaneous rupture of membranes. The precise mechanism of membrane and decidual membrane activation remains to be elucidated, but extracellular matrix-degrading enzymes such as MMP type 1 (MMP-1), interstitial collagenase, MMP-8 (neutrophil collagenase), MMP-9 (gelatinase B), neutrophil elastase, and plasmin have been implicated. These enzymes degrade extracellular matrix proteins (e.g., collagens and fibronectins), thereby weakening the membranes, which eventually leads to the rupture of membranes. Some MMPs, such as MMP-9, may induce apoptosis in the amnion.

Phase 3: Involution

Phase 3 begins with the third stage of labor and involves placental separation and uterine contraction. Placental separation occurs by cleavage along the plane of the decidua basalis. Uterine contraction is essential to prevent bleeding from the large venous sinuses that are exposed after delivery of the placenta and is primarily affected by oxytocin.

Summary of Human Parturition

Parturition in women involves a progressive cascade of events initiated by HPA activation and increased placental CRH expression, leading to a functional progesterone withdrawal and estrogen activation, which in turn results in the expression and activation of CAPs (including oxytocin receptors), oxytocin, and prostaglandins. This biological cascade eventually leads to a common pathway involving cervical ripening, uterine contractility, decidual and fetal membrane activation, and, in the second stage, increases in maternal oxytocin. It has been hypothesized that both preterm and term labor share this common pathway and that the pathologic stimuli of parturition, as described in the following sections, may act in concert with the normal physiological preparation for labor, especially after 32 weeks of gestation. Before 32 weeks of gestation, a greater degree of pathologic stimulus may be required to initiate labor. One fundamental difference between spontaneous parturition at term and preterm labor is that whereas term labor results from physiological activation of the components of the common pathway, preterm labor arises from pathologic processes that activate one or more of the components of the common pathway of parturition. However, further research is necessary to answer fundamental questions, including the following:

- What role do implantation errors have in the pathogenesis of preterm delivery?
- What are the cellular, endocrine, and paracrine mechanisms that maintain uterine quiescence?
- What are the mechanisms involved in the switch from the quiescent uterus to uterine activation and stimulation?
- What is the basis for disparities in gestational length between ethnic groups? Does it have a biological basis, or can it be accounted for by environmental and social factors?

PATHWAYS TO SPONTANEOUS PRETERM PARTURITION

Until recently, obstetricians and epidemiologists have had a tendency to combine, for statistical purposes, all preterm births occurring between 22 and 37 weeks of gestation. The traditional empirical approach to preterm labor presupposed a single pathologic process for which treatment could be uniform.

It is now clear that the causes of preterm labor are multifactorial and vary according to gestational age. They include systemic and intrauterine infections (which are responsible for a majority of extremely preterm births), stress, uteroplacental thrombosis and intrauterine vascular lesions

TABLE 6-1 Commonly Recognized Etiologies and Pathways Leading to Spontaneous Preterm Birth

Maternal-fetal HPA activation	Stress	Maternal-fetal HPA activation
Infection and inflammation	Intrauterine Lower genital tract Systemic	Proinflammatory cytokine and prostaglandin cascade Matrix metalloproteinases
Decidual hemorrhage	Thrombophilias, Abruptio placentae Autoantibody syndromes	Thrombin Matrix metalloproteinases
Pathologic uterine overdistension	Multifetal gestation Polyhydramnios	Expression of gap junctions proteins Prostaglandins Oxytocin receptors

associated with fetal stress or decidual hemorrhage, uterine overdistension, and cervical insufficiency. Each pathway may be influenced by gene-environment interactions, as discussed in Chapter 7 (Table 6-1 and Figure 6-2). It is also noted that these pathways or their relative impact may differ for ART patients. The causes for preterm birth among ART patients are multifactorial and poorly understood, except for uterine overdistension resulting from multiple gestations. The reader is referred to Chapter 5 for discussion of the impact of infertility and infertility treatment on preterm birth. Nevertheless, there is strong evidence that despite different etiologies and initiators, preterm and term labor share many common pathways in the activation of common downstream cellular and molecular effectors. This may include stimulation of the fetal HPA axis (by maturation, infection, or ischemia), in addition to endocrine, paracrine, and immune system interactions, which were summarized in the preceding section. Commonly occurring pathways of preterm parturition are described below.

Stress and the Placental Clock

Stress is increasingly being recognized as an important risk factor for preterm delivery. Stress may be simply defined as any challenge—psychological or physical—that threatens or that is perceived to threaten homeostasis (i.e., the stability of the internal milieu of the organism). The epidemiological evidence linking maternal psychological stress to prematurity is reviewed in Chapter 3. Several pathways linking maternal psychological stress and prematurity have been proposed, including neuroendocrine, immune-inflammatory, vascular, and behavioral processes.

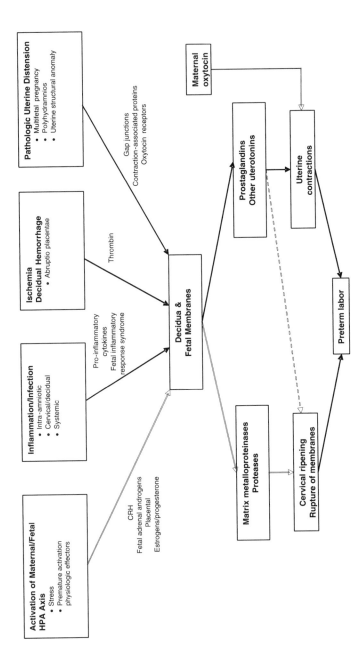

FIGURE 6-2 Overview of commonly occurring pathways to preterm birth. Although the causes of preterm birth are multiple and there are many unique upstream regulatory initiators of preterm birth, there are few downstream effectors that lead to preterm birth. These include prostaglandins or other uterotonins, MMPs, and oxytocin. This suggests that interventions for the prevention of preterm birth can be directed either to the inhibition of specific upstream initiators of a given pathway or to the blocking of down-stream effectors in general.

Neuroendocrine Processes

The neuroendocrine processes linking stress to prematurity are mediated by placental CRH (reviewed by Wadhwa et al. [2001]). Placental CRH is responsive to stress. In vitro studies of human placental cells have shown that CRH is released from cultured human placental cells in a dose-response manner in response to all the major biological effectors of stress, including cortisol, catecholamines, oxytocin, angiotension II, and IL-1. In vivo studies have also found significant correlations between maternal psychosocial stress and the levels of CRH, ACTH, and cortisol in maternal plasma. Several studies have related early increases in maternal plasma CRH levels to the timing of birth. Hobel and colleagues (1999) conducted serial assessments of CRH levels over the course of gestation and found that women delivering preterm had significantly elevated CRH levels compared with those in women delivering at term, as well as a significantly accelerated rate of increase in CRH levels over the course of their gestations. In addition, they found that maternal psychosocial stress levels at midgestation significantly predicted the magnitude of increase in maternal CRH levels between midgestation and later times of gestation.

These data suggest that the relationship between maternal psychological stress and prematurity may be mediated by prematurely increased levels of expression of placental CRH. As discussed earlier in this chapter, in term parturition placental CRH activation is largely driven by the fetal HPA axis in a forward-feedback loop upon fetal maturation. In preterm parturition it may be the maternal HPA axis (as well as the sympathoadrenal-medullary [SAM] system) that drives placental CRH expression (Wadhwa et al., 2001). Maternal stress results in increased levels of biological effectors of stress, including cortisol and epinephrine, which could activate placental CRH gene expression. Placental CRH, in turn, can stimulate fetal secretion of cortisol and DHEA-S (by activation of the fetal HPA axis) and placental release of estriol and prostaglandins, thereby precipitating preterm delivery (reviewed by Hobel et al., 1998).

Immune and Inflammatory Processes

Stress can also alter neuroendocrine modulation of immune function, leading to increased susceptibility to intra-amniotic infection or inflammation. Extensive interconnections exist among the SAM system, the HPA axis, and the immune system. Under physiological conditions, the SAM system and the HPA axis suppress the body's immunoinflammatory responses. A negative-feedback loop exists between the HPA axis and the immune system; proinflammatory cytokines (e.g., IL-1β, TNF-α, and IL-6) stimulate the HPA axis, resulting in the secretion of glucocorticoids. These glucocorticoids, in turn, down-regulate proinflammatory cytokines and also suppress other aspects of the inflammatory response (reviewed by McEwen et al. [1997]).

During acute stress, glucocorticoids primarily suppress inflammation; but with repeated or chronic stress, glucocorticoids can enhance inflammation, including the expression of proinflammatory cytokine expression. Excessive secretion of proinflammatory and T-helper cell type 1 (Th1)-type cytokines is found in subjects undergoing life stress, and this immune activation is associated with a loss of nonspecific and specific cellular immune responses (Irwin, 1999). These cytokines, in turn, can down-regulate glucocorticoid receptors (Norbiato et al., 1997) and decrease glucocorticoid receptor affinity (Pariante et al., 1999). Evidence suggests that this cycle of immune activation, together with insufficient HPA axis restraint of cytokine secretion, is a major component of inflammatory disease progression. Thus, repeated or chronic stress could lead to a dysregulation of proinflammatory and Th1 cytokine expression, thereby predisposing an overreactive inflammatory response to stress or infection. The role of these mechanisms in contributing to preterm birth, however, has not been well studied, and may represent a fertile area for further investigation.

Behavioral Processes

Stress may induce maternal risk behaviors as a means of coping with stress. These behavioral processes may be mediated by altered neurochemistry. In animal studies, CRH and related neuropeptides play a central role in mediating motor and psychic activation, stimulus avoidance, and threat recognition responses to aversive stimulus exposure (Heinrichs and Koob, 2004). CRH may also mediate some of the neuroendocrine and behavioral effects of cocaine addiction (Sarnyai, 1998). In rhesus monkeys, strong correlations were found between behavioral hyperactivity and the CRH-dependent elements of pulsatile activity of the HPA axis. Acute cocaine administration induced dose- and time-dependent alterations in hypothalamic and extrahypothalamic-limbic CRH concentrations in rats. Cocaine withdrawal elicited anxiety-like behavior and alterations of CRH concentration in the hypothalamus, amygdala, and basal forebrain (Sarnyai, 1998).

Despite the accumulating data from animal studies, the question of whether stress increases maternal risk behaviors has not been clearly addressed in human studies. Most epidemiological studies of maternal stress and birth outcomes have treated risk behaviors as confounders, although a few clinic-based studies have found that behaviors may play a mediating role between maternal psychosocial stress and lower birth weight (see Chapter 3). A recent population-based study (Whitehead et al., 2003) found maternal stressful life events were significantly associated with cigarette smoking during pregnancy and late entry into prenatal care, although stressful life events were not significantly associated with preterm delivery.

Uterine Overdistension

Uterine overdistension plays a key role in the onset of preterm labor associated with multiple gestations, polyhydramnios, and macrosomia. The mechanisms by which uterine overdistension might lead to preterm labor are not well understood. Uterine stretch induces the expression of gap junction proteins, such as CX-43 and CX-26 (Ou et al., 1997), as well as other contraction-associated proteins, such as oxytocin receptors (Terzidoo et al., 2005). In vitro stretch of myometrial strips also increases PGHS-2 and PGE (Sooranna et al., 2004). Stretching the muscle of the lower uterine segment has been shown to increase the levels of IL-8 and collagenase production, which in turn facilitates cervical ripening (Loudon et al., 2004; Maradny et al., 1996). The increased myometrial expression of PGHS-2 and IL-8 from uterine stretch appears to be mediated by activation of the MAPK system (Sooranna et al., 2005). An interaction between mechanical and endocrine signals during myometrial activation may exist; in vivo studies have shown increased levels of expression of CX-43 in response to mechanical stretch in an ovariectomized rat uterus, an effect that could be blocked by progesterone administration (Ou et al., 1998). Similarly, in rats uterine stretch has no effect on myometrial CX-43 expression in midpregnancy, probably as a result of the high levels of progesterone that are present at that time; progesterone withdrawal before the onset of labor allows stretch-induced CX-43 expression (Wathes and Porter, 1982).

The effect of uterine stretch on myometrial expression of G proteins (e.g., Gsα), which mediate myometrial relaxation, is not known. Human studies of uterine overdistension are lacking. One recent study found no difference between singleton and multiple gestations in the levels of expression of Gsα, PGE2 receptors, CX-43, and CX-26 in myometrium taken from nonlaboring women undergoing elective cesarean delivery at term (Lyall et al., 2002). Moreover, mechanical stretch did not alter the levels of Gsα expression in vitro, and Gsα expression was unaffected by steroid hormones. These findings suggest that the mechanisms by which uterine stretch can promote myometrial contractions in humans are complex and may involve additional factors or that multiple gestations that do not result in preterm labor may have compensatory mechanisms for the increased uterine stretch by preventing aberrant CAP expression.

Uteroplacental Thrombosis and Decidual Hemorrhage

Vascular lesions of the placenta are commonly associated with preterm birth and preterm premature rupture of membranes (PPROM) (PROM refers to premature rupture of membranes, meaning before the onset of labor at any gestational age; hence, although "preterm PROM" is apparently redundant, it is not, given the definition of PROM, and is abbreviated here PPROM). Vascular lesions of the placenta have been reported in 34 percent of women with preterm delivery, 35 percent of women with PPROM, and 12 percent of uncomplicated deliveries at term (Arias et al., 1993). These lesions may be characterized as failure of the physiological transformation of the spiral arteries, atherosis, and maternal or fetal arterial thrombosis. The proposed mechanism linking vascular lesions to preterm birth is related to uteroplacental ischemia. Although the pathophysiology remains unclear, thrombin is thought to play a central role.

Independent of its critical role in coagulation, thrombin is a multifunctional protease that elicits the contractile activity of vascular, intestinal, and myometrial smooth muscle. Thrombin activates a unique set of receptors, including protease-activated receptor 1, protease-activated receptor 3, and protease-activated receptor 4 (Bohm et al., 1998; Grand et al., 1996). These transmembrane receptors are members of the heptahelical G-protein-coupled superfamily. Interaction with thrombin results in conformational changes that produce G-protein coupling and phospholipase C activation (Bohm et al., 1998; Grand et al., 1996). Phospholipase C activation initiates the biochemical reactions that lead to the release of intracellular calcium from the endoplasmic reticulum. The combination of intracellular calcium release and the influx of extracellular calcium cause cytosolic calcium oscillations that activate calmodulin, MLCK, actin, and myosin, resulting in phasic uterine contraction (Phillippe and Chien, 1998). Through these intracellular signaling events, thrombin acts as a classic uterotonic agonist.

Thrombin stimulates increases in basal tone and phasic contractions in longitudinal myometrial smooth muscle in vitro in a dose-dependent manner (Elovitz et al., 2000). Recently, these in vitro observations have been confirmed with in vivo models by using thrombin, whole blood, and thrombin inhibitors (Elovitz et al., 2000). Both thrombin and whole blood increased myometrial contractions in a dose-dependent fashion. However, myometrial contractility was significantly reduced by the addition of heparin, a known thrombin inhibitor. These in vitro and in vivo experiments provide a possible mechanistic explanation for the increased uterine activity clinically observed in abruptio placentae and preterm birth following first- or second-trimester bleeding.

A relationship between thrombin and PPROM may also exist. MMPs break down the extracellular matrix of the fetal membranes and the choriodecidua and contribute to PPROM, as discussed below. In vitro, thrombin significantly increases the levels of MMP-1, MMP-3, and MMP-9 protein expression in decidual cells and fetal membranes collected from uncomplicated term pregnancies (MacKenzie et al., 2004; Rosen et al., 2002; Stephenson et al., 2005). Thrombin also elicits a dose-dependent increase in decidual interleukin-8, a chemoattractant cytokine responsible for neutrophil recruitment (Lockwood et al., 2005). Overt abruptio placentae, an example of decidual hemorrhage, is also associated with a marked decidual infiltration of neutrophils, a rich source of proteases and matrix metalloproteinases (Lockwood et al., 2005). This may provide a mechanism for premature rupture of the membranes in the setting of decidual hemorrhage. Taken together, these investigations provide a mechanism for the relationship between increased intrauterine thrombin levels and PPROM.

However, confirmation of these in vitro observations in women has been difficult, largely because the direct measurement of thrombin levels is very difficult. Instead, the levels of thrombin-antithrombin III (TAT) complexes are usually measured as an indirect measurement of thrombin activation. In pregnant women TAT levels increase throughout gestation. TAT levels continue to increase with labor and reach a peak with the delivery of the placenta. A prospective cohort study found that pregnant women with preterm labor who delivered within 3 weeks of admission had significantly elevated TAT levels compared with those in control subjects (Elovitz et al., 2001). A receiver-operator-curve analysis generated in that study demonstrated that a TAT level of greater than 8.0 nanograms per milliliter had a sensitivity of 50 percent, a specificity of 91 percent, a positive predictive value of 80 percent, and a negative predictive value of 71 percent for the prediction of preterm delivery. These results add credence to the hypothesis that a significant portion of the cases of idiopathic preterm labor or PPROM may be caused by subclinical decidual bleeding. Subclinical decidual bleeding would provide the small quantities of thrombin that would significantly stimulate uterine activity. The recognition that thrombin plays an important role in contractility and in membrane degradation may help explain the association between vaginal bleeding, retroplacental hematomas, and preterm birth.

The relationship between elevated TAT levels and PPROM has also been explored in a nested case-control study in which plasma samples from women with eventual PPROM were examined in the second and third trimesters (Rosen et al., 2001). In both the second and the third trimesters, plasma TAT levels were significantly increased among women who experienced PPROM compared with the levels among women at term without PPROM.

Infection and Inflammation

Genital tract infections are strongly associated with preterm birth (Andrews et al., 2000; Goldenberg et al., 2000). These generally represent bacterial infections that ascend from the lower genital tract; viral infections have not been implicated as a significant cause of preterm birth. The sources of infection that have been linked to preterm birth include intrauterine infections, lower genital tract infections, systemic maternal infections, asymptomatic bacteruria, and maternal periodontitis.

Intrauterine infections are recognized as one of the most important and potentially preventable causes of preterm birth. These infections are thought to be responsible for up to 50 percent of extreme preterm births of less than 28 weeks of gestation, in which the rates of both neonatal mortality and neonatal morbidity are high. The prevalence of microbial invasion of the chorioamnion is 73 percent in women with a spontaneous preterm birth before 30 weeks of gestation and only 16 percent among women with indicated preterm delivery without labor (Hauth et al., 1998). The prevalence of histologic chorioamnionitis is inversely related to gestational age and occurs in 60 to 90 percent of gestations ending at between 20 and 24 weeks; microbial infection of the chorioamnion occurs in 60 percent of patients with preterm delivery (Hillier et al., 1988). Furthermore, the infections in a high proportion of women in preterm labor with evidence of microbial invasion of the amniotic fluid are refractory to standard tocolytic therapy and result in rapid preterm delivery (in 62 percent of women with evidence of microbial invasion but only 13 percent of women with sterile amniotic fluid) (Romero et al., 1991). This suggests that the pathophysiology of infection-associated preterm labor differs from that of idiopathic preterm labor.

Considerable evidence now suggests that the proinflammatory cytokine-prostaglandin cascade plays a central role in the pathogenesis of infection-associated preterm birth (Romero et al., 2005). These inflammatory mediators are produced by macrophages, decidual cells, and fetal membranes in response to bacteria or bacterial products. A role for selected cytokines in preterm labor is based on the following observations (see Gravett and Novy (1997) for a concise review of this literature): elevated concentrations of cytokines and prostaglandins in amniotic fluid are found in patients with intra-amniotic infection and preterm labor; in vitro, bacterial products stimulate the production of proinflammatory cytokines by human decidua; these cytokines, in turn, stimulate the production of prostaglandins by the amnion and the decidua; the administration of IL-1 to pregnant mice or nonhuman primates induces preterm labor, which can be prevented by the administration of IL-1 receptor antagonist protein.

Another complementary mechanism by which intrauterine infection leads to preterm birth is by activation of the fetal HPA axis. Increases in fetal cortisol and fetal adrenal androgen levels have been reported among the fetuses of women with intrauterine infections (Gravett et al., 2000; Yoon et al., 1998) and in nonhuman primates with experimental intra-amniotic infections (Gravett et al., 1996).

Gravett and colleagues (1994) have demonstrated in nonhuman primates that after experimental intra-amniotic infection with group B streptococci there are sequential increases in the levels of proinflammatory cytokines (IL-1β, TNF-α, IL-6, and IL-8), prostaglandins, and MMPs in amniotic fluid that precede increases in uterine contractility by 24 to 48 hours and that result in preterm delivery. This model provides a characterization of the temporal relationships among infection, inflammation, and labor. In complementary work with knockout mice, Hirsch and Wang (2005) have demonstrated that IL-6 is neither a sufficient nor a necessary component of this cascade to stimulate preterm labor but that IL-1β is sufficient. Thus, animal models, as discussed below, have contributed greatly to providing an understanding of the pathophysiology of infection-induced preterm birth.

The observations presented above suggest that infection-associated preterm birth is an acute event that occurs proximal to delivery. Recent evidence, however, suggests that midtrimester amniotic fluid infection with *Ureaplasma urealyticum* may result in preterm birth many weeks later (Greber et al., 2003; Gray et al., 1992). Furthermore, elevated midtrimester concentrations of IL-6, a proinflammatory cytokine, in amniotic fluid have been associated with preterm birth at 32 to 34 weeks of gestation (Wenstrom et al., 1996).

Although the strongest evidence associating preterm birth with infection is derived from intrauterine infections, considerable evidence also suggests that lower genital tract infections, especially bacterial vaginosis, contribute to prematurity. Bacterial vaginosis has been associated with preterm labor or delivery, amniotic fluid infection, chorioamnionitis, and postpartum endometritis. These associations have been reviewed extensively elsewhere (Kimberlin and Andrews, 1998) and are based on the findings of case-control and cohort studies that consistently demonstrate an approximate twofold increase in the rates of preterm labor or delivery among women with bacterial vaginosis (Kimberlin and Andrews, 1998); the recovery of bacterial vaginosis-associated microorganisms from the amniotic fluid of 30 percent of women with intact fetal membranes in preterm labor and subclinical amniotic fluid infection (Martius and Eschenbach, 1990); and the frequent recovery of bacterial vaginosis-associated microorganisms from the amniotic fluid of women with overt clinical amniotic fluid infection or from the chorioamnions of women with histological chorioamnionitis or preterm delivery (Hillier et al., 1988).

Although the magnitude of the increased risk for prematurity noted in these studies is modest (an approximately twofold increased risk compared with that for women without bacterial vaginosis), the total impact upon prematurity may be much greater given the high prevalence (20 percent) of bacterial vaginosis during pregnancy. It has been estimated that up to 6 percent of the cases of preterm delivery of infants with low birth weights may be attributable to bacterial vaginosis (Hillier et al., 1995).

Thus, bacterial vaginosis represents an important and potentially preventable cause of prematurity. However, trials of antibiotic treatment for bacterial vaginosis during pregnancy have met with mixed results (see Chapter 9 for a full review). Several studies have demonstrated reductions in the rates of preterm delivery or pregnancy loss among women at increased risk of prematurity by antibiotic treatment and eradication of bacterial vaginosis, whereas others have not (Hauth et al., 1995; McDonald et al., 1997b; Morales et al., 1994; Ugwumadu et al., 2003). However, a recent meta-analysis of all trials of antibiotic treatment for bacterial vaginosis during pregnancy did not reveal a consistent reduction in the rates of preterm birth or pregnancy morbidities, in part because of heterogeneity of the data (McDonald et al., 2005; Varma and Gupta, 2006). (An analysis of these treatment trials is discussed in detail in Chapter 9.)

Preterm birth has also been associated with maternal systemic infection (and is largely attributable to the severity of maternal illness) and, more recently, with maternal periodontal disease. Periodontal disease is an anaerobic bacterial infection of the mouth that affects up to 50 percent of the population, including pregnant women. Maternal periodontal disease has been associated with several adverse pregnancy outcomes, including preterm birth, preeclampsia, and fetal loss (Boggess et al., 2003; Jeffcoat et al., 2001a,b; Offenbacher et al., 1996). In a recent review of 25 studies, 18 found an association between periodontal disease and adverse outcomes of pregnancy, with odds ratios for preterm birth or low birth weight of 1.1 to 20 (Xiong et al., 2005). Further, three clinical trials of periodontal treatment suggested a 50 percent reduction in the risk of preterm birth.

The mechanisms responsible for preterm birth in association with periodontal disease are not completely understood. Experimental evidence from studies with rabbits suggests that the oral pathogens associated with periodontitis can gain access to the systemic circulation and can be recovered from amniotic fluid or the organism's DNA can be recovered from the placenta (Boggess et al., 2005a). Additionally, the gram-negative anaerobes associated with periodontitis may serve as a source of the lipopolysaccharide endotoxin that increases the levels of proinflammatory mediators, including cytokines and prostaglandins.

One conundrum for infection-associated preterm birth is that the majority of women who have lower genital tract infections, systemic infections, or periodontal disease do not deliver prematurely. Hence, the host inflammatory response to a potential pathogen must play a critical role in preterm birth. Cytokines (and some Toll-like receptors) are genetically very pleomorphic. It is likely that genetic differences in inflammatory responsiveness play a major role in determining whether or not a preterm birth occurs. (This concept of the gene-environment interaction is discussed in detail in Chapter 7.)

Implantation Errors

Traditionally, preterm delivery was thought to result from events that occurred at about the time of labor onset. The finding of elevated CRH levels before midgestation in association with preterm delivery suggests that some events triggering preterm delivery may be set in motion earlier in pregnancy than was previously thought (Hobel et al., 1999; Leung et al., 1999; McLean and Smith, 1999; McLean et al., 1999). A growing body of evidence now suggests that complications that become apparent relatively late in pregnancy, including preterm delivery, may actually reflect errors that occurred much earlier in placental development, beginning with implantation of the blastocyst in the uterus.

Implantation occurs approximately 6 or 7 days after conception and consists of three stages: apposition, adhesion, and invasion (reviewed by Norwitz et al. [2001]). Successful implantation is the end result of complex synchronized interactions between a receptive uterus and an activated blastocyst. Ovarian estrogen and progesterone transform the prereceptive uterus to a receptive state via a number of locally expressed growth factors, cytokines, transcription factors, vasoactive mediators in the uterus, whereas uterine-derived catecholestrogen and embryonic chorionic gonadotrophin are involved in implantation (Cameo et al., 2004). However, many of these data are derived from animal studies, and it is difficult to determine precisely what factors are critical in human implantation. Once implantation begins, a brief interval of stable adhesion involving adhesion molecules and other proteins is followed by a much longer period during which trophoblasts invade the uterus. The molecular mechanisms that regulate trophoblastic invasion are not well understood but probably involve multiple growth factors and cytokines, including leukemia-inhibiting factor, a heparin-binding epidermal growth factor, IL-1 and its receptors, and vascular endothelial growth factor (Dey et al., 2004; Kayisli et al., 2004; Norwitz et al., 2001). IL-1 appears to play a key role in implantation. For example, IL-1 induces the expression of COX-2 and MMP-9, both of which are central to implantation and decidualization (Fazleabas et al., 2004). Additionally, IL-1α also stimulates the production of uterine IL-10, a Th2-type cytokine that plays a crucial role in the maintenance of pregnancy, in part by inhibiting the synthesis of Th1-type cytokines and suppressing the activities of natural killer-like cells and other inflammatory cells at the uteroplacental interface (Kelly et al., 2001; Vigano et al., 2003). However, data derived from humans remains incomplete, and there is a need for more research in this area.

A direct causal link between implantation problems and spontaneous preterm delivery has not been established in animal or human studies; nonetheless, indirect evidence suggests that this may be an important area for further research. The nonpregnant endometrial cavity is frequently colonized by microorganisms (Arechavaleta-Velasco et al., 2002; Romero et al., 2004b), and subclinical endometrial infection or inflammation may impair implantation or placentation, possibly by eliciting an antitrophoblast immune response that results in apoptosis, reduced trophoblast invasion and remodeling of the deciduas and uterine arterial vessels, and the arrest of early embryonic development (Romero et al., 2004b). This raises the possibility that inflammation in the endometrium around the time of implantation may contribute to subsequent preterm delivery. Furthermore, a normal pregnancy is characterized by a shift from a proinflammatory Th1-type response toward an anti-inflammatory Th2-type response (Marzi et al., 1996). One untested hypothesis is that women with microbial invasion of the endometrium may develop a persistent proinflammatory response in the endometrium (a Th1-type bias). This, in turn, could predispose the woman toward damage of the conceptus, implantation failure, spontaneous abortion, and preterm delivery. Of note, pregnancies complicated by preeclampsia, an important cause of indicated preterm delivery, also show reduced trophoblastic invasion and spiral artery remodeling as well as increased trophoblast apoptosis. No study, however, has directly linked preeclampsia to peri-implantation endometrial infection or inflammation. A recent study showed that modest undernutrition (defined as caloric restriction) in sheep commencing before conception and continuing for only 30 days thereafter induces premature delivery (Bloomfield et al., 2003). The undernourished ewes had higher ACTH levels throughout gestation, with a precocious rise in cortisol levels in half of them. This raises the possibility that the placental clock can be set by undernutrition at about the time of conception, resulting in accelerated maturation of the fetal HPA axis, leading to preterm birth.

Summary of the Pathways to Preterm Birth

Preterm birth has many potential pathways (Figure 6-2). In the past, obstetricians and epidemiologists have had a tendency to combine, for statistical purposes, all preterm births occurring between 22 and 37 weeks of gestation. This has obscured the opportunity to study preterm birth as a final common end point and has led to uniform, largely empirical, and unsuccessful treatment strategies. It is now clear that the causes of preterm labor and multifactorial and vary according to gestational age. Each pathway to preterm labor can be characterized by its own unique upstream initiators of preterm parturition. Nonetheless, all share common downstream effectors of preterm contractions. For example, whether it is related to stress or infection, fetal HPA activation plays a role. Similarly, whether they are related to infection, uterine overdistension, or PPROM, MMPs play a role. Finally, regardless of the unique initiating circumstances myometrial contractility is mediated by prostaglandins. The recognition that preterm delivery is the common end result of a myriad of unique initiators provides an opportunity for research into unique upstream and common downstream interventions that can be used to reduce the risks of preterm birth.

Important areas of research on the pathways to preterm birth remain

- the need for better understanding of human implantation and placentation,
- the need for improved early diagnostic tests to better discriminate between the many pathways to preterm birth,
- recognition that preterm birth is multifactorial and represents only a common end point for a myriad of unique, independent etiologies, and
- the development of rational intervention strategies that target unique upstream initiators and common downstream effectors of preterm birth.

Finding 6-1: Preterm parturition has heterogeneous origins that result in common biological pathways and that lead to relatively few clinical presentations (e.g., preterm labor, preterm rupture of membranes, and cervical insufficiency).

PREMATURE RUPTURE OF MEMBRANES

Regardless of the etiology or mechanistic pathway to spontaneous preterm labor, preterm birth is usually preceded by PPROM. PPROM accounts for approximately 40 percent of preterm births (Shubert et al., 1992) and represents a final common pathway to preterm birth. Thus, an understanding of the mechanistic pathways leading to PPROM is important in understanding the biological basis of prematurity. Preterm prelabor rupture of membranes has been associated with intrauterine infection, tobacco use, abruption, multiple gestations, previous PPROM, previous cervical surgery or laceration, a short cervix as detected by ultrasound, genetic connective tissue disorders, and vitamin C deficiency (Asrat, 2001; Asrat et al., 1991;

Barbaras, 1966; Major et al., 1995; Odibo et al., 2002; Sadler et al., 2004; Spinello et al., 1994; Wideman et al., 1964).

Potential Mechanisms of PPROM

The fetal membranes (amnion and chorion) abut the maternal decidua and rest upon a collagenous basement membrane of type II and IV collagen. Beneath this layer is a fibrous layer that contains collagen types I, III, V, and VI. Thus, collagen provides major structural strength for the membranes. Membrane rupture is a process similar to wound healing, a process in which collagen is degraded (Malak and Bell, 1994). MMPs are the only family of enzymes that act to degrade collagen and play a major role in tissue remodeling. MMP-1 and MMP-8 are collagenases that act to degrade collagen types I, II, and III. MMP-2 and MMP-9 are gelatinases that degrade collagen types IV and V.

The activities of MMPs are regulated at several levels but, most importantly, are regulated by tissue inhibitors of MMPs (TIMPs). A balance between activators and tissue inhibitors of metalloproteinases controls metalloprotease activity. An increased ratio of MMP-9 to TIMP type 1 (TIMP-1) is associated with a decrease in the tensile strength of fetal membranes. Menon and Fortunato (2004) reviewed the role of MMPs in PPROM, with the overall hypothesis that a host inflammatory response inappropriately activates MMPs in the (ECM). Specifically, MMP type 1 to 3, 8, 9, and 14 messenger RNAs are detected in the amnion and chorion; and their levels increase in the amniotic fluid in PPROM (Menon and Fortunato, 2004). MMP-9 concentrations are increased in the amniotic fluid of patients with PPROM and to a lesser extent in patients with preterm birth (Fortunato et al., 2000a). Increased levels of pro-MMP-9 are found overlying the cervix in term gestation. MMP types 2 and 9 degrade type IV collagen, which is found in the basement membranes of the extracellular matrix (ECM).

Epidemiological, histological, and microbiological studies indicate that changes in fetal membrane production of MMP may be caused by infection or inflammation (reviewed by Menon and Fortunato [2004]). In vitro studies demonstrate an increase in MMP levels and a decrease in TIMP levels when the amniochorion is exposed to bacterial products (Fortunato et al., 1999). Several species of bacteria produce collagenases and decrease the bursting load and elasticity and work to rupture the membranes in vitro (MacGregor et al., 1987). Infection has been associated with an increase in MMP levels and a decrease in TIMP levels in the amniotic cavity. MMP-9 levels are increased in the amniotic fluid of women with intrauterine infections (Fortunato et al., 1999). MMP-2 levels are increased in membranes exposed to lipopolysaccharide in vitro (Fortunato et al., 2000b).

The mechanisms by which infection causes PPROM are likely multifactorial. Bacteria may directly secrete proteases that degrade collagen (MacGregor et al., 1987). Some bacterial species produce phospholipase A_2, which acts to increase the levels of arachidonic acid, a prostaglandin precursor (Bejar et al., 1981). PGE2 decreases collagen synthesis in fetal membranes. Prostaglandin increases MMP-1 and MMP-3 levels in fibroblasts. Proinflammatory cytokines such as IL-1 and TNF-α also increase MMP levels and decrease TIMP levels in cultured amniocytes (So, 1993). In nonhuman primates, intrauterine infection with group B streptococci stimulates both proinflammatory cytokine and MMP-9 production (Vadillo-Ortega et al., 2002). Reactive oxygen species (ROS) resulting from immune cell signaling may also increase MMP levels and contribute to PPROM (Woods, 2001). Many clinical risk factors for PPROM, such as smoking, vaginal bleeding, cocaine use, and intra-amniotic infection, may also increase ROS levels by a variety of mechanisms. Exposure to superoxide increases MMP-9 activity and stimulates the release of arachidonic acid, a precursor to PGE2.

Amniotic fluid concentrations of MMP may also be increased in PPROM in the absence of infection. In vitro data indicate that both thrombin and thrombin receptor agonist peptide type 14 also increase MMP-9 concentrations (Stephenson et al., 2005). Thrombin increases MMP-9 levels in cultures with amniochorion. Thrombin also increases MMP-3 levels, and progesterone decreases this effect in decidual cell cultures (MacKenzie et al., 2004). Stretching of the membranes in multifetal gestations or hydramnios may result in PPROM by increasing PGE2, IL-8, and MMP-1 activities (Maradny et al., 1996).

The mechanisms by which decreased collagen content causes rupture of the fetal membranes are unknown. Rupture of the membranes may be mediated by apoptosis or programmed cell death following degradation of the extracellular matrix. Human fetal membranes have more apoptotic cells near the rupture site in women with premature rupture of membranes (Leppert et al., 1996). MMP-2 gene activation coincides with increased apoptosis in fetal membranes in PPROM (Fortunato et al., 2000a). The MMP-2 gene promoter has a transcription factor binding site that can be bound by protein p53, an intracellular regulator of apoptosis (Bian and Sun, 1997). Fetal membranes have high levels of expression of several components of the FAS-caspase apoptosis pathway. Women with PPROM had higher levels of proapoptotic proteins such as p53, Bax, and caspase, whereas the membranes of women with preterm labor had higher levels of Bcl2, an antiapoptotic protein. Investigators have also found that FAS and TNF-α-mediated apoptotic pathways are up-regulated in PPROM but not in preterm labor without premature rupture of membranes (reviewed by Menon and Fortunato, 2004).

ANIMAL MODELS FOR PRETERM BIRTH AND NEONATAL SEQUELAE

Although most animal species do not have significant rates of spontaneous preterm birth, there is much interest in the use of relevant animal models to elucidate the mechanisms of preterm birth and the neonatal sequelae of prematurity and to develop rationale and efficacious treatment and prevention strategies. However, in choosing an appropriate animal model, a necessary caveat is that many species differ from humans in the length of gestation and the number of fetuses, the type of placentation, the hormonal control of parturition, and the timing of fetal organ maturation (Figure 6-3 and Table 6-2). For example, lower mammalian species such as rats, rabbits, and mice have short gestational periods with multiple fetuses and delayed maturation of the fetal brain. Sheep, another commonly used experimental model, have a longer gestation and a singleton pregnancy, similar to humans, but have different placentation; and parturition is initiated by abrupt increases in cortisol levels, which is not seen in humans. In all of these species, parturition is preceded by systemic progesterone withdrawal, which is not seen in humans (refer to the works of Challis et al. [2000] and Elovitz and Mrinalini [2004] for reviews). Finally, there may be species differences in implantation and placentation. Further research in this area is critical. Recent research with nonhuman primates suggests that they have a reproductive biology that is the most similar to that of humans and represent the most appropriate model with which to study preterm birth; however, the cost and restricted availability of nonhuman primates limit their use (Elovitz and Mrinalini, 2004).

Despite their differences in reproductive biology, mice continue to play a major role in prematurity-related research. Their ready availability, low cost, and ability to be genetically manipulated (i.e., gene-knockout models are available) make the mouse model appealing. However, their short length of gestation (19 to 20 days) and delayed fetal maturation, especially of the central nervous system, limit the ability to generalize observations for mice to humans.

Much can be learned about the mechanisms of preterm birth by use of appropriate animal models. However, each species has distinct advantages and disadvantages that must be carefully considered in asking and answering important research questions relevant to preterm birth and neonatal sequelae.

Animal Models of Preterm Birth

Spontaneous preterm birth occurs infrequently in most species. This has limited research in this area to specific pharmacological or environmen-

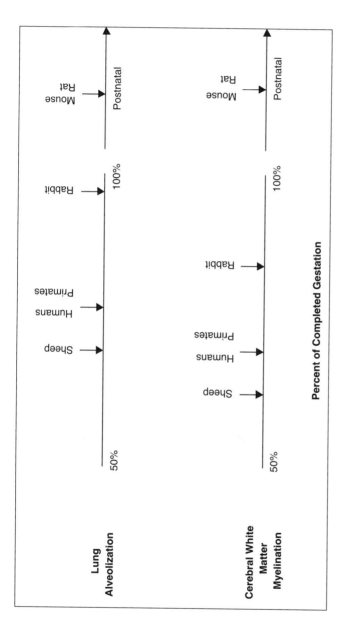

FIGURE 6-3 Comparative gestational ages at critical maturational steps in fetal development among different species relevant to neonatal morbidity. Vertical arrows indicate when lung alveolar development or preoligodendrocyte development (oligodendrocytes are responsible for myelination) begins. This schema indicates that maturation of the lungs and cerebrum, two organs with important contributions to neonatal morbidity and mortality, in sheep and nonhuman primates most closely parallel development in humans. In contrast, rabbits and rodents experience equivalent maturational sequences only near term or postnatally, limiting their role in ascertaining the relationships among the causes of prematurity and its consequences.

TABLE 6-2 Reproductive Characteristics of Animal Models Used to Study Parturition

Species	Gestational Length (days)	Placentation	Fetus
Mouse	18	Nonvillous hemochorial	Multiple fetuses; delayed myelination of cerebral white matter
Rat	21	Nonvillous hemochorial	Multiple fetuses; delayed myelination of cerebral white matter
Rabbit	31	Discoid hemoendothelial	Multiple fetuses
Sheep	150	Cotyledonary syndesmochorial	Single fetus; myelination of cerebral white matter similar to that in humans; fetal growth similar to that in humans
Nonhuman primate	167	Discoid hemochorial	Most similar to humans; single fetus; myelination of cerebral white matter similar to that in humans; fetal growth similar to that in humans

NOTE: For reference, human parturition is characterized by a single fetus with a gestational length of 280 days and discoid hemochorial placentation; fetal hypothalamic adrenal axis activation, which is possibly influenced by placental CRH, occurs before parturition; fetal

tal interventions that result in preterm birth. Pharmacological administration of RU-486, a progesterone antagonist, leads to preterm delivery in rodents but not in nonhuman primates (Dudley et al., 1996; Garfield et al., 1987; Haluska et al., 1994). Administration of cortisol (Grigsby et al., 2000) or maternal starvation (protein and caloric restriction) (Kumarasamy et al., 2005) leads to preterm delivery in sheep.

Reproductive Biology	Advantages	Disadvantages
Corpus luteum is source of progesterone; progesterone withdrawal precedes parturition	Inexpensive and readily available; genetic manipulationis possible (knockout variants are available)	Progesterone dependence; delayed cerebral maturation; short gestation
Corpus luteum is source of progesterone; progesterone withdrawal precedes parturition	Inexpensive and readily available	Progesterone dependence; delayed cerebral maturation; short gestation
Corpus luteum is source of progesterone; progesterone withdrawal precedes parturition	Transcervical inoculation of infectious stimuli possible	Intermediate expense; progesterone dependence
Cortisol surge precedes parturition	Continuous access to intrauterine environment and myometrial contractility by chronic instrumentation	Expense; cortisol and progesterone dependence
Fetal HPA activation	Most similar to human parturition; continuous access to intrauterine environment and myometrial contractility by chronic instrumentation	Expense; limited availability

cerebral white matter maturation occurs at about 70 percent of the length of gestation; and no systemic progesterone withdrawal occurs.

SOURCE: Modified, with permission, from Elovitz and Mrinalini (2004).

The most compelling data from animal models are derived from studies of the role of infection and inflammation in preterm birth. Research with nonhuman primates has demonstrated that following experimental intra-amniotic fluid infection, sequential increases in the levels of proinflammatory cytokines, prostaglandins, and MMPs precede the onset of preterm labor by 24 to 48 hours (Gravett et al., 1994; Vadillo-Ortega et al., 2002).

This research has also shown that pregnancy can be significantly prolonged by treatment with antibiotics and immunomodulators but not with antibiotics alone (Gravett et al., 2003).

Mice, rats, rabbits, sheep, and nonhuman primates have all been used as models for infection-induced preterm delivery. Regardless of the inciting stimuli (e.g., lipopolysaccharide, live microorganisms, or cytokines) or the route of administration, all of these models have confirmed the central role of the inflammatory response and proinflammatory cytokines in infection-induced preterm birth (see the review by Elovitz and Mrinalini [2004]).

The inflammatory system is redundant; that is, many proinflammatory cytokines act to up-regulate other proinflammatory cytokines. Hence, the role of individual cytokines in preterm labor has been difficult to ascertain. Recent work by Hirsch and Wang (2005), however, with genetically altered gene-knockout mice has demonstrated a central role for IL-1α but not IL-6, in infection-induced preterm labor. That important work demonstrates the utility of animal models in elucidating the mechanisms of preterm labor and points the way to effective intervention strategies.

Animal Models of Neonatal Sequelae

Two of the most important neonatal sequelae of preterm birth, especially in the setting of infection and inflammation, are periventricular white matter disease (PWMD) and neonatal lung disease (Dammann et al., 2005). Animal models have been particularly useful in elucidating the role of prematurity in these adverse neonatal outcomes.

Periventricular Leukomalacia and Cerebral White Matter Lesions

PWMD is detected in a significant proportion of premature infants and is strongly associated with adverse outcomes, including motor, perceptual, visual, behavioral, and cognitive disorders (see Chapter 10 for a further discussion of PWMD). The incidence of PWMD in preterm infants ranges from 3 to 20 percent, depending on the method of diagnosis and the extent of prematurity (Blumenthal, 2004). Approximately 10 percent of very low birth weight infants develop cerebral palsy, and 90 percent of these cases are thought to be due to PWMD (Blumenthal, 2004; Hack and Taylor, 2000; Wood et al., 2000).

PWMD includes a spectrum of cerebral injuries, ranging from focal cystic necrotic lesions (periventricular leukomalacia) to extensive, diffuse white matter lesions. Focal lesions occur in the deep white matter and are characterized by the necrosis of all cellular elements (axons, oligodendrocytes [OLs], and astrocytes), with subsequent cyst formation. Diffuse lesions, on the other hand, are characterized by more widespread, cell-specific injury to OL precursors (pre-OLs), with the subsequent impairment of myelinogenesis.

The pathogenesis of PWMD in the premature brain has been studied extensively in both in vitro and in vivo models (Back and Rivkees, 2004; Hagberg et al., 2002; Inder et al., 2004). A complex interplay of factors related to cerebrovascular immaturity appears to predispose the preterm periventricular white matter to injury. The major interacting factors include an underdeveloped vascular system, impaired cerebrovascular regulation, and pre-OL populations that are more vulnerable to oxidative stress and injury (Back and Rivkees, 2004).

Underdeveloped Vascular System

The vascular supply to the brain principally consists of the long and short penetrating arteries, neither of which is fully developed in the premature brain. Any decrease in cerebral blood flow can therefore lead to ischemia in the "watershed" areas of the white matter. Decreased blood flow to the long penetrating arteries results in severe ischemia and subsequent focal damage to the deep white matter, whereas decreased blood flow to the short penetrating arteries leads to moderate ischemia and subsequent diffuse pre-OL-specific damage in the border zones between the long penetrating arteries and at the end zones of the short penetrating arteries (subcortical areas).

A number of different animal models have been developed to evaluate the role of hypoperfusion in PWMD. These models have used transient or permanent unilateral or bilateral carotid artery ligation, combined hypoxia-ischemia, umbilical cord occlusion, or hemorrhagic hypotension. In the vast majority of these models, however, both the white matter and the gray matter are affected. Two models in which the distribution and the morphology of PWMD more closely resemble those in the brains of human infants born preterm include a neonatal dog model in which bilateral ligation of the common carotids is used (Yoshioka et al., 1994) and a fetal sheep model in which hemorrhagic hypotension is used (Matsuda et al., 1999).

A physiological correlate of these anatomic factors is the observation of extremely low level of blood flow to the cerebral white matter in premature infants compared with that in term infants and adults (Altman et al., 1988; Greisen, 1986). This suggests that there is a minimal margin for safety for blood flow to cerebral white matter in such infants. Direct experimental evidence that human periventricular white matter is selectively susceptible to hypotension and ischemic injury, however, is lacking.

Impairment of Cerebrovascular Regulation

Studies have indicated that a significant proportion of ventilated premature infants (up to 53 percent) have impairment of cerebrovascular regulation (Tsuji et al., 2000). In these infants the cerebral circulation is pressure passive, and therefore, as the blood pressure falls, so, too, does cerebral blood flow. Again, a minimal margin of safety may exist, leading to ischemia in the watershed areas of the white matter. In a child or an adult, an intact cerebrovascular regulation system is in place that keeps the cerebral blood flow constant over a wide range of blood pressures through appropriate compensatory vessel dilation and vasoconstriction (Volpe, 2001).

Studies with preterm lambs indicate that at an early stage during maturation of the cerebrovascular autoregulatory system, the range of blood pressures over which cerebral blood flow is maintained constant, although present, is particularly narrow (Papile et al., 1985; Szymonowicz et al., 1990). This indicates that even premature infants with newly intact cerebrovascular autoregulation would be vulnerable to modest declines in blood pressure.

The relationship between cerebral blood flow and PWMD is further supported by clinical studies that demonstrate a correlation between PWMD and neonatal events expected to cause cerebral ischemia (severe hypotension, marked hypocarbia, hypoplastic left heart syndrome, patent ductus arteriosus with retrograde cerebral diastolic flow, and severe illness requiring extracorporeal membrane oxygenation) (Volpe, 2001).

Pre-OL Vulnerability

Before 32 weeks of gestation in humans, 90 percent of OLs are in an early stage of development and are known as pre-OLs (Back et al., 2001). Several lines of evidence from both in vitro and in vivo experimental models, outlined below, support the role of targeted pre-OL death in the pathogenesis of PWMD. Pre-OLs are exquisitely sensitive to injury and death by a number of different mechanisms.

Studies with neonatal and fetal rats, rabbits, and sheep have provided both direct and indirect evidence of increases in the levels of oxygen free radicals in the developing brain following hypoxia-ischemia (Bagenholm et al., 1997, 1998; Hasegawa et al., 1993; Rosenberg et al., 1989). The generation of free radicals is most pronounced during the initial period of reperfusion. The type of free radical involved varies somewhat by experimental model but principally involves superoxide anion and hydrogen peroxide. In vitro and in vivo neonatal rodent models of hypoxia-ischemia have demonstrated that pre-OLs are highly susceptible to free radical attack, whereas mature OLs are resistant (Back et al., 2002). Studies with neonatal piglets subjected to hypoxia-ischemia have shown that the mechanism of pre-OL death from free radical attack is apoptosis (Yue et al., 1997). This has been confirmed in in vitro studies and has been suggested by autopsy studies of the brains of human infants born preterm (Back et al., 1998; Gilles et al., 1983).

In addition to being more vulnerable to free radicals, pre-OLs tend to accumulate free radicals, whereas mature OLs do not. Information derived from animal models (mouse, rat, and lamb models) and limited analyses of autopsied brains of human infants born preterm suggest that there is a delay in the development and the reactivity of antioxidant defenses, especially those involving glutathione peroxidase and catalase (Juurlink, 1997; Volpe, 2001). These enzymes are involved in the detoxification of hydrogen peroxide. If hydrogen peroxide accumulates and iron ions (Fe^{2+}) are present, the Fenton reaction will take place, producing the deadly hydroxyl radical.

Glutamate has also been implicated in rodent models of PWMD (Deng et al., 2004; Follett et al., 2000; Liu et al., 2002). Hypoxia-ischemia in the preterm infant brain leads to coagulation necrosis and the disruption of axons. Axon disruption leads to the leakage of glutamate into the extracellular space. In addition, with an altered brain energy supply, the level of glutamate uptake by astrocytes and neurons is reduced. Additional sources of glutamate include the reversal of glutamate transporter function in astrocytes and OLs and cytokine effects on astrocytes, among other factors.

Glutamate can cause the destruction of pre-OLs by either receptor-mediated or non-receptor-mediated mechanisms (Volpe, 2001). Activation of the α-amino-3-hydroxy-5-methyl-4-isoxazole propionate (AMPA) and kainite type of glutamate receptor has been shown to lead to pre-OL death in culture and in rodent models of PWMD (Follett et al., 2000; Gan et al., 1997). This occurs only in developing OLs and not in mature OLs. In an immature rat model, Follet and colleagues (2000a,b) showed that such injuries could be prevented by the administration of a receptor antagonist such as 6-nitro-7-sulfamoylbenzo(f)quinoxaline-2,3-dione or topiramate, an anticonvulsant drug.

In a non-receptor-mediated mechanism, glutamate causes glutathione depletion in pre-OLs, leading to free radical generation and subsequent cell death. This is mediated by activation of a glutamate-cystine exchange transporter, whereby glutamate uptake results in the efflux of cystine, intracellular cystine depletion, and impaired glutathione synthesis (Oka et al., 1993).

Maternal or Fetal Infection or Inflammation and Cerebral White Matter Lesions

Recently, the role of intrauterine infections in the pathogenesis of periventricular leukomalacia and cerebral palsy has become a major focus of research (Dammann and Leviton, 1998; Grether and Nelson, 1997; Leviton, 1993). A growing body of evidence suggests that maternal genital tract infections, particularly intrauterine and intra-amniotic infections, may be important and potentially preventable causes of periventricular white matter damage and cerebral palsy. The association between intrauterine infection and cerebral palsy is supported by human observational studies and animal experimental studies. Bejar and colleagues (1988) observed that the risk of cerebral white matter damage was 9.4-fold greater among preterm neonates with purulent amniotic fluid than among those with nonpurulent fluid. Similarly, Grether and Nelson (1997) observed cerebral white matter damage in association with maternal intrapartum fever or chorioamnionitis. A recent meta-analysis of 30 human observational studies by use of a random-effects model reported that clinical chorioamnionitis was significantly associated with both cerebral palsy (relative risk [RR] 1.9; 95% confidence interval [CI] 1.4–2.5) and periventricular leukomalacia (RR 3.0; 95% CI 2.2–4.0) in preterm infants (Wu and Colford, 2000). Among term infants, a significant association was also found between clinical chorioamnionitis and cerebral palsy (RR 4.7; 95% CI 1.3–16.2) Clinical studies have reported elevated concentrations of proinflammatory cytokines, including IL-6, IL-1, and TNF-α, in amniotic fluid and elevated concentrations of IL-6 in umbilical cord plasma among neonates with periventricular leukomalacia or cerebral palsy (Nelson et al., 1998; Yoon et al., 1996, 1997a); increased expression of IL-6 and TNF-α within the brain lesions of infants who died with periventricular leukomalacia has also been reported (Yoon et al., 1997b).

Animal models consisting of pregnant rabbits with experimental intrauterine infection have demonstrated brain white matter lesions characterized by increased karyorrhexis, rarefaction, disorganization of the white matter, and increased apoptosis in the cerebral cortex (Yoon et al., 1997c). Finally, in a feline model of *Escherichia coli* endotoxin-induced cerebral white matter injury, daily intraperitoneal injections of endotoxin resulted in injury of the telencephalic white matter of newborn kittens (Gilles et al., 1976). One shortcoming of these animal studies is a lack of detailed monitoring of adverse systemic events associated with endotoxin, including hypoglycemia, acidosis, and hypotension. Subsequent studies with rabbit pups (Ando et al., 1988) and neonatal dogs (Young et al., 1983) demonstrated that cerebral white matter lesions occurred within 1 to 3 days of endotoxin exposure in the setting of transient acute arterial hypotension. Hence, the diverse forms of white matter pathology induced by endotoxin or infection might be due, at least in part, to systemic vascular effects.

Neonatal Lung Disease

The premature infant faces primarily two lung-related injuries: acute injury (respiratory distress syndrome [RDS]) and chronic or progressive lung injury (bronchopulmonary dysplasia [BPD]) (also see Chapter 10 for a discussion). A complex interplay of factors plays into the risk of these injuries, including incomplete development (immaturity), mechanical ventilation, oxidative stress, and inflammation (Zoban and Cerny, 2003).

Neonatal RDS is an acute lung process due to a deficiency in surfactant. It ranks as the sixth most common cause of death among newborns in the United States and occurs almost exclusively in premature infants, occurring in excess of 80 percent of infants born before 27 weeks of gestation (Bancalari, 2002; Lemons et al., 2001). The incidence and severity are dependent on the infant's gestational age at birth and birth weight. Although the outcome of RDS has improved in recent years, the incidence and severity of complications continue to present significant morbidities. Complications may include pneumothorax; intraventricular hemorrhage; chronic lung disease (BPD); or even respiratory failure, leading to death.

BPD, also known as neonatal chronic lung disease, is another important cause of respiratory illness in preterm newborns. BPD is usually defined by the requirement of oxygen at 36 weeks since the mother's last menstrual period and is characterized by small airway injury, dilated alveolar ducts, and decreased alveolarization. The incidence of BPD is directly related to birth weight, with rates of 7 percent in infants weighing 1,241 to 1,500 grams, 15 percent in infants weighing 1,001 to 1,240 grams, 34 percent in infants weighing 751 to 1,000 grams, and 52 percent in infants weighing 501 to 750 grams (Lemons et al., 2001).

Normal Lung Development

Fetal lung development is divided into the pseudoglandular, canalicular, and saccular-alveolar stages on the basis of histological appearance (Cardoso and Williams, 2000; Zeltner and Burri, 1987). The pseudoglandular stage takes place at between 7 and 17 weeks of gestation, the canalicular stage takes place at between 16 and 24 weeks of gestation, and the saccular-alveolar stage takes place at between 24 and 40 weeks of gestation. The saccular and alveolar stages overlap beginning at approximately 32 weeks of gestation, when secondary septation begins the process of alveolarization. Microvascular development occurs in parallel with alveolarization and continues for several months after term birth. Alveolarization and the associated vascularization are the critical terminal stages of lung development. The increase in alveoli, lung volume, and lung surface area establishes the anatomic potential for gas exchange and thus the potential for fetal viability.

Surfactant production by type II alveolar cells begins at about 34 weeks of gestation. Normal production is achieved by the time that the fetal lungs are mature, at about 37 weeks of gestation. Pulmonary surfactant is a complex lipoprotein made up of six phospholipids and four apoproteins (Jobe and Ikegami, 2001). Functionally, dipalmitoylphosphatidylcholine, or lecithin, is the principal phospholipid. The components of surfactant are synthesized in the Golgi apparatus of the endoplasmic reticulum of type II alveolar cells. The surfactant is then secreted by exocytosis, ultimately forming monolayers in the air-liquid interface inside the alveoli. Surfactant is necessary for reducing the surface tension of the liquid lining and therefore decreasing the pressure needed to keep the alveoli inflated. A deficiency in surfactant leads to high surface tension, making it difficult to inflate the alveoli. Alveolar collapse subsequently occurs, leading to diffuse atelectasis and decreased compliance. Any disruption in the process of lung development can lead to both short-term and long-term effects on lung function in newborns, as described below.

Surfactant Deficiency

Surfactant deficiency is the primary cause of RDS and has been demonstrated in both animals (sheep) and humans. Studies with preterm rabbits have found that surfactant-deficient lungs do not accumulate much gas on inflation until pressures exceed 25 centimeters of water (cm H_2O) (Jobe, 1993). Surfactant treatment results in a striking decrease in the opening pressure to about 15 cm H_2O. This decrease in opening pressure allows more units to open and therefore leads to more uniform inflation and a decreased risk of overdistension.

Neonatal surfactant therapy reduces the rate of mortality from RDS and overall infant mortality rates (Soll and Morley, 2001). In addition, surfactant treatment decreases the incidence of pneumothorax, oxygen requirements, and ventilatory requirements during the first several days of life. Although neonatal surfactant therapy has had an impressive effect on the incidence of RDS, it has not been seen to have an effect on BPD. Presumably, infants who survive RDS with surfactant treatments are those who are more likely to go on to develop BPD. Further studies are necessary to test this hypothesis.

Disruption of Alveolarization

Recent pathologic analyses of very low birth weight human infants who have died of BPD demonstrate an arrest of alveolar development, with the lungs containing fewer and larger alveoli (Thibeault et al., 2000). Numerous exposures common to the care of the premature infant have been shown to disrupt normal alveolarization. These exposures include hypoxia or hyperoxia, mechanical ventilation, nutritional deficits, glucocorticoids, and inflammatory mediators.

Both hypoxia and hyperoxia disrupt septation and therefore reduce the surface area for gas exchange. Rats exposed to increased oxygen concentrations are found to have severely disrupted alveolarization (Randell et al., 1989; Thibeault et al., 1990). Abnormalities, including decreased pulmonary septation, increased terminal space diameter, and decreased surface area, persist even after recovery.

Mechanical ventilation can also interfere with alveolar and vascular development, as has been demonstrated in preterm baboons and sheep (Jobe and Bancalari, 2001). Coalson and colleagues (1999) studied preterm baboons and found that mechanical ventilation with 100 percent oxygen severely reduced the number of alveoli. The same interference with septation was noted after surfactant treatment and ventilation but without exposure to large amounts of supplemental oxygen.

Glucocorticoid treatment can cause a profound arrest in alveolarization, as seen in many animal models, including rodents, monkeys, and sheep. In preterm mice and rats, glucocorticoid treatment has been found to cause permanent abnormalities in alveolar and vascular development (Massaro and Massaro, 2000). In preterm monkeys, glucocorticoid administration during the saccular stage of lung development leads to a decrease in the mesenchyme, a lower gas volume, and fewer alveoli (Johnson et al., 1978). In preterm sheep, glucocorticoid treatment is associated with a decrease in the numbers of alveoli; however, the alveoli increase in size (Ikegami et al., 1996, 1997; Willet et al., 2001).

Maternal glucocorticoid treatment has both an acute and a chronic effect on the fetal monkey lung (Johnson et al., 1978, 1981). Glucocorticoid treatment in preterm monkeys causes mesenchynal thinning and a large increase in maximal lung gas volumes. In term monkeys, however, the alveolar number, lung surface area, and lung gas volumes are decreased with glucocorticoid treatment. These results suggest that glucocorticoids are associated with an acute increase in lung gas volume (early lung maturation) but have an adverse effect on subsequent alveolarization and lung growth (Johnson et al., 1981).

Mechanical Ventilation and Lung Injury

Diffuse atelectasis and decreased compliance lead to alveolar hypoventilation and an imbalance in ventilation-perfusion. The ultimate outcome is worsening hypoxemia, requiring aggressive mechanical ventilation. Studies done with preterm animal models (predominantly baboons and lambs) have demonstrated that the strategy of ventilation plays an important role in the development of the progression of lung injury (Albertine et al., 1999; Coalson et al., 1999; Yoder et al., 2000). Ventilatory factors that have been found to increase lung injury include high tidal volumes, a lack of surfactant before the institution of ventilation, and inadequate end-expiratory pressure.

High tidal volumes lead to regional overinflation of alveoli and airways (volutrauma). In neonates with RDS, only a small portion of the lung may be recruited and available for ventilation. If only a small portion of the lung is being ventilated, a normal tidal volume for weight will be too large and will result in the disruption of structural elements, such as the pulmonary capillary endothelium, the alveolar and airway epithelia, and the basement membrane.

This concept has been tested in studies with preterm lambs, in which as few as six manual inflations of 35 to 40 milliliters per kilogram of body weight before surfactant treatment and mechanical ventilation led to increased lung injury and a decrease in the response to surfactant therapy (Bjorklund et al., 1997). In contrast, Wada and colleagues (1997) found, again in studies with preterm lambs, that surfactant treatment before the institution of assisted ventilation decreased the degree of lung injury, presumably by promoting more uniform lung inflation.

The premature lung, which is deficient in surfactant, is prone to collapse (atelectasis). Ventilation below a normal functional residual capacity leads to cyclic opening and closing of lung units, which adds to lung injury. This type of injury can be minimized by recruiting lung volumes with positive end-expiratory pressure (PEEP) and then maintaining a higher than normal functional residual capacity with high-frequency oscillatory ventilation. The combination of PEEP and oscillatory ventilation has been shown to improve surfactant function, decrease lung injury, and improve survival in rats (Chiumello et al., 1999).

Oxidative Stress and Lung Injury

The premature lung is particularly susceptible to free radical-induced injury because of the delay in the development and the reactivities of anti-oxidant defenses (Bracci, 1997; Saugstad, 1990). Oxygen-induced injury is caused by the overproduction of free radicals, such as superoxide, hydrogen peroxide, and perhydroxyl. The presence of free radicals overwhelms the immature antioxidant system, leading to the oxidation of enzymes, the inhibition of proteins and DNA synthesis, decreased surfactant production, and lipid peroxidation, all of which play a role in lung injury.

Multiple pathways of ROS generation have been found both in humans and in animal models. These include ischemia-reperfusion and hypoxanthine oxidase reactions, the metabolism of catecholamines, the arachidonic acid cascade, and mitochondrial metabolism. An additional source of free radicals in the lungs is thought to be phagocyte activation. The increases in phagocyte numbers and interleukin concentrations and the increased levels of free radical release seen in the bronchoalveolar fluid of premature infants with both acute and chronic lung disease indicate that oxygen toxicity and inflammation are involved in the development of lung injury (Zoban and Cerny, 2003).

Infection-Inflammation and Lung Injury

Increasing evidence indicates that infection and inflammation may play a role in the development of lung injury. The role of inflammation in RDS is suggested by several studies with preterm animal models. Infection-inflammation is also associated with a disruption in alveolus formation. This has been demonstrated in studies with both mice and sheep. In an experimental model of chorioamnionitis in sheep, a single dose of endotoxin given 7 days before preterm delivery or a continuous 28-day intra-amniotic infusion of endotoxin significantly decreased the numbers of alveoli (Willet et al., 2000). In transgenic mouse models, the overexpression of proinflammatory cytokines during the period of postnatal alveolarization has been found to disrupt alveolus formation (Jobe, 1999).

Studies done with preterm lambs have found that atelectasis (which is due to surfactant deficiency) initiates a cytokine-mediated inflammatory cascade that promotes the recruitment of neutrophils into the lung and that leads to endothelial cell damage and subsequent pulmonary edema. The depletion of neutrophils, however, prevents the pulmonary edema (Carlton et al., 1997; Naik et al., 2001). Proteins in the edema fluid are thought to worsen the lung injury by inactivating surfactant and exacerbating the surfactant deficiency.

Mechanical ventilation plays an important role in the inflammatory response of the preterm lung. Ventilation affects the numbers of inflammatory cells and the expression of soluble mediators within the lungs. This has been demonstrated with several animal models.

In rabbits subjected to saline lavage, injurious mechanical ventilation increased the levels of lung neutrophil accumulation and chemiluminescence (an indicator of neutrophil priming), increased the levels of inflammatory mediators (platelet-activating factor and thromboxane B_2) in bronchoalveolar lavage fluid, and increased the levels of TNF-α expression by alveolar macrophages (Clark et al., 2001).

Summary of Pathophysiological Mechanisms

An understanding of the relevant pathophysiological mechanisms of preterm birth is necessary to develop rationale and efficacious intervention strategies in preventing and treating preterm birth and its sequelae in neonates. Animal models provide a unique opportunity to study longitudinally the causes and consequences of preterm birth in a controlled experimental environment that cannot be created in women. However, many animal models have important limitations based on the length of gestation, the endocrine events of parturition, the presence of multiple fetuses, and fetal developmental milestones. Experimental animal models must be developed that address specific questions on the basis of their similarities or relevance to the research questions important in human preterm birth. These include the use of

- nonhuman primates to describe the temporal or longitudinal relationships among the mediators of preterm labor;
- genetically altered mice to ascertain the roles that putative mediators of preterm birth has in leading to prematurity; and
- sheep or nonhuman primates to ascertain the relationships among the various pathways to preterm birth and their sequelae in neonates, such as cerebral white matter injury and bronchopulmonary dysplasia.

7

Role of Gene-Environment Interactions in Preterm Birth

ABSTRACT

Until recently, the role of genetic susceptibility and gene-environment interactions in preterm birth has largely been unexplored. Growing evidence indicates that familial or intergenerational factors influence preterm birth. This influence may reflect shared environmental factors or genetic factors, or both. With recent advances in human genetics and molecular biology, assessment of genetic contributions to human diseases has progressed significantly, but the number of studies in this area is limited. These genetic studies have been mostly association studies, not corrected for population admixture using state of the art methods, and based on small sample sizes. Most sophisticated methodology and technology in genomics and proteomics has not been applied to preterm birth research. Epigenetics (the study of how gene regulatory information that is not expressed in DNA sequences is transmitted from one generation to the next) and proteomics (identification of the expression of proteins within biological fluid, tissue, or cells at a certain point in time under conditions of health or disease) have the potential to provide a greater understanding of the pathways to preterm birth but have not been adequately investigated. There is considerable room for improvement in the search for new biomarkers predicting preterm birth. While there are compelling reasons to examine gene-environment interactions, there are a limited number of published studies. Those those that have been con-

ducted suggest that individual genotypes may modify the risk of preterm birth associated with certain enviornmental exposures. Racial and ethnic differences in preterm birth have been discussed extensively throughout this report. This question remains largely unanswered. New tools for high-throughput genotyping, coupled with very-large-scale population-based studies that use sensitive biomarkers, comprehensive exposure assessment, and advanced biotechnology and analytical strategies, are needed to unravel the complex environmental and genetic factors, and gene-gene, and gene-environment interactions responsible for preterm birth. Understanding these factors and their interactions could lead to major improvements in the diagnosis, prevention, and treatment of preterm birth.

The completion of the first draft of the human genome sequence (Lander et al., 2001) and increasing information about the genome's function have provided new opportunities for the investigation of human health and disease. Likewise, results from the exploration of human genetic variation through the International HapMap Project, spearheaded by The National Human Genome Research Institute (The International HapMap Consortium, 2003), will furnish researchers with a powerful tool for identifying variants that contribute to common diseases. This information will be especially useful when it is combined with reliable, cost-effective, high-throughput methods that can be used to genotype these variants in large population samples (Shi, 2002).

In parallel, there is a growing recognition that changes in the earth's environment, in combination with genetic susceptibility, may contribute to many chronic diseases and may hold the key to reversing the course of some diseases (Chakravarti and Little, 2003). The improved methods for measuring nongenetic factors and environmental exposures promise to extend the scope of epidemiological investigation (Weaver et al., 1998).

Together, these developments present an exciting opportunity to address unanswered questions related to the complex contributions of genes, the environment, and gene-gene and gene-environment interactions to complex human diseases, including preterm birth. This chapter provides a review of recent progress in understanding the genetics of preterm birth, summarizes important methodological issues, and highlights areas for future research.

EVIDENCE OF GENETIC INFLUENCES ON PRETERM DELIVERY

The available literature has provided some evidence of familial and intergenerational influences on low birth weight or preterm birth (Bakketeig et al., 1979; Carr-Hill and Hall, 1985; Khoury and Cohen, 1987; Porter et al., 1997; Varner and Esplin, 2005). A population-based cohort study of data from birth certificates and fetal death certificates from the state of Georgia between 1980 and 1995 suggest that the recurrence of preterm delivery contributes to a notable portion of all preterm births, especially for the shortest gestations (Adams et al., 2000). Analysis of the data from the live birth cohort of the 1988 U.S. National Maternal and Infant Health Survey demonstrated a strong familial aggregation of low birth weight and preterm birth in both white and African American populations (Wang et al., 1995).

Familial and intergenerational influences on preterm birth may be attributable to shared environmental factors or genetic factors, or both. Studies with twins are a powerful approach to detecting the environmental and genetic components of a given disease or trait, but very few studies of preterm birth in human twins have been performed. The heritability of preterm birth was found to be 17 to 27 percent in an Australian population (Treloar et al., 2000), the heritability of gestational length was found to be 25 to 40 percent in a Swedish population (Clausson et al., 2000). The limited number of twin studies was in part due to the difficulty of assembling such a study population (i.e., female twins and their babies). The large registries of twins have the potential of probing not only concordance of preterm birth among female twins, but also the contributions of males and intergenerational effects.

As detailed below, with recent advances in human genetics and molecular biology, assessment of the contributions of genetics to human diseases has progressed from indirect measurements based on family history to direct measures of an individual's genotype (genome sequence) at particular gene loci. Nevertheless, it should be emphasized that family history and a woman's past medical history remain valuable tools in assessments of a woman's risk for preterm birth.

Genetic Association Studies

Disorders found to be associated with changes in the sequence of a single gene have been associated with an increased risk of preterm birth, often as a result of a predisposition to polyhydramnios in pregnancies with fetuses with changes in the sequence of that single gene. Among these conditions are myotonic dystrophy, Ehlers-Danlos syndrome, Smith-Lemli-Opitz syndrome, and neurofibromatosis. However, like many other complex human diseases, such as obesity, hypertension, diabetes, and asthma, preterm birth is a complex trait and possesses the following features: non-Mendelian transmission, the involvement of multiple genes, and gene-gene and gene-environment interactions. Research on the genetics of preterm birth thus faces significant challenges. The approaches available for the identification of genes that may be associated with a particular trait include positional cloning, the identification of positional candidate genes, whole-genome association analysis, and functional candidate gene analysis. Positional cloning requires extended pedigrees or sibling pairs. It has been successful for the analysis of disease transmitted by Mendelian genetics but has not been so successful for the study of more complex diseases and conditions. The identification of positional candidate genes requires linkage information, which is not possible for the genetic analysis of preterm birth. Scanning of the whole genome requires the identification of more than 100,000 single-nucleotide polymorphism (SNPs), which are single-base-pair substitutions in the DNA sequence; but this procedure is costly. The functional candidate gene approach, that is, the study of carefully selected candidate genes associated with major pathogenic pathways of preterm birth, is feasible and is commonly used. Relevant genetic association studies are summarized below.

One characteristic of the human genome with medical and social relevance is that each person's genome, except those of monozygotic twins, is unique. A persons' genotype represents the blending of parental genotypes. In addition, the human genome undergoes natural mutation. On average, the DNA sequences of two unrelated humans vary by millions of bases. Nearly all human genes are capable of causing disease if they are altered substantially. Mutations known to cause disease have been identified in about 1,000 genes. About 90 percent of all DNA sequence variations occur as SNPs (Brookes, 1999). The human genome contains about 10 million SNPs. A haplotype, on the other hand, represents a considerably longer sequence of nucleotides (an average of 25,000 nucleotides, which are the building blocks of DNA and genes), as well as any variants, that tend to be inherited together. Analysis of both SNPs and haplotypes is thus necessary to identify the genetic factors associated with complex diseases and syndromes, including preterm birth.

Two organizations have focused on the analysis of SNPs to identify the genes that may be associated with particular diseases and syndromes. The SNP Consortium Ltd. is a nonprofit foundation whose mission was to identify up to 300,000 SNPs distributed evenly throughout the human genome and to make the information related to those SNPs available to the public without intellectual property restrictions. Eventually, however, the SNP Consortium Ltd. discovered many more SNPs (1.5 million in total) than it had originally planned. The National Institute of Environmental Health

Sciences initiated the Environmental Genome Project (EGP) in 1998 to identify polymorphisms in the genes involved in environment-induced diseases (Olden and Wilson, 2000). In addition to the identification of polymorphisms, EGP aims to characterize the functions of these polymorphisms and supports epidemiological studies of gene-environment interactions.

Studies Involving One or a Few Candidate Genes

To date, most published studies on the genetics of preterm birth have examined only one or a few genes in a given study sample. The frequent association of spontaneous preterm labor and preterm birth with histological infection-inflammation and elevated concentrations of inflammatory cytokines in body fluids has focused investigations on single gene polymorphisms in the genes for these cytokines in both the mother and the fetus (Varner and Esplin, 2005), as it has been well established that upper genital tract infections and inflammation are associated with spontaneous preterm labor and preterm birth (Goldenberg and Andrews, 1996). The polymorphisms examined include those in the genes for the cytokines tumor necrosis factor alpha (TNF-α) nucleotide 308 (Dizon-Townson et al., 1997; Roberts et al., 1999), interleukin-1β (IL-1β) nucleotides 3953 and 3954 (Genc et al., 2002), and IL-6 nucleotide 174 (Jamie et al., 2005; Simhan et al., 2003); but the findings of an association of polymorphisms in these genes and preterm birth have been inconsistent.

Other studies have examined the roles of SNPs in preterm labor and preterm birth. Toll-like receptors, which are important components of the innate immune system, have been linked to spontaneous preterm labor and preterm birth (Lorenz et al., 2002). Gene polymorphisms in matrix metalloproteineases (MMPs) and preterm premature rupture of membranes (PPROM) were examined in African Americans. The breakdown of the interstitial collagens is mediated by MMPs. A fetal genotype of a mutation in the gene for matrix metalloproteinease type 1 (MMP-1) was found in association with PPROM (Fujimoto et al., 2002). Three SNPs located at positions −799 C to T), −381 (A to G), and +17 (C to G) (where C, T, A, and G represent the nucleotides cytosine, thymine, adenine, and guanine, respectively) from the major transcription start site in the MMP-8 gene have been identified; and the functional significance of SNP haplotypes in the MMP-8 gene and associations with PPROM has been demonstrated (Wang H et al., 2004). MMP-8 is an enzyme that degrades fibrillar collagens and that imparts strength to the fetal membranes; it is expressed by leukocytes and chorionic cytotrophoblast cells. There are cell host-dependent differences in MMP-9 promoter activity related to CA-repeat number and fetal carriage of the 14 CA-repeat allele is associated with PPROM in African Americans (Ferrand et al., 2002). Finally, a study (Ozkur et al., 2002) found that a mutation in the β_2-adrenergic receptor, the predominant β-adrenergic receptor subtype that relaxes myometrial muscle fibers at term (Liu et al., 1998), changed the amino acid glutamic acid to glutamine at codon 27 and is associated with preterm labor.

Multiple Candidate Gene Study

Investigators generally agree that the "one gene, one risk factor" approach to understanding the etiology of complex human diseases will not likely yield great progress in understanding the causes of human diseases and syndromes, and as mentioned earlier in this report, preterm birth is increasingly recognized as a syndrome with multiple etiologies. Therefore, because of the heterogeneous nature of preterm birth, it is necessary to study a large number of candidate genes to better understand genetic influences on preterm birth. However, the numbers of published studies of this kind are limited. One study simultaneously investigated the relationships of polymorphisms in six cytokine genes associated with inflammation (IL-1α, IL-1β, IL-2, IL-6, TNF-α, and lymphotoxin alpha [LTA]) with spontaneous preterm birth and the birth of infants who are small for gestational age in a nested case-control study with women from a prospective pregnancy cohort (Engel et al., 2005a). Two haplotypes spanning the TNF-α and LTA-α genes were associated with an increased risk for spontaneous preterm birth in white subjects (for the AGG haplotype, odds ratio [OR] 1.5; 95% confidence interval [CI] 0.8–2.6; for the GAC haplotype, OR 1.6; 95% CI 0.9–2.9). Additionally, carriers of the GAG haplotype were found to have a decreased risk of spontaneous preterm birth (OR 0.6; 95% CI 0.3–1.0). The TNF-α and LTA variants TNF-α(−488)A and LTA(IVS1-82)C, constituents of the AGG and GAC haplotypes, respectively, were also strongly associated with an increased risk of spontaneous preterm birth.

A large-scale case-control study explored the associations of 426 SNPs with preterm birth in 300 mothers with preterm deliveries (cases) and 458 mothers with term deliveries (controls) (Hao et al., 2004). Twenty-five candidate genes were included in the final haplotype analysis, and a significant association of the Factor V (F5) gene haplotype with preterm birth was revealed and remained significant after Bonferroni correction for multiple testing (p = 0.025). That study also performed exploratory ethnicity-specific analyses, which confirmed the findings that the association of the F5 gene haplotype with preterm birth is consistent across ethnic groups.

Until now, the discovery of genes found to be associated with preterm birth has been limited to studies of candidate genes. Although it is not possible for this report to cover all candidate genes, a list of potential candidate genes affecting preterm birth is provided in Table 7-1. On the other hand, the availability of SNP gene microarrays and high-throughput genotyping

TABLE 7-1 Potential Candidate Genes for Preterm Births

Gene No. and Pathway	Gene Name	Gene	Chromosome Location
Inflammatory pathway			
1	Colony-stimulating factor 1	CSF1	1p21-p13
2	Colony-stimulating factor 1 receptor	CSF1R	5q33-q35
3	Colony-stimulating factor 2	CSF2	5q31.1
4	Colony-stimulating factor 2 receptor alpha	CSF2RA	Xp22.32 and Yp11.3
5	Colony-stimulating factor 2 receptor beta	CSF2RB	22q13.1
6	Colony-stimulating factor 3	CSF3	17q11.2-q12
7	Colony-stimulating factor 3 receptor	CSF3R	1p35-p34.3
8	Interferon gamma receptor 1	IFNGR1	6q23-q24
9	Interleukin-1α	IL1A	2q14
10	Interleukin-1 receptor type I	IL1R1	2q12
11	Interleukin-1 receptor type II	IL1R2	2q12-q22
12	Interleukin-1 receptor antagonist	IL1RN	2q14.2
13	Interleukin-1β	IL1b	2q14
14	Interleukin-2	IL2	4q26-q27
15	Interleukin-2 receptor alpha	IL2RA	10p15-p14
16	Interleukin-2 receptor beta	IL2RB	22q13.1
17	Interleukin-4	IL4	5q31.1
18	Interleukin-4 receptor	IL4R	16p11.2-12.1
19	Interleukin-5	IL5	5q31.1
20	Inteleukin-6	IL6	7p21
21	Interleukin-6 receptor	IL6R	1q21
22	Interleukin-8	IL8	4q13-q21
23	Interleukin-8 receptor alpha	IL8RA	2q35
24	Interleukin-10	IL10	1q31-q32
25	Interleukin-10 receptor alpha	IL10RA	11q23
26	Interleukin-10 receptor beta	IL10RB	21q22.11
27	Interleukin-11	IL11	19q13.3-q13.4
28	Interleukin-12A	IL12A	3p12-q13.2
29	Interleukin-13	IL13	5q31
30	Interleukin-15	IL15	4q31
31	Interleukin-17	IL17	6p12
32	Interleukin-18	IL18	11q22.2-q22.3
33	Lymphotoxin alpha	LTA	6p21.3
34	Lymphotoxin beta	LTB	6p21.3
35	Nitric oxide synthase 2A	NOS2A	17q11.2-q12
36	Nitric oxide synthase 3	NOS3	7q36
37	Tumor necrosis factor alpha	TNFA	6p21.3
38	Type 1 tumor necrosis factor alpha receptor	TNFR1	12p13.2
39	Type 2 tumor necrosis factor alpha receptor	TNFR2	1p36.3-p36.2
40	Tumor necrosis factor receptor superfamily member 6	TNFRSF6	10q24.1

continued

TABLE 7-1 Continued

Gene No. and Pathway	Gene Name	Gene	Chromosome Location
41	Type 1 tumor necrosis factor receptor shedding aminopeptidase regulator	*ARTS-1*	5q15
42	Gamma interferon	*IFN-?*	12q14
43	Gamma interferon receptor 1	*IFNGR1*	6q23-q24
44	Neurotrophin-3	*NT-3*	12p13
45	Neurotrophin-5	*NT-5*	19q13.3
46	Triggering receptor expressed on myeloid cells 1	*TREM-1*	6p21.1
47	Migration inhibitory factor	*MIF*	22q11.23
48	Pre-B-cell colony-enhancing factor 1	*PBEF1*	7q22.3
49	Nuclear factor kappa B	*NF-Kb*	4q24
50	B-cell activating factor	*BAFF*	13q32-34
51	Toll-like receptor 2	*TLR2*	4q32
52	Toll-like receptor 3	*TLR3*	4q35
53	Toll-like receptor 4	*TLR4*	9q32-q33
54	Toll-like receptor 5	*TLR5*	1q41-q42
55	Toll-like receptor 7	*TLR7*	Xp22.3
56	Toll-like receptor 8	*TLR8*	Xp22
57	Toll-like receptor 9	*TLR9*	3p21.3
58	CC chemokine receptor 5	*CCR5*	3p21
59	T-cell immunomodulatory protein	*CDA08*	16q12.1
60	Monocyte chemoattractant protein 1	*MCP-1*	17q11.2-q12
61	Monocyte chemoattractant protein 2	*MCP-2*	17q11.2
62	Macrophage inflammatory protein-1α	*MIP-1a*	17q11-q21
63	Macrophage inflammatory protein-1β	*MIP-1b*	17q12
64	Intercellular adhesion molecule-1	*ICAM-1*	19p13.3-p13.2
65	Prolactin	*PRL*	6p22.2-p21.3
66	Prolactin receptor	*PRLR*	5p14-p13
67	Transforming growth factor β1	*TGFB1*	19q13.1
68	Transforming growth factor β2	*TGFB2*	1q41
69	Transforming growth factor β3	*TGFB3*	14q24
70	Transforming growth factor receptor beta receptor I	*TGFBR1*	9q22
71	Transforming growth factor receptor beta receptor II	TGFBR2	3P22
72	Platelet-activating factor	*PTAF*	
73	Platelet-activating factor receptor	*PTAFR*	1p35-p34.3
74	Guanine nucleotide binding protein, beta polypeptide 3	*GNB3*	12p13

Uteroplacental pathway

1	Coagulation factor II	*F2*	11p11-q12
2	Coagulation factor V	*F5*	1q23
3	Protein C	*PROC*	2q13-q14

TABLE 7-1 Continued

Gene No. and Pathway	Gene Name	Gene	Chromosome Location
4	β₂-Adrenergic receptor	Beta2-AR	5q31-q32
5	Vascular endothelial growth factor	VEGF	6p12
8	Angiotensinogen	AGT	1q42-q43
9	Apolipoprotein E	APOE	19q13.2
10	Methylenetetrahydrofolate reductase	MTHFR	1p36.3
11	Methylenetetrahydrofolate homocysteine methyltransferase	MTR	1q43
Endocrine pathway			
1	Corticotropin-releasing hormone binding protein	CRHBP	5q11.2-q13.3
2	Adrenocorticotropin	ACTH	2p23.3
3	Corticotropin-releasing hormone	CRH	8q13
4	Corticotropin-releasing hormone receptor 1	CRHR1	17q12-q22
5	Corticotropin-releasing hormone receptor 2	CRHR2	7p14.3
6	Estrogen receptor 1	ESR1	6q25.1
7	Estrogen receptor 2	ESR2	14q23.2
8	Brain-derived neurotrophic factor	BDNF	11p13
9	Dopamine receptor D2	DRD2	11q23
10	Progesterone receptor	PGR	11q22-q23
Uterine contraction			
1	Prostaglandin E receptor 2	PTGER2	14q22
2	Prostaglandin E receptor 3	PTGER3	1p31.2
3	Prostaglandin E synthase	PTGES	9q34.3
4	Prostaglandin F receptor	PTGFR	1p31.1
5	Cyclooxygenase 1	COX-1	9q32-q33.3
6	Cyclooxygenase 2 (inducible)	COX-2	1q25.2-q25.3
7	Oxytocin	OXT	20p13
8	Oxytocin receptor	OXTR	3p25
9	Matrix metalloproteinase 1	MMP1	11q22.3
10	Matrix metalloproteinase 2	MMP2	16q13-q21
11	Matrix metalloproteinase 3	MMP3	11q22.3
12	Matrix metalloproteinase 8	MMP8	11q22.3
13	Matrix metalloproteinase 9	MMP9	20q11.2-q13.1
14	Relaxin 1	RLN1	9p24.1
15	Relaxin 2	RLN2	9p24.1
16	Relaxin 3	RLN3	19p13.2
Metabolic pathway			
1	Glutathione S-transferase θ	GSTT1	
2	Opioid receptor, mu 1	OPRM1	6q24-q25
3	N-Acetyltransferase 1	NAT1	8p23.1-p21.3
4	N-Acetyltransferase 2	NAT2	8p22

continued

TABLE 7-1 Continued

Gene No. and Pathway	Gene Name	Gene	Chromosome Location
5	Cytochrome P450, family 1, subfamily A, polypeptide 1	CYP1A1	15q22-q24
6	Cytochrome P450, family 2, subfamily A, polypeptide 6	CYP2A6	19q13.2
7	Cytochrome P450, family 2, subfamily D, polypeptide 6	CYP2D6	22q13.1
8	Cytochrome P450, family 2, subfamily E, polypeptide 1	CYP2E1	10q24.3-qter
9	Heat shock protein 70	Hsp-70	6p21.3
10	Alcohol dehydrogenase 1A	ADH1A	4q21-q23
11	Alcohol dehydrogenase 1B	ADH1B	4q21-q23
12	Alcohol dehydrogenase 1C	ADH1C	4q21-q23
13	Aldehyde dehydrogenase	ALDH2	12q24.2

technologies makes it possible to conduct studies of the association of genes with preterm birth by use of the entire genome. Gene microarrays consist of microscope-sized slides on which the sequences of thousands of genes can be placed. Hybridization of those sequences with the gene sequence to be tested can be used to determine the genotypes of the test gene. Recently, a 500,000-SNP microarray became available. In this way, the discovery of genes associated with preterm birth will not be limited to known or suspected candidate genes. Although these technologies are costly, they represent means for the systematic identification of the genes associated with preterm birth.

GENE-ENVIRONMENT INTERACTIONS

The goal of gene-environment studies in epidemiology is to advance knowledge of how genetic and environmental factors combine to affect the risk of disease and, more specifically, how the variations in the human genome (polymorphisms) can modify the effects of exposures to environmental health hazards (Kelada et al., 2003). There are compelling reasons to examine the association of gene-environment interactions with preterm birth. The data presented in the previous chapters and in this chapter suggested that both socioenvironmental factors and genetic factors may influence preterm birth. Given individual genetic variations and differential environmental exposures, stratification of study subjects by genotype may allow the detection of risk of preterm birth among individuals exposed to a particular environmental toxicant (Rothman et al., 2001). Furthermore, enhanced understanding of pathologic mechanisms may allow the development of drugs or interventions that can be used to prevent or treat preterm birth. To date, however, only a relatively few studies on the association of gene-environment interactions with preterm birth have been published (Genc et al., 2004; Macones et al., 2004; Nukui et al., 2004; Wang et al., 2000, 2002). Two of these studies are described below.

Gene-Genital Tract Infection Interaction

Given the association between genital tract infections such as bacterial vaginosis (BV) and preterm birth, a case-control study of 375 women examined the interactions among BV, the TNF-α genotype, and preterm birth (Macones et al., 2004). Maternal carriers of the rarer allele (TNF-α-2) were found to be at a significantly increased risk of spontaneous preterm birth (OR 2.7; 95% CI 1.7–4.5). The association between carriage of the TNF-α-2 allele and preterm birth was found to be modified by the presence of BV, such that those with a genotype that made them susceptible to preterm birth and BV had an increased odds of preterm birth compared with the odds for those who did not (OR 6.1; 95% CI 1.9–21.0). The study thus provides evidence that an interaction between genetic susceptibility (i.e., carriage of TNF-α-2) and an environmental factor (i.e., BV) is associated with an increased risk of spontaneous preterm birth.

Gene-Smoking Interaction

In the United States, about 13 percent of all pregnant women smoke cigarettes, which is a recognized risk factor for preterm birth. A study of 741 U.S. mothers investigated whether maternal genotypes can modify the association between maternal cigarette smoking and infant birth weight, gestational age, and intrauterine growth retardation (Wang et al., 2002). The study found that without consideration of genotype, the OR of preterm birth in association with maternal smoking was 1.8. When the mothers were stratified by their CYP1A1 genotypes, the mothers with variant genotypes had a higher risk of preterm birth. Similarly, when the mothers were stratified by their GSTT1 genotypes, the mothers with variant genotypes had a higher risk of preterm birth. More strikingly, the mothers with both CYP1A1 and GSTT1 variant genotypes had the highest risk of preterm birth (OR = greater than 10). This study provides additional evidence that individual genotypes may modify the risk of preterm birth in association with an environmental exposure.

EPIGENETICS

DNA is not freely floating within the cell cytoplasm or nucleus; it is organized with proteins called histones to form a complex substance known as chromatin (see Box 7-1 for definition of terms). Biostructural modifications to the DNA or the histones alter chromatin without changing the actual nucleotide sequence of the DNA. These modifications are described as epigenetic. The two main sources of epigenetic modification are DNA methylation and histone deacetylation (Haig, 2004). DNA methylation is a chemical modification of the DNA proper by an enzyme known as DNA methyltransferase. Methylation can directly switch off gene expression by preventing transcription factors from binding to promoters. However, a more general effect of methylation is the attraction of methyl-binding domain proteins. Methyl-binding domain proteins can activate histone deacetylases, which function to chemically modify histones and change chromatin structure. Chromatin containing acetylated histones is open and accessible to transcription factors, and, thus, the genes contained within that chromatin are potentially active. Histone deacetylation causes the condensation of the chromatin. When chromatin is condensed, the genes therein are unable to be expressed. In this manner, genes may be "switched off" or silenced (Haig, 2004; Henikoff et al., 2004). Thus, broadly considered, epigenetic changes to DNA or to histones can alter the expression of genes within the genome. Even in the setting of identical genetics, differences in epigenotype may account for important phenotype differences. For example, epigenetic differences may account for disease discordance among monozygotic twins (Wong et al., 2005). Epigenetics has been hypothesized to play a major role in human health and disease in a wide variety of areas, from psychoneurodevelopment (Abdolmaleky et al., 2005; Hong et al., 2005) to

---

BOX 7-1
Definition of Terms in Epigenetics

Chromatin—DNA organized by histones
DNA methyltransferase—The enzyme responsible for methylating DNA
Histone deacetylases—A class of enzymes that structurally modifies histones
Epigenetic modification—Biostructural modifications to DNA or histones that alter chromatin without changing the actual nucleotide sequence of DNA
Epigenotype—The pattern of epigenetic modifications of a genome

cancer (Laird, 2005) to heart disease (Muskiet, 2005). Epigenetic modification of genes may be influenced by environmental exposure, such as nutritional micronutrients. Folate, biotin, niacin, and tryptophan may all influence gene silencing (Oommen et al., 2005).

The pattern of epigenetic modifications of a genome may be termed an epigenotype (Jiang et al., 2004). Epigenotypes are, by definition, more plastic than genotypes, and are highly context dependent; that is, epigenotypes vary between cells within the same organism and are modifiable by the environment in critical windows of exposure (Henikoff et al., 2004; Jiang et al., 2004; Wang Y et al., 2004). Extreme examples of pregnancy disorders related to epigenetics are choriocarcinoma and hydatidiform moles (Xue et al., 2004). However, the consequences of epigenetic influences on pregnancy course may be much more subtle. Van Dijk and coworkers (2005) noted that epigenetic modification of the *STOX1* gene might be of importance in preeclampsia. While there are no data regarding the possibility of epigenetic influences on spontaneous preterm parturition, it is important to recognize the possible influence that epigenotype may have gene expression and, thus, on the functional consequences that it may have on the length of gestation.

PROTEOMICS

Despite the many advantages and advances in knowledge attributable to genomics and microarray analysis, these approaches have several limitations. Although the human genome contains approximately 30,000 genes, many more messenger RNA transcripts potentially coding for different proteins exist because of the alternate splicing of genes. Depending on codon bias, there is only a limited relationship between the expression of a gene and the amount of protein expression directed by that gene. The expression or function of proteins is modulated at many points from transcription to posttranslation, and protein expression or function cannot be reliably predicted merely by analysis of the nucleic acid sequences. Extensive posttranslational protein modification (e.g., phosphorylation, methylation, and compartmentalization) may occur and may dramatically alter the function of a protein. Because of the wide variety of posttranslational modifications, it is estimated that as many as 1 million distinct proteins derived from the 30,000 genes in the human genome may exist. This has important implications in the understanding of biological mechanisms and pathways, as well as in the development of disease-specific biomarkers, because the flow of information between cells and tissues is mediated by protein-protein interactions in both health and disease.

Recent advances in protein chemistry and the identification of peptide fragments by two-dimensional gel electrophoresis and mass spectrometric analysis have led to the emerging field of proteomics (McDonald and Yates, 2002). Proteomics refers to the identification of the global expression of proteins within a biological system (biological fluid, tissue, or cell) at a certain point in time under given conditions of health or disease. Because the expression and concentrations of many proteins depend on complex regulatory systems, the proteome, unlike the genome, is highly dynamic. The dynamic nature of the proteome complements genomics both in providing an understanding of pathophysiological processes such as preterm birth and in the discovery of protein biomarkers that may be uniquely associated with certain conditions and therefore useful as diagnostic biomarkers.

Proteomic strategies are based on the description of protein expression or protein function. Expression proteomics involves the identification or cataloguing of all proteins present within a biological system under given conditions. The differential expression of some proteins can link dynamic changes in protein expression to physiological conditions or disease states. Thus, expression profiling is uniquely suited to the identification of potential diagnostic biomarkers or to the description of biological changes that occur under certain conditions (e.g., labor). Functional proteomics places these proteins within their proper context by mapping their intracellular localization and their interactions with other proteins. Both genomics and proteomics allow for a comprehensive evaluation of proteins or messenger RNA transcripts that may provide valuable insights into the complex etiologies of preterm birth, and may facilitate potential biomarker for preterm birth (see Shankar et al., 2005 for review).

To date scientists in reproductive medicine have not vigorously used the field of proteomics in reproductive medicine. No research reported thus far has used a proteomics approach in the study of preterm labor or preterm birth. Several reports, however, have emphasized the potential importance of proteomics in pregnancy-related research (Page et al., 2002; Shankar et al., 2005); and others have addressed factors that are directly relevant to preterm birth, including implantation (Daikoku et al., 2005), preeclampsia (Koy et al., 2005; Myers et al., 2004; Sawicki et al., 2003), premature rupture of fetal membranes (Vuadens et al., 2003), and intra-amniotic fluid infection (Buhimschi et al., 2005; Gravett et al., 2004). For example, novel biomarkers discovered by proteomic profiling of amniotic fluid, including defensins, calgranulins, and specific proteolytic fragments of insulin growth factor binding protein-1, have recently been identified in intra-amniotic fluid infection, an important and potentially preventable cause of preterm birth. Two recent reports suggest that the detection of these peptides by proteomic analysis yields a sensitivity and a specificity in excess of 90 percent each for the detection of subclinical intra-amniotic fluid infection associated with preterm labor (Buhimschi et al., 2005; Gravett et al., 2004).

Proteomic profiling has also identified a unique protein expression profile in women with severe preeclampsia that precedes the clinical onset of symptoms (Koy et al., 2005; Myers et al., 2004). An improved understanding of the early events in preeclampsia and the ability to provide an early diagnosis of this and other pregnancy-related conditions are necessary to develop rational and efficacious intervention strategies that may reduce the risks of preterm birth.

Two initiatives that may lead to significant contributions of proteomics to pregnancy-related research have been instituted. The Human Proteomics Organization (www.hupo.org) was organized in 2001 to facilitate proteomic research in humans. More recently, the National Institute of Child Health and Human Development initiated the Genomic and Proteomic Network for Premature Birth Research. The aim of this network is to accelerate the pace of research on preterm birth by focusing on global genomic and proteomic strategies and the dissemination of genomic and proteomic data to the scientific community. Specifically, the network will (1) design and implement hypothesis-driven, mechanistic studies based on large-scale, high-output genomic and proteomic approaches and (2) provide a public, web-based, genomic and proteomic database that the research community can use to mine and deposit data. It is anticipated that the creation of this network will hasten a deeper understanding of the pathophysiology of premature birth, discover novel target molecules and diagnostic biomarkers, and ultimately, aid in the formulation of more effective interventions for the prevention of preterm birth.

GENETICS AND RACIAL-ETHNIC DISPARITIES IN PRETERM BIRTH RATES

The significance of the racial and ethnic differences of human populations is frequently debated in clinical, epidemiological, and molecular research (Ioannidis et al., 2004). The undeniable evidence of health disparities between individuals of different races and ethnicities indicates that in some cases a correlation exists between race and health or disease. However, this relationship is complex and poorly understood. First, it is essential to point out that there are no generally agreed upon definitions of race. By and large, racial categories are social defined and are associated with certain social, cultural, educational, and economic dimensions. However, racial categories are also associated, to varying degrees, with genetic inferences of ancestry, the frequency of gene variants, and genetic effects (Bamshad, 2005). There is considerable controversy regarding the existence and importance of genetic influences on racial differences in complex diseases influenced by a large number of genes (Cooper et al., 2003).

Preterm birth is an example of a condition in which disparities among individuals of different races and ethnicities exist, with the largest and most persistent disparity occurring between Asian or Pacific Islanders and non-Hispanic black women, who have overall rates of preterm birth of 10.5 and 17.9 percent, respectively (CDC, 2005i). As discussed in Chapter 4, some evidence suggests that genetic factors may play a role in the disparities in preterm birth rates by race-ethnicity. However, the evidence by no means proves that genetic factors contribute to these disparities. The most direct way to study whether genetic factors vary among racial-ethnic groups is to find variants that influence susceptibility to the risk of preterm birth and then to assess whether these variants differ in frequency or effect across populations.

Allele Frequency

One possible reason for a genetic influence on racial disparities in preterm birth is that susceptibility variants may be present in one population but absent in others or may vary in frequencies across diverse populations. This may affect the number of individuals at increased risk for preterm birth. One obvious example is the unequal distribution of disease-associated alleles for certain recessive disorders, such as sickle cell disease or Tay-Sachs disease. One study examined a total of 179 African American women and 396 white women for the presence of functionally relevant allelic variants in cytokine genes (Hassan et al., 2003). African American women were found to be significantly more likely to carry allelic variants known to up-regulate proinflammatory cytokines, and the ORs increased with the allele dose. The ORs for African American women compared with those for white women to have genotypes that up-regulate the proinflammatory cytokine variantss IL-1, IL1A-4845G/G, IL1A-889T/T, IL1B-3957C/C, and IL1B-511A/A ranged from 2.1 to 4.9. The proinflammatory cytokine genotype IL6-174G/G variant was 36.5 times (95% CI 8.8–151.9) more common among African American women than white women. The frequencies of genotypes known to down-regulate the antiinflammatory cytokine genotypes IL10-819T/T and IL10-1082A/A were elevated 3.5-fold (95% CI 1.8–6.6) and 2.8-fold (95% CI 1.6–4.9), respectively, in African American women compared with those in white women. Except for the gamma interferon genotype, cytokine genotypes found to be more common in African American women were consistently those that up-regulate inflammation (Hassan et al., 2003; Ness et al., 2004).

Genetic Effects

Another possible reason for a genetic influence on racial-ethnic disparities in preterm birth rates is the variation in the effect of a given genetic variant between racial groups. However, data that can be used to either support or disprove this hypothesis are limited. One study examined the genetic effects of 43 validated gene-disease associations among 697 study populations of various descents (Ioannidis et al., 2004). The frequencies of the genetic marker of interest in the control populations often (in 58 percent of the studies) showed large heterogeneity (statistically significant variability) between people of different races. Conversely, large heterogeneity in the genetic effects (ORs) between races was found for only 14 percent of the studies. This finding suggests that the frequencies of genetic markers of complex diseases often vary among populations, but their biological effects may usually be consistent across traditional racial-ethnic boundaries.

Gene-Environment Interactions

Because the constellation of socioenvironmental variables known to affect the risk of preterm birth is not equitably distributed across racial-ethnic groups, the interaction of these factors with genetic predispositions may also produce highly disparate clinical outcomes. As discussed in the previous section, this area needs to be further investigated.

In summary, the question of whether genetics explains a substantial proportion of health disparities in preterm birth, is largely unanswered. It is anticipated that as populations increasingly become admixed (that is, as populations increasingly comprise couples of different ancestries), race and ethnicity will become even more inaccurate proxies for health risk. Without discounting self-identified race or ethnicity as a variable correlated with health, researchers must move beyond these weak and imperfect relationships. We need to understand not only what is downstream from race or ethnicity, but also upstream factors that explain how and why a racial-ethnic group's disparity exists in health or disease. Such information may shed light on the pathways and mechanisms explaining why race-ethnicity are associated with health or disease. Furthermore, future genetic epidemiological studies need to employ advanced methodology in dealing with admixed populations (see section on Methodological Issues below).

METHODOLOGICAL ISSUES

Although multiple genetic markers have been identified to be potentially associated with preterm birth, preterm labor, or PPROM, none of the markers has been adequately validated as a cause of preterm birth in studies with various populations and no single marker appears to be highly sensitive or specific to preterm birth, preterm labor, or PPROM. Although many gene-environment interaction studies have been conducted with human populations in the past decade, the number of studies that have demonstrated important and consistent positive relationships between genes and the environment is remarkably small. Key methodological issues that need to be carefully addressed in future molecular genetic epidemiological studies of preterm birth are highlighted below.

Definition of Preterm Birth Phenotypes

Despite considerable research efforts, limited progress has been made in understanding the etiology of preterm birth. One important problem is the definition of the preterm birth phenotypes. The current approaches for defining and assessing preterm birth phenotypes are inadequate for etiological research and for making the optimal use of genomic data. Most previous studies have relied exclusively on the conventional definition of preterm birth (less than 37 weeks of gestation). Cases of preterm birth so defined, however, constitute a highly heterogeneous group; and even subgroups of preterm births, defined as very preterm births (less than 32 weeks of gestation), preterm labor, and preterm rupture of membranes, constitute heterogeneous groups. As such, standard genetic or epidemiological analysis may lack the power to detect the causative genes and the environmental risk factors because of the dilution effect.

One way to overcome this challenge is to divide preterm birth into more homogeneous subgroups according to the underlying pathogenic pathways to preterm birth. This will require the incorporation of detailed clinical information (for example, pregnancy complications), pathological examination of the placenta, as well as genetic or nongenetic markers to stratify preterm birth into pathogenically meaningful subgroups. Although division into more homogeneous subgroups increases the complexity of the scientific endeavor and requires much larger sample sizes, it helps to reduce genetic heterogeneity and to enhance the ability to identify genetic associations and the gene-environment interactions that are specific to pathogenic pathways of preterm birth. It also raises the possibility that the specific causes of preterm birth in a specific woman may be identifiable, preventable, or treatable. The availability of such information will be important so that interventions can be targeted to women and their infants with different underlying etiologies for preterm birth in the future.

Analytical Challenges

Analytically, in a simplistic case, a case-control study in which exposure and genotype are dichotomized, the conventional analysis of exposure and disease by use of a two-by-two table needs to be expanded to include genotype, which yields a two-by-four table. In this manner, the raw exposure and genotype data are displayed in such a way that relative risk estimates for each factor alone and their joint effect can be easily generated

(Botto and Khoury, 2001). Regression models of interactions can also be used (Neter et al., 1996). However, the burgeoning volume of genetic data provides both unprecedented opportunities and unprecedented challenges for dissecting the genetics of preterm birth. It requires the development and application of innovative statistical methods, which will be further elaborated in the following section.

Testing of Multiple Genes

The testing of multiple genes is almost inevitable in large-scale studies of candidate genes that play a role in preterm birth. Traditional gene testing approaches study SNPs one at time, which ignores gene-gene interactions or the linkage disequilibrium among linked SNPs. Such an approach has an inherent low power, because the results of testing of multiple genes need to be adjusted by use of a Bonferroni correction to protect against an inflated Type I error. Many researchers argue that the multiplicity problems encountered in genetic epidemiology research require the use of a new paradigm to handle the problem. Haplotype analysis is advantageous, in that more information about variation in a gene can be captured (Nebert, 2002). Haplotype analysis has been applied in two recent studies of candidate gene that may play a role in preterm birth. In one study haplotypes were inferred by use of the EM algorithm and the Bayesian method (Engel et al., 2005b). In another study, both Gibbs sampling and expectation-maximization were used to reconstruct haplotype phases (Hao et al., 2004). These studies demonstrated the utility of the haplotype-based approach in a large-scale study of candidate genes that may play a role in preterm birth.

Methods are evolving to include adjustment for covariates in the analysis (Annells et al., 2004; Engel et al., 2005a,b; Hao et al., 2004; Schaid et al., 2002; Wang H et al., 2004). Although tests that incorporate haplotypes (especially within a haplotype block with limited haplotype diversity) are suggested to be more powerful than tests that incorporate only single markers, the block structure of haplotypes may not always be evident. It has been shown that under some circumstances the single-marker test is more powerful than the haplotype test. What remains unclear are the effects of haplotyping error because of the uncertainty of the inference drawn from the results of the derivation of the SNP block structure and subsequent association tests obtained with unrelated diploid subjects.

Population Admixture

A source of potential confounding in genetic tests is a hidden population genetic structure. The population sampled may consist of several genetically distinct subpopulations that are incompletely mixed. If those populations differ by both the prevalence of a variant allele at the candidate locus and the prevalence or magnitude of a trait, an apparent association between the allele and the trait may simply reflect confounding of the allele's effect by subpopulation identity. Because exposure prevalences may also vary among genetically distinct subpopulations, exposure and gene-exposure interaction effects can also be biased by the subpopulation structure. For a diverse population such as that of the United States, admixture-induced bias may be relatively small for common variants (Wacholder et al., 2000). Concerns about the possible effects of population admixture have stimulated the development of family-based association tests, which essentially eliminate the potential bias from population stratification (Schaid and Sommer, 1993; Spielman et al., 1993) and gene-environment interactions (Schaid, 1999; Umbach, 2000).

In addition to conventional stratified analysis by maternal subgroups such as ethnicity, various methods were used to address population admixture, including the use of a within-population permutation procedure in the association analysis (Hao et al., 2004); use of ancestry-informative genetic markers to infer and control population admixture in genetic association study (Reiner et al., 2005); and admixture-matched cases and controls for genetic association study (Tasi et al., 2006).

The Role of Maternal Versus Fetal Genes

Children receive half of their alleles from their mother and half from their father. Diseases that develop during gestation may be influenced by the genotype of the mother and the inherited genotype of the embryo-fetus. Understanding of the separate, joint, and synergistic effects of the two relevant genotypes is important to obtaining an understanding of the etiology of the disease. Understanding of these effects may also allow recurrence risk counseling. However, given the correlation between maternal and offspring genotypes, the relative importance of these two interrelated risk factors (or of their interactions with exposures) may be difficult to assess by studies with the commonly used case-control or cohort designs (Umbach, 2000).

The two-step transmission disequilibrium test was the first family-based test proposed for the differentiation of maternal and offspring genetic effects (Mitchell, 1997). However, this approach, which requires data from "pents," which comprise data for the affected child and the child's mother, father, and maternal grandparents, provides biased tests for maternal genetic effects when the genotype of the offspring is associated with disease. An alternative approach based on transmissions from grandparents provides unbiased tests for maternal and offspring genetic effects but requires genotype information for the paternal grandparents, in addition to that for the pents (Mitchell and Weinberg, 2005).

Sample Size and Power

In studies of gene-environment interactions, it is difficult to obtain the correct sample size and power estimate, and there are no well-established methods for doing so. Efforts to study complex gene-environment interactions are also tempered by the difficulty of obtaining adequate sample sizes. Two primary factors to be considered are the prevalence of the polymorphism in the population and the magnitude of the effect modification detected, because there is a trade-off between the prevalence of a polymorphism and the magnitude of the effect that may be detected. On the one hand, common variants are less likely to exhibit a strong effect. On the other hand, there is more statistical power in studying these variants because they are more common. Furthermore, the population-attributable risk of common variants will be greater, even if the penetrance in the population is modest.

At present, there are two approaches to the study of gene polymorphisms and their effects: the analytical method and the simulation method. Analytical methods require knowledge of the underlying distributions and genetic models. The available methods usually handle one exposure and one genetic marker at a time. Use of this method is difficult in higher-order interactions. In comparison, simulation methods estimate power by simulated random sampling. This method is able to deal with higher-order interactions, but it is computationally intensive.

Data Management and Integration

With major advances in genotyping technologies, it has become practical and affordable to screen biological samples for multiple polymorphisms for which there is more or less knowledge about their functional relevance in relation to exposure to toxicological agents or disease. Investigators have had increasing interest in and discussions about the development of an integrated database that links new findings on exposures, etiologic pathways, relevant genes, the polymorphisms in those genes, and their functions.

This database would guide the design of new studies as well as data analysis and interpretation of results (De Roos et al., 2004). The National Institutes of Health has funded the Pharmacogenetics Research Network and Knowledge Base (PharmGKB; http://www.pharmgkb.org and http://www.nigms.nih.gov/funding/pharmacogenetics.html). PharmGKB will become a national resource containing high-quality structured data linking genomic information, molecular and cellular phenotype information, and clinical phenotype information (Klein et al., 2001).

Reporting and Replication of Results

Negative results should have a venue for publication, and an unbiased collection of all results will have considerable value when meta-analyses are conducted (Romero et al., 2002). There has been considerable concern about the lack of ability to replicate the findings of gene-disease association studies. "The literature is full of reports of genetic linkage or association that do not hold up under scientific scrutiny." "Replication of findings remains a critical step to confirming the presence of such effects" (Vogler and Kozlowski, 2002).

Nevertheless, progress is being made in defining quality standards for genetic-epidemiological research. On the basis of the findings presented at the Human Genome Epidemiology workshop, a checklist for the reporting and appraisal of studies of the prevalence of genotypes and studies of gene-disease associations was developed (Little et al., 2002). This checklist focuses on the selection of study subjects, the analytical validity of genotyping, population stratification, and statistical issues. Use of the checklist should facilitate the integration of evidence from genetic and epidemiological studies of preterm birth (Little et al., 2002). Ongoing evaluation is needed to make sure that such guidelines are refined and are suitable for research on the genetics of preterm birth.

CONCLUSION

For many years, research on the etiology of preterm birth has primarily focused on demographic, social-behavioral, and environmental risk factors. Until recently, the roles of genetic susceptibility and gene-environment interactions in preterm birth have largely been unexplored. The use of molecular genetic epidemiology represents a promising approach to understanding the role and biological mechanisms of the genetic and environmental factors involved in preterm birth and their interactions in the pathogenesis of preterm birth. New tools for high-throughput genotyping, coupled with very-large-scale population-based studies that use sensitive biomarkers, comprehensive exposure assessment, and advanced biotechnology and analytical strategies, are needed to unravel the complex multiple gene-environment interactions responsible for preterm birth. Understanding these factors and their interactions could lead to major improvements in the diagnosis, prevention, and treatment of preterm birth.

8

The Role of Environmental Toxicants in Preterm Birth

ABSTRACT

Few environmental pollutants have been investigated for their potential to increase the risk for preterm birth. Among those pollutants that have been studied, however, only limited information is available for most of them. Because of this general lack of information, the potential contribution of environmental chemical pollutants to preterm birth is poorly understood. Possible exceptions are lead and environmental tobacco smoke, for which the weight of evidence suggests that maternal exposure to these pollutants increases the risk for preterm birth. In addition, a number of epidemiological studies have found significant relationships between exposures to air pollution and preterm birth, particularly for sulfur dioxide and particulates, suggesting that exposure to these air pollutants may increase a woman's risk for preterm birth. Studies to date suggest that agricultural chemicals deserve greater attention as potential risk factors for preterm birth. Other studies suggest that follow-up investigations that examine exposures to nitrates and arsenic in drinking water are warranted. In addition, despite persistent racial-ethnic disparities in the rates of preterm birth and increased awareness of racial-ethnic disparities in the levels of exposure to environmental toxicants, few studies have considered the interactions among race-ethnicity, environmental chemical exposure, and preterm birth. Nevertheless, the vast numbers of pollutants to which a woman may be exposed have never been consid-

ered in an investigation of preterm birth. Because of the large number of potential exposures, an efficient and effective research program that will serve public health needs is required.

Various environmental chemical pollutants are recognized as risk factors for numerous diseases and pathophysiological responses, and with the recognition that these pollutants pose a risk, policies have been instituted to protect the public health. Lead is perhaps the most renowned toxicant for which such actions have been taken, with national policies and programs established to protect children from neurotoxicity by removing lead from gasoline and paint. However, the potential risk for preterm birth as a result of exposure to environmental pollutants is poorly understood. This lack of knowledge presents a potentially significant shortcoming in the design of public health preventive strategies.

The present discussion specifically considers epidemiological studies that have analyzed the associations between exposure to environmental chemical pollutants and preterm birth. For this review, preterm birth is defined as the delivery of a live infant before 37 completed weeks of gestation, unless an alternative definition was used by a particular study. Analyses and findings of associations between environmental chemical exposures and low birth weight are not discussed. Because differences in mean gestational age at birth may or may not be relevant for preterm birth, depending on whether or not the distribution is affected at the lower gestational ages, studies in which gestational age was used as a continuous variable are discussed only as they contribute to the understanding of preterm birth.

Studies for consideration were identified on the basis of a PubMed Boolean search that crossed various terms for preterm birth (e.g., "premature birth," "prematurity," and "preterm delivery") or the term "birth outcomes" with general terms for toxicants (e.g., "air pollutants," "water pollutants," and "pesticides") and terms for selected specific pollutants (e.g., "dioxin," "polychlorinated biphenyls," and "DDT" [dichlorodiphenyltrichloroethane]). If the results of the studies evaluated were adjusted for confounders, only the adjusted statistics were considered in the final review. If adjustments were not made for potential confounders, the crude odds ratio (OR), crude relative risk (RR; risk ratio), or the most relevant statistical result was considered. The results were considered significant if they achieved statistical significance in the particular study and the confidence interval of the statistical estimate of adjusted OR or RR did not include unity (1.0). Although an attempt has been made to be thorough, some studies in this area may have been overlooked.

EXPOSURE ASSESSMENT CHALLENGES

A variety of approaches have been used to estimate exposures and to investigate the associations between environmental chemical exposures and preterm birth. A common approach has been to use employment or location of residence as a proxy for exposure, such as working with pesticides, proximity to a pollution source, or residence in a polluted locality. In those studies, exposure is typically estimated from measurement of the levels of contamination of common environmental media, such as drinking water sources and ambient air. However, such studies usually lack information about individual exposures and confounders, among other limitations.

Different approaches have been used to obtain information on individual levels of exposure. Perhaps the most conventional approach is to obtain self-reported data on exposures collected by survey or interview, but this method has the potential for reporting bias. Alternatively, measurements of the levels of chemical exposure have been used. These typically involve measurement of the levels of selected pollutants or their metabolites in body fluids or tissues, such as maternal blood, umbilical cord blood, and the placenta. However, the tissue or body fluid selected for toxicant level analysis has implications for the study, depending on the distribution of the toxicant in the body during pregnancy and the expected tissue or body fluid target for the action of the toxicant. Information on individual exposures provides potential advantages, such as controlling or adjusting for confounding variables and minimizing exposure misclassification.

The timing of the assessment may also influence the exposure measure. For example, if the toxicant concentration in the tissue changes over the course of gestation, the toxicant concentrations at the time of birth for preterm births may differ from those for term births simply as a function of gestational age. Similarly, if self-reporting or geographical-ecological assessments are used, the results may vary depending on whether the exposure is assessed for the last month of pregnancy, the entire pregnancy, or even for a period before the pregnancy. Co-exposures are common for environmental pollutants and pose another exposure assessment challenge. For example, cigarette smoke contains thousands of chemicals, many with known toxicity. Sulfur dioxide and particulates are typical co-pollutants of air, and many of the fat soluble toxicants are co-pollutants of food. Few studies have addressed potential impacts of co-pollutants in studies of preterm birth.

A major challenge is the assessment of cumulative exposures. Some pollutants are stored in the body, such as lead in bone or the pesticide DDT in fat. Metabolic changes of pregnancy cause increased metabolism of bone and fat tissues, such that toxicants are released from these sites to the blood and general circulation. Moreover, the impact of cumulative exposure may be important for preterm birth, but has been largely unexplored. However, cumulative exposure assessments face many challenges, in part because individuals are often unaware of exposure levels. Consequently, the development of biological markers for estimating cumulative exposure (e.g., k-x-ray fluorescence measurements of lead in bones) is needed for studies to assess impacts of cumulative exposures.

AIR POLLUTION

A significant and relatively recent effort has been made to link environmental air pollution exposures with preterm birth. Recent reviews examined a subset of articles on this topic in detail and drew different conclusions (Maisonet et al., 2004; Sram et al., 2005). Sram et al. (2005) reported that the evidence was insufficient to derive conclusions about an association between air pollution exposure and preterm birth and that further studies were justified. In contrast, Maisonet et al. (2004) reported that air pollution has an apparent effect on the rates of preterm birth, although the effects are relatively small, and that the conclusions were limited by the small number of studies and differences in the measurements of outcome, exposure, and confounders. The reviews by Sram et al. (2005) and Maisonet et al. (2004) included only 4 studies each, however, whereas the committee located 21 studies in the scientific literature for the present discussion on this topic. This section provides a brief review of the approaches, major findings, and challenges that is more inclusive than those provided in the reviews by Sram et al. (2005) and Maisonet et al. (2004). Moreover, some exposures that may have had an air pollution component but that fit better in other categories, such as lead exposure, are discussed elsewhere in this chapter in the discussion of the specific toxicant.

Different approaches have been used to assess exposure to air pollution. The most common approach has been to use residential proximity to air pollution sources, such as highways or oil refineries, as a proxy for exposure. An alternative exposure assessment approach relied on fixed air-monitoring stations to estimate the levels of air pollution exposure in the study population. An advantage of the latter approach is that specific pollutants were analyzed for their associations with preterm birth. However, estimates of the health effects of air pollutants tend to be smaller when exposure is assessed by using fixed-site air-monitoring station data rather than individual exposure data obtained by sampling individual women (Navidi and Lurmann, 1995). Moreover, the proximity of an individual's residence to a monitoring station was shown to influence the statistical association with preterm birth, further illustrating the heterogeneity of exposure as a limitation of this approach (Wilhelm and Ritz, 2005). Additionally, studies showed that pregnant women who were socioeconomically disadvantaged and of a nonwhite race were more likely to live in neighborhoods with more air pollution (Ponce et al., 2005; Woodruff et al., 2003). Because socioeconomic disadvantage and African American race are risk factors for preterm birth (see Chapter 4), geographical or ecological assessments of exposure to pollutants may be confounded by socioeconomic condition and race.

A variety of comparison strategies have been used. Many studies compared women who resided in a more polluted community with women who resided in a less polluted community. Some studies that used stationary air-monitoring station data to estimate exposures evaluated exposure-response relationships by analyzing the trends in preterm birth rates with respect to the exposure level on the basis of the woman's residence. Another approach has been to study the same population over time, because air pollutant levels vary significantly due to short-term fluctuations and the seasons (Sagiv et al., 2005; Sram et al., 1996; Wilhelm and Ritz, 2005). Moreover, the air concentrations of certain pollutants are known to correlate with one another. Because of this potential confounding, some studies that monitored exposure to multiple air pollutants also analyzed or adjusted for copollutant effects (Sagiv et al., 2005; Xu et al., 1995).

Sulfur Dioxide and Particulates

The most consistent relationships between specific air pollutants and preterm birth have been reported for sulfur dioxide and particulates. Of particular relevance to the United States is a study of births in Vancouver, British Columbia, Canada, conducted between 1985 and 1998, which reported an association between sulfur dioxide air pollution and preterm birth with an adjusted OR of 1.09 (95% confidence interval [CI] = 1.01–1.19) per 5.0 parts per billion (ppb) (14.3 micrograms per cubic meter [$\mu g/m^3$]) of sulfur dioxide (Liu et al., 2003). The mean daily concentration of sulfur dioxide during the study period was 4.9 ppb, with a maximum peak concentration (over 1 hour) of 128.5 ppb. Studies of women in the Czech Republic and Beijing, China, who were exposed to sulfur dioxide pollutant concentrations higher than usual for those in the United States reported concentration-dependent relationships between ambient air sulfur dioxide concentrations and preterm birth, with adjusted ORs of 1.27 (95% CI 1.16–1.39) per 50-$\mu g/m^3$ increase in the sulfur dioxide concentration (Bobak, 2000) and 1.21 (95% CI 1.01–1.45) for each ln natural log unit $\mu g/m^3$ increase in the sulfur dioxide concentration (Xu et al., 1995). The rates of preterm births also increased among women living in the vicinity of a coal-burning power plant in Croatia during a period of high-intensity power plant operation with higher sulfur dioxide emissions compared with those during a period of lower-intensity power plant operation (RR = 1.76; p = 0.026) (Mohorovic, 2004).

Similar to sulfur dioxide, associations between exposure to airborne particulates and preterm birth have been reported. Airborne particulates have been measured as total suspended particulates and particulates equal to or less than 10 micrometers (μm) in diameter (PM_{10}). In a study of women in Southern California, PM_{10} exposure in the 6-week period before birth increased the risk for preterm birth by vaginal delivery (adjusted RR 1.19 per 50 μg of total suspended particulates/m^3; 95% CI 1.10–1.40) and preterm birth by delivery by cesarean section (adjusted RR 1.35 per 50 μg of total suspended particulates/m^3; 95% CI 1.06–1.69) (Ritz et al., 2000). Concentration-dependent responses were observed in populations of women in the Czech Republic (adjusted OR 1.18; 95% CI 1.05–1.31 per 50 μg of total suspended particulates/m^3) (Bobak, 2000) and Beijing (adjusted OR 1.10 μg/m^3; 95% CI 1.01–1.20 per 100 μg of total suspended particulates/ m^3) (Xu et al., 1995) who were exposed to concentrations of particulate air pollution higher than those usually found in the United States.

In contrast, a time-series study of four Pennsylvania counties found suggestive, but not significant, associations between exposure to sulfur dioxide or PM_{10} and preterm birth (Sagiv et al., 2005). Likewise, the linkage of medical registries with air pollution data on sulfur dioxide, hydrocarbons, and nitrogen oxides in southern Sweden found no differences in the rates of preterm birth in comparisons of the municipalities with pollutant levels above and below the mean level and when the rate of preterm birth in the municipality with the highest pollutant level was compared with the rates in all other municipalities (Landgren, 1996).

Carbon Monoxide, Nitrogen Oxides, and Ozone

The relationship of the rates of preterm birth to exposure to carbon monoxide, nitrogen oxides, and ozone pollution is less certain. Exposure to carbon monoxide in ambient air in the last month of pregnancy was associated with preterm birth in a population of women in Vancouver, British Columbia, Canada (Liu et al., 2003), with an adjusted OR of 1.08 (95% CI 1.01–1.15) for each 1.0-part-per-million increase in the carbon monoxide level. In contrast, the relationship between carbon monoxide pollutant levels and preterm birth was inconsistent in a study of pregnancies in Southern California: exposure to carbon monoxide in the 6-week period before birth was associated with increased rates of preterm birth for inland regions (RR 1.12; 95% CI 1.04–1.21) but with decreased rates of preterm births for coastal regions (RR 0.77; 95% CI 0.64–0.91) (Ritz et al., 2000).

Disparate results have also been reported for nitrogen oxides. Maroziene and Grazuleviciene (2002) reported increased rates of preterm birth among Lithuanian women in association with exposure to nitrogen dioxide in ambient air (adjusted ORs for medium and high tertile exposures to nitrogen dioxide were 1.14 [95% CI 0.77–1.68] and 1.68 [95% CI 1.15–2.46], respectively). However, other studies failed to find a significant association between the levels of nitrogen oxide exposure and the rates of preterm birth (Bobak, 2000; Liu et al., 2003; Ritz et al., 2000).

Likewise, ozone was not significantly associated with preterm birth in two studies (Liu et al., 2003; Ritz et al., 2000).

Location of Residence

Several studies found that women who live in an area with high levels of air pollution are more likely to deliver preterm than women who live in less polluted areas. Women who live near petroleum refinery plants (Lin et al., 2001; Yang et al., 2004a), petrochemical industrial complexes (Yang et al., 2002a,b), or industrial districts with increased levels of emission of air contaminants from multiple sources (including petrochemical, petroleum, steel, and shipbuilding industries) (Tsai et al., 2003) had an increased risk for delivery of preterm infants, with ORs ranging from 1.03 to 1.41. Women living in a mining district of the Czech Republic had nearly twice the prevalence of preterm birth compared with that of women living in a less polluted district ($p < 0.01$), although that study was confounded by cigarette smoking and racial differences that stratified with the districts (Dejmek et al., 1996; Sram et al., 1996). Residential proximity to highways was also found to be related to the risk for preterm birth, with ORs or RRs ranging from 1.08 to 1.30 (Ponce et al., 2005; Wilhelm and Ritz, 2003, 2005; Yang et al., 2003a).

Exposure by Stage of Gestation

Several studies specifically analyzed whether a stage of gestation for exposure to air pollutants is the most strongly associated with preterm birth. The results have been inconsistent, with some studies reporting significant associations early or late in gestation. Exposure to sulfur dioxide (Bobak, 2000; Mohorovic, 2004), total suspended particulates (Bobak, 2000), and nitrogen dioxide (Maroziene and Grazuleviciene, 2002) in the first trimester, but not the second or the third trimester, of pregnancy was associated with preterm birth. Among women living in a mining district of the Czech Republic who smoked cigarettes during pregnancy, there was an increased prevalence of preterm births for pregnancies conceived in the winter compared with pregnancies conceived in summer. Because winter in this study was characterized by weather inversions that resulted in unusually high concentrations of fine particles dominated by acidic sulfates, genotoxic organic compounds, and toxic trace elements (Dejmek et al., 1996; Sram et al., 1996), a relationship between conception, exposure and preterm birth is suggested..

In contrast, other studies have reported associations between preterm birth and exposures to toxicants later in pregnancy. Specifically, Liu et al. (2003) found that the rates of preterm birth increased with exposure to sulfur dioxide and carbon monoxide during the last but not the first month of pregnancy. In addition, the most significant elevation in the rates of preterm birth among women who lived near roadways in Los Angeles County with heavy traffic occurred for women whose third trimester fell during the fall and winter months, when the level of traffic-related air pollution was the highest (Wilhelm and Ritz, 2003). In one study, preterm birth was associated with exposure to particulate air pollution (PM_{10}) in the last 6 weeks but not the first month of pregnancy (Ritz et al., 2000). Bobak (2000) found no differences in the odds of preterm birth among the trimesters of gestation (adjusted OR range = 1.24 to 1.27 per 50 μg of increase in the sulfur dioxide concentration/m^3). A detailed time-series analysis of exposure to sulfur dioxide and fine particulates (PM_{10}) found suggestive, although not significant, associations of preterm birth with the levels of PM_{10} and sulfur dioxide exposures in the last 6 weeks and the last 1 week of gestation (Sagiv et al., 2005).

Significance of Overall Findings for Air Pollution

It should be noted that the adjusted ORs or RRs in all of the studies were relatively low (less than 1.68), with many estimates being much lower. The relatively small increased risk of preterm birth reflected by the relatively low ORs or RRs may represent a truly marginal increased risk or may be a consequence of the exposure assessment complexities discussed earlier. In addition, several of the studies analyzed multiple air pollutants, and the tendency to focus on positive findings should be balanced by consideration of the entire context of the study. Nonetheless, given the number of studies that have found significant relationships between exposures to air pollution and preterm birth, the epidemiological findings suggest that air pollution contributes to a woman's risk for preterm birth. Moreover, several studies reported exposure-response relationships of significance, particularly for sulfur dioxide and particulates (Bobak, 2000; Liu et al., 2003; Maroziene and Grazuleviciene, 2002; Ritz et al., 2000; Sagiv et al., 2005; Xu et al., 1995). Inconsistent findings that were regionally dependent were reported for carbon monoxide, and contradictory results were reported for nitrous oxides. Consequently, conclusions about the risk for preterm birth from ambient air exposures to carbon monoxide and nitrous oxides cannot be made at this time. Moreover, the two studies that evaluated ozone found that ozone exposure has no significant association with preterm birth, suggesting that ozone may not be a significant contributor to preterm birth. Likewise, the contradictory findings do not allow conclusions regarding a critical gestational stage for exposure to air pollutants and an increased risk of preterm birth.

Finally, the analysis by Xu et al. (1995) deserves further comment. Those investigators found that exposure to sulfur dioxide and total suspended particles modified the distribution of gestational age at birth, such that the largest effects were observed with exposures at the youngest gestational ages. Those researchers calculated an attributable risk (the proportion of cases of preterm delivery in the sample attributable to air pollution) of 33.4 percent. This high attributable risk indicates that exposure to elevated levels of sulfur dioxide and particulate air pollution poses a significant public health concern for pregnant women. Although the concentrations of sulfur dioxide and particulate air pollution that Xu and colleagues (1995) measured in Beijing air are not anticipated in the United States, the study nonetheless illustrates the potential and preventable impacts that air pollutants can have on preterm birth.

AGRICULTURAL CHEMICALS

A variety of agricultural chemicals are manufactured and widely applied in the United States and worldwide to control pests and enhance agricultural productivity. Human exposures may result from occupational manufacture or use or may be indirect as a result of contamination of environmental media, such as water, air, and food. Among the agricultural chemicals, pesticides have been the most intensively studied for their association with preterm birth. Some of the most notorious pesticides, such as the insecticide DDT, persist in the environment, are poorly excreted, and (biomagnify) in the food chain, thereby increasing potential for human exposure.

Exposure to agricultural chemicals has been assessed by a variety of methods in epidemiological studies of preterm birth. The most common approach has been measurement of the pollutant concentrations in maternal blood, umbilical cord blood, or neonatal blood. Other approaches have used residence on a farm, survey assessment of occupational exposure, and retrospective surveys of exposures of the mother.

DDT has been examined more than any other pesticide in epidemiological studies of preterm birth. DDT is an environmentally persistent insecticide that biomagnifies in the food chain, with known disastrous reproductive consequences for certain wildlife. Although the use of DDT in the United States has been discontinued since 1972, it continues to be applied worldwide to kill mosquitoes for the control of malaria, and environmental residues persist because of its poor ability to degrade biologically in the environment. DDT is applied as a technical grade of isomers, of which p,p'-DDT is the most abundant. Much of the interest in the o,p'-DDT isomer has been due to its affinity for estrogen receptor alpha. Human excretion of DDT is nominal, although it is metabolized to its persistent metabolite, (p,p'-DDE), which is also poorly excreted. Consequently, studies of DDT have monitored for p,p'-DDT, o,p'-DDT, p,p'-DDE, and, less frequently, various other isomers of DDT. A recent publication includes a comparison table of published reports of studies that analyzed for an association between DDT exposure and preterm birth (Farhang et al., 2005).

Two studies examined the associations between DDT exposure and preterm birth for similar exposure measures over a similar time period and used logistic regression analysis that adjusted for similar confounding variables. The most comprehensive assessment of the association between exposure to DDT and preterm birth included 2,380 women (361 of whom delivered prematurely) who had participated in the U.S. Collaborative Perinatal Project between 1959 and 1965 (Longnecker et al., 2001). By using a logistic regression analysis of third-trimester maternal serum DDE concentrations, Longnecker and colleagues (2001) found that the odds of preterm birth increased steadily and significantly with increasing concentrations of serum DDE ($p < 0.0001$), with adjusted ORs of 2.5 (95% CI 1.5–4.2) when levels in serum were 45 to 59 µg of DDE/liter and 3.1 (95% CI 1.8–5.4) when levels in serum were ≥60 µg of DDE/liter. The same study failed to find a significant association between preterm birth and either third-trimester maternal serum DDT concentrations or the ratios of maternal serum DDT levels to serum DDE levels.

In contrast, a logistic regression analysis failed to detect an association between preterm birth and maternal serum concentrations of DDE or DDT or the DDT:DDE ratio among 420 women who had participated in the Child Health and Development Studies of the San Francisco Bay Area from 1959 to 1967 (Farhang et al., 2005). However, that study had significant limitations, such as the inclusion of only 33 preterm births; the inclusion of only infants who had survived until 2 years of age; and the use of maternal blood samples, the majority of which were taken at an unspecified time in the postpartum period, with the untested assumption that the postpartum and pregnancy serum DDT and DDE concentrations would be interchangeable.

Other studies used a case-control approach and relatively small sample sizes (4 to 24 cases of preterm birth). Those studies compared the tissue DDT concentrations and the concentrations of other pesticides in women who delivered preterm with those in women who delivered at term. Many of these studies analyzed for multiple persistent toxicants and emphasized the positive results. Nonetheless, the findings deserve consideration, albeit with some attention to the context of the study.

Berkowitz and colleagues (1996) reported the only case-control study that matched for potential confounding variables (maternal age, race, and prepregnancy body mass index) and analyzed other potential confounders in a group of New York women who gave birth between 1990 and 1993. They found no significant differences in first-trimester maternal serum DDE levels for women who delivered preterm ($n = 20$) compared with those for women who delivered at term ($n = 20$).

Three case-control studies that did not control for potentially confounding variables reported that increased tissue concentrations of several pesticides were associated with preterm birth. In two studies of pregnant women from Lucknow, India, Saxena et al. (1980, 1981) found elevated concentrations of three major isomers of DDT (including DDE), as well as the pesticides lindane, aldrin, and hexachlorobenzene, in the blood and placentas of women who went into preterm labor (defined as labor during 12 to 32 weeks of gestation in the first study; preterm labor was not defined in the second study) compared with those in the blood and placentas of women who delivered at term ($p < 0.001$). Likewise, a study of Israeli women who delivered preterm reported elevated maternal blood concentrations of the pesticides lindane, dieldrin, heptachlor, and several isomers of DDT, including DDE, at the time of delivery compared with the concentrations in women who delivered at term ($p < 0.02$) (Wassermann et al., 1982).

In a study of Brazilian births, elevated concentrations of DDT and DDE were observed in the umbilical cord blood of preterm infants compared with those in term infants, even though there were no differences in maternal blood DDT concentrations (Procianoy and Schvartsman, 1981). A study of births in Flix, Spain, of women exposed to extremely high levels of atmospheric pollution from an electrochemical plant found umbilical cord blood DDE concentrations that were three times higher for preterm births ($n = 4$) than for term births ($n = 66$) ($p < 0.05$) (Ribas-Fito et al., 2002), but no significant differences in the concentrations of the pesticide β-hexachlorocyclohexane were detected.

Although they do not tend to persist in the environment, organophosphate insecticides comprise another category of pesticides with potential for human exposure because of their widespread use. By using inhibition of cholinesterase enzyme activity in umbilical cord blood as a biomarker of exposure to organophosphates, Eskenazi et al. (2004) reported an increased odds for preterm birth in association with organophosphate pesticide exposure (adjusted OR 2.3; 95% CI 1.1–4.8; $p = 0.02$). Although the concentrations of metabolites of organophosphate pesticides in maternal urine were not associated with preterm birth in the latter study, the urine samples were collected before parturition, whereas the umbilical cord blood was collected at the time of delivery. In a population of primarily Hispanic, low-income women assessed for exposure to organophosphate pesticides through analysis of maternal blood cholinesterase activity and exposure history by self-report, no differences in the risk of preterm birth were observed between exposed and unexposed women (Willis et al., 1993).

By using employment in the floriculture industry as a proxy for exposure to pesticides and self-reported data on pregnancy outcomes, Restrepo et al. (1990) compared the prevalence of preterm birth before and after employment for floriculture industry workers in Colombia. They reported an increased odds of preterm birth after working in floriculture for female workers (OR 1.86; 95% CI 1.59–2.17; $p < 0.01$) and the wives of male workers (OR 2.75; 95% CI 2.01–3.76; $p < 0.01$).

Paternal exposure, but not maternal exposure, to pesticides was associated with preterm birth in a study of U.S. Navy women that used the mother's retrospective self-report to assess the father's occupational exposure to pesticides (Hourani and Hilton, 2000). Exposure to the widely applied herbicide atrazine via drinking water was not significantly associated with preterm birth in logistic regression analyses (Villanueva et al., 2005).

Application of inorganic and organic fertilizer (e.g., manure) to crops is a potential source of nitrate contamination of drinking water supplies. A population-based case-control study with 321 cases found that women in Prince Edward Island, Canada, who lived in regions on the island with higher concentrations of nitrates in the drinking water were more likely than women who lived in the region on the island with the lowest nitrate water levels to deliver the infants preterm (Bukowski et al., 2001a). This association of nitrates in drinking water with preterm birth was exposure dependent, with adjusted ORs increasing from 1.82 (95% CI 1.23–2.69) at the median nitrate concentration of 3.1 milligrams per liter (mg/liter) to ORs of 2.33 (95% CI 1.46–3.68) and 2.37 (95% CI 1.07–4.08) at median nitrate concentrations of 4.3 and 5.5 mg/liter, respectively (Bukowski et al., 2001a). In contrast, a study of 486 West African infants found no association between preterm birth and living in a region with very high nitrate levels in the drinking water, when regions with low and high nitrate were compared according to whether the well water nitrate concentration was below or above 20 mg/liter (Super et al., 1981).

Another study compared Norwegian farmers with a nonfarmer reference group ($n = 192,417$ births) and found no significant relationship between owning a farm and the risk for preterm birth if all births before 37 completed weeks of gestation were included in the analysis (Kristensen et al., 1997). However, among farmers there was an increase of extremely early, midgestation preterm births (between 21 and 24 weeks of gestation), with an adjusted OR of 1.54 (95% CI 1.23–1.93) for singleton births and a much higher adjusted OR of 3.75 (95% CI 1.72–8.20) for multiple gestations. Moreover, that study found significant associations with grain farming in particular (OR 1.58; 95% CI 1.19–2.09) and also found a pattern of association with the season of the year and a poor grain harvest quality, which led the authors to speculate that mycotoxins produced by molds may induce midpregnancy preterm labor, with the strongest effect on multiple-fetus pregnancies.

Although the epidemiological findings do not present a consensus on whether exposures to particular agricultural chemicals increase the risk for preterm birth, the studies that have been performed to date suggest that agricultural chemicals deserve greater attention as potential risk factors for preterm birth. In particular, the report by Longnecker et al. (2001) provides the strongest evidence for an association of DDT exposure with preterm birth because of the large sample size, the significant exposure-response relationship, and adjustment for confounders. Although DDT exposure may continue to be significant elsewhere in the world, it should be noted that the latter study used blood samples collected from women in the United States between 1959 and 1967, when exposures to DDT were substantially greater in the United States than they are today. Other studies of DDT and its association with preterm birth are compromised by small sample sizes, a lack of subject demographic information, or a lack of consideration for confounders.

Early reports that associated preterm birth with elevated tissue levels of other persistent organochlorine pesticides (lindane, aldrin, dieldrin, heptachlor, and hexachlorobenzene) have not been pursued. The report that preterm birth was significantly associated with a biomarker in umbilical cord blood for exposure to organophosphate pesticides (Eskenazi et al., 2004) requires follow-up. Given the potential for exposure from contaminated drinking water, further examination of the risk for preterm birth from nitrates is also warranted. Finally, the potential for mycotoxins to contribute to early preterm births is intriguing (Kristensen et al., 1997) and deserves further analysis by the use of individual-specific exposure assessments.

POLYCHLORINATED BIPHENYLS

Polychlorinated biphenyls (PCBs) are industrial chemicals that were manufactured and used commercially as mixtures of congeners, with each congener distinguished by the number and pattern of chlorination of the biphenyl rings. Certain PCB congeners persist in the environment, are poorly metabolized, and biomagnify in the food chain. These characteristics result in increased opportunities for human exposure. The production and commercial use of PCBs were discontinued in most countries in the late 1970s, although there is evidence that production continued in some countries until recently.

An early study reported that the concentration of total PCBs in the blood of 17 women who delivered prematurely was 3.7-fold higher than that observed in 10 women with normal third-trimester pregnancies ($p <$ 0.025) and found that penta- and hexachlorinated biphenyl congener levels were specifically elevated in the maternal blood of women who delivered preterm (Wassermann et al., 1982). However, no demographic information on the women in the latter case-control study was available. Longnecker et al. (2005) failed to find a significant association between PCBs and preterm birth in a logistic regression analysis of 1,034 historical maternal blood samples collected between 1959 and 1965 that included potential confounding factors. Likewise, a case-control study failed to find differences in maternal serum levels of PCBs (total or individual congeners) between New York City women who delivered preterm ($n = 20$) or full term ($n = 20$) between 1990 and 1993 in a study that matched the women for potential confounding variables (maternal age, race, and prepregnancy body mass index) and that analyzed for other potential confounders (Berkowitz et al., 1996). Furthermore, there were no significant differences between PCB concentrations in umbilical cord serum from preterm births compared with those from full-term births in a Spanish population exposed to extremely high levels of air pollution (Ribas-Fito et al., 2002).

Because PCBs biomagnify in the food chain, two studies examined relationships between the consumption of Great Lakes fish, PCB exposure and preterm birth. In a study conducted in Michigan, women who reported eating the equivalent of about two salmon or lake trout meals per month had decreased gestational lengths (an average of 4.9 days shorter) compared with those of women who ate less Great Lakes fish, and infants with higher concentrations of PCBs in the umbilical cord serum were born an average of 8.8 days earlier than infants with lower cord serum PCB concentrations (Fein et al., 1984). In contrast, a later study conducted in Green Bay, Wisconsin, found no significant associations between maternal reports of Lake Michigan fish consumption or maternal serum concentrations of PCBs and any adverse reproductive outcome (Dar et al., 1992).

In an analysis of a population of women who worked in two capacitor manufacturing facilities in upstate New York, women with higher levels of occupational exposure to PCBs had significantly decreased gestational durations (an average of 6.6 days shorter) (Taylor et al., 1984). A follow-up study of the women in the capacitor manufacturing facilities found that the differences in infant birth weights between women exposed to high levels of PCBs and women with low levels of exposure to PCBs was explained, at least in part, by differences in gestational duration (Taylor et al., 1989).

The largest and most rigorous studies (with respect to control for confounding factors) failed to establish a significant association between exposure to PCBs and preterm birth. Because of the epidemiological findings and the fact that environmental contamination from PCBs is declining in environmental media in most regions of the world, the studies do not support the possibility that exposure to PCBs is likely a significant risk factor for preterm birth in women currently residing in the United States.

DIOXIN

Chlorinated dioxins comprise a class of compounds made up of 75 structurally related congeners that are distinguished by the number and position of chlorine atoms on the dibenzo-*p*-dioxin molecule. The most toxic and well known chlorinated dioxin is 2,3,7,8-tetrachlorodibenzo-*p*-dioxin (TCDD), commonly referred to as dioxin. Although TCDD and other dioxins are produced naturally by forest fires or volcanic activity from the incomplete combustion of organic matter, it is the anthropomorphic production as unintended by-products of incineration or combustion that contributes the greatest amount of pollution of chlorinated dioxins in the environment. TCDD was also an unintended by-product in the production of the defoliating herbicide Agent Orange, which was widely applied in southeastern Asia during the Vietnam War.

Several studies have examined whether exposure to dioxin is associated with preterm birth, but the findings are contradictory. Serum TCDD levels of women living in Seveso, Italy, near the site of a major industrial accident that released TCDD into the air, were not significantly associated with an increased odds of preterm delivery (Eskenazi et al., 2003). In a survey study of cancer and reproductive outcomes in the TCDD-contaminated Russian town of Chapvaevsk, the average rate of preterm labor was reported to be significantly higher in women who lived in Chapvaevsk than in women who lived in other towns in the region (Revich et al., 2001). However, preterm birth was not defined, and statistical comparisons were not provided.

In a pilot qualitative study conducted in the year 2000, higher numbers of preterm births were reported among 30 Vietnamese women whose husbands or who themselves were exposed to TCDD through the herbicide Agent Orange (Le and Johansson, 2001). Because TCDD mediates most, if not all, of its toxicity by the binding and activation of the Ah receptor, one study measured the placental concentration of Ah receptor sites, the affinity of TCDD for the Ah receptor, and aryl hydroxylase activity (a cytochrome P450 CYP1A1 enzyme regulated by the Ah receptor) but found no significant differences between normal and preterm births (Okey et al., 1997).

Consequently, despite the general toxicity and notoriety of TCDD, epidemiological studies have failed to find a significant relationship between maternal exposure to TCDD and preterm birth. Consequently, the epide-miological reports do not provide support the possibility that maternal exposure to TCDD is an important risk factor for preterm birth.

CHLORINATION DISINFECTION BY-PRODUCTS

Because of the widespread use of chlorination as a means to disinfect drinking water supplies, there is considerable interest in the potential health risks from the by-products that are formed because of chlorination disinfection. The principal by-products are trihalomethanes (e.g., chloroform, bromodichloromethane, and dichlorobromomethane), haloacetic acids (e.g., trichloroacetic acid and dichloroacetic acid), and 3-chloro-4-(dichloromethyl)-5-hydroxy-2(5H)-furanone.

Studies of the health effects of chlorination disinfection by-products are complicated by exposure assessment challenges. Specifically, the levels of trihalomethanes increase during the summer and autumn months, when organic material from leaves and other sources increasingly infiltrate surface water supplies and thereby favor the formation of trihalomethanes during chlorination disinfection. Additionally, the concentrations of disinfection by-products vary depending on their location in the distribution system, such that the levels of some by-products (e.g., bromodichloromethane) in the supply system increase over time but the levels of haloacetic acids seem to decrease over time. Moreover, individual behaviors can significantly affect exposure. For example, bathing habits and whether a woman drinks tap water or bottled water can significantly modify individual exposures. Studies that rely on geographical or ecological exposure assessments of community drinking water samples are limited by the inability to account for individual exposure variations.

Epidemiological studies of associations between chlorination disinfection by-products and preterm birth or gestational age published before 2002 have been reviewed in detail by Bove et al. (2002) and Graves et al. (2001). The conclusions of those reviews are summarized here, but the individual studies included in those recent reviews are not discussed in detail. Rather, the reader is referred to these reviews for details on the specific studies.

Bove et al. (2002) reviewed eight studies and Graves et al. (2001) reviewed seven studies that analyzed for associations between preterm birth and contamination of drinking water with chlorination disinfection by-products. Among the studies reviewed by Bove et al. and Graves et al., only a single study (Yang et al., 2000) found a significantly increased odds for preterm birth (adjusted OR 1.34; 95% CI 1.1–1.6) in a comparison of births in municipalities in Taiwan that chlorinated the drinking water supply with births in municipalities that did not. Consequently, the conclusion of both reviews was that exposure to disinfection by-products was not likely associated with preterm birth. Additional studies found no associations between chlorination disinfection or chlorination disinfection by-products and an increased risk for preterm birth, including a study published in 1982 (Tuthill et al., 1982) but not included in the reviews by Bove et al. (2002) and Graves et al. (2001), as well as more recent studies (Aggazzotti et al., 2004; Wright et al., 2003, 2004). In fact, Wright et al. (2004) reported a slight but significantly reduced odds of preterm delivery with maternal exposure to the chlorination disinfection by-products total trihalomethanes, chloroform, and bromodichloromethane.

The only study to identify a positive association between exposure to chlorination disinfection by-products and preterm birth based its exposure assessment on the method used to chlorinate the drinking water supply rather than the amounts of by-products in the water. Consequently, the only positive study is limited by the potential for exposure misclassification. In contrast, many of the studies that reported a lack of a relationship or even a positive relationship between exposure to chlorination disinfection by-products and preterm birth relied on specific measures of exposure. Thus, the general result is that the studies fail to support a relationship between preterm birth and exposure to disinfection by-products.

ENVIRONMENTAL TOBACCO SMOKE

Environmental tobacco smoke constitutes passive exposure to cigarette smoke in the ambient air as opposed to active exposure through cigarette smoking. Risks to preterm birth from active cigarette smoking are covered in Chapter 3. A handful of studies have analyzed for an association between environmental tobacco smoke and preterm birth. Among those studies, maternal self-reporting was the most commonly used exposure assessment measure, although two studies used biomarkers of exposure (the maternal serum concentration of the nicotine metabolite cotinine and the concentration of nicotine in maternal hair). Each of the studies reported a positive association between exposure to environmental tobacco smoke and an increased risk for preterm birth. However, the studies have specific nuances that distinguish the findings.

Among women interviewed a few days after delivery for retrospective self-assessment of exposure to environmental tobacco smoke, daily exposure to environmental tobacco smoke of 7 hours or more was significantly associated with an increased risk for preterm birth (OR 1.86; 95% CI 1.05–3.45) (Hanke et al., 1999). In another study that relied on maternal self-reporting, exposure to environmental tobacco smoke for 7 hours or more daily was associated with an increased odds for preterm birth (less than 35 weeks of gestation; adjusted OR 2.4; 95% CI 1.0–5.3) but not with an increased risk for preterm birth before 37 weeks of gestation (Windham et al., 2000). However, the latter study was prospective and assessed exposure based on maternal self-reporting of estimated exposure to environmental tobacco smoke in the 1 week before an interview during early to midpregnancy.

Using maternal self-reporting of exposure to the cigarette smoke of a household member during pregnancy as the index of exposure, Ahluwalia et al. (1997) reported a significantly increased risk for preterm birth for women age 30 years or older (adjusted OR 1.88; 95% CI 1.22–2.88) but not younger women. Also relying on maternal self-reports of exposure, Ahlborg and Bodin (1991) found that exposure to environmental tobacco smoke in the workplace but not in the home was associated with an increased risk of preterm birth. As assessed by questionnaire information in another study, the odds of preterm birth were increased with exposure to environmental tobacco smoke at work only (adjusted OR 2.35; 95% CI 0.50–11.1) and, to a greater extent, with exposure at both work and home (adjusted OR 8.89; 95% CI 1.05–75.3) but not with home exposure only (Jaakkola et al., 2001).

Two studies assessed exposure to environmental tobacco smoke on the basis of a combination of interviews of the mother and biomarkers of exposure. Jaakkola et al. (2001) used the nicotine concentration in hair samples obtained after delivery to assess environmental tobacco smoke exposure and found that there was a concentration-dependent association, with the adjusted OR increasing 1.22 (95% CI 1.07–1.39) with each 1 μg of nicotine/gram of hair. In the high-exposure group in the latter study, the odds of preterm delivery were about sixfold higher in comparison with that for the reference group (adjusted OR 6.12; 95% CI 1.31–28.7) (Jaakkola et al., 2001). A second study relied on the concentrations of the nicotine metabolite cotinine in maternal serum at midpregnancy as an index of exposure to environmental tobacco smoke (Kharrazi et al., 2004). The authors of that study reported an increased odds for preterm birth at the highest quintile level of exposure (0.236 to 10 nanograms [ng] of cotinine/milliliter [ml]) compared with that at the lowest quintile (<0.026 ng/ml) (adjusted OR 1.78; 95% CI 1.01–3.13) in a study of 2,777 births (Kharrazi et al., 2004).

Despite differences in exposure assessment and study design, the six published reports show general agreement that exposure to environmental tobacco smoke is associated with an increased risk for preterm birth. The finding by Ahluwalia et al. (1997) of an interaction between exposure to environmental tobacco smoke and maternal age is particularly interesting and deserves further analysis. The adjusted ORs of the studies on the risk of preterm birth as a result of exposure to environmental tobacco smoke ranged from 1.2 to 2.4, with the exception of the study by Jaakkola et al. (2001), which found adjusted ORs of 6.12 and 8.89. Exempting the study Jaakkola et al. (2001), the magnitude of the increase in the odds for preterm birth as a result of exposure to environmental tobacco smoke is similar to or somewhat higher than that observed for active cigarette smoking (see Chapter 3). Although speculative at this time, one possible explanation for the latter observation may be that environmental tobacco smoke exposures tend to be more constant and longer in duration whereas active cigarette smoking is more episodic. Regardless, the studies suggest that environmental tobacco smoke deserves greater attention as a risk factor for preterm birth. Overall, the published reports indicate that exposure to environmental tobacco smoke should be considered a potential risk factor for preterm birth.

METALS AND METALLOIDS

Metals and metalloids are elements that are found in nature and that can form a variety of chemical moieties. This review considers all chemical forms of a metal or metalloid evaluated in studies that analyzed for associations between exposures and preterm birth. Furthermore, several of the metallic elements constitute the so-called nutritional micronutrients, and deficiencies of these micronutrients have been associated, in some cases, with an increased risk for preterm birth (see Chapter 3). However, this section of the report deals only with excess environmental exposure to metals and metalloids.

Among the metals and metalloids, lead exposure has been studied the most intensively for an association with preterm birth. A thorough review by Andrews et al. (1994) discusses epidemiological studies published before 1994 that analyzed for associations between lead exposure and preterm birth, as well as other birth outcomes. Although noting the weaknesses and the shortcomings of particular studies, Andrews et al. concluded that an adverse effect of lead exposure on preterm delivery was supported because (1) mean lead levels were elevated in women with preterm births compared with those in women with term births in all studies reviewed, and (2) the prevalence of preterm births increased with an increase in the level of maternal exposure to lead in most of the studies reviewed. The specific studies that Andrews et al. reviewed will not be described here; rather, the reader is referred to that review for a detailed discussion (Andrews et al., 1994).

Similar to the results noted by Andrews et al. (1994), Falcon et al. (2003) found that mean placental lead concentrations were significantly (1.5-fold) higher for 18 women who delivered preterm or who had premature rupture of the membranes than for 71 women who delivered at term (Falcon et al., 2003). The latter study of Spanish women found no significant differences in age, parity, smoking habits, or location of residential for the women who delivered term and those who delivered preterm.

Torres-Sanchez et al. (1999) found that mean umbilical cord lead levels were marginally significantly higher ($p < 0.051$) for preterm births than for term births, but only for primiparous women. However, Torres-Sanchez et al. (1999) also analyzed their data by separate logistic regression analyses for the primiparous and multiparous women using quartile groupings of umbilical cord lead concentrations and adjusting for various known preterm birth risk factors. Using the lowest quartile group (that with a mean umbilical cord blood concentration of < 5.1 µg of lead/deciliter) as the reference group, they found a significantly increased odds ratio for preterm birth for the primiparous women but not the multiparous women at the three higher lead exposure levels, with adjusted ORs ranging from 2.60 to 2.82 (Torres-Sanchez et al., 1999). In contrast, a small case-control study that compared Swedish and Polish women who delivered preterm ($n = 17$) or at term ($n = 13$) found no significant differences in maternal blood, myometrium, or placenta concentrations of lead at the time of delivery (Fagher et al., 1993).

Studies of historical occupational records conducted in Norway found that women who worked during pregnancy in jobs classified as having high levels of lead exposure were at increased risk for preterm birth compared with the risk for women who worked at jobs classified as having nominal levels of lead exposure (adjusted OR 1.93; 95% CI 1.09–3.28) (Irgens et al., 1998).

Many of the preceding studies used lead concentrations in blood as a measure of exposure. However, the lead in whole blood may not reflect bioavailable lead, because the majority of lead in blood (more than 95 percent) is bound to red blood cells and is thus not available to cause harm (Manton and Cook, 1984; Smith D et al., 2002).

Contradictory results were obtained in pairs of studies on exposures to cadmium and arsenic in drinking water. Cadmium concentrations at the time of delivery were significantly higher in maternal blood but not in the myometriums or the placentas of women who delivered preterm ($n = 13$) than in those of women who delivered at term ($n = 11$) (Fagher et al., 1993). In a study of women ($n = 44$) living in a cadmium-contaminated region of China in which the median concentrations were used to form the comparison groups, there were no significant differences in preterm birth rates between women with higher cadmium concentrations and women with lower cadmium concentrations in maternal blood, umbilical cord blood, or the placenta (Zhang et al., 2004).

In a study of women in Bangladesh, the rate of preterm births was 2.5-fold higher among women in a village serviced by arsenic-contaminated drinking water ($n = 96$) than among women matched for age, socioeconomic condition, level of education, and age at marriage who lived in a village with much lower concentrations of arsenic in the drinking water ($\leq$0.02 mg of arsenic/liter; $n = 96$) ($p < 0.02$) (Ahmad et al., 2001). Moreover, the rates of preterm births were significantly higher for those Bangladeshi women who relied on arsenic-contaminated drinking water for more than 15 years than for Bangladeshi women who drank arsenic-contaminated water for less than 15 years ($p < 0.02$) (Ahmad et al., 2001). In contrast, maternal arsenic exposure from drinking well water was not significantly associated with a risk of preterm delivery in a study that compared women who lived in an arsenic-contaminated area with women who lived in an area without a history of arsenic contamination in Taiwan, with the townships matched for degree of urbanization (Yang et al., 2003b).

No excess numbers of preterm birth were observed in a community in which there was an accidental spill of aluminum sulfate into the drinking water than in neighboring communities (Golding et al., 1991). However, the population size of the exposed pregnant women in the latter study was relatively small (4 preterm births among 88 exposed pregnant women).

Overwhelmingly, lead has been investigated in more studies than any other metal or metalloid for associations with preterm birth or decreased gestation length. Although the evidence is not unanimous, there is sufficient evidence to suggest that maternal exposure to lead results in an increased risk for preterm delivery. The current level of knowledge is inadequate to determine if there may be a risk for paternal exposure to lead for preterm birth. Studies of associations between preterm birth and exposures to other metals, such as aluminum and cadmium, or to the metalloid arsenic are too limited to draw even tentative conclusions at this time.

PATERNAL EXPOSURES TO ENVIRONMENTAL TOXICANTS

A few studies have considered the role of toxicant exposures of the father in preterm birth. Each of these studies involved exposures in the workplace.

Two studies of Norwegian historical occupational records examined the role of paternal occupational exposure and preterm birth. In the first study, paternal employment in the printing industry, which results in increased occupational exposure to lead and solvents, was not associated with preterm birth of less than or equal to 37 completed weeks of gestation but was significantly associated with an increased odds for early preterm birth at between 16 and 27 weeks of gestation (adjusted OR 8.6; 95% CI 2.7–27.3) (Kristensen et al., 1993). A second study found that fathers who worked at jobs with moderate to low levels of exposure to lead but not with high levels of exposure had slightly decreased odds for fathering a pregnancy that delivered preterm (adjusted OR 0.89; 95% CI 0.86–0.93) (Irgens et al., 1998).

A study conducted by the U.S. National Institute for Occupational Safety and Health found no relationship between paternal occupational exposure to the dioxin TCDD and preterm birth. That study used a pharmacokinetic model to estimate worker's serum TCDD concentration at the time of conception (Lawson et al., 2004). Similarly, a study of veterans of Operation Ranch Hand, who were responsible for spraying herbicides during the Vietnam War, failed to find consistent effects of paternal exposure to TCDD (which is present in Agent Orange) on the rates of preterm birth (Michalek et al., 1998). In the latter study, the paternal dioxin level measured in 1987 or 1992 was extrapolated to the time of conception of the child to estimate the level of TCDD exposure.

In summary, the few studies that have assessed paternal toxicant exposure failed to find evidence of an increased risk for preterm birth as a result of paternal occupational exposure to lead or TCDD.

RACIAL DISPARITIES IN ENVIRONMENTAL EXPOSURES

As discussed more extensively elsewhere in this report, preterm births are more prevalent among African American women than among women of other racial-ethnic groups, and this pattern has persisted over the years. The terms "environmental justice" and "environmental racism" describe the disproportionate burden of environmental pollution on poor and minority populations (Brown, 1995; Silbergeld and Patrick, 2005). A recent review by Silbergeld and Patrick (2005) discusses in detail the disproportionate exposures of those populations to environmental pollutants and the effects on birth outcomes. Although the latter review emphasizes birth outcomes other than preterm birth, its discussion includes reports of racial-ethnic differences in environmental exposures that are relevant to preterm birth. Silbergeld and Patrick (2005) concluded that, "exposures to these toxicants may explain part of the socioeconomic disparity that is observed in terms of risks of adverse pregnancy outcomes" (Silbergeld and Patrick, 2005).

Despite the persistent racial-ethnic disparities in the rates of preterm birth and the increased awareness of racial-ethnic disparities in environmental exposures, few studies have considered the interactions among race-ethnicity, environmental chemical exposures, and preterm birth. Woodruff et al. (2003) reported increased levels of air pollution in neighborhoods consisting predominantly of minority populations and, after adjusting for maternal risk factors that included race-ethnicity, found a small increase in the odds of preterm delivery (OR 1.05; 95% CI 0.99–1.12) in association with high levels of air pollution.

Other factors that may influence exposure in racially and ethnically distinct patterns include behavioral, cultural, and sociological characteristics and practices. In a case-control study (188 preterm births and 304 normal births), use of a chemical hair straightener (relaxer) or chemical curl products by African American women just before or during pregnancy had no effect on the risk for preterm birth (Blackmore-Prince et al., 1999).

More research is needed obtain an improved understanding of environmental pollution with respect to race-ethnicity and preterm birth. Because exposure to environmental chemicals may be codependent with race-ethnicity, examination of racial-ethnic differences in environmental exposures during pregnancy may provide new insight into the racial-ethnic disparities in the rates of preterm birth.

BIOLOGICAL MECHANISMS

There has been little research on mechanisms by which pollutants may stimulate preterm birth. Conceivably, pollutants could increase risk for preterm birth by prematurely activating physiologic mechanisms of parturition or by activating pathologic mechanisms that prematurely initiate parturition. Consequently, biological mechanisms by which pollutants may stimulate preterm birth could include disruption of the endocrine systems that regulate parturition, activation of cell signaling pathways that stimulate uterine muscle contraction, and activation of the inflammatory pathway, among others (see Chapters 6 for discussion of these mechanisms in preterm birth). Moreover, toxicants may be considered as potential tools to uncover previously unknown aspects of parturition, as has been the case for the nervous system.

Mechanisms of direct stimulation of uterine contraction frequency have been studied in rat uteri exposed to DDT isomers and polychlorinated biphenyls (PCBs). These studies suggest that stimulation of uterine contraction frequency by a DDT isomer and a commercial PCB mixture (Aroclor 1254) involves increased intracellular calcium due to activation of voltage-sensitive calcium channels in the uterine smooth muscle cells (Bae et al., 1999b; Juberg and Loch-Caruso, 1992; Juberg et al, 1995). Moreover, stimulation of uterine contraction by the PCB mixture is dependent on activation of a calcium-independent phospholipase A_2 and increased release of arachidonic acid (Bae et al., 1999a). A PCB congener (PCB 50) was shown to stimulate rat uterine contractions by activating an endometrial calcium-independent phospholipase A_2 that was differentially expressed in late gestation (Brant et al., 2006a). Furthermore, Brant and colleagues showed that PCB 50 activation of phospholipase A_2 is mediated by p38 mitogen activated protein kinase (MAPK) (Brant and Caruso, 2005). Although increased intracellular calcium of uterine muscle cells, arachidonic acid release, prostaglandin release, and increased uterine contraction frequency are characteristics of parturition, it is not known if these responses measured in rat cells and tissues in vitro have relevance for human preterm birth.

Recent studies suggest that some toxicants may stimulate an intrauterine inflammatory response. Xu et al. (2005) showed that a phthalate (plasticizer and fragrance stabilizer) and its metabolites increase the expression of peroxisome proliferator-activated receptors (PPARs) in a rat placental trophoblast cell line. Latini and colleagues have proposed that induction of an inflammatory response via PPAR could be a mechanism by which phthalates decrease gestation length (Latini et al., 2003, 2005). Brant and colleagues reported that polybrominated diphenyl ethers (used as flame retardants), stimulate the release of pro-inflammatory cytokines from human gestational membranes (Brant et al., 2006b). Although intrauterine inflammation is associated with preterm birth (see Chapter 6), it remains to be shown whether toxicant-induced inflammation is a mechanism for preterm birth in women. Clearly, there is need for improved understanding of toxicant modification of mechanisms of normal and preterm birth.

CONCLUSIONS

Few environmental pollutants have been investigated for their potential to increase the risk for preterm birth, and among those pollutants that have been studied, the information available for most of them is limited. Because of this general lack of information, the potential contribution of environmental chemical pollutants to preterm birth is poorly understood. Possible exceptions are lead and environmental tobacco smoke, for which the weight of evidence suggests that maternal exposure to these pollutants increases the risk for preterm birth. In addition, a number of epidemiological studies have found significant relationships between exposures to air pollution and preterm birth, particularly for sulfur dioxide and particulates, suggesting that exposure to these air pollutants may increase a woman's risk for preterm birth.

Studies to date suggest that exposures to agricultural chemicals deserve greater attention as potential risk factors for preterm birth. In particular, the report by Longnecker et al. (2001) provides the strongest evidence for an association of DDT exposure with preterm birth, although it should be noted that the exposure levels were substantially higher for the samples used in that study compared with the current levels of DDT exposure in the United States. Other studies suggest that follow-up investigations that examine exposures to nitrates and arsenic in drinking water are warranted.

Although particular pollutants are cited here as deserving further scientific inquiry, it should be noted that the vast numbers of pollutants to which a woman may be exposed have never been considered in an investigation of preterm birth. It would be shortsighted to limit future research on the basis of the paucity of information on pollutants for which some information is already available. However, because of the large number of potential exposures, a strategy for an efficient and effective research program that will serve public health needs is required. Such strategies may be based on pathophysiological mechanisms or chemical structure-activity approaches to investigate related toxicants. Alternative strategies might target the most common pollutants identified, for example, pollutants listed in the National Health and Nutrition Examination Survey or Toxics Release Inventory databases. For example, we know from the NHANES study that phthalates are found in urine of most women and are high in women of childbearing age (Silva et al., 2004). New strategies from investigative lines of research involving proteomics, genomics, and metabolomics will likely evolve.

The studies currently available raise important questions. For example, when is the critical window for pollutant exposure during pregnancy? This question has been addressed only recently in investigations of air pollutants, with no clear answer, and has not been examined for other pollutants. It is likely that the critical period would depend, in part, on the pathway through which the environmental pollutant initiates its action. Because pollutants have widely diverse chemical structures and biological activities, there may not be a single best time during gestation to assess exposure for all environmental pollutants. Furthermore, there may not be a single critical exposure period if multiple mechanisms can be activated. For some pollutants, critical exposures may occur before pregnancy or even during prenatal development or well after birth, say, during adolescence. The exposure assessment methodology will therefore require some understanding of the biological plausibility by which the pollutant under study would be hypothesized to affect preterm birth.

Another important question concerns the methodology used to assess exposure. So-called ecological exposure assessments that rely on the measurement of the levels of pollutants in certain geographical areas are limited by the inability to account for the heterogeneity of exposures and individual confounding factors. Methodologies that assess individual exposures through survey or interview instruments are subject to various biases and may suffer from imprecision. However, individual exposure assessments that use biological or chemical markers also present challenges specific to investigations related to preterm birth. Foremost among those challenges is the selection of the appropriate measurement technique and the fluid or tissue to be sampled. For example, several studies found significant associations by using one biomonitoring technique but not another or by measurement of toxicant concentrations in one tissue or body fluid but not another. Moreover, if a pollutant's concentration in the tissue or fluid sampled changes as a function of gestational age because of the physiological changes that occur during pregnancy, the concentrations in samples taken at the time of delivery may reflect the gestational age rather than actual differences in levels of exposure.

Progress in understanding the biological basis for associations between exposures to environmental pollutants and preterm birth have been limited, in part, by the significant limitations of current laboratory animal models (see Chapter 6). Additionally, few studies have examined mechanisms by which pollutants may stimulate preterm birth. Because pollutants may increase risk for preterm birth by prematurely activating physiologic mechanisms of parturition or by activating pathologic mechanisms that prematurely initiate parturition, toxicant mechanisms need to consider. Consequently, biological mechanisms by which pollutants may stimulate preterm birth could include disruption of the endocrine systems that regulate parturition, activation of cell signaling pathways that stimulate uterine muscle contraction, and activation of the inflammatory pathway, among others. Clearly, there is need for improved understanding of toxicant modification of mechanisms of normal and preterm birth.

Understanding the potential impact of exposure to environmental pollutants on preterm birth is inherently a complex proposition. However, the challenge posed by its complexity should not negate the importance of the task. By and large, women's exposures to environmental pollutants are unavoidable and unintended. Furthermore, there is the potential for very large numbers of women to be exposed to particular pollutants, such that an increased risk presented by such exposures could have a significant impact on the population as a whole. Public health therefore plays an important role in regulating such exposures. However, regulatory actions to protect the health of pregnant women and their unborn children cannot be made in a vacuum of information.

As the discussion in this chapter indicates, there is a need to increase and improve research in this area to provide the knowledge foundation needed to design effective public health preventive strategies to minimize the risk of preterm birth as a result of environmental exposures.

Finding 8-1: Limited data suggest that some environmental pollutants, such as lead and tobacco smoke, and air pollution may contribute to the risk of preterm birth; but most environmental pollutants have not been investigated. In addition, the interactions between environmental toxicant exposures with other behavioral, psychosocial, and sociodemographic attributes have been understudied.

Section II

Causes of Preterm Birth

RECOMMENDATIONS

The committee finds that the lack of success of public health and clinical interventions to date is due, in large measure, to the limited understanding of the heterogeneous etiologies of preterm birth.

Recommendation II-1: *Support research on the etiologies of preterm birth. Funding agencies should be committed to sustained and vigorous support for research on the etiologies of preterm birth to fill critical knowledge gaps.*

Areas to be supported should include the following:

- The physiological and pathologic mechanisms of parturition across the entire gestational period as well as the pregestational period should be studied.
- The role of inflammation and its regulation during implantation and parturition should be studied. Specifically, perturbations to the immunologic and inflammatory pathways caused by bacterial and viral infections, along with the specific host responses to these pathogens, should be addressed.
- Preterm birth should be defined as a syndrome of multiple pathophysiological pathways, with refinement of the phenotypes of preterm birth that recognizes and accurately reflects the heterogeneity of the underlying etiology.

• Animal models, in vitro systems, and computer models of human implantation, placentation, parturition, and preterm birth should be studied.
• Simple genetic and more complex epigenetic causes of preterm birth should be studied.
• Gene-environment interactions and environmental factors should be considered broadly to include the physical and social environments.
• Biological targets and the mechanisms and biological markers of exposure to environmental pollutants should be studied.

The committee finds that psychosocial, behavioral, and sociodemographic risk factors for preterm birth tend to cooccur; and the potentially powerful and complex interactions among these factors have been understudied. When they are studied independently, each of these risk factors tends to have a weak and inconsistent association with the risk of preterm birth. The committee acknowledges that with each additional potential interaction sought, the sample size required to retain an adequate statistical power to reveal meaningful differences increases.

Recommendation II-2: *Study multiple risk factors to facilitate the modeling of the complex interactions associated with preterm birth. Public and private funding agencies should promote and researchers should conduct investigations of multiple risk factors for preterm birth simultaneously rather than investigations of the individual risk factors in isolation. These studies will facilitate the modeling of these complex interactions and aid with the development and evaluation of more refined interventions tailored to specific risk profiles.*

Specifically, these studies should achieve the following:

• Develop strong theoretical models of the pathways from psychosocial factors, including stress, social support, and other resilience factors, to preterm delivery as a basis for ongoing observational research. These frameworks should include plausible biological mechanisms. Comprehensive studies should include psychosocial, behavioral, medical, and biological data.
• Incorporate understudied exposures, such as the characteristics of employment and work contexts, including work-related stress; the effects of domestic or personal violence during pregnancy; racism; and personal resources, such as optimism, mastery and control, and pregnancy intendedness. These studies should also investigate the potential interactions of these exposures with exposure to environmental toxicants.

• Emphasize culturally valid measures in studies of stress and preterm delivery to consider the unique forms of stress that individuals in different racial and ethnic groups experience. Measurement of stress should also include specific constructs such as anxiety.

• Expand the study of neighborhood-level effects on the risk of preterm birth by including novel data in multilevel models. Data that address this information should be made more available to researchers for such activities. Interagency agreements for the sharing of data should be reached to support the development of cartographic modeling of neighborhoods.

• Work toward the development of primary strategies for the prevention of preterm birth. When there is evidence of modest effects of multiple causes, interventions that address all of these factors should be considered.

• Have designs that are common enough to allow for pooling of data and samples, and consider studying high-risk populations to increase the power of the study.

Recommendation II-3: *Expand research into the causes and methods for the prevention of the racial-ethnic and socioeconomic disparities in the rates of preterm birth. The National Institutes of Health and other funding agencies should expand current efforts in and expand support for research into the causes and methods for the prevention of the racial-ethnic and socioeconomic disparities in the rates of preterm birth. This research agenda should continue to prioritize efforts to understand factors contributing to the high rates of preterm birth among African-American infants and should also encourage investigation into the disparities among other racial-ethnic subgroups.*

Recommendation II-4: *Investigate the causes of and consequences for preterm births that occur because of fertility treatments. The National Institutes of Health and other agencies, such as the Centers for Disease Control and Prevention and the Agency for Healthcare Research and Quality, should provide support for researchers to conduct investigations to obtain an understanding of the mechanisms by which fertility treatments, such as assisted reproductive technologies and ovulation promotion, may increase the risk for preterm birth. Studies should also be conducted to investigate the outcomes for mothers who have received fertility treatments and who deliver preterm and the outcomes for their infants.*

Specifically, those conducting work in this area should attempt to achieve the following:

• Develop comprehensive registries for clinical research, with particular emphasis on obtaining data on gestational age and birth weight, whether the preterm birth was indicated or spontaneous, the outcomes for the newborns, and perinatal mortality and morbidity. These registries must distinguish multiple gestations from singleton gestations and link multiple infants from a single pregnancy.

• Conduct basic biological research to identify the mechanisms of preterm birth relevant to fertility treatments and the underlying causes of infertility or subfertility that may contribute to preterm delivery.

• Investigate the outcomes for preterm infants as well as all infants whose mothers received fertility treatments.

• Understand the impact of changing demographics on the use and outcomes of fertility treatments.

• Assess the short- and long-term economic costs of various fertility treatments.

• Investigate ways to improve the outcomes of fertility treatments, including ways to identify high-quality gametes and embryos to optimize success through the use of single embryos and improve ovarian stimulation protocols that lead to monofollicular development.

Recommendation II-5: *Institute guidelines to reduce the number of multiple gestations. The American College of Obstetricians and Gynecologists, the American Society for Reproductive Medicine, and state and federal public health agencies should institute guidelines that will reduce the number of multiple gestations. Particular attention should be paid to the transfer of a single embryo and the restricted use of superovulation drugs and other nonassisted reproductive technologies for infertility treatments. In addition to mandatory reporting to the Centers for Disease Control and Prevention by centers and individual physicians who use assisted reproductive technologies, the use of superovulation therapies should be similarly reported.*

SECTION III

DIAGNOSIS AND TREATMENT OF PRETERM LABOR

9

Diagnosis and Treatment of Conditions Leading to Spontaneous Preterm Birth

ABSTRACT

The diagnosis and treatment of preterm labor is currently based on an inadequate literature. Not only is there a paucity of well-designed and adequately powered clinical trials, but there is incomplete understanding of the sequence and timing of events that precede clinical evidence of preterm labor. To date, there is no single test or sequence of assessment measures to accurately predict preterm birth. Prevention of preterm birth has primarily focused on the treatment of the woman with symptomatic preterm labor. Treatment has been directed toward the inhibition of contractions. This approach has not decreased the incidence of preterm birth but can delay delivery long enough to allow administration of antenatal steroids and to transfer the mother and the fetus to an appropriate hospital, two interventions that have consistently been shown to reduce the rates of perinatal mortality and morbidity. Preterm birth has historically not been emphasized in prenatal care, in the belief that the majority of preterm births are due to social rather than medical or obstetric causes or are the appropriate result of pathological processes that would benefit the mother or the infant, or both. Because preterm labor or premature rupture of membranes may occur in response to conditions that threaten fetal or maternal well-being, whether preterm birth is appropriately preventable is a topic that regularly influences clinical decision making. The ultimate goal of treatment for preterm labor is to eliminate or reduce perinatal morbidity and mortality. Thus, despite several interventions designed to inhibit preterm labor and prolong pregnancy, the frequency of preterm birth continues to pose a major barrier to the health of newborns worldwide. Although current obstetric and neonatal strategies have resulted in improved rates of neonatal survival and an earlier threshold for viability, effective strategies for the prevention of preterm birth are urgently needed. As basic and translational research continues to reveal more of the complex endocrinological and immunological aspects of parturition, investigators must continue to search for biologically plausible new therapies to prevent preterm birth and develop markers or multiple markers to diagnose the disease accurately in its early stages.

Nearly 75 percent of the cases of perinatal mortality and approximately half of the cases of long-term neurologic morbidity occur in infants born preterm. Preterm births have been organized into two broad categories, spontaneous and indicated, based on the presence or absence of factors that place the mother or the fetus at risk (Meis et al., 1987, 1995, 1998). Spontaneous preterm births occur as a result of preterm labor or preterm premature rupture of fetal membranes before 37 weeks of gestation and account for the majority of preterm births in developed countries. Preterm births that are the result of conditions that directly threaten the health of the mother or fetus, such as preeclampsia, placenta previa, and fetal growth restriction, are categorized as indicated preterm births and account for the remaining 25 to 30 percent of preterm deliveries (Meis et al., 1987, 1995, 1998). Although categorization of preterm births as indicated versus spontaneous allows analysis of preterm births according to those that might be prevented versus those that might be beneficial, there is increasing recognition that this distinction may understate the contribution of factors such as vascular compromise or fetal stress to the pathogenesis of preterm labor. This is suggested by reports that infants born after spontaneous preterm labor in the absence of apparent maternal disease have a higher than expected rate of poor intrauterine growth (Bukowski et al., 2001b; Gardosi, 2005). Figure 9-1 shows the negative skew in birth weights for fetuses destined for preterm birth versus the range of fetal weights of fetuses ultimately born at term. Efforts to prevent preterm birth must therefore be applied and evaluated primarily for their effects on perinatal mortality and morbidity.

The care of infants born preterm and their mothers may be described as primary (prevention and reduction of risk in the population), secondary (identification of and treatment for individuals with an increased risk), and tertiary (treatment aimed at reducing morbidity and mortality after the

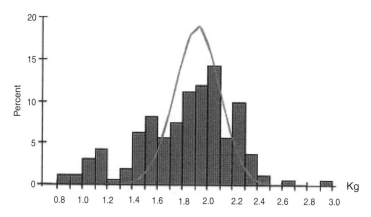

FIGURE 9-1 Ultrasound versus birth weight standard at 32 weeks of gestation. SOURCE: Gardosi et al. (2005). Reprinted with permission from *Early Human Development*, Vol. 81, Pg. 45, © 2004 by Elsevier.

preterm parturitional process has begun). In the past 30 years, important strides in obstetric and neonatal tertiary care have been made to reduce the rates of infant morbidity and mortality related to preterm birth. However, the primary and secondary interventions used to date have not reduced the rate of spontaneous preterm birth. This chapter describes and assesses the success of secondary- and tertiary-care practices. As will become evident as these are recounted, there are major impediments to the appropriate application of reasonable interventions for the risk factors for preterm birth. Many risk factors have been identified and removed without affecting the rate or morbidity of preterm birth. Cofactors, both exogenous and innate, that might contribute to or impede the success of an intervention are not well understood. Because clinically overt evidence of preterm labor is often preceded by weeks or months of activation of the parturitional process, the optimal timing for effective interventions is not always clear. Figure 9-2 presents these interactions.

Remarkably, current prenatal care is focused on risks other than preterm birth. Birth defects, adequate fetal growth, preeclampsia, gestational diabetes, selected infections (urinary tract, group B streptococcus, and rubella virus infections), and complications of postdate pregnancy are emphasized in the prenatal record (see Attachment 9-1). Preterm birth has historically not been emphasized in prenatal care in the belief that the majority of preterm births are due to social rather than medical or obstetrical causes (Main et al., 1985; Taylor, 1985) or are the appropriate result of pathological processes that would benefit the mother or the infant, or both. More recently, the failure of repeated efforts to prevent preterm birth (see

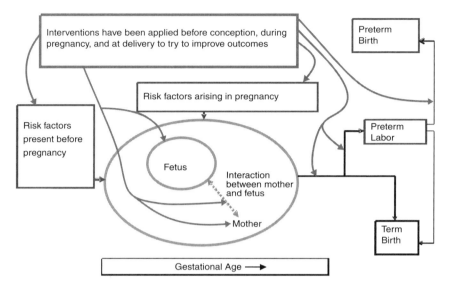

FIGURE 9-2 Interventions for preterm birth.

below) has lent support to the historical view. Because preterm labor or preterm premature rupture of membranes may occur in response to conditions that threaten fetal or maternal well-being, whether preterm birth is appropriately preventable is a topic that regularly influences clinical decision making.

Thus, efforts to prevent preterm birth have increasingly focused on early pregnancy and preconceptional care. Some risks are amenable to intervention, whereas others serve primarily to inform theories of causation or to identify at-risk groups for further study.

> Finding 9-1: Prenatal care was designed to address one complication of pregnancy; namely, preeclampsia. The proper timing of visits and the appropriate content of prenatal care for the detection or management of preterm delivery are not known.

PREDICTION AND ASSESSMENT OF RISK OF PRETERM BIRTH

The rationale for prediction of spontaneous preterm birth is threefold. First, by delineating factors predictive of preterm birth, the mechanisms and biological pathways that lead to spontaneous preterm parturition may be better understood. Second, the use of predictors of spontaneous preterm birth permits identification of a group of women at the highest risk for whom an intervention may be tested and for whom intervention is most needed. The third motivation for prediction of spontaneous preterm birth is a corollary of the second: by identifying women at low risk for preterm birth, unnecessary, costly, and sometime hazardous interventions might be avoided. To date, no single test or sequence of tests has an optimal sensitivity or predictive value. This section reviews clinical, biophysical, and biochemical tests that can be used as predictors for preterm birth.

CLINICAL PREDICTORS

Clinical risk factors alone or in combination most frequently report a sensitivity of about 25 percent for prediction of preterm birth (Goldenberg et al., 1998; Mercer et al., 1996). Low prepregnancy weight (body mass index less than 19.8), genitourinary bacterial colonization or infection, and African American ethnicity have relative risks (RRs) of about twofold but contribute significant attributable risk because of their prevalence in the population. African American women deliver before 37 weeks of gestation twice as often as women of other races and ethnicities and deliver before 32 weeks of gestation three times as often as white women. The strongest risk factors in all racial-ethnic groups are multiple gestation (RR = five- to sixfold), a history of preterm birth (RR = three- to fourfold), and vaginal bleeding (RR = threefold).

The risk of preterm and low-birth-weight delivery rises in direct proportion to the number of fetuses, as can be seen Table 9-1.

Vaginal bleeding in pregnancy is a risk factor for preterm birth because of placenta previa, because of placental abruption, and when the origin is unclear (Ekwo et al., 1992; Meis et al., 1995; Yang et al., 2004b). Unexplained vaginal bleeding is particularly associated with preterm birth if it is persistent and if it occurs in white women (Yang et al., 2004b).

The risk of recurrent preterm birth rises with the number of prior preterm births, with maternal African American ethnicity, and as the gestational age of the prior preterm birth decreases (Adams et al., 2000; Mercer et al., 1999). The effect of a woman's prior obstetrical history on the risk of preterm birth is shown in Table 9-2.

The data in Table 9-2 describe a homogeneous population from Norway. Data from the United States show the same phenomenon, with markedly increased rates of preterm birth for African Americans, reaching 50 percent or more for an African American woman with two or more prior preterm deliveries (Adams et al., 2000; Mercer et al., 1996). Other reported risk factors include the use of assisted reproductive technology, poor nutrition, periodontal disease, absent or inadequate prenatal care, age less than 18 years or over 35 years, strenuous work, high levels of personal stress,

TABLE 9-1 Risks of Preterm and Low Birth Weight Births by Number of Fetuses

Births	Twin	Triplet	Quadruplet	Quintuplet
<32 wk	12 percent	36 percent	60 percent	78 percent
<37 wk	58 percent	92 percent	97 percent	91 percent
Mean GA	35 wk	32 wk	30 wk	28 wk
<1.5 kg	10 percent	34 percent	61 percent	84 percent
<2.5 kg	55 percent	94 percent	99 percent	94 percent

	Risk of Preterm Birth or Low Birth Weight (%)			
No. of Births	<32 wk of Gestation	<37 wk of Gestation	Birth Weight <1.5 kg	Birth Weight <2.5 kg
Twin	12	58	10 (35 wk)[a]	55 (35 wk)
Triplet	36	92	34 (32 wk)	94 (32 wk)
Quadruplet	60	97	61 (30 wk)	99 (30 wk)
Quintuplet	78	91	84 (28 wk)	94 (28 wk)

[a]Times in parentheses are mean gestational age.

SOURCE: CDC (2002c).

TABLE 9-2 Risk of Preterm Delivery by Obstetrical History

Outcome of First Birth	Outcome of Second Birth	Number of Women	Likelihood of Peterm Birth in Next Pregnancy	
			Percent	RR
Term		25,817	4.4	1.0
Preterm		1,860	17.2	3.9
Term	Term	24,689	2.6	.6
Preterm	Term	1,540	5.7	1.3
Term	Preterm	1,128	11.1	2.5
Preterm	Preterm	320	28.4	6.5

SOURCE: Bakketeig and Hoffman (1981).

anemia, cigarette smoking, cervical injury or abnormality, and uterine anomaly (Meis et al., 1995; Mercer et al., 1996). As discussed in Chapter 5, the increased number of pregnancies conceived after the use of assisted reproductive technologies is associated with a rise in preterm birth not only because of multiple gestations but also because the singleton gestations that occur after the use of assisted reproductive technologies have a twofold increased risk of preterm birth (Jackson et al., 2004; Schieve et al., 2004; Van Voorhis, 2006).

Biophysical Predictors

Uterine Contractions

The detection of uterine contractions through maternal self-perception (Mercer et al., 1996) and electronic monitoring (Iams et al., 2002; Main et al., 1993; Nageotte et al., 1988) has been studied to predict preterm delivery. The threshold number of contractions most often studied is four per hour. An increased frequency of self-reported contractions is associated with preterm delivery before 35 weeks of gestation in both nulliparous women (RR 2.41; 95% interval [CI] 1.47–3.94; $p < 0.001$) and parous women (RR 1.62; 95% CI 1.20–2.18; $p = 0.002$) women (Mercer et al., 1996). In a study of 306 women in whom uterine contraction frequency was electronically recorded for 2 or more hours a day at least twice weekly between 22 and 37 weeks of gestation, contraction frequency was significantly greater in women who delivered before 35 weeks of gestation than in women who delivered after 35 weeks of gestation (Table 9-3) (Iams et al., 2002). Con-

TABLE 9-3 Prediction of Spontaneous Preterm Birth before 35 Weeks of Gestation (22 to 24 and 27 to 28 Weeks of Gestation) in 306 Women at Risk of Preterm Birth

Gestational Length and Test	Sensitivity (%)	Specificity (%)	Predictive Value (%)	
			Positive	Negative
22 to 24 wk				
UC ≥4/h	6.7	92.3	25.0	84.7
Bishop score ≥4	32.0	91.4	42.1	87.4
CL ≤25 mm	40.8	89.5	42.6	88.8
Fibronectin level ≥50 ng/ml	18.0	95.3	42.9	85.6
27 to 28 wk				
UC ≥4/h	28.1	88.7	23.1	91.1
Bishop score ≥4	46.4	77.9	18.8	92.9
CL ≤25 mm	53.6	82.2	25.0	94.1
Fibronectin level ≥50 ng/ml	21.4	94.5	30.0	91.6

NOTE: UC = uterine contractions; CL = cervical length.

SOURCE: Iams et al. (2002).

tractions increased significantly as gestational age advanced and were more frequent between 4 p.m. and 4 a.m. Although the difference in contraction frequency was statistically significant, contraction frequency was not a clinically efficient predictor of preterm birth at 24 or 28 weeks of gestation. The threshold of four or more contractions per hour at 24 and 28 weeks of gestation for prediction of the risk of preterm birth had sensitivities of 8.6 and 28 percent, respectively, and positive predictive values of 25 and 23 percent, respectively (Iams et al., 2002).

Clinical studies of the symptoms of preterm birth (Hueston, 1998; Macones et al., 1999b) confirm the poor performance of contraction frequency as a test for acute preterm labor as well.

Cervical Examination

Manual examination Cervical dilatation, effacement, consistency, position, and station of the presenting part as determined by manual examination have been related to an increased risk of preterm birth (Copper et al., 1990; Iams et al., 1996; Mercer et al., 1996; Newman et al., 1997). However, even when these features are combined in composite scores (e.g., Bishop scores [Bishop, 1964] or cervical scores [Newman, 1997]) of cervical readiness for labor, the sensitivity is low. The RRs for birth before 35 weeks of gestation were increased at 24 weeks of gestation: 5.3 (95% CI 3.4–8.5) for the cervical score (defined as cervical length in centimeters minus the cervical dilatation in centimeters) and 3.5 (95% CI 2.4–5.0) for the Bishop score. The sensitivities of both scores for prediction of the risk of preterm birth in a general obstetrical population were low, however: 13.4 and 27.6 percent, respectively (Iams et al., 1996; Newman et al., 1997).

Sonographic evaluation A decreased cervical length as measured by endovaginal ultrasound examination has also been related to an increased risk of preterm birth. The RR of preterm birth before 35 weeks of gestation was about sixfold higher (95% CI 3.84–9.97) among women whose cervical length was less than the 10th percentile (25 millimeters [mm]) than that among women with a cervical length above the 75th percentile (40 mm), but the absolute risk of birth before 35 weeks of gestation and the sensitivity were both only 40 percent in two studies performed in the United States (Iams et al., 1996, 2002). A study of cervical length in low-risk women found an eightfold increased risk of preterm birth when the cervix was less than 29 mm at 18 to 22 weeks of gestation, but the sensitivity and positive predictive value were low: 19 and 6 percent, respectively (Taipale and Hiilesmaa, 1998). Finally, the likelihood ratio for prediction of birth before 34 weeks of gestation for a cervical length of 25 mm or less when the length was measured before 20 weeks of gestation was estimated to be +6.3 (95%

CI 3.3–12.0), indicating that the risk of preterm birth is 6.3 times greater for women whose cervical length is < 25 mm than for those whose cervical length is >25 mm (Honest et al., 2003).

Biological Predictors

Biological markers may be collected from maternal blood or urine, cervicovaginal fluid secretions, or amniotic fluid. Maternal blood and vaginal fluids have been the most studied. Table 9-4 summarizes the myriad efforts used to identify the risk of preterm birth based on biomarkers from asymptomatic women (Vogel et al., 2005).

Serum Biomarkers

Maternal serum is routinely drawn several times during prenatal care. Screening of serum biomarkers for various conditions, such as open neural tube defects and aneuploidy, is already part of routine prenatal care (Canick et al., 2003; Cheschier, 2003). The use of serum biomarkers of spontaneous preterm birth to identify several pathways to preterm birth have been investigated, as described by Romero and colleagues (1994) and Lockwood and Kuczynski (2001) and described in Chapter 6, including (1) activation of maternal or fetal hypothalamic-pituitary-adrenal axis (e.g., corticotropin-releasing hormone) and (2) inflammation due to upper genital tract infection (e.g., defensins and tumor necrosis factor alpha) or decidual hemorrhage or ischemia (e.g., thrombin-antithrombin III complex). No serum biomarkers of pathologic uterine overdistension have been described.

Lower Genital Tract Markers

Bacterial vaginosis (BV) is an alteration of the maternal vaginal flora in which normally predominant lactobacilli are largely replaced by gram-negative anaerobic bacteria, such as *Gardnerella vaginalis* and *Bacteroides*, *Prevotella*, *Mobiluncus*, and *Mycoplasma* species. BV in pregnancy is consistently associated with a twofold increased risk of spontaneous preterm birth (Hillier et al., 1995; Meis et al., 1995). The association of BV with preterm birth has been reported to be stronger when the condition is present in the first half of pregnancy (Hay et al., 1994), but a recent analysis of the relationship between gestational age at the time of detection of BV and pregnancy outcome in 12,937 women found "the odds ratio of preterm birth among BV-positive versus -negative women raged from 1.1 to 1.6 and did not vary significantly according to the gestational age at which BV was screened" (Klebanoff et al., 2005, p 470). Despite the consistency of the reports relating BV to preterm birth, the clinical utility of tests for BV to

TABLE 9-4 Ability of Selected Biomarkers to Predict Preterm Delivery in Asymptomatic Women

Biomarker	No. of Subjects	Compartment	GA (wk) at Sampling	End Point (GA [wk])	LR+	SENS (%)	FP (%)	Reference[a]
Multiple gestations (≥2 of 5)	177	S/P, C, V+C	24	<32	24	59	2	58
Ureaplasma urealyticum	254	Amniotic fluid	<17	<37	10	88	9	9
Relaxin	176	S/P	<24	<34	6.8	27	4	64
Cervical length	Meta-analysis	Cervix	<24	<34	6.3			29
Alkaline phosphatase	1,868	S/P	<20	<37	4.6	14	3	69
CRH	860	S/P	<30	<37	3.0	39	13	40
G-CSF	388	S/P	24	<32	3.3	49	15	16
Interleukin-6	250	V+C	24	<32	3.3	20	6	15
Interleukin-6	580	Amniotic fluid	<20	<34	2.8	14	5	14
Fetal fibronectin	Meta-analysis	V+C	>20	<37	2.9			22
α-Fetoprotein	254	S/P	24	<35	2.6	35	13	58
Chlamydia	380	U	24	<37	2.5	16	6	10
Ferritin	100	S/P	34	<37	2.2	75	33	70
C-reactive protein	484	S/P	<21	<37	1.8	26	15	75
Bacterial vaginosis	Meta-analysis	V+C	<24	<37	1.6			8
Ferritin	364	V+C	<25	<37	1.4	35	25	71

NOTE: LR+ = likelihood ratio; SENS = sensitivity; FP = false-positive rate; CRH = corticotropin-releasing hormone; G-CSF = granulocyte colony-stimulating factor; U = uterine; V = vaginal secretions; C = cervical secretions; S/P = serum or plasma; GA = gestational age.
[a]Citations in the paper by Vogel et al. (2005).

SOURCE: Vogel et al. (2005).

identify women at risk is low, owing to the modest strength of the association, the high prevalence of BV in some populations, and the high degrees of variation in the accuracies of the tests used to detect BV (Honest et al., 2004).

Testing of the cervicovaginal secretions of asymptomatic women have been screened for markers of preterm birth, including fetal fibronectin (Goldenberg et al., 1996b,c, 1998), interleukins 6 and 8 (Goepfert et al., 2001; Kurkinen-Raty et al., 2001), and tumor necrosis factor alpha and matrix metalloproteinases (Vogel et al., 2005). The biochemical test for fetal fibronectin is the one about which the most data are available and is the only one marketed in the United States for that purpose.

Fetal Fibronectin

Fetal fibronectin is a glycoprotein of fetal origin that normally resides at the decidual-chorionic interface within the uterus but is present in cervicovaginal secretions in 3 to 4 percent of pregnant women at between 21 and 37 weeks of gestation (Goldenberg et al., 1996c; Lockwood et al., 1991). Evaluation of fibronection levels in asymptomatic women at 24 weeks of gestation has a sensitivity of 20 to 30 percent for the prediction of spontaneous preterm birth at before 35 weeks of gestation (Goldenberg et al., 1996c; Iams et al., 2002). The sensitivity of determination of fibronectin levels for prediction of early preterm births before 28 weeks of gestation was found to be 63 percent (Goldenberg et al., 1996c). Determination of fibronectin levels is a better test for screening for the risk of delivery within 2 weeks of sampling than for delivery before a specific gestational week of pregnancy (Goldenberg et al., 1997).

Combination of Markers

Given the pathophysiological heterogeneity of the causes of spontaneous preterm birth, the clinical utility of any individual biomarker for predicting preterm birth is limited. Combinations of markers can increase the sensitivity of the prediction by combining risk predictors that address diverse causes of spontaneous and indicated preterm birth (Goldenberg et al., 2001). The positive predictive value can also be increased (at the sacrifice of sensitivity) by combining selected markers such as the woman's obstetric history and cervical length; for example, a sonographic cervical length less than 25 mm predicted recurrent preterm birth in 100 percent of African American women with a prior preterm birth (Yost et al., 2004).

Goldenberg and colleagues (1998) sought to develop a multiple-marker test for preterm birth with data collected in the Preterm Prediction Study of the Maternal-Fetal Medicine Units (MFMU) Network of the National Institute of Child Health and Human Development (NICHD). They performed a nested case-control study with a cohort of 2,929 women with singleton gestations recruited from the general obstetric populations of the 10 participating centers (Goldenberg et al., 2001). The women in that study underwent serial assessment of serum, cervical, vaginal, ultrasound, and historical markers or risk factors. The serum markers associated with spontaneous preterm birth at less than 32 weeks of gestation were α-fetoprotein, alkaline phosphatase, granulocyte-macrophage colony-stimulating factor, and defensins. The only serum markers related to spontaneous preterm birth at less than 35 weeks of gestation were α-fetoprotein and alkaline phosphatase. Importantly, the overlap between the biomarkers was small, supporting the concept that there are several heterogeneous pathways to spontaneous preterm birth. Use of the markers in concert improved the predictive ability. No individual serum biomarker of spontaneous preterm birth was useful when used alone; but when the woman was positive for any one of markers alkaline phosphatase, maternal serum α-fetoprotein, and granulocyte colony-stimulating factor, these three tests had a collective sensitivity of 81 percent and a specificity of 78 percent for prediction of spontaneous preterm birth at less than 32 weeks of gestation and 60 percent sensitivity and 73 percent specificity for prediction of spontaneous preterm birth at less than 35 weeks of gestation. Because this was a nested case-control study, the true-positive and negative predictive values are uncertain.

Despite the enhanced sensitivity of a multiple-marker approach, no prediction model to date provides adequate utility for justification of its routine clinical use, especially in the absence of an effective intervention for women with a positive screening test result. Development of an effective prediction model may permit the evaluation of targeted therapies, such as the provision of supplemental progesterone (described below). Interventions directed at women with a single marker, for example, a positive test for BV (Carey et al., 2000), fetal fibronectin (Andrews et al., 2003), or a short cervix (Rust et al., 2001; To et al., 2004), have been unsuccessful. Future directions for research in this area will involve the development and validation of multiple markers with diverse prospective cohorts. Research to develop novel markers for premature labor is crucial and may be facilitated by the use of high-throughput proteomic and metabolomic technologies and the use of more complex modeling techniques, such as those involving neural networks and artificial intelligence.

Finding 9-2: Current methods for the identification of women at risk for preterm birth by the use of demographic, behavioral, and biological risk factors have low sensitivities. Although the sensitivities increase as pathways and clinical syndromes are identified, the

efficacies of interventions decline as the parturitional process progresses.

PREVENTION STRATEGIES

The prevention of preterm birth has been attempted by the use of interventions aimed at each of the risk factors described in the previous chapters, largely without success (Table 9-5).

Most interventions are based on the traditional medical model of identifying and correcting each potential cause or risk factor for preterm birth, with the expectation that the rate of preterm births would decline in accordance with the contribution of that factor to the prematurity rate. Intervention trials have thus addressed the early identification of preterm labor through patient education, pharmacologic suppression of uterine contractions, antimicrobial therapy of vaginal microorganisms, the use of cerclage sutures to bolster the cervix, reduction of maternal stress, improved nutrition and improved access to prenatal care, and reduced physical activity. Some trials enrolled women with the risk factor in question without regard to obstetric history (e.g., antibiotics for women with a positive culture for a genital microorganism), whereas others were limited to women with a prior preterm delivery (e.g., the European cerclage trials or the recent progesterone supplementation studies [Da Fonseca et al., 2003; Meis et al., 2003]). Although successful elimination of single risk factors has been accomplished, for example, by antibiotic treatment of a targeted vaginal organism or suppression of contractions with tocolytic compounds (labor-inhibiting agents), successful removal of a risk factor has not produced a decrease in preterm birth rates. In fact, the overall rate of preterm birth has continued to increase.

Future studies of the etiology and means of prevention of preterm birth should recognize the implications of these findings to develop a more sophisticated understanding of preterm birth as a syndrome in which multiple physiological pathways operate simultaneously to initiate preterm parturition. The common complex disorder model currently used in cardiovascular disease and neoplasia may be an appropriate replacement for the more unifactorial approach that has dominated the last two decades of research. The findings of studies of prevention strategies described below reinforce this recommendation.

Medical Interventions

Early Detection of Preterm Labor

Early diagnosis of preterm labor has been pursued with the expectation that the use of tocolytic drugs to stop labor would be more effective if they

TABLE 9-5 Summary of Studies of Medical Interventions to Prevent Preterm Birth

Risk Factor or Population Studied	Interventions Tested in RCT	Outcome	Reference(s)
Nutritional deficiencies	Nutritional supplements Vitamins C and E	No benefit, vitamin C-CPEP Trial, inadequate data	Rumbold and Crowther, 2005
Prior preterm birth and bacterial vaginosis	Antibiotics during pregnancy	Mixed results	McDonald et al., 1994; Carey et al., 2000; Hauth et al., 1995; Carey, 2000; Lamont et al., 2003; Guise et al., 2001; Okun et al., 2005
Prior preterm birth	Cervical cerclage	Mixed but mostly negative	Berghella et al., 2005; see also Odibo et al., 2003; Harger, 2002; Owen et al., 2003; Bachmann et al., 2003; Belej-Rak et al., 2003; Drakeley et al., 2003
Positive risk score	Education and self-detection of contractions	No benefit	Collaborative Group on Preterm Birth Prevention, 1993; Mueller-Heubach and Guzick, 1989
Prior preterm birth (singletons)	Progesterone suppository and intramuscular 17α-hydroxyprogesterone caproate	33 percent reduction in preterm birth rates	Da Fonseca et al., 2003; Meis et al., 2003; see also meta-analyses by Dodd et al., 2005; Sanchez-Ramos et al., 1999
Prior preterm birth and increased contractions (singletons)	Nurse contact and/or contraction monitor	No benefit meta-analyses	CHUMS, 1995; Dyson et al., 1998
Positive vaginal swab cultures for various organisms	Antibiotics during pregnancy	No benefit; mixed if also positive cultures VIP	Brocklehurst et al., 2000; Gibbs et al., 1992; Carey and Klebanoff, 2003; Riggs and Klebanoff, 2004; Klebanoff et al., 2005

TABLE 9-5 Continued

Risk Factor or Population Studied	Interventions Tested in RCT	Outcome	Reference(s)
Positive fetal fibronectin	Metronidazole and erythromycin at 24–27 wk	No benefit; some (?) increased risk in antibiotic group	Andrews et al., 2003
Prior PTD and positivity for fetal fibronectin	Metronidazole at 24–27 wk	Increased preterm birth in metronidazole group	Shennan et al., 2006
Short cervix without a prior PTD	Cerclage (usually with antibiotics at surgery)	Mixed results, but mostly negative	Rust et al., 2001; Berghella et al., 2005
Short cervix in women with prior preterm birth	Cerclage (usually with antibiotics at surgery)	Mixed results	Berghella et al., 2005
Prior preterm birth	Antibiotics before next pregnancy	No benefit	Andrews et al., 2006
Preterm labor in current pregnancy	Nurse contact or contraction monitor	No benefit	Berkman et al., 2003; Iams et al., 1990; Brown et al., 1999; Nagey et al., 1993
Preterm labor in current pregnancy	Maintenance tocolysis (oral and subcutaneous infusion)	No benefit	Berkman et al., 2003; Sanchez-Ramos et al., 1999
Singletons at risk and Twins	Prophylactic bed rest	Inadequately studied (Sosa et al., 2004); no benefit (Goldenberg et al., 1994)	Sosa et al., 2004; Goldenberg et al., 1994
Twins	Prophylactic tocolytic drugs	No benefit	Marivate et al., 1977
Twins and increased contractions	Nurse contact or contraction monitor	No benefit	Dyson et al., 1998

NOTE: RCT = randomized controlled trial; PTD = preterm delivery.

are given early, before significant cervical changes occur. The results of an initial experience that used a program of preterm labor risk assessment and education of at-risk women about preterm labor were favorable (Herron et al., 1982), but larger trials of similar interventions with diverse populations found no benefit (Collaborative Group on Preterm Birth Prevention, 1993; Mueller-Heubach and Guzick, 1989). This approach was expanded by using sensitive electronic monitoring of uterine contractions at home accompanied by daily nursing contact, but the intervention had no effect on eligibility for tocolysis, the rate of preterm birth, or neonatal outcomes in large randomized controlled trials conducted with women at risk (CHUMS, 1995a,b; Dyson et al., 1998; Hueston et al., 1995). The largest such trial (Dyson et al., 1998) enrolled 2,422 women with an increased risk of preterm birth, including 844 women with twins, in a three-armed trial in which the participants were assigned to receive (1) education plus weekly nursing contact, (2) daily nursing contact, or (3) daily nursing contact and daily electronic uterine contraction monitoring. The women in the last two groups were seen and treated more frequently, but the group assignment had no effect on the preterm birth rate or eligibility for tocolysis.

Antibiotics to Prevent Preterm Birth

The serendipitous observation (Elder et al., 1971) of a reduced frequency of preterm birth in women who received tetracycline as prophylaxis for urinary tract infection has been followed by a mixed literature describing the successes and failures of this intervention, as shown in Table 9-6.

TABLE 9-6 Randomized Trials of Antibiotics to Prevent Preterm Birth

Reference	Entry Criteria	Antibiotics	Outcome
Elder et al., 1971	Bacteriuria	Oral tetracycline	↓ LBW
Romero et al., 1989	Bacteriuria	Meta-analysis	↓ LBW
Smaill, 2001	Bacteriuria	Meta-analysis	↓ LBW
Eschenbach et al., 1991	_U. urealyticum_ infection	Oral erythromycin	No effect
Klebanoff et al., 1995	Group B streptococcus infection	Oral erythromycin	No effect
Hauth et al., 1995	Prior PTD or maternal weight <50 kg	Oral metronidazole and erythromycin	No effect if BV negative, ↓ PTD if BV positive
Joesoef et al., 1995	BV	Vaginal clindamycin	No effect
McDonald et al., 1997	BV	Oral metronidazole	None if no Hx PTD, benefit if Hx PTD
Gichangi et al., 1997	Poor obstetric Hx[a]	Cefetamet-pivoxil	↓ LBW

TABLE 9-6 Continued

Reference	Entry Criteria	Antibiotics	Outcome
Vermeulen and Bruinse, 1999	Prior preterm birth	Vaginal 2 percent clindamycin versus placebo at 26 and 32 wk of gestation	No benefit; greater PTD rate and infections in compliant clindamycin group
Carey et al., 2000	BV	Oral metronidazole	No effect in Asx women or Hx PTD
Klebanoff et al., 2001	*Trichomonas*	Oral metronidazole	↑ PTD
Rosenstein, 2000	BV	Vaginal clindamycin	No difference in PTD
Kurkinen-Raty et al,. 2001	BV at 12 wk of gestation	Vaginal 2 percent clindamycin	No difference in PTD
Kekki et al., 2001	BV at 10–17 wk of gestation	Vaginal 2 percent clindamycin versus placebo at 10–17 wk of gestation	No difference in rates of PTD
Ugwumadu et al., 2003	BV	Oral clindamycin	↓ PTD
Lamont et al., 2003	BV	Vaginal clindamycin	↓ PTD, no change in rate of rate of LBW infants
Andrews et al., 2003	Positive fibronectin	Oral metronidazole + erythromycin	No effect
Kiss, 2004	Gram stain for BV, *Trichomonas*, yeast	Treatment of the organism detected	↓ PTD
Shennan et al., 2006	Clinical risk of PTB and positive fFN at 24–27 wk of gestation	Metronidazole	Study stopped due to 2× increase in numbers of births at <37 wk of gestation in metronidazole group

NOTE: ↓ LBW = decrease in low birth weight infants; PTD = preterm delivery; ↓ PTD = decrease in rates of preterm delivery; ↑ PTD= increase in rates of preterm delivery; fFN = fetal fibronection.
*a*African population.

Metronidazole and erythromycin treatment (Hauth et al., 1995) and metronidazole treatment (McDonald et al., 1997) were reported to reduce the risk of recurrent preterm delivery in women with BV who also had had a prior preterm birth, but metronidazole treatment had no effect on the rate of preterm birth in a placebo-controlled trial with 1,900 women with asymptomatic BV (Carey et al., 2000). Analysis by obstetric history of preterm birth, race-ethnicity, gestational age at the initiation of treatment, eradication of BV, and prepregnancy weight in that study did not reveal any subgroup in which treatment improved the perinatal outcome. Trials of clindamycin administered orally (*n* = 485) (Ugwumadu et al., 2003) or vaginally (*n*= 409) (Lamont et al., 2003) to women with BV reported reductions in the rates of preterm birth, especially if treatment was administered early in pregnancy, but two other studies of vaginal clindamycin found no benefit. One found no difference in preterm birth rates, despite the successful elimination of BV in treated women (*n* = 601) (Joesoef et al., 1995), and the other found an increased rate of preterm birth before 34 weeks of gestation in women who were fully compliant with clindamycin treatment compared with the rate in the placebo group (9 versus 1.4 percent) (Vermeulen and Bruinse, 1999).

A review of seven randomized clinical trials of screening and antibiotic treatment of BV in pregnancy to reduce preterm birth found no benefit in low-risk women or in women with an unspecified "increased risk" of preterm birth (Guise et al., 2001; Okun et al., 2005). The most recent American College of Obstetricians and Gynecologists (ACOG) Practice Bulletin (ACOG, 2001) specifically noted "There are no current data to support the use of . . . BV screening as a strategy to identify or prevent preterm birth." McDonald and colleagues (2005) concluded in a recent *Cochrane Review*, "Antibiotic treatment can eradicate bacterial vaginosis in pregnancy . . . [but there is] little evidence that screening and treating all pregnant women with asymptomatic bacterial vaginosis will prevent preterm birth and its consequences. For women with a previous preterm birth, there is some suggestion that treatment of bacterial vaginosis may reduce the risk of preterm prelabour rupture of membranes and low birthweight." The failure of antibiotics to reduce the rates of preterm birth, despite successful eradication of the genital tract organisms linked to preterm birth, is an urgent research issue that will require sophisticated studies of the host response to infection and inflammation and environmental influences on infection and inflammation.

The disappointing results of studies of the use of antibiotic treatment to reduce the risk of preterm birth have prompted investigation of the preconceptional use of antibiotics for women with a history of preterm birth, under the theory that relatively benign microorganisms colonizing the upper genital tract might produce intrauterine inflammation after conception (Andrews and Goldenberg, 2003). In a study of women with a prior preterm birth who were treated with metronidazole and azithromycin or placebo at 3-month intervals between pregnancies, Andrews et al. (in press) found no reduction in the rates of preterm birth in those who received antibiotic treatment. Of concern, that report included data that suggested that antibiotic use might actually increase the likelihood of preterm birth, a finding similar to the NICHD Network trial of metronidazole treatment for women infected with *Trichomonas vaginalis* (Klebanoff et al., 2001). Although the data from these two studies are preliminary, they argue against the clinical use of antibiotics solely to prevent preterm birth until future research explains these findings. Therefore, investigation of strategies that can be used to prevent infection-related preterm birth is justified and, indeed, urgent.

Although genital tract colonization and infection are frequent in women who deliver preterm, most women with BV do not deliver preterm, and most preterm births are not accompanied by evidence of infection. Thus, studies of the use of antibiotics in women with infection or prior preterm birth, or both, are likely to include many women for whom antibiotics have no potential benefit (Romero et al., 2003). Future research should therefore emphasize the identification of the particular subset of women with BV for whom antimicrobial or anti-inflammatory therapies might prove beneficial. The pathways by which genital tract infection is related to early delivery merits renewed research efforts so that more sophisticated interventions might be developed.

Infections outside the genital tract are also related to preterm birth, most commonly to urinary tract and intra-abdominal infections, for example, pyelonephritis and appendicitis (Romero et al., 1989). The presumed mechanism is inflammation of the nearby reproductive organs; but infections at remote sites, especially if the infection is chronic, have also been associated with an increased risk of spontaneous preterm birth. The recent literature provides information that links maternal periodontal disease to preterm birth (Goepfert et al., 2004; Jeffcoat et al., 2001a,b; Offenbacher et al., 2001) and to "late miscarriage" (loss of a pregnancy at between 12 and 24 weeks of gestation) and stillbirth (Moore et al., 2004). This association remains after confounding covariables are controlled for and suggests that the effect may be mediated by the systemic induction of cytokines in response to chronic inflammation (Boggess et al., 2005b).

Interestingly, periodontitis is characterized by an altered host flora and is thus similar to BV. A study of periodontal screening and treatment in pregnant women to reduce the rate of preterm birth (Jeffcoat et al., 2003) enrolled 366 women who were randomized at 21 to 25 weeks of gestation to one of three treatment groups: routine dental care plus placebo medication, scaling and root planing (intensive physical treatment of periodontal plaque) plus metronidazole (250 milligrams [mg] three times a day for 1 week), or scaling and root planing plus placebo medication. The rates of preterm birth (before 35 weeks of gestation) in the three groups were 4.9, 3.3, and 0.8 percent, respectively. Although good dental care is important for all pregnant women, there is insufficient evidence to conclude that dental care will reduce the occurrence of preterm birth (Khader and Ta'ani, 2005). Periodontal disease and other causes of systemic inflammation and their relationship to preterm birth are thus promising areas of research that merit funding for interdisciplinary investigations.

Other Prophylactic Medications

Tocolytic Prophylaxis

Studies of the use of tocolytic agents as prophylaxis for preterm birth have shown no evident benefit (Berkman et al., 2003; King et al., 1988; Sanchez-Ramos et al., 1999). Evidence that the parturitional process begins well in advance of coordinated uterine activity (Challis et al., 2000) may explain the inability of contraction suppression to prevent preterm birth in randomized trials.

Progesterone

Investigations summarized and reanalyzed by Keirse (1990) suggested that supplemental administration of progesterone might reduce the rate of preterm birth in women at increased risk. Two randomized placebo-controlled trials whose findings were published in 2003 found that progesterone, administered as either weekly intramuscular injections of 250 mg of 17α-hydroxprogesterone caproate (Meis et al., 2003) or daily progesterone vaginal suppositories (Da Fonseca et al., 2003), reduced the rate of recurrent preterm delivery by about a third. When these data were combined with data from earlier trials of supplemental progesterone in meta-analyses (Dodd et al., 2005; Sanchez-Ramos et al., 2005), the risk of recurrent preterm birth was reduced by 40 to 55 percent (in the study of Dodd et al. [2005] the RR was 0.58 and the 95 percent CI was 0.48 to 0.70; in the study of Sanchez-Ramos et al. [2005] the RR was 0.45 and the 95 percent CI was 0.25 to 0.80). Unlike strategies targeted at a specific risk factor such as infection, supplemental progesterone treatment was effective at reducing the rates of preterm birth in women chosen only because of a prior preterm birth. This suggests three possibilities: (1) that progesterone is effective in inhibiting a pathway shared by diverse causes of preterm birth, (2) that progesterone has diverse effects that act on several different pathways, or

(3) that progesterone is very effective against one highly prevalent pathway or cause.

Although progesterone supplementation is promising, several questions about its use remain incompletely answered:

1. How does progesterone work? The original rationale for progesterone prophylaxis was that it is a uterine relaxant, but some studies (Elovitz and Mrinalini, 2005; Kelly, 1994; Ragusa et al., 2004; Szekeres-Bartho, 2002) suggest it may act through an effect on the inflammatory response. The optimal dose, interval, and duration of treatment have also not been determined. Pharmacokinetic, pharmacodynamic, and pharmacogenetic studies of progesterone are urgently needed.

2. Is supplemental progesterone safe? There is little evidence from studies with humans that progesterone presents a teratogenic risk (Meis, 2005), but theoretical concern remains that it may blunt a fetal signal for labor generated by an in utero risk.

3. Who should receive supplemental progesterone? Data showing that progesterone provides a benefit are available only for women with a prior preterm birth at between 18 and 36 weeks of gestation. There is evidence that progesterone offers the greatest benefit for women with a prior preterm birth before 34 weeks of gestation (Spong et al., 2005).

Petrini et al. (2005) projected that use of 17P in women with a prior pretem birth would have a small but significant effect on the rate of preterm birth in the US (12.1% to 11.8% [$p < .001$]).

No studies of 17α-hydroxyprogesterone have been conducted with women with other risk factors, such as a multiple gestation, short cervix, positive fibronectin, a history of cervical insufficiency or cerclage, or preterm labor in the current pregnancy.

Surgical Interventions

Prophylactic Cerclage for Women with a Risk of Preterm Birth

Recognition that some early preterm births may be due to variant clinical presentations of cervical insufficiency led to consideration of cervical cerclage treatment for women with such a history. A randomized trial of cerclage for women with a prior preterm birth (MacNaughton et al., 1993) found that cerclage resulted in fewer preterm births before 33 weeks of gestation in women with multiple prior early births but that it had no effect on the overall rate of preterm birth in women treated with cerclage.

The introduction of cervical sonography in the early 1990s produced strong evidence that a short cervix in midpregnancy is associated with an increased risk of early delivery (see above), but the basis for this association remains inadequately understood. There is evidence that a cervical length below the 10th percentile in the second trimester may represent at the short end of a biological continuum of inherent cervical function (Goldenberg et al., 1998; Iams et al., 1995) or result as well from biochemical (inflammatory) or biophysical (stretch or contraction) processes. It is likely that all of these factors are operative to various degrees in an individual, but to date there is no satisfactory method to determine the contributions of physical and biochemical influences on the cervix and, thus, no way to select an appropriate therapy.

The literature on the use of cerclage includes the findings of trials with women with a prior preterm birth and current ultrasound evidence of cervical effacement (Althuisius et al., 2001; Berghella et al., 2004) and of trials with women with ultrasound findings alone (To et al., 2004; Rust et al., 2001). The evidence of a benefit of cerclage is the strongest from studies of women who have a history of preterm birth and who have a short cervix in the current pregnancy. Data from these four trials were reanalyzed by the original authors (Berghella et al., 2005). When data for women with singleton pregnancies enrolled in four trials were combined, the risk of birth before 35 weeks of gestation was significantly reduced with cerclage treatment for women with a prior preterm birth and a short cervix (defined as <2.0 centimeters [cm]) in the current pregnancy (RR 0.63; 95% CI 0.48–0.85), but there was no advantage of cerclage for women with a short cervix who did not have a prior preterm birth (RR 0.84; 95% CI 0.60–1.17).

Evidence indicates that the efficacy of cerclage may vary according to the cause of the short cervix. In the meta-analysis by Berghella and colleagues (2005), cerclage was not effective at reducing the rates of preterm birth in women with twin gestations, in which uterine stretch is an important factor. In this group, cerclage for a short cervix was associated with increased rates of preterm birth (RR 2.15; 95% CI 1.15–4.01). A recent study found evidence that intracervical inflammation was related to the success or failure of cerclage in women with a short cervix. Sakai et al. (2006) studied women treated with cerclage for a short cervix and found reduced rates of preterm birth in women with low levels of the inflammation-related marker interleukin-8 in their cervical fluid and increased rates of preterm birth when the level of interleukin-8 was high. Further research to identify appropriate candidates for cerclage is thus needed.

Nonmedical Interventions

Nonmedical interventions, such as social support, reduction of stress, improved access to prenatal care, and reduced physical activity, can be used to reduce the rates of preterm birth and were reviewed in Chapter 3. A recent study examined the rates of low birth weight among participants in a Medicaid-funded prenatal program for high-risk women (Ricketts et al., 2005). The results indicated that the infants of women who stopped smoking had a rate of low birth weight of 8.5 percent, whereas the rate was 13.7 percent among the infants of women in the program who did not stop smoking. The infants of women with adequate weight gain had a rate of low birth weight rate of 6.7 percent, whereas the rate was 17.2 percent among the infants of women with inadequate weight gain. Finally, the infants of women who eliminated all risks had a low birth weight rate of 7.0 percent, whereas the rate was 13.2 percent among the infants of women who eliminated none of their risks. Those who attended at least 10 program visits were more likely to eliminate their risks than women who attended fewer visits.

Although many nonmedical efforts have had limited success to date, considerable opportunity for further research on nonmedical efforts at reducing the rates of preterm birth exists. Activity modification is widely practiced, but the evidence of a benefit does not exist. Most studies of nonmedical interventions have been conducted with women identified as being at risk, as defined by their ethnicity, socioeconomic condition, or medical and obstetric history (e.g., prior preterm birth and multiple gestations). Future studies of nonmedical interventions to reduce the rates of preterm birth with women who are defined by specific criteria for risk are needed. These could include, for example, studies of social interventions in women with measurable evidence of stress and studies of activity restriction in women with short cervical lengths.

Finding 9-3: Studies of intervention strategies for the prevention of preterm birth have had preterm birth as their only outcome variable. The study samples have not been large enough for sufficient investigations of morbidity, mortality, and neurological morbidity.

DIAGNOSIS AND TREATMENT OF PRETERM LABOR

The methods for the diagnosis and treatment of preterm labor are based on an inadequate literature that is compromised not only by the oft-cited paucity of well-designed and adequately powered clinical trials but also, even more, by an incomplete understanding of the sequence and timing of events that precede clinical evidence of preterm labor, such as progressive cervical dilatation and ruptured membranes. Because the progression from subclinical preterm parturition to overt preterm labor is often gradual, standard criteria for the diagnosis of preterm labor (uterine contractions accompanied by cervical change) lack precision. Consequently, preterm labor is often overdiagnosed so that women with frequent contractions who are not in labor are enrolled in studies of tocolytic drugs (King et al., 1988). Women treated to prevent or arrest preterm labor may therefore have been treated successfully or may not have required treatment at all. The true result of treatment is known with confidence only for those whose treatment was unsuccessful.

Useful studies of methods for the prevention or arrest of preterm labor therefore depend on the development of more accurate methods for the diagnosis of preterm labor. The current uncertainty is reflected by the division of clinicians into two camps: those who believe that nothing works and others who claim great success with various interventions. The truth likely falls somewhere in between but will emerge only if additional resources are devoted to improving the means of diagnosis of preterm labor.

Diagnosis of Preterm Labor

Preterm labor must be considered whenever abdominal or pelvic symptoms occur after 18 to 20 weeks of gestation. Symptoms like pelvic pressure, increased vaginal discharge, backache, and menstrual-like cramps are common with advancing pregnancy and suggest preterm labor more by their persistence than by their severity. Contractions may be painful or painless, depending on the resistance offered by the cervix. Contractions against a closed, uneffaced cervix are likely to be painful, but recurrent pressure or tightening may be the only symptoms, as often occurs when cervical effacement precedes the onset of contractions (Olah and Gee, 1992). The traditional criteria for labor, persistent uterine contractions accompanied by dilatation or effacement of the cervix, or both, are reasonably accurate when the frequency is six or more contractions per hour, cervical dilatation is 3 cm or more, effacement is 80 percent or greater, and membranes rupture or bleeding occurs (Hueston, 1998; Macones et al., 1999a). When lower thresholds for contraction frequency and cervical change are used, a false-positive diagnosis of labor is common (in up to 40 percent of cases) (King et al., 1988) but the sensitivity of the diagnosis does not necessarily increase (Peaceman et al., 1997).

The accurate diagnosis of early preterm labor is difficult because the symptoms (Iams et al., 1994) and signs (Moore et al., 1994) of preterm labor commonly occur in healthy women who do not deliver preterm and because digital examination of the cervix in early labor (less than 3 cm of dilatation and less than 80 percent effacement) is not highly reproducible (Berghella et al., 1997; Jackson et al., 1992). Women whose symptoms are cervical dilatation of less than 2 cm or effacement of less than 80 percent, or both, present a diagnostic challenge. In a clinical trial to identify women with true preterm labor, Guinn et al. (1997) randomly assigned 179 women with preterm contractions and minimal cervical dilatation to receive intravenous hydration, observation without intervention, or a single dose of 0.25 mg of subcutaneous terbutaline (a tocolytic agent). Intravenous hydration did not decrease preterm contractions. Women whose contractions recurred despite transient cessation after terbutaline treatment were more often found to be in preterm labor; those whose contractions stopped and did not recur were sent home. The authors concluded that a single dose of subcutaneous terbutaline was an efficient method of identifying those with actual preterm labor.

Other means of enhancing diagnostic accuracy in preterm labor include transvaginal sonographic measurement of cervical length and testing for fetal fibronectin in cervicovaginal fluid (ACOG, 2003; Leitich et al., 1999a,b). Both of these tests improve the diagnostic accuracy by reducing the possibility of a false-positive diagnosis of labor. Transabdominal sonography, however, has a poor reproducibility for cervical length measurement (Mason and Maresh, 1990) and the findings should not be used clinically without confirmation of the findings by transvaginal ultrasound. A cervical length of 30 mm or more by endovaginal sonography, however, suggests that preterm labor is unlikely in symptomatic women if the examination is properly performed (Iams, 2003). Similarly, a negative fibronectin test in women with symptoms before 34 weeks of gestation with cervical dilatation of less than 3 cm can also reduce the rate of a false-positive diagnosis of labor if the result is returned promptly and the clinician is willing to act on a negative test result by not initiating treatment (Chien et al., 1997; Leitich et al., 1999b). The combined use of tests for cervical length and fibronectin identifies a group of patients with a very high risk of preterm birth when the fibronectin test is positive and the sonographic cervical length is less than 30 mm (Table 9-7).

Despite evidence that the overdiagnosis of preterm labor in women with frequent contractions is common and results in unnecessary treatment, the clinical use of the fibronectin test and cervical sonography is not widespread.

Barriers to improved accurate diagnosis before treatment is initiated include a lack of professional and public education about the parturitional process and the risks of preterm birth for the infant (Massett et al., 2003), inadequate training of medical professionals other than physicians to perform the appropriate examinations (speculum examination of the cervix, endovaginal cervical sonography), and medicolegal fears that failure to treat a pregnant woman who may be in labor may invite lawsuits. Research and educational programs should aim to address these problems and to identify the most appropriate point(s) at which parturition should be arrested once it has begun.

TABLE 9-7 Frequency of Spontaneous Preterm Delivery According to Cervical Length (cutoff 30 mm) and Vaginal Fibronectin Results

Cervical Length <30 mm	Fetal Fibronectin +	Delivery Within 48 Hours	Delivery Within 7 Days	Delivery Within 14 Days	Delivery ≤32 Weeks	Delivery ≤35 Weeks
No	No	2.2% (2/93)	2.2% (2/93)	3.2% (3/93)	0% (0/47)	1.1% (1.93)
No	Yes	0% (0/14)	7.1% (1/14)	14.3% (2/14)	0% (0/5)	21.4% (3/14)
Yes	No	7.1% (5/70)	11.4% (8/70)	12.9% (9/70)	6.5% (2/31)	17.1% (12/70)
Yes	Yes	26.3% (10/38)	44.7% (17/38)	52.6% (20/38)	38.9% (7/18)	47.4% (18/38)
Prevalence of the outcome		7.9% (17/215)	13.0% (28/215)	15.8% (34/215)	8.9% (9/101)	15.8% (34/215)

SOURCE: Gomez et al. (2005). Reprinted from American Journal of Obstetrics and Gynecology, Vol. 192, Pg. 354, © 2005, with permission from Elsevier.

Finding 9-4: Current methods for the diagnosis and treatment of women at risk of an imminent preterm birth are not sufficiently evidence based.

Information Informing Decisions Surrounding Perinatal Interventions

Obstetricians are taught that their first obligation and priority is the mother's health but that women and families are willing to accept some degree of increased risk to the mother if it will benefit her fetus (see Appendix C for a discussion of ethical issues). A decision to arrest preterm labor may increase the risk to both the mother and the fetus if the pregnancy is complicated by bleeding, hypertension, or infection. A lesser risk usually attends uncomplicated preterm labor; but intrauterine fetal stress or compromise may contribute to the onset of preterm labor, and tests of fetal well-being are imperfect. Tocolytic drugs, which are used to arrest labor, can have serious maternal and fetal side effects, especially if they are used in increasing doses, for prolonged periods, or in combination with one another. The decision about whether to arrest preterm labor, to transfer the mother and the fetus in utero to another hospital, or to administer antenatal glucocorticoids is made against this background in an environment of spoken and unspoken assumptions about their wisdom, according to current information and beliefs. The quality of this information necessarily varies with the dissemination and local application of advancements in perinatal and neonatal care. Beliefs about the anticipated rates of morbidity and mortality for preterm infants according to gestational age are the foundation for decisions regarding obstetric and perinatal care.

Reports of improved perinatal outcomes for preterm infants could be expected to and do apparently result in an increased willingness to choose delivery and neonatal care over the uncertainties of continuing the pregnancy. The mortality and morbidity of prematurely born infants are discussed in Chapter 10. Recent data from one center are shown in Figure 9-3 to illustrate how improved outcomes for infants born after 32 weeks of gestation might lead to a decision to allow preterm delivery rather than initiate treatment with drugs that may prolong the pregnancy for only a few days (Mercer, 2003).

Finding 9-5: The goal of prevention of preterm birth is subordinate to the goal of improved perinatal morbidity and mortality outcomes. This goal is important, because the continuation of pregnancy in women with preterm parturition in some instances may increase the health risk for the mother or the fetus, or both.

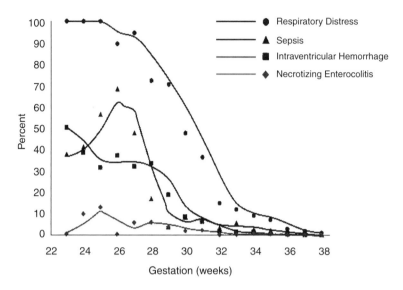

FIGURE 9-3 Perinatal mortality and gestational age.
SOURCE: Mercer (2003). Reprinted with permission from *Obstetrics & Gynecology*, Vol. 101, Pg. 180, © 2003 by the American College of Obstetricians and Gynecologists.

Although the expectations of obstetric and neonatal doctors and nurses about neonatal and infant outcomes are known to influence decision making in perinatal care (Bottoms et al., 1997), these same practitioners' assessments are not necessarily accurate. Morse et al. (2000) found that both obstetric and neonatal care providers' predictions of neonatal survival and survival without handicap were substantially below the actual rates, indicating a need for improved information before and after delivery (Figures 9-4 and 9-5). Finally, the medical-legal environment may also be a consideration; however, the extent of its influence on this decision-making process is unknown.

Finding 9-6: The knowledge and beliefs of health care providers influence their attitudes toward and their management of mothers with threatened preterm delivery and their infants.

Treatment Strategies and Effectiveness

The prevention of preterm birth has primarily been focused on the treatment of the woman with symptomatic preterm labor. This strategy is based

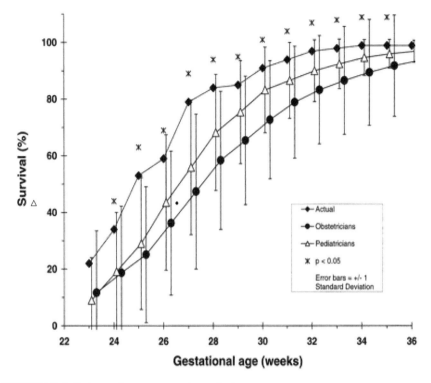

FIGURE 9-4 Estimated versus actual survival rates.
SOURCE: Morse et al. (2000). Reproduced with permission from *Pediatrics*, Vol.
105, Pg. 1047, © 2000 by the American Academy of Pediatrics.

on the assumption that clinically apparent labor is commensurate with the
initiation of the parturitional process and that successful inhibition of labor
should prevent delivery. Thus, treatment has been directed toward the inhibition of myometrial contractions. This approach has not decreased the
incidence of preterm birth but can delay delivery long enough to allow
administration of antenatal steroids and to transfer the mother and fetus to
an appropriate hospital, two interventions that have consistently been
shown to reduce the rates of perinatal mortality and morbidity.

Labor inhibition has not prevented preterm birth because arresting
myometrial contractions does not address the specific initiators of preterm
labor. In addition, few medications can inhibit uterine contractions safely
and effectively for more than a few days. Research to find tocolytic drugs is
hampered by the inaccurate diagnosis of preterm labor, such that many
women with preterm labor are not detected early enough to expect success,
whereas others are treated for preterm contractions that do not result in

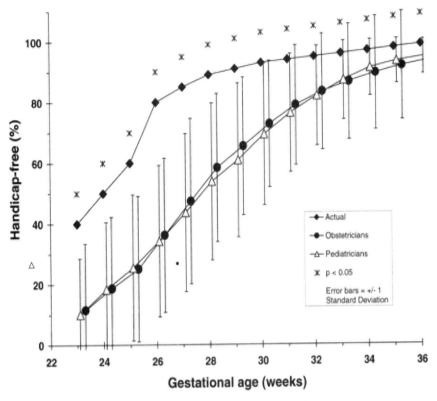

FIGURE 9-5 Estimated versus rates of freedom from handicap.
SOURCE: Morse et al. (2000). Reproduced with permission from *Pediatrics*, Vol. 105, Pg. 1047, © 2000 by the American Academy of Pediatrics.

labor. The treatment strategies used to treat women diagnosed with preterm labor are reviewed below.

Tocolytics

Labor-inhibiting agents are commonly referred to as tocolytic drugs, after the Greek *tokos*, meaning childbirth, and *lysis*, meaning to release. The purpose of tocolytic agents is to inhibit myometrial contractions. The labor-inhibiting agents used today abrogate myometrial contractility by one of two major pathways. These drugs affect either the contractile proteins (usually the phosphorylation of myosin) by generation or alteration of an intracellular messenger or inhibit the synthesis or block the action of a known myometrial stimulant. The first group includes the β-adrenergic receptor agonists, nitric oxide donors, and magnesium sulfate and the calcium channel blockers. The second group includes prostaglandin synthesis inhibitors and oxytocin antagonists.

Randomized, controlled trials of tocolytics have shown that they successfully inhibit contractions for 2 to 7 days. They have not been useful for long-term maintenance of contraction inhibition and in most studies have not improved perinatal outcomes, although their use does allow time for the administration of corticosteroids and maternal transfer to an appropriate hospital.

Magnesium sulfate The precise mechanism by which magnesium affects uterine contractions has not been completely elucidated. Magnesium likely competes with calcium at the level of plasma membrane voltage-gated channels. It hyperpolarizes the plasma membrane and inhibits myosin light-chain kinase activity by competing with intracellular calcium at this site. Interference with the activity of myosin light-chain kinase reduces myometrial contractility (Cunze et al., 1995; Lemancewicz et al., 2000; Mizuki et al., 1993). In two randomized, placebo-controlled trials of magnesium sulfate, magnesium sulfate did not lead to improved birth outcomes, although the cessation of contractions for a short interval was demonstrated (Cox et al., 1990; Fox et al., 1993). Three of four randomized clinical trials that compared magnesium sulfate with terbutaline found no difference in perinatal outcomes (Berkman et al., 2003). Meta-analysis also indicates that magnesium sulfate is ineffective for the treatment of preterm labor (Crowther et al., 2002). Potential adverse effects of magnesium sulfate include respiratory depression, flushing, nausea, and pulmonary edema.

Beta-mimetic drugs The β-adrenergic receptor agonists cause myometrial relaxation by binding with β_2-adrenergic receptors and increasing intracellular adenyl cyclase. An increase in intracellular cyclic adenosine monophosphate levels activates protein kinase, which results in the phosphorylation of intracellular proteins. The resultant drop in intracellular free calcium levels interferes with the activity of myosin light-chain kinase, which inhibits the interaction between actin and myosin, and thus, myometrial contractility is diminished (Caritis et al., 1979, 1987, 1991).

Beta-sympathomimetic drugs, including terbutaline and ritodrine, have been widely used as tocolytics for many years. The most commonly used beta-mimetic in the United States is terbutaline (marketed in the United States as a drug for the treatment of asthma); but others, including albuterol, fenoterol, hexoprenaline, metaproterenol, nylidrin, orciprenaline, and salbutamol, are used in other countries. Ritodrine hydrochloride, the only drug ever approved for use as a parenteral tocolytic by the Food and Drug Administration (FDA), never achieved widespread use because of frequent maternal side effects. It is no longer marketed in the United States. Terbutaline is more commonly used because clinicians are familiar with it and it has a rapid onset of action (3 to 5 minutes) when it is given subcutaneously. Published protocols often use subcutaneous administration, with a usual dose of 0.25 mg (250 micrograms) every 3 to 6 hours.

Once frequently prescribed for acute and maintenance therapy of women with suspected preterm labor, beta-mimetic drugs are less commonly used because of reports of their limited efficacy for this syndrome and because of concern about their cardiovascular and metabolic side effects. The Cochrane database includes data for 1,332 women enrolled in 11 randomized, placebo-controlled trials of beta-mimetic drugs. Those data indicate that treated subjects were less likely to deliver within 48 hours (RR 0.63; 95% CI 0.53–0.75) but not within 7 days (Anotayanonth et al., 2004). Although a 48-hour delay in delivery allows sufficient time for in utero transfer to an appropriate hospital and treatment with steroids, the rates of perinatal and neonatal death and perinatal morbidity were not reduced in that analysis. Side effects requiring a change or a cessation of treatment were frequent. Previous reviews have found similar results (Berkman et al., 2003, Gyetvai et al., 1999).

Long-term or maintenance use of beta-mimetic drugs has been advocated to suppress contractions to prevent preterm labor, but tachyphylaxis or desensitization of the adrenergic receptor occurs after prolonged exposure to beta-agonists, so that increasing dosages are required to sustain a response. After animal studies suggested that the myometrium remains quiescent longer with pulsatile administration of lower doses of beta-mimetics (Casper and Lye, 1986), a protocol that used a continuous subcutaneous infusion of terbutaline at lower doses was reported to result in fewer side effects than the numbers of side effects encountered with oral administration (Lam et al., 2001; Perry et al., 1995). Although these protocols suppress contractions, they had no effect on the rates of preterm birth or perinatal morbidity in randomized, placebo-controlled trials (Guinn et al., 1998; Wenstrom et al., 1997), and the use of beta-mimetic compounds is not recommended by ACOG (ACOG, 2001). A 2002 *Cochrane Review* also concluded that current evidence does not support terbutaline infusion to prolong pregnancy (Nanda et al., 2002).

Calcium channel blockers Calcium channel blockers directly block the influx of calcium ions through the cell membrane. They also inhibit the release of intracellular calcium from the sarcoplasmic reticulum and increase the level of calcium efflux from the cell. The ensuing decrease in intracellular free calcium levels leads to inhibition of calcium-dependent myosin light-chain kinase phosphorylation and results in myometrial relaxation. One study compared nifedipine, the most commonly studied calcium channel blocker, with magnesium but showed no difference between nifedipine and magnesium in prolonging pregnancy or improving the perinatal outcome (Floyd et al., 1995). Use of the combination of magnesium and calcium channel blockers could, in theory, cause respiratory depression and extreme hypotension; so use of this combination is best avoided.

Eight randomized clinical trials and one nonrandomized trial have compared calcium channel blockers with beta-mimetics. In two trials, women treated with nifedipine had a longer interval between treatment and delivery and their infants had a greater mean estimated gestational age at delivery (Jannet et al., 1997; Papatsonis et al., 1997), but five other trials showed no significant differences in perinatal outcomes (Berkman et al., 2003). Side effects of nifedipine include dizziness, headache, flushing, and edema.

Cyclooxygenase inhibitors Cyclooxygenase (COX; prostaglandin synthase) is the enzyme responsible for the conversion of arachidonic acid to prostaglandins, which are critical in parturition. Prostaglandins enhance the formation of myometrial gap junctions and increase the amount of intracellular calcium available by raising transmembrane influx and the sarcolemmal release of calcium (Challis et al., 2002). COX exists in two isoforms, COX-1 and COX-2. COX-1 is constitutively expressed in gestational tissues, whereas COX-2 is the inducible form. COX-2 is the isoform whose levels dramatically increase in the decidua and the myometrium during term and preterm labor. COX inhibitors decrease prostaglandin production by either general inhibition of COX or specific inhibition of COX-2, depending on the agent. These inhibitors include indomethacin, sulindac, and ibuprofen.

The first randomized placebo control trial of indomethacin involved 30 patients with preterm labor. One of 15 patients who received indomethacin but 9 of 15 patients in the placebo group began labor after 24 hours (Niebyl et al., 1980). Although the maternal adverse effects of COX inhibitors are largely limited to mild gastrointestinal upset, fetal effects of concern include oligohydramnios and premature closure of the ductus arteriosus. Limiting indomethacin therapy to 24 to 48 hours of treatment before 32 weeks of gestation avoids these concerns (Moise et al., 1988).

Oxytocin receptor antagonists In normal parturition, oxytocin stimulates contractions by inducing the conversion of phosphatidylinositol to inositol triphosphate, which binds to a protein in the sarcoplasmic reticulum that causes the release of calcium into the cytoplasm. Oxytocin receptor antagonists compete with oxytocin for binding to receptors in the myometrium and decidua, thus preventing the increase in intracellular free calcium levels that occurs with receptor binding (Goodwin et al., 1996; Phaneuf et al., 1994). Atosiban is a selective oxytocin-vasopressin receptor antagonist that inhibits spontaneous and oxytocin-induced contractions but not prostaglandin-induced contractions. Because oxytocin receptors are mostly confined to the uterus and myoepithelial cells of the breast, maternal side effects are minimal (Romero et al., 2000). Oxytocin antagonists cross the placenta, but fetal cardiovascular status and acid-base status are not affected.

In a placebo-controlled trial, the duration of pregnancy after the initiation of therapy with atosiban was not different (26 days for treated women and 21 days for women in the placebo group; $p = 0.6$) when the entire group of women was evaluated (gestational age, 20 to 33 weeks 6 days; $n = 531$), but atosiban treatment prolonged pregnancy significantly more often than placebo for up to 48 hours and for up to 7 days in women treated at 28 weeks of gestation or later ($n = 424$) (Romero et al., 2000). In a randomized trial ($n = 733$) in which atosiban was compared with intravenous beta-mimetic drug (Moutquin et al., 2001), the rates of delivery within 48 hours and 7 days after the initiation of therapy were not different, but women treated with atosiban had fewer and less severe side effects.

Despite these results, FDA did not approve atosiban for use because adverse outcomes were noted in fetuses of less than 28 weeks of gestation. It is not clear whether these outcomes were related to the drug or to greater numbers of pregnancies treated before 28 weeks of gestation in the atosiban arm. Atosiban is available for clinical use in Europe, where it is the most commonly used tocolytic drug in many countries (personal communication, H.P. van Geijn and D. Papatsonis, Free University Hospital, Amsterdam, the Netherlands, December 16, 2005).

Nitric oxide donors Nitric oxide (NO) is produced in a variety of cells and is essential for maintenance of normal smooth muscle tone. NO is synthesized during the oxidation of L-arginine (an essential amino acid) to L-citrulline, which then diffuses from the source cell. This reaction is catalyzed by the enzyme nitric oxide synthase. The interaction between NO and soluble guanylyl cyclase, which is present in nearby effector cells, represents a widespread signal transduction mechanism that couples the diverse extracellular stimuli of NO formation to the synthesis of cyclic guanosine 3',5'-monophosphate (cGMP) in target cells. The increase in cGMP content in smooth muscle cells activates myosin light-chain kinases, leading to smooth muscle relaxation (Yallampalli et al., 1998). NO donors such as nitroglycerin inhibit spontaneous and oxytocin- and prostaglandin-induced activity in vitro and effectively inhibit postsurgical uterine contractility in pregnant monkeys and humans. A randomized study comparing intravenous nitroglycerin and magnesium sulfate found that magnesium therapy was more likely to successfully delay delivery for at least 12 hours (El-Sayed et al., 1999). Two other randomized trials comparing transdermal nitroglycerin with placebo or ritodrine found no difference in their abilities to prolong pregnancy for 48 hours (Lees et al., 1999; Smith et al., 1999). There is thus insufficient evidence at this time to recommend the use of NO donors for the inhibition of preterm labor.

Summary of tocolytic drug treatment The ultimate goal of treatment for preterm labor is to eliminate or reduce perinatal morbidity and mortality. No trials of the efficacies of tocolytics of sufficient sample size are available to assess these outcomes. The surrogate or secondary outcomes used instead of neonatal morbidity are pregnancy prolongation, frequency of preterm birth, and gestational age at birth. Few placebo-controlled trials of tocolytic drugs have been conducted. β-Adrenergic receptor agonists, indomethacin, and atosiban have demonstrated superiority over placebo in achieving limited pregnancy prolongation. The findings of other of the efficacies of tocolytics have been less persuasive and have included those that have compared two active agents, that enroll women at a very low risk of preterm delivery, and that have had an inadequate power to demonstrate any statistically significant difference between agents. Meta-analyses address the issue of sample size but do not overcome problems with poor study design, selection criteria, and the use of intermediate outcomes. Delaying the time to delivery to allow maternal transfer to the most appropriate hospital and the administration of corticosteroids antenatally is clearly supported by the available evidence and is the strongest argument for the short-term use of tocolytic drugs.

Antibiotics and Preterm Labor

Abundant evidence supports an association between subclinical infection and preterm labor. The mechanism of this association has not been elucidated. Among 14 randomized controlled trials performed between 1986 and 2001 to evaluate the benefit of antibiotic treatment of women with preterm labor and intact membranes, only 2 showed a prolongation of pregnancy and a decreased rate of preterm delivery by the use of antibiotic therapy. In a meta-analysis of seven trials that enrolled 795 patients treated with broad-spectrum antibiotics or placebo, the length of pregnancy was unchanged by antibiotic administration (Egarter et al., 1996). Although the rates of occurrence of some neonatal outcomes such as pneumonia and necrotizing enterocolitis were reduced, the risk of neonatal mortality was increased (odds ratio = 3.25; 95% CI 0.93–1.38). Antibiotic administration had no effect on neonatal sepsis or intraventricular hemorrhage.

The largest study to date randomized 6,295 women in spontaneous preterm labor to receive (1) erythromycin, (2) co-amoxicillin–clavulanic acid (co-amoxiclav), (3) erythromycin and co-amoxiclav, or (4) placebo (Kenyon et al., 2001a). None of the antibiotic treatments was associated with a prolongation of pregnancy or improvements in perinatal outcomes. Maternal infections were reduced in women exposed to antibiotics.

Despite the association of various infections with preterm labor, the use of broad-spectrum antibiotics for women in preterm labor has not improved any outcome. Most authors have explained this by noting that the timing of antibiotic treatment after preterm labor is clinically manifest is too late to influence any outcomes other than acute neonatal or maternal infection.

Antibiotics for Preterm Premature Rupture of Fetal Membranes

Although antibiotics have been unsuccessful for the treatment of women with intact membranes, adjunctive antibiotic therapy is recommended for women who are managed expectantly after preterm premature rupture of membranes (PPROM). (PROM refers to premature rupture of membranes, meaning before the onset of labor at any gestational age; hence, although "preterm PROM" is apparently redundant, it is not, given the definition of PROM, and is abbreviated here PPROM.) Evidence from appropriately conducted placebo-controlled trials has shown that antibiotic treatment can reduce morbidity for infants born after PPROM and prolong the interval from rupture to delivery. A study that compared ampicillin plus erythromycin and placebo (Mercer et al., 1997) demonstrated improved neonatal outcomes (risk of death, respiratory distress syndrome, sepsis, severe intraventricular hemorrhage, and severe necrotizing enterocolitis) in the infants of women receiving antibiotics compared with the neonatal outcomes in women receiving placebo. Another study of 4,826 women with PPROM showed that erythromycin was associated with a prolongation of pregnancy and improved neonatal outcomes (Kenyon et al., 2001b). That trial showed a significant increase in the occurrence of necrotizing enterocolitis in those infants exposed to co-amoxiclav.

A meta-analysis of 14 randomized clinical trials that included more than 6,000 women found that treatment with broad-spectrum antibiotics prolonged latency and led to significant decreases in neonatal infections, positive neonatal blood cultures, the need for surfactant treatment and oxygen therapy, and abnormal ultrasounds before hospital discharge. Although the rate of neonatal mortality was reduced, it was not statistically significant. Antibiotic treatment was also found to be associated with a statistically significant reduction in maternal infection and chorioamnionitis (Kenyon et al., 2004).

Antenatal Corticosteroids

The one intervention that reduces perinatal morbidity and mortality and that is firmly supported by the findings of research is the antenatal administration of glucocorticoids to women at risk of preterm birth. A 1994 National Institutes of Health Consensus Conference recommended the administration of corticosteroids to women with preterm labor before 34 weeks of gestation and women with PPROM before 32 weeks of gestation by the use of a single course of either betamethasone (two doses of 12 mg intramuscularly administered 24 hours apart) or dexamethasone (four doses of 6 mg intramuscularly administered 12 hours apart). Studies have shown conclusively that the antepartum administration of the glucocorticoids betamethasone or dexamethasone to the mother reduces the risk of death, respiratory distress syndrome, intraventricular hemorrhage, necrotizing entercolitis, and patent ductus arteriosus in the preterm neonate (Crowley, 1999). Other morbidities of preterm birth reduced by antenatal glucocorticoid administration include necrotizing enterocolitis, patent ductus arteriosus, and bronchopulomary dysplasia.

Betamethasone and dexamethasone are apparently equally effective in reducing perinatal morbidity, but there may be some advantage to the use of betamethasone. In a study of infants born between 24 and 31 weeks of gestation, the rate of periventricular leukomalacia was 4.4 percent among 361 infants who were treated antenatally with betamethasone, 11.0 percent among 165 infants who received dexamethasone, and 8.4 percent among 357 infants who were not treated with antenatal corticosteroids (Baud et al., 1999).

Other fetal effects of glucocorticoids have been reported. Transient reductions in fetal breathing and body movements sufficient to affect the interpretation of the biophysical profile have been described after the administration of both drugs but are more common after administration of betamethasone and typically last for 48 to 72 hours after administration of the second dose (Mulder et al., 1997; Rotmensch et al., 1999; Senat et al., 1998). Transient suppression of neonatal cortisol levels has been reported, but the neonatal response to adrenocorticotropin stimulation was unimpaired (Teramo et al., 1980; Terrone et al., 1997, 1999). Neonatal leukocyte counts are not affected by antenatal steroid administration (Zachman et al., 1988). Although maternal adrenal suppression has been described with repeated courses of antenatal steroids, the adrenal suppression had no clinical consequences (Wapner et al., 2005).

Concern about whether corticosteroids given to women with ruptured membranes might increase the risk of neonatal infection has been addressed by reports that found no such association (Harding et al., 2001; Lewis et al., 1996). Harding and colleagues (2001) found no evidence of increased maternal infections (RR 0.86; 95% CI 0.61–1.2) or neonatal infections (RR 1.05; 95% CI 0.66–1.68) in a meta-analysis of steroid treatment of women with PPROM.

The duration of the beneficial effects on the fetus after the administration of a single course of glucocorticoids is not clear. The issue is difficult to study because the interval between treatment and delivery in clinical trials varies and because some effects may be transient, whereas others are permanent. The benefit to the neonate has been most easily observed when the interval between the first dose and delivery exceeds 48 hours, but some benefit is evident after an incomplete course. One large multicenter trial (Gamsu et al., 1989) found evidence of a benefit for as long as 18 days after the initial course of treatment.

The increasing use of repeated courses of antenatal steroid treatment prompted animal and human studies that have raised concerns about the effects of prolonged exposure to steroids on fetal growth and neurological function. The animal studies showed reduced fetal growth and adverse brain and neurological development and a pattern of decreased fetal growth in several species (Aghajafari et al., 2002; Cotterrell et al., 1972; Huang et al., 1999; Jobe et al., 1998; Quinlivan et al., 2000; Stewart et al., 1997).

Human studies also found reduced growth in fetuses exposed to multiple courses of antenatal steroids. An Australian study found a twofold increase in the numbers of infants with birth weights below the 10th percentile and a significantly reduced head circumference in infants exposed to more than three antenatal courses of steroids (French et al., 1999). A reduced head circumference was also reported in other studies (Abbasi et al., 2000). These reports led NICHD to reconvene the Consensus Conference Panel in August 2000 to review the available information about repeated courses of steroids. That panel reemphasized the benefit and safety of a single course of antenatal corticosteroids (given either as two intramuscular doses of 12 mg 24 hours apart or four doses of dexamethasone every 12 hours) for women between 24 and 34 weeks of gestation who are deemed to be at risk of preterm delivery within 7 days. The panel noted data suggesting a benefit for repeat courses of steroids, but in the absence of appropriate clinical studies, the panel recommended that "repeat courses of corticosteroids . . . should not be used routinely . . . [but] should be reserved for patients enrolled in randomized controlled trials" (NIH, 2001, p. 146).

Five prospective, randomized, clinical trials of repeat antenatal corticosteroids in humans have been performed. Three (Guinn et al., 2001; Mercer et al., 2001a,b; Wapner, 2003) have been reported in articles or abstracts, and two (Australian and Canadian trials) are ongoing or have not yet been described. Guinn and colleagues (2001) enrolled 502 women who had received one course of steroids to receive betamethasone once weekly or no further treatment. There was no difference in the composite rates of morbidity (defined as severe respiratory distress syndrome, bronchopulmonary dysplasia, severe intraventricular hemorrhage, periventricular leukomalacia, sepsis, necrotizing enterocolitis, or death) in the two groups (22.5 and 28.0 percent, respectively; $p = 0.16$). There was a reduction in the rate of severe respiratory distress syndrome (15.3 and 24.1 percent, respectively; p = 0.01) and composite morbidity (96.4 and 77.4 percent, respectively; p = 0.03) in infants treated repeatedly if they were delivered at between 24 and 27 weeks of gestation.

Another trial (Mercer et al., 2001a,b) compared weekly betamethasone to rescue treatment from enrollment through 34 weeks of gestation. Notably, only 37 percent of women assigned to receive rescue steroids were so treated, indicating the difficulty in predicting imminent preterm delivery. More than 75 percent of the women in the weekly treatment group received corticosteroids within a week of preterm birth (p = 0.001) (Mercer et al., 2001a). The NICHD MFMU Network Study (Wapner, 2003) randomized 495 women, of whom 492 (591 infants) were available for analysis and 252 received repetitive steroids. The trial was stopped by the independent data and safety monitoring board before the planned sample size was reached because of slow enrollment. The investigators found no difference in the primary (composite) outcome for infants who were exposed to multiple courses compared with that for infants who received placebo (7.7 and 9.2 percent, respectively; p = 0.67). Trends toward improvement were seen in the group receiving multiple courses of steroids for each component of the primary outcome and for secondary outcomes related to lung function: use of surfactant (12.5 and 18.4 percent, respectively; p = 0.02), mechanical ventilation (15.5 and 23.5 percent, respectively; p = 0.005), and treatment for hypotension (5.7 and 11.2 percent, respectively; p = 0.02). Among infants delivered before 32 weeks of gestation, the composite morbidities[1] included in the primary outcome were less common in the group receiving multiple courses of steroids (21.3 and 38.5 percent, respectively; p = 0.083). Multiple courses of steroid treatment were associated with insignificant trends toward reduced infant weight (2,194 and 2,289 grams for the treatment and placebo groups, respectively; p = 0.09) and length (44.2 and 44.7 cm for the treatment and placebo groups, respectively; p = .09). Infants exposed to four or more courses of steroids had a significant decrease in birth weight (2,396 and 2,561 grams for the treatment and placebo groups, respectively; p = 0.01) (Wapner, 2003).

Other Antenatal Treatments to Reduce Fetal Morbidity

Respiratory distress Several alternative approaches to reducing the rate of occurrence of neonatal respiratory distress syndrome that are used before

---

[1]Defined as stillbirth, neonatal death, severe respiratory distress syndrome, grade III or IV intraventricular hemorrhage, periventricular leukomalacia, or chronic lung disease (Wapner, 2003).

and after birth have been studied. Neonatal treatment with surfactant is an effective adjunctive therapy that adds independently and synergistically to the benefit offered by corticosteroids in reducing respiratory distress syndrome-related morbidity (St. John and Carlo, 2003). The use of antenatal thyrotropin-releasing hormone (TRH) to reduce neonatal lung disease has been studied in trials that enrolled more than 4,600 women. TRH did not improve any neonatal outcome when TRH treatment was compared with corticosteroid treatment alone and actually increased the risk of poor outcomes for the infants in some trials (Crowther et al., 2004).

Neurological morbidity Antenatal maternal treatment with phenobarbital, vitamin K, and magnesium sulfate has been studied as a means of reducing or preventing neonatal neurological morbidity. Phenobarbital did not decrease intraventricular hemorrhage when it was given alone (Shankaran et al., 1997) or in combination with vitamin K (Thorp et al., 1995). Antenatal maternal treatment with magnesium has also been studied after observational reports found reduced rates of intraventricular hemorrhage, cerebral palsy, and perinatal mortality in premature infants exposed to antenatal magnesium (Grether et al., 1998, 2000; Mittendorf et al., 1997; Nelson and Grether, 1995; Paneth et al., 1997; Schendel et al., 1996). A randomized placebo-controlled trial of antenatal magnesium conducted with 1,062 women who delivered before 30 weeks of gestation found that magnesium-treated infants had significantly improved gross motor dysfunction and a trend suggesting a lower rate of cerebral palsy at 2 years of age (Crowther et al., 2003). No significant adverse effects were noted in infants exposed to antenatal magnesium sulfate in this study. The NICHD- and National Institute of Neurological Disorders and Stroke-Sponsored MFMU Network's BEAM Trial (Randomized Clinical Trial of the Beneficial Effects of Antenatal Magnesium Sulfate) has concluded enrollment and will report on the outcomes for the infants in 2007, when the infants will be 2 years old.

Maternal Transfer

Many states have adopted systems of regionalized perinatal care, in recognition of the advantages of concentrating care for preterm infants, especially those born before 32 weeks of gestation. Hospitals and birth centers caring for healthy mothers and infants are typically designated Level I. Larger hospitals that care for the majority of maternal and infant complications are designated Level II centers; these hospitals have neonatal intensive care units staffed and equipped to care for most infants with birth weights between 1,250 and 1,500 grams. Level III centers typically provide care for the sickest and the smallest infants and for maternal complications requiring intensive care. The use of this approach has been associated with improved outcomes for preterm infants (Towers et al., 2000; Yeast et al., 1998) (see Chapters 10 and 14 for further discussion).

FUTURE DIRECTIONS

Despite several interventions designed to inhibit preterm labor and prolong pregnancy, the frequency of preterm birth continues to pose a major barrier to the health of newborns worldwide. Although current obstetric and neonatal strategies have resulted in improved rates of neonatal survival and an earlier threshold for viability, effective strategies for prevention of preterm birth are urgently needed. As basic and translational research continues to reveal more of the complex endocrinological and immunological aspects of parturition, investigators must continue to search for biologically plausible new therapies to prevent preterm birth and develop markers or multiple markers to diagnose the syndrome accurately in its early stages.

ATTACHMENT 9-1
(SAMPLE)

NAME: _____
      LAST   FIRST   MIDDLE

ID # _____ HOSPITAL OF DELIVERY _____

NEWBORN'S PHYSICIAN _____ REFERRED BY _____

FINAL EDD _____   PRIMARY PROVIDER/GROUP _____

BIRTH DATE	AGE	RACE	MARITAL STATUS	ADDRESS		
MONTH DAY YEAR			S M W D SEP			
OCCUPATION			EDUCATION (LAST GRADE COMPLETED)	ZIP	PHONE	(H) (O)
LANGUAGE				INSURANCE CARRIER/MEDICAID #		
HUSBAND/DOMESTIC PARTNER		PHONE		POLICY #		
FATHER OF BABY		PHONE		EMERGENCY CONTACT		PHONE

TOTAL PREG	FULL TERM	PREMATURE	AB. INDUCED	AB. SPONTANEOUS	ECTOPICS	MULTIPLE BIRTHS	LIVING

MENSTRUAL HISTORY

LMP ☐ DEFINITE ☐ APPROXIMATE (MONTH KNOWN) MENSES MONTHLY ☐ YES ☐ NO FREQUENCY Q_____ DAYS MENARCHE _____ (AGE ONSET)
   ☐ UNKNOWN ☐ NORMAL AMOUNT/DURATION PRIOR MENSES _____ DATE ON BCP AT CONCEPT ☐ YES ☐ NO hCG + __/__/__
   ☐ FINAL _____

PAST PREGNANCIES (LAST SIX)

DATE MONTH/ YEAR	GA WEEKS	LENGTH OF LABOR	BIRTH WEIGHT	SEX M/F	TYPE DELIVERY	ANES.	PLACE OF DELIVERY	PRETERM LABOR YES/NO	COMMENTS/ COMPLICATIONS

MEDICAL HISTORY

	O Neg. + Pos.	DETAIL POSITIVE REMARKS INCLUDE DATE & TREATMENT		O Neg. + Pos.	DETAIL POSITIVE REMARKS INCLUDE DATE & TREATMENT
1. DIABETES			17. D (Rh) SENSITIZED		
2. HYPERTENSION			18. PULMONARY (TB, ASTHMA)		
3. HEART DISEASE			19. SEASONAL ALLERGIES		
4. AUTOIMMUNE DISORDER			20. DRUG/LATEX ALLERGIES/ REACTIONS		
5. KIDNEY DISEASE/UTI					
6. NEUROLOGIC/EPILEPSY			21. BREAST		
7. PSYCHIATRIC			22. GYN SURGERY		
8. DEPRESSION/POSTPARTUM DEPRESSION			23. OPERATIONS/ HOSPITALIZATIONS (YEAR & REASON)		
9. HEPATITIS/LIVER DISEASE					
10. VARICOSITIES/PHLEBITIS			24. ANESTHETIC COMPLICATIONS		
11. THYROID DYSFUNCTION			25. HISTORY OF ABNORMAL PAP		
12. TRAUMA/VIOLENCE			26. UTERINE ANOMALY/DES		
13. HISTORY OF BLOOD TRANSFUS.			27. INFERTILITY		
	AMT/DAY PREPREG	AMT/DAY PREG	# YEARS USE		28. RELEVANT FAMILY HISTORY		
14. TOBACCO						
15. ALCOHOL				29. OTHER		
16. ILLICIT/RECREATIONAL DRUGS						

COMMENTS _____

SYMPTOMS SINCE LMP

GENETIC SCREENING/TERATOLOGY COUNSELING
INCLUDES PATIENT, BABY'S FATHER, OR ANYONE IN EITHER FAMILY WITH:

	YES	NO			YES	NO
1. PATIENT'S AGE ≥ 35 YEARS AS OF ESTIMATED DATE OF DELIVERY			12. HUNTINGTON'S CHOREA			
2. THALASSEMIA (ITALIAN, GREEK, MEDITERRANEAN, OR ASIAN BACKGROUND): MCV <80			13. MENTAL RETARDATION/AUTISM			
			IF YES, WAS PERSON TESTED FOR FRAGILE X?			
3. NEURAL TUBE DEFECT (MENINGOMYELOCELE, SPINA BIFIDA, OR ANENCEPHALY)			14. OTHER INHERITED GENETIC OR CHROMOSOMAL DISORDER			
4. CONGENITAL HEART DEFECT			15. MATERNAL METABOLIC DISORDER (EG, TYPE 1 DIABETES, PKU)			
5. DOWN SYNDROME			16. PATIENT OR BABY'S FATHER HAD A CHILD WITH BIRTH DEFECTS NOT LISTED ABOVE			
6. TAY-SACHS (EG, JEWISH, CAJUN, FRENCH CANADIAN)			17. RECURRENT PREGNANCY LOSS, OR A STILLBIRTH			
7. CANAVAN DISEASE			18. MEDICATIONS (INCLUDING SUPPLEMENTS, VITAMINS, HERBS OR OTC DRUGS)/ILLICIT/RECREATIONAL DRUGS/ALCOHOL SINCE LAST MENSTRUAL PERIOD			
8. SICKLE CELL DISEASE OR TRAIT (AFRICAN)						
9. HEMOPHILIA OR OTHER BLOOD DISORDERS			IF YES, AGENT(S) AND STRENGTH/DOSAGE			
10. MUSCULAR DYSTROPHY						
11. CYSTIC FIBROSIS			19. ANY OTHER			

COMMENTS/COUNSELING _____

INFECTION HISTORY	YES	NO			YES	NO
1. LIVE WITH SOMEONE WITH TB OR EXPOSED TO TB			4. HISTORY OF STD, GONORRHEA, CHLAMYDIA, HPV, SYPHILIS			
2. PATIENT OR PARTNER HAS HISTORY OF GENITAL HERPES						
3. RASH OR VIRAL ILLNESS SINCE LAST MENSTRUAL PERIOD			5. OTHER (See Comments)			

COMMENTS _____

INTERVIEWER'S SIGNATURE _____

INITIAL PHYSICAL EXAMINATION

DATE ____ / ____ / ____   HEIGHT _____   BP _____

	NORMAL	ABNORMAL				NORMAL		CONDYLOMA		LESIONS
1. HEENT	☐ NORMAL	☐ ABNORMAL	12. VULVA		☐ NORMAL		☐ CONDYLOMA		☐ LESIONS	
2. FUNDI	☐ NORMAL	☐ ABNORMAL	13. VAGINA		☐ NORMAL		☐ INFLAMMATION		☐ DISCHARGE	
3. TEETH	☐ NORMAL	☐ ABNORMAL	14. CERVIX		☐ NORMAL		☐ INFLAMMATION		☐ LESIONS	
4. THYROID	☐ NORMAL	☐ ABNORMAL	15. UTERUS SIZE	____ WEEKS					☐ FIBROIDS	
5. BREASTS	☐ NORMAL	☐ ABNORMAL	16. ADNEXA		☐ NORMAL		☐ MASS			
6. LUNGS	☐ NORMAL	☐ ABNORMAL	17. RECTUM		☐ NORMAL		☐ ABNORMAL			
7. HEART	☐ NORMAL	☐ ABNORMAL	18. DIAGONAL CONJUGATE		☐ REACHED		☐ NO		____ CM	
8. ABDOMEN	☐ NORMAL	☐ ABNORMAL	19. SPINES		☐ AVERAGE		☐ PROMINENT		☐ BLUNT	
9. EXTREMITIES	☐ NORMAL	☐ ABNORMAL	20. SACRUM		☐ CONCAVE		☐ STRAIGHT		☐ ANTERIOR	
10. SKIN	☐ NORMAL	☐ ABNORMAL	21. SUBPUBIC ARCH		☐ NORMAL		☐ WIDE		☐ NARROW	
11. LYMPH NODES	☐ NORMAL	☐ ABNORMAL	22. GYNECOID PELVIC TYPE		☐ YES		☐ NO			

COMMENTS (Number and explain abnormals) _____

EXAM BY _____

ACOG ANTEPARTUM RECORD (FORM B)

NAME _____
LAST   FIRST   MIDDLE

| DRUG ALLERGY | LATEX ALLERGY |

IS BLOOD TRANSFUSION ACCEPTABLE IN AN EMERGENCY? ☐ YES ☐ NO | ANESTHESIA CONSULT PLANNED ☐ YES ☐ NO

PROBLEMS/PLANS

1. _____
2. _____
3. _____
4. _____
5. _____
6. _____

MEDICATION LIST   Start date   Stop date

1. _____ ___/___/___ ___/___/___
2. _____ ___/___/___ ___/___/___
3. _____ ___/___/___ ___/___/___
4. _____ ___/___/___ ___/___/___
5. _____ ___/___/___ ___/___/___
6. _____ ___/___

EDD CONFIRMATION

INITIAL EDD
LMP ___/___/___ = EDD ___/___/___
INITIAL EXAM ___/___/___ = ___ WKS = EDD ___/___/___
ULTRASOUND ___/___/___ = ___ WKS = EDD ___/___/___
INITIAL EDD ___/___/___ INITIALED BY _____

18–20-WEEK EDD UPDATE

QUICKENING ___/___/___ +22 WKS = ___/___/___
FUNDAL HT.
AT UMBIL ___/___/___ +20 WKS = ___/___/___
ULTRASOUND ___/___/___ = ___ WKS = ___/___/___
FINAL EDD ___/___/___ INITIALED BY _____

PREPREGNANCY WEIGHT _____

Column headers: WEEKS GEST (BEST EST), FUNDAL HEIGHT (CM), PRESENTATION, FHR, FETAL MOVEMENT, PRETERM LABOR SIGNS/SYMPTOMS **PRESENT □ ABSENT, CERVIX EXAM (DIL/EFF/STA) ULTRASOUND LENGTH, BLOOD PRESSURE, WEIGHT, URINE (ALBUMIN/GLUCOSE), NEXT APPOINTMENT, PROVIDER (INITIALS)

COMMENTS

PROBLEMS _____

COMMENTS _____

ACOG ANTEPARTUM RECORD (FORM C)

LABORATORY AND EDUCATION

INITIAL LABS	DATE	RESULT	REVIEWED
BLOOD TYPE	/ /	A B AB O	
D (Rh) TYPE	/ /		
ANTIBODY SCREEN	/ /		
HCT/HGB	/ /	_____ % _____ g/dL	
PAP TEST	/ /	NORMAL/ABNORMAL/_____	
RUBELLA	/ /		
VDRL	/ /		
URINE CULTURE/SCREEN	/ /		
HBsAg	/ /		
HIV COUNSELING/TESTING*	/ /	POS. NEG. DECLINED	

OPTIONAL LABS	DATE	RESULT	
HGB ELECTROPHORESIS	/ /	AA AS SS AC SC AF $1A_2$	
PPD	/ /		
CHLAMYDIA	/ /		
GONORRHEA	/ /		
GENETIC SCREENING TESTS (SEE FORM B)	/ /		
OTHER			

8–18-WEEK LABS (WHEN INDICATED/ ELECTED)	DATE	RESULT	
ULTRASOUND	/ /		
MSAFP/MULTIPLE MARKERS	/ /		
AMNIO/CVS	/ /		
KARYOTYPE	/ /	46,XX OR 46,XY/OTHER_____	
AMNIOTIC FLUID (AFP)	/ /	NORMAL_____ ABNORMAL_____	

24–28-WEEK LABS (WHEN INDICATED)	DATE	RESULT	
HCT/HGB	/ /	_____ % _____ g/dL	
DIABETES SCREEN	/ /	1 HOUR_____	
GTT (IF SCREEN ABNORMAL)	/ /	_____FBS _____1 HOUR	
		_____2 HOUR _____3 HOUR	
D (Rh) ANTIBODY SCREEN	/ /		
ANTI-D IMMUNE GLOBULIN (RhIG) GIVEN (28 WKS)	/ /	SIGNATURE	

32–36-WEEK LABS	DATE	RESULT	
HCT/HGB	/ /	_____ % _____ g/dL	
ULTRASOUND (WHEN INDICATED)	/ /		
VDRL (WHEN INDICATED)	/ /		
GONORRHEA (WHEN INDICATED)	/ /		
CHLAMYDIA (WHEN INDICATED)	/ /		
GROUP B STREP	/ /		

COMMENTS/ADDITIONAL LABS

*Check state requirements before recording results.

PROVIDER SIGNATURE (AS REQUIRED)_____

ACOG ANTEPARTUM RECORD (FORM D)

NAME _____
          LAST   FIRST   MIDDLE

PLANS/EDUCATION
(COUNSELED ☐)—BY TRIMESTER. INITIAL AND DATE WHEN DISCUSSED.

FIRST TRIMESTER	COMPLETED	NEED FOR FURTHER DISCUSSION
☐ HIV AND OTHER ROUTINE PRENATAL TESTS		
☐ RISK FACTORS IDENTIFIED BY PRENATAL HISTORY		
☐ ANTICIPATED COURSE OF PRENATAL CARE		
☐ NUTRITION AND WEIGHT GAIN COUNSELING		
☐ TOXOPLASMOSIS PRECAUTIONS (CATS/RAW MEAT)		
☐ SEXUAL ACTIVITY		
☐ EXERCISE		
☐ ENVIRONMENTAL/WORK HAZARDS		
☐ TRAVEL		
☐ TOBACCO (ASK, ADVISE, ASSESS, ASSIST, AND ARRANGE)		
☐ ALCOHOL		
☐ ILLICIT/RECREATIONAL DRUGS		
☐ USE OF ANY MEDICATIONS (INCLUDING SUPPLEMENTS, VITAMINS, HERBS, OR OTC DRUGS)		
☐ INDICATIONS FOR ULTRASOUND		
☐ DOMESTIC VIOLENCE		
☐ SEAT BELT USE		
☐ CHILDBIRTH CLASSES/HOSPITAL FACILITIES		
SECOND TRIMESTER		
☐ SIGNS AND SYMPTOMS OF PRETERM LABOR		
☐ ABNORMAL LAB VALUES		
☐ INFLUENZA VACCINE		
☐ SELECTING A PEDIATRICIAN		
☐ POSTPARTUM FAMILY PLANNING/TUBAL STERILIZATION		
THIRD TRIMESTER		
☐ ANESTHESIA/ANALGESIA PLANS		
☐ FETAL MOVEMENT MONITORING		
☐ LABOR SIGNS		
☐ VBAC COUNSELING		
☐ SIGNS AND SYMPTOMS OF PREGNANCY-INDUCED HYPERTENSION		
☐ POSTTERM COUNSELING		
☐ CIRCUMCISION		
☐ BREAST OR BOTTLE FEEDING		
☐ POSTPARTUM DEPRESSION		
☐ NEWBORN CAR SEAT		
☐ FAMILY MEDICAL LEAVE OR DISABILITY FORMS		
REQUESTS		

TUBAL STERILIZATION CONSENT SIGNED   DATE   INITIALS
                                            __/__/__   _____

HISTORY AND PHYSICAL HAS BEEN SENT TO HOSPITAL, IF APPLICABLE.   DATE   INITIALS
                                                                 __/__/__   _____

ACOG ANTEPARTUM RECORD (FORM E)

NAME _____
    LAST   FIRST   MIDDLE

ID # _____

EDD _____

Supplemental Visits

PREPREGNANCY WEIGHT _____

Column headers (angled): WEEKS GEST. (BEST EST.), FUNDAL HEIGHT (CM), PRESENTATION, FHR, FETAL MOVEMENT, PRETERM LABOR SIGNS/SYMPTOMS: + PRESENT 0=ABSENT, CERVIX EXAM (DIL/EFF STA.) ULTRASOUND LENGTH, BLOOD PRESSURE, WEIGHT, URINE (ALBUMIN/GLUCOSE), NEXT APPOINTMENT, PROVIDER (INITIALS)

COMMENTS

Progress Notes

PROVIDER SIGNATURE (AS REQUIRED) _____

Version 5. Copyright © 2002 The American College of Obstetricians and Gynecologists, 409 12th Street, SW, PO Box 96920, Washington, DC 20090-6920   AA198   1 2 3 4 5 / 7 6 5 4 3

ACOG ANTEPARTUM RECORD (FORM F)

SAMPLE

Section III

Diagnosis and Treatment of Preterm Labor

Recommendation III-1: *Improve methods for the identification and treatment of women at increased risk of preterm labor. Researchers should investigate ways to improve methods to identify and treat women with an increased risk of preterm labor.*

Specifically:

• The content and structure of prenatal care should include an assessment of the risk of preterm labor.

• Improved methods for the identification of women at increased risk of preterm labor both before pregnancy and in the first and second trimesters are needed.

• Combinations of known markers of preterm labor (e.g., a prior preterm birth, ethnicity, a short cervix, and biochemical and biophysical markers) and potential new markers (e.g., genetic markers) should be studied to allow the creation of an individualized composite assessment of risk.

• More accurate methods are needed to
  o diagnose preterm labor,
  o assess fetal health to identify women and fetuses that are and that are not candidates for the arrest of labor, and
  o arrest labor.

• The success of perinatal care during preterm birth should be based primarily on perinatal morbidity and mortality rates as well as the rate of preterm birth, the numbers of infants born with low birth weights, or neonatal morbidity and mortality.

SECTION IV

CONSEQUENCES OF PRETERM BIRTH

10

Mortality and Acute Complications in Preterm Infants

ABSTRACT

Although the mortality rate for preterm infants and the gestational age-specific mortality rate have dramatically improved over the last 3 to 4 decades, infants born preterm remain vulnerable to many complications, including respiratory distress syndrome, chronic lung disease, injury to the intestines, a compromised immune system, cardiovascular disorders, hearing and vision problems, and neurological insult. Infants born at the lower limit of viability have the highest mortality rates and the highest rates of all complications. Few studies have reported mortality and morbidity rates in gestational age-specific categories, which limits the information available for counseling of parents before a preterm delivery and for making important decisions on the timing and the mode of preterm delivery. Although much progress in the treatment of infants born preterm has been made, many of the medications and treatment strategies used in the neonatal intensive care unit have not been adequately evaluated for their efficacies and safety. The high rates of neurological injury in preterm infants highlight the need for better neuroprotective strategies and postnatal interventions that support extrauterine neuromaturation and the neurodevelopment of infants born preterm.

The significance of preterm birth lies in the complications of prematurity sustained by the infant and the impacts of these complications on the infant's survival and subsequent development. Many clinical research studies of infants born preterm limit their outcomes to neonatal mortality and morbidity. Complications and the disturbance of normal development may result from factors that influence prenatal development and the etiology of preterm birth, but the extent to which this happens is often unknown. Although this chapter is by no means a complete catalog of complications of preterm birth, this chapter discusses how these various complications reflect immaturity; the impact that they have on survival, organ maturation, and health; and the efficacies of a number of intervention strategies designed to prevent and mitigate the effects of these complications. As outlined in Chapter 2, information based on gestational age is preferred over information based on birth weight because of the value of knowledge of gestation age in making decisions regarding preterm delivery and prenatal counseling of the parent.

The complications of preterm birth arise from immature organ systems that are not yet prepared to support life in the extrauterine environment. The risk of acute neonatal illness decreases with gestational age, reflecting the fragility and immaturity of the brain, lungs, immune system, kidneys, skin, eyes, and gastrointestinal system. In general, more immature preterm infants require more life support. There is controversy about how infants at the border of viability should be managed (see also Chapter 2 for discussion of Perinatal Mortality of Infants Born at the Limit of Viability). Neonatologists may vary in terms of how conservative they are with regard to treatment of these infants and some may regard treatment of infants at these very early gestational ages as experimental. The reader is referred to Appendix C for further discussion of ethical aspects of decision-making at the threshold of fetal viability.

The response of the infant's organ systems to the demands of the extrauterine environment and the life support provided have an important impact on the infant's short and long-term health and neurodevelopmental outcomes (Chapter 11). These outcomes are also influenced by the etiology of the preterm birth; maternal and family risk factors; and the extrauterine environment, including the neonatal intensive care unit (NICU), home, and community.

MORTALITY

Infants born preterm are more likely than infants born full term to die during the neonatal period (first 28 days) and infancy (first year), and mortality rates increase proportionally with decreasing gestational age or birth weight (Alexander et al., 1999; Allen et al., 2000; Lemons et al., 2001;

CDC, 2005i) (see also Figures 9-2 and 9-3 in Chapter 9 and Appendix B). The leading causes of infant mortality in the United States are preterm birth, low birth weight, and birth defects; so preterm birth and low birth weight are major contributors to infant mortality (Alexander et al., 2003; CDC, 2005i; Petrini et al., 2002). Dramatic declines in infant and neonatal mortality and gestational-age specific mortality over the last several decades have been attributed to improvements in obstetric and neonatal intensive care, especially for infants born preterm and small for gestational age (Allen et al., 2000; Alexander and Slay, 2002). However, the United States most recently had an increase in infant mortality from 6.8 to 7.0 per 1,000 live births in 2002 and an increase in the preterm birth rate to 12.3 percent in 2003 (CDC, 2005i) (see also Chapter 1 for discussion of mortality rates and variations in mortality by race and ethnicity).

Intranational and International Comparisons

Large variations in infant mortality rates exist among different geographical regions as well as among racial and ethnic groups (Alexander et al., 1999; Allen et al., 2000; Carmichael and Iyasu, 1998; Joseph et al., 1998) (Chapters 1 and 2 and Appendix B). The United States ranked 28th of 37 industrialized nations in infant mortality in 2001 and has a higher rate of low birth weight. Although increasing preterm birth rates and racial and ethnic disparities in the rates of preterm birth have been implicated, methodological factors are contributors to these differences (Chapter 2 and Appendix B). For example, efforts at resuscitating infants born at the lower limit of viability, thereby classifying them as live births (not stillbirths), increases the rate of infant mortality because so many infants born before 24 weeks of gestation die (Alexander et al., 2003; CDC, 2005i; MacDorman et al., 2005). The dearth of international comparisons of preterm birth rates is due to similar methodologic concerns about how gestational age, live births, and fetal deaths are recorded and reported (Appendix B).

The rate of infant mortality among African American populations in the United States in 2000 was 14.1 per 1,000 live births, more than twice the national average of 6.9 per 1,000 live births (NCHS, 2002). The rate of access to high-quality neonatal intensive care varies by race and ethnicity (Alexander et al., 2003; Morales et al., 2005; Wise, 2003). Preterm birth rates for African Americans are more than twice those for of Hispanic or white infants (Alexander et al., 2003). Although African American infants born preterm have had a survival advantage over white infants born preterm, this gap is narrowing, and the higher proportion of African American infants born preterm and the higher mortality rate among African American infants born full term play a greater role in the disparity in African American and white infant mortality rates (Allen et al., 2000) (Appendix B).

Effects of Regionalization and NICUs on Mortality

Access to neonatal intensive care was recognized as an important issue in the 1970s. Schlesinger (1973) was the first to report differences in the rates of neonatal survival among hospitals. The dearth of physicians and nurses skilled in the new techniques and support services needed to care for sick neonates led to the development of regional programs with NICUs with prescribed structures and functions, formalized arrangements for obstetric referrals, and transportation systems for sick neonates (Blackwell et al., 2005) (see Chapter 14). Regionalization initially involved transporting sick newborns from community hospitals to regional medical centers and outreach community education on the stabilization of acutely ill newborns.

The main arguments in favor of regionalized care rested largely on improved neonatal survival after its introduction into a geographically defined region (McCormick and Richardson, 1995). Low birth weight infants born in hospitals without a NICU had higher risk-adjusted mortality rates than those born in hospitals with an intermediate- or high-level NICU, and the mortality rate only marginally improved with subsequent transfer of the infant to an NICU (Cifuentes et al., 2002). The advantage of the earlier identification of high-risk pregnancies and referral to tertiary perinatal centers before delivery is supported by the more favorable outcomes for infants whose mothers were transported to perinatal centers before delivery compared with the outcomes for infants transported after birth (Doyle et al., 2004a; Kollée et al., 1988; Levy et al., 1981).

The concept of regionalized services has evolved to include the prenatal period and a fully integrated system of consultation, referral, and transport (McCormick et al., 1985).

Guidelines for designating levels of perinatal care (Level I, II, or III, depending on the resources available, the delivery volume, and geographic need) have been developed. As the proportion of infants with birth weights of less than 1,000 grams born at Level III perinatal centers has increased, their survival has improved, and the gap in survival between infants born in and out of such centers has increased (Saigal et al., 1989). In addition to gains in safety and expertise, the development of highly integrated vertical networks is inherently cost-effective because of the elimination of fragmented and redundant services.

This level of integration of regionalized perinatal services is difficult to achieve. In Georgia, the rate of delivery of infants with birth weights of less than 1,500 grams at recommended perinatal centers was better for urban mothers than for rural mothers who lived farther away from regional centers (Samuelson et al., 2002). Other factors associated with a lack of access to subspecialty care include content of prenatal care (e.g., risk assessment, education about signs and symptoms of labor, and communication and transportation plans), delays in assessment of labor, the adequacy of emergency transport for pregnant women, and the willingness to transfer mothers before delivery. Samuelson et al. (2002) speculated that 16 to 23 percent of neonatal deaths among infants with birth weights of less than 1,500 grams could be prevented if 90 percent of infants born outside hospitals with subspecialty care were delivered at the recommended hospitals (assuming that mortality differences were due to the level of care). As advances in health care improve the rates of survival of infants born preterm, access to care in regionalized subspecialty centers becomes increasingly important in determining infant mortality rates.

COMPLICATIONS OF PRETERM BIRTH

Developmental immaturity affects a wide range of organ systems. This section describes the short-term complications of preterm birth in terms of fetal development as well as injury to fragile organ systems during the perinatal and neonatal periods. Many of these complications have lifelong consequences for the health, growth, and development of infants born preterm. As described in Chapter 6, the complex interplay of the mechanisms involved in preterm delivery, including inflammation and cytokine injury, has also been implicated in the pathogenesis of chronic lung disease, necrotizing enterocolitis, retinopathy of prematurity (ROP), and brain white matter injury in the preterm infant. Although some randomized, controlled trials demonstrate the safety and effectiveness of a few treatments for neonates, most standard NICU treatments and interventions have not been adequately investigated. The role that defining and treating the complications resulting from preterm birth plays in the health and neurodevelopmental outcomes of children born preterm argues for more long-term outcome studies and more rigorous studies of new therapies and medications before they are widely adopted.

Lungs and Respiratory System

The primary function of the lung is gas exchange (i.e., they inhale oxygen and exhale carbon dioxide). Fetal breathing movements begin as early as 10 weeks of gestation, and the breathing of amniotic fluid in and out is essential for the stimulation of lung development. Fetal breathing movements tend to be erratic and occur only 30 to 40 percent of the time up to 30 weeks of gestation. The failure of fetal breathing movements or a lack of amniotic fluid that can be breathed in and out results in underdeveloped lungs (i.e., pulmonary hypoplasia), which can be incompatible with extrauterine life. By approximately 30 to 32 weeks of gestation, the lungs make surfactant, a soaplike substance that helps keep the air sacs (alveoli) open. Infants born before 28 to 30 weeks gestation lack alveoli and breath with their terminal bronchioles and primitive air sacs. After delivery, the breathing pattern generally becomes more regular and continuous, but immature regulatory systems can lead to brief episodes of not breathing (apnea) (see Chapter 6 for discussion of normal lung development and respiratory distress syndrome).

Respiratory Distress Syndrome

About 24,000 infants a year and 80 percent of infants born before 27 weeks of gestation will develop respiratory distress syndrome (RDS). RDS is associated with surfactant deficiency. The incidence of RDS increases with decreasing gestational age and is higher among white infants than African American infants at each week of gestation (Hulsey et al., 1993). Although respiratory distress is less common in infants born at 33 to 36 weeks of gestation and is rare in full-term infants, it can be severe, with a 5 percent mortality rate (Clark et al., 2004; Lewis et al., 1996). Antenatal administration of glucocorticoids to women at risk for preterm delivery reduces the incidence and severity of RDS as well as the rate of mortality (NIH, 1994) (see Chapter 9). Soon after birth, preterm infants with RDS develop rapid breathing, grunting, poor color, and crackling or diminished breath sounds breathing requires increased work. Respiratory failure because of fatigue, apnea, hypoxia, or an air leak (from alveolar injury) results from stiff lungs that need high pressures for ventilation.

RDS is an acute illness treated with respiratory support (oxygen, positive airway pressure, ventilator, or surfactant) as needed and improves in 2 to 4 days and resolves in 7 to 14 days. The optimal methods of providing respiratory support and even the safe and optimal blood levels of oxygen and carbon dioxide in very preterm infants remain quite controversial (Collins et al., 2001; Phelps, 2000; Saugstad, 2005; Thome and Carlo, 2002; Tin, 2002; Tin and Wariyar, 2002; Woodgate and Davies, 2001). The provision of exogenous surfactant through an endotracheal tube improves pulmonary gas exchange and reduces mortality (by 40 percent), air leak (by 30 to 65 percent), and chronic lung disease but does not influence neurodevelopmental or long-term pulmonary outcomes (Courtney et al., 1995; Dunn et al., 1988; Gappa et al., 1999; Ho and Saigal, 2005; Morley, 1991; Soll, 2002a,b,c; Stevens et al., 2002; Ware et al., 1990). A few randomized controlled trials have addressed the effectiveness of high-frequency ventilation or the use of an inhaled gas (nitric oxide) on survival and the severity of lung injury in severely ill preterm infants (Bhutta and

Henderson-Smart, 2002; Henderson-Smart and Osborn, 2002; Mestan et al., 2005; Van Meurs et al., 2005).

Not all acute respiratory illnesses in preterm neonates are RDS. Because congenital pneumonia is difficult to distinguish from RDS, infants with respiratory distress are generally treated with antibiotics. Some infants also have difficulty transitioning from the type of circulation that they have in utero, where gas exchange occurs in the placenta. When they breathe at birth, their circulatory pattern should change to send blood through their lungs. The retention of fetal lung fluid can also cause respiratory distress, but the condition improves as the fluid is reabsorbed.

Bronchopulmonary Dysplasia and Chronic Lung Disease

The chronic lung disease (CLD) that sometimes follows RDS in preterm infants is also called bronchopulmonary dysplasia (BPD). BPD/CLD is a chronic disorder that results from inflammation, injury, and scarring of the airways and the alveoli. It is associated with growth, health, and neurodevelopmental problems during childhood (see Chapter 11). Positive-pressure ventilation, high oxygen concentrations, infection, and other inflammatory triggers all contribute to lung injury; but the primary cause of BPD/CLD is lung immaturity. Especially for infants born at less than 28 to 30 weeks of gestation, the lung tissue is very fragile and the injured lung tissue tends to trap air, collapse, or fill with mucus and other fluids, which further compromise lung growth and development.

Various definitions of BPD/CLD have been used and are based on the respiratory support that an infant requires, but the most commonly used definition is a requirement for oxygen at 36 weeks of postmenstrual age (gestational age plus chronological age). Its incidence varies with gestational age at birth: in a study of infants born in 2002, 28 percent of infants born before 29 weeks of gestation and 5 percent of infants born 29 to 32 weeks gestation required oxygen at 36 weeks of postmenstrual age (Smith et al., 2005). By using this same definition, the incidence of BPD/CLD varies widely among centers:, from 3 to 43 percent among infants with birth weights of less than 1,500 grams (Lee et al., 2000; Lemons et al., 2001).

Infants with BPD/CLD have nutritional and fluid problems because of fluid sensitivity and increased metabolic needs, have difficulties with reactive airways (wheezing), and are quite vulnerable to infections, especially respiratory infections (Vaucher, 2002). Surprisingly few studies of the standard medications used to treat infants with BPD/CLD have been conducted, including diuretics and bronchodilators (Walsh et al., 2006). Modest improvements in survival and BPD/CLD rates have been reported with intramuscular injections of vitamin A (Darlow and Graham, 2002).

The most controversial treatment for preterm infants with BPD/CLD is systemic postnatal corticosteroids (especially dexamethasone), which arrest alveolar and lung growth but allow the pulmonary system to mature (see Chapter 6). Two studies in the 1980s reported that long courses of relatively high doses of corticosteroids reduced the duration of time that oxygen and mechanical ventilation were needed in preterm infants (Avery et al., 1985; Mammel et al., 1983). More than 40 randomized, controlled trials of postnatal systemic steroids have been published, with most reporting improved gas exchange, fewer days of mechanical ventilation, and a lower incidence of BPD/CLD; but side effects, including glucose problems, high blood pressure, and growth failure were reported (Bhutta and Ohlsson, 1998; Halliday, 1999; Halliday and Ehrenkranz, 2001a,b,c).

Years after systemic steroids were widely adopted for the treatment of BPD/CLD, follow-up studies reported higher rates of cerebral palsy and cognitive impairment in infants randomly assigned to steroids than in those assigned to placebo, and systematic reviews of the available data have expressed similar concerns (Barrington et al., 2001a,b; Bhutta and Ohlsson, 1998; Halliday, 2004; Kamlin and Davis, 2004; O'Shea et al., 1999; Shinwell et al., 2000; Yeh et al., 1998). Two large trials of lower doses of hydrocortisone for the prevention of BPD/CLD were stopped because of adverse side effects (including gastrointestinal perforation) (Stark et al., 2001; Watterberg et al., 1999). One review calculated that for every 100 neonates given steroids within 96 hours of birth, BPD/CLD would be prevented in 9, while 6 would develop gastrointestinal hemorrhage and 6 would develop cerebral palsy.

Inhaled steroids are also frequently used, despite trials that show that they provide no significant benefits (Shah et al., 2004).

Whether corticosteroids should be used to treat the sickest infants with severe BPD/CLD (many of whom may die) remains controversial, especially if lower doses and much shorter courses are used (Doyle et al., 2005; Jones et al., 2005). Whether a drug that provides a short-term gain (and sometimes dramatic results) but increases the likelihood of serious long-term consequences should be used and how one decides between benefit to one organ system (the lungs) but adverse effects on another organ system (the brain) are serious dilemmas.

The likelihood of persistent respiratory problems during infancy is higher in preterm infants with BPD/CLD than in those without BPD/CLD. They may develop significant wheezing with respiratory infections (viral broncholitis) and may need to be rehospitalized, placed back on a ventilator, or even given exogenous surfactant (Kneyber et al., 2005). Preterm infants are especially vulnerable to respiratory syncytial virus (RSV) infection. The American Academy of Pediatrics recommends RSV prophylaxis for 6 months for infants born at 29 to 32 weeks of gestation and for 12 months for infants born at less than 28 weeks of gestation (AAP, 2006). BPD/CLD often results in residual effects on pulmonary function later in life: children who had had BPD/CLD as infants are particularly vulnerable to the effects of secondhand smoke and have higher rates of asthma, persistent growth problems, and neurodevelopmental disabilities (Hack et al., 2000; Jacob et al., 1998; Jones et al., 2005; Thomas et al., 2003; Vohr et al., 2005).

Apnea

Another complication of preterm birth is apnea, in which infants may stop breathing for 20 seconds or more, sometimes accompanied by a slow heart rate (bradycardia). Immaturity of the control of breathing is the major cause of apnea and bradycardia, although sometimes preterm infants have obstructive apnea (an obstruction to the movement of air in their airways). They require constant monitoring but generally respond quickly to stimulation (or in the case of obstructive apnea, repositioning). They may occasionally need to be given some positive-pressure breaths to get them breathing again. There is no agreement as to what constitutes pathologic apnea or the threshold of apnea that requires treatment (Finer et al., 2006).

A number of strategies have been used to treat preterm apnea. The primary drugs used to treat apnea are the methylxanthines. Both theophylline and caffeine are effective, but caffeine has less toxicity (Henderson-Smart and Steer, 2004). Another drug, doxapram, has been associated with increases in cognitive delay (Henderson-Smart and Steer, 2004; Sreenan et al., 2001). The provision of vestibular stimulation is not as effective as treatment with methylxanthines for the prevention or treatment of apnea (Henderson-Smart and Osborn, 2002). There is no evidence that treatment of gastroesophageal reflux decreases the frequency or severity of apnea (Finer et al., 2006). Frequent apnea unresponsive to medications is treated with nasal positive airway pressure or mechanical ventilation.

Apnea generally resolves as the preterm infant matures. Occasionally, preterm infants continue to have apnea beyond term, and some are discharged on home apnea monitors. The long-term beneficial effects of the treatment of apnea in preterm infants in an NICU have not been demonstrated (Finer et al., 2006). Acute respiratory infections (especially RSV infections) may cause a recurrence of apnea. Although there is relationship between preterm birth and sudden infant death syndrome, the mechanisms are poorly understood and probably do not include apnea of prematurity (Baird, 2004).

Gastrointestinal System

The gastrointestinal (GI) tract digests and absorbs food, but it also has immune and endocrine functions and receives a good deal of input from the nervous system. It begins to form as early as the fourth week of gestation, and the stomach and the intestines are fully formed by 20 weeks of gestation (Berseth, 2005). The intestines double in length in the last 15 weeks of gestation (to 275 cm at term). The intestinal absorptive cells form as early as 9 weeks of gestation, and endocrine and immune functions also begin early. Taste buds form at between 7 and 12 weeks of gestation. However, preterm infants have difficulty with digesting nutrients because many specialized cells are not fully functional.

The earliest coordinated reflexes are related to stimulation around the mouth, with mouth opening in response to perioral stimulation occurring at 9.5 weeks of gestation and head turning occurring by 11.5 weeks of gestation (Hooker, 1952; Hooker and Hare, 1954; Humphrey, 1964). The fetus swallows by 10 to 12 weeks of gestation and can suck by 20 weeks of gestation. After birth, the newborn's GI tract becomes colonized with bacteria, which aids with food digestion. Antibiotics alter this process. The safety and efficacy of giving preterm infants favorable bacteria (i.e., probiotics) for GI tract colonization is being studied (Bin-Nun et al., 2005).

Feeding intolerance is a common complication of preterm birth. The immature GI tract has difficulty digesting food necessary for ongoing growth and development. Very immature and sick infants receive parenteral (intravenous) nutrition with amino acids, glucose, electrolytes, and lipids. Preterm infants below 34 to 35 weeks of postmenstrual age require tube feeding because they cannot coordinate sucking, swallowing, or breathing. Providing the preterm infant with sufficient nutritional requirements for growth and development can complicate the treatment of other conditions.

Necrotizing enterocolitis (NEC) is an acute injury of the small or large intestines that causes inflammation and injury to the bowel lining and that primarily affects preterm infants. NEC occurs in 3 percent of infants born before 33 weeks of gestation and in 7 percent of infants with birth weights less than 1,500 grams (Lee et al., 2000; Lemons et al., 2001; Smith et al., 2005). It typically occurs within 2 weeks of birth and presents as feeding difficulties, abdominal swelling, hypotension, and other signs of sepsis. When NEC is suspected, infants are treated with antibiotics and bowel rest (i.e., no feedings).

The exact cause of NEC is unknown and, like most other complications of prematurity, is multifactorial. The preterm infant's intestinal lining is fragile, and stresses (infections and insufficient oxygen or blood flow) can injure it. Inflammation is important in terms of both the etiology and the outcomes. Injury to the GI tract lining can progress through the wall of the intestines, causing perforation and spilling of the intestinal contents into the abdomen, which causes peritonitis and sepsis. The gram-negative bacteria that colonize the GI tract secrete toxins that can cause severe systemic illness and death. Infants with perforated intestines require blood pressure support, surgery for removal of dead or dying bowel, and frequently, an ostomy until the bowel is healed. The damage may affect only a short segment of the intestine, or it may progress quickly to involve a much larger portion. Around the time of surgery, the infant's nutritional intake is generally severely limited and the infant may require large amounts of blood products, fluids, and drugs (pressors) for the treatment of hypotension.

Survivors can experience significant short-term and long-term morbidities. Patients cannot be fed until the GI tract recovers, so they require parenteral nutrition and fluid. Although intravenous access is difficult in many infants, prolonged parenteral nutrition requires the placement of central venous catheters, which has attendant risks and complications of its own. Prolonged hyperalimentation and the absence of enteral nutrition can also cause liver damage with cholestasis. In addition, patients with significant disease can develop a stricture (narrowing of the bowel as it heals), which may require surgical intervention and which further compromises successful enteral feeding. Infants with extensive involvement of the GI tract are critically ill, and removal of large portions of the bowel results in malabsorption even after they have recovered. Occasionally, the injury is so extensive, that the small amount of intestines left is insufficient for growth and development or incompatible with life. Long-term morbidities can include ileostomy, colostomy, repeated surgical procedures, prolonged parenteral nutrition, liver failure, poor nutrition, malabsorption syndromes, failure to thrive, and multiple hospitalizations.

Because of the devastating nature of NEC, neonates are not fed during an acute illness. Feedings are introduced gradually, with each increase in the volume or the concentration of feedings carefully monitored, and feedings are stopped at the earliest signs of feeding intolerance. This situation creates a tension for the clinician: balancing the complications of the administration of intravenous fluids and parenteral nutrition against the complications of increasing enteral feedings too fast. If difficulty with digestion is anticipated, the infant may initially be given more elemental formulas. The provision of very small amounts of feedings initially stimulates the GI tract to produce the enzymes needed to digest larger volumes and concentrations of subsequent feedings. Attention to feeding regimens may improve feeding tolerance and reduce the incidence of NEC in NICUs (Patole and de Klerk, 2005).

Gastroesophageal reflux (GER) is common in preterm and full-term infants, often presents as regurgitation, and may adversely affect growth and health. It may also be manifested by aspiration pneumonia, wheezing, or worsening of BPD/CLD because of an inability to protect the airway when refluxing. The presence of a nasogastric feeding tube increases the likelihood of reflux. Severe GER with aspiration of the stomach contents into the lungs is life threatening. GER is often treated with medications, including H_2 blockers or protein pump inhibitors, which neutralize gastric acidity (and which may increase vulnerability to infection via the GI tract), and prokinetic compounds, which increase GI motility. The efficacies and safety of these medications have not been established, however. Occasionally, severe cases may require surgery, especially in infants with severe BPD/CLD. There is no convincing evidence that the medications currently available for the treatment of GER are efficacious in treating or preventing apnea (Walsh et al., 2006).

Skin

Skin, which begins to form as early as 6 weeks of gestation, is an important barrier between the fetus or infant and the environment (Cohen and Siegfried, 2005). Skin plays important roles in fluid balance, temperature regulation, and the prevention of infection. The skin of infants born at the lower limit of viability (i.e., 22 to 25 weeks of gestation) is generally gelatinous, is easily injured when touched, allows tremendous loss of fluids, and does not provide an adequate barrier to infection. Fluid and electrolyte (i.e., salt) needs are often difficult to predict and are quite variable during the first several days after birth, until the skin toughens. Frequent procedures and significant infiltrates from intravenous lines lead to multiple scars in preterm infants. At the limit of viability, skin can scar from the removal of chest monitor leads. Covering the skin of preterm infants born before 26 weeks of gestation with a barrier ointment does not prevent but actually increases the risks of infection (Conner et al., 2003).

Infections and the Immune System

The interactions between the fetal and the maternal immune systems during pregnancy are complex (Taeusch et al., 2005). Carefully regulated changes in the fetal immune system are programmed to retain the pregnancy and reduce the likelihood of being attacked by the maternal immune system (i.e., as in an allogeneic graft) yet to prepare the fetus for birth and survival in the extrauterine environment. Many of the mother's antibodies cross the placenta to protect the growing fetus beginning at 20 weeks of gestation, but most transfer during the third trimester.

Abnormalities of this delicate and complex interplay between the fetal and the maternal immune systems and infections can result in fetal compromise, maternal or fetal death, or preterm birth. Although the mechanism is not well understood, many data support the association between subclinical infection and preterm birth (see Chapter 9). Infections with the rubella virus, cytomegalovirus, *Toxoplasma*, the syphilis spirochete, the malaria parasite, and human immunodeficiency virus during pregnancy can have devastating consequences for the fetus and infant (Beckerman, 2005; Pan et al., 2005; Sanchez and Ahmed, 2005). Other maternal infections and subsequent inflammation in the fetus have been implicated as causes of fetal brain injury (including white matter injury, disruption, and programmed neuronal cell death) and, later, neurodevelopmental disabilities (Dammann et al., 2002; Hagberg et al., 2005; Walther et al., 2000).

Preterm infants have immature immune systems that are inefficient at fighting off the bacteria, viruses, and other organisms that can cause infections. The most serious manifestations of infections with these agents commonly seen in preterm infants include pneumonia, sepsis, meningitis, and urinary tract infections. As many as 65 percent of infants with birth weights of less than 1,000 grams have at least one infection during their initial hospitalization (Stoll et al., 2004). Neonates contract these infections at birth from their mothers or after birth through their immature skin, lungs, or GI tract, which lack fully developed immunoprotective functions. They have difficulty confining infections to where they arise and forming abscesses, so sepsis (i.e., a blood-borne infection) frequently develops. Septic infants are generally critically ill, and infection can spread to other parts of the body (resulting in, for example, meningitis, an infection of the membranes that surround the brain). In addition to intravenous antibiotics, septic infants often require support for other organ systems that break down (e.g., respiratory and blood pressure support). Neonates with birth weights of less than 1,000 gram and infections have been found to have poorer head growth, more cognitive impairment, and higher rates of cerebral palsy than those who did not have infections as neonates (Stoll et al., 2004).

Invasive fungal infections occur in 6 to 7 percent of infants in an NICU, and the rates of such infections increase with decreasing gestational age and birth weight (Hofstetter, 2005; Stoll et al., 1996). *Candida* is the most common fungal species that causes infections in preterm infants and colonizes approximately 20 percent of infants with birth weights of less than 1,000 grams (Kaufman et al., 2001). Disseminated fungal infection, in which the infection is spread throughout the body, has a mortality rate of 30 percent. Prompt treatment with antifungal medication can prevent dissemination and improve survival, but side effects are frequent. Intravenous administration of the antifungal fluconazole as prophylaxis against fungal infections in infants with birth weights of less than 1,000 grams can reduce the rates of colonization and fungal infection (Kaufman et al., 2001).

The immune system has many component parts, and there are significant differences between the immune systems of neonates and adults and their responses to inflammation and infections with pathogens. Inflammation is implicated in many of the complications of prematurity, including BPD/CLD, NEC, intracranial and especially white matter injury, and ROP. The complex relationships among pathogens, stress, the cytokine system, tissue injury, hormones, and multiple gene-environment interactions in producing or reducing inflammation have important implications for preterm birth, survival, health, brain injury, and neurodevelopmental outcomes (see Chapter 6).

Cardiovascular System

Preterm infants can experience a variety of cardiovascular disorders, ranging from major morphological defects to dysfunctional autoregulation of blood vessels (hypotension). By embryonic day 20, the cells that will form the heart begin to differentiate (Maschoff and Baldwin, 2005; Schultheiss et al., 1995). The primitive heart beats by 4 weeks of gestation and is fully formed at the end of the 6th week. Because gas exchange occurs in the placenta, most of the fetal blood flow bypasses the lungs through the ductus arteriosus.

The ductus arteriosus normally closes after birth, when the lungs expand; air enters the lungs; and blood is redirected from the right side of the heart, through the lungs, back to the left side of the heart, and out to the body. In preterm infants, the duct may not close properly, which results in a patent (open) ductus arteriosus, which can lead to heart failure and reduced blood flow to vital body organs (e.g., the kidney and the GI tract). Heart murmur, active precordium, and bounding pulses are clinical signs; and an echocardiography performed at the bedside can confirm the presence of a patent ductus arteriosus and an otherwise normal anatomy. A patent ductus arteriosus can be asymptomatic and may close spontaneously in the first week of life, or it can complicate a preterm infant's clinical course and increase the risks of intraventricular hemorrhage (IVH), NEC, BPD/CLD, and death (Shah and Ohlsson, 2006).

Approximately 5 percent of infants with birth weights of less than 1,500 grams are treated for patent ductus arteriosus (Lee et al., 2000). Medication and surgery are equally effective at closing a patent ductus arteriosus, and each has significant side effects and outcomes (Malviya et al., 2006). The most common medication used, indomethacin, has significant side effects because of the decreasing blood flow to the lower body (which results in decreased urine output and gastrointestinal perforation). Ibuprofen is effective and may have fewer side effects, but it has not been as well studied (Shah and Ohlsson, 2006). The value of indomethacin for the prevention of patent ductus arteriosus or the treatment of a patent with asymptomatic ductus arteriosus remains controversial (Cooke et al., 2003; Fowlie, 2005).

Although the focus has been on closing the patent ductus arteriosus, lower rates of mortality or morbidity (BPD/CLD, NEC, or neurodevelopmental disability) have not been demonstrated (Fowlie, 2005).

Hypotension is a frequent concern in preterm infants, but there is no consensus as to what the blood pressure readings should be in preterm infants with gestational ages of less than 26 or 27 weeks. The administration of boluses of normal saline and pressors is used to support blood pressure. Although preterm infants with severe refractory hypotension are often treated with physiological doses of hydrocortisone, its safety or efficacy has not been established.

Apnea and bradycardia are common in premature infants and are manifestations of immature cardiorespiratory control (Veerappan et al., 2000). However, preterm infants and, indeed, some term infants can have bradycardia during feeding, despite the absence of other cardiorespiratory symptoms and a lack of clinical reflux. The nature of the autonomic nervous system's contribution to these symptoms is not well understood (bradycardia could be due to increases in reflex parasympathetic autonomic nervous system activity).

Hematologic System

Hematopoiesis is the generation of blood cells from stem cell progenitors. It begins in the embryo 7 days after conception (Juul, 2005). Stem cells are active in the aortogonadomesonephron at 10 days and then shift to the liver and, finally, the bone marrow. There are developmental changes in the numbers and functions of hematopoietic stem cells and in the various differentiated blood cells (e.g., red blood cells, white blood cells, and platelets). Red blood cells in the fetus contain fetal hemoglobin, which is necessary for intrauterine gas exchange because it has a higher affinity for oxygen. Fetal hemoglobin levels decrease after birth.

Fetal blood loss, fetomaternal hemorrhage, and hemolysis can all result in congenital anemia, but the most common hematologic complication in preterm infants is anemia of prematurity. Anemia of prematurity is an exaggeration of the physiological anemia of infancy because of suppressed hematopoiesis for 6 to 12 weeks after birth and is earlier in onset and symptomatic. Its causes are multifactorial and include blood loss from frequent blood sampling, the shorter survival of red blood cells in preterm infants, a suboptimal response to anemia, and a greater need for red blood cells with growth. Preterm infants often need red blood cell transfusions, and many of the sickest and most immature infants need multiple transfusions. A meta-analysis of a number of randomized controlled trials documented a modest reduction in the number of red blood cell transfusions required after the administration of recombinant human erythropoietin and iron (Vamvakas and Strauss, 2001).

Auditory System and Hearing

The ear begins to develop at the end of 6 weeks of gestation and is fully developed by 20 weeks of gestation. A response to sound can be demonstrated in fetuses and infants born at 23 and 24 weeks of gestation, and auditory brainstem-evoked responses can be recorded this early in preterm infants (Allen and Capute, 1986; Birnholz and Benacerraf, 1983; Starr et al., 1977). The shape of the waveform changes and the conduction time decreases with increasing gestational or postmenstrual age.

One to two of 1,000 newborns suffer from congenital or perinatally acquired hearing disorders. The prevalence of neonatal hearing disorders has been reported to be increased 10- to 50-fold in infants at risk, which includes preterm infants. In addition to hearing impairment as a result of heredity, which is the cause of the largest percentage of hearing disorders, a number of in utero and neonatal complications (e.g., infections, immaturity, asphyxia, ototoxic medications, and hyperbilirubinemia) have been described to be risk factors for neonatal hearing disorders. Ventilated infants are at increased risk for otitis media. Significant hearing impairment, often requiring hearing aides, occurs in 1 to 5 percent of infants born at gestational ages of less than 25 or 26 weeks (Hintz et al., 2005; Vohr et al., 2005; Wood et al., 2000) (see Chapter 11).

Moderate to severe bilateral hearing impairment can distort the developing child's perception of speech and may interfere with his or her attempt at speech production. If the hearing impairment remains undetected through the critical period of language acquisition, that is, within the first 2 years of life, a profound impairment of receptive and expressive speech and language development can result. Early detection of hearing impairment facilitates early remediation (e.g., hearing aides or cochlear implants) and early intervention for speech and language acquisition (Gabbard and Schryer, 2003; Gravel and O'Gara, 2003; Niparko and Blankenhorn, 2003). The prognosis for functional speech and language skills improves with the early detection and treatment of hearing impairment (Yoshinaga-Itano, 2000).

Most communities are moving toward universal hearing screening for all newborns (White, 2003). The most widely used methods to screen newborns for their hearing abilities are auditory brainstem responses and otoacoustic emissions (Hayes, 2003). Both methods detect the infant's response to sounds. The auditory brainstem response provides an electrical recording of the brainstem's response to sound. The otoacoustic emissions test evaluates the integrity of the cochlea (inner ear) by detecting the low sounds that the cochlea emits in response to sound perception. These tests are sensitive but have low specificity rates. Neonates who fail a hearing test should have a repeat test and then be referred for confirmatory audiological testing and medical evaluation.

Progressive hearing impairment has been reported in infants with cytomegalovirus infection and persistent pulmonary hypertension of the newborn. These infants and infants who demonstrate a delay in language milestone acquisition should have a follow-up hearing test during the first year of life.

Ophthalmic System and Vision

Preterm infants are more likely than term infants to have significant abnormalities of all parts of the visual system, leading to reduced vision (Repka, 2002). The optic vesicles that will become the eyes form during the fifth and sixth weeks after conception (Back, 2005). The eyeball is well formed by the lower limit of viability (22 to 25 weeks gestation). However, a pupillary membrane covers the anterior vascular capsule of the lens and gradually disappears between 27 and 34 weeks of gestation (Hittner et al., 1977). The retina is a vascular layer in the back of the eye that translates light into electrical messages to the brain. The retina is the one of the last organs to be vascularized in the fetus (Madan and Good, 2005). Blood vessel-forming cells originate near the optic disc (where the optic nerve enters the retina) from spindle cell precursors at 16 weeks of gestation and gradually spread across the surface of the retina, from the center to the periphery. Vessels cover only 70 percent of the retina by 27 weeks of gestation, but in most cases the retina is completely vascularized to the nasal side by 36 weeks of gestation and to the temporal side by 40 weeks of gestation (Palmer et al., 1991).

The visual system functions very early, with the preterm infant blinking in response to bright light by 23 to 25 weeks of gestation and with papillary constriction in response to light by 29 to 30 of weeks gestation (Allen and Capute 1986; Robinson, 1966). By 30 to 32 weeks of postmenstrual age, the preterm infant begins to differentiate visual patterns (Dubowitz, 1979; Dubowitz et al., 1980; Hack et al., 1976, 1981; Morante et al., 1982). Visual acuity progressively improves with increasing postmenstrual age. The full-term neonate sees shapes (approximate visual acuity of 20/150) and colors and has a fixed focal length of 8 in. (anything closer or farther away becomes more blurry).

ROP is the most common eye abnormality in preterm infants. It is a neovascular retinal disorder, and its incidence increases with decreasing gestational age and decreasing birth weight. It is multifactorial in etiology, with the primary determinant being immaturity with an avascular retina (Madan et al., 2005). Environmental factors, including hypoxia, hyperoxia, variations in blood pressure, sepsis, and acidosis, may injure the endothelia (the cells that line) of the immature retinal blood vessels. The retina then enters a quiescent phase for days to weeks and forms a pathognomonic ridge-like structure of mesenchymal cells between the vascularized and the avascular regions of the retina by 33 to 34 weeks of postmenstrual age. In some infants, this ridge regresses, and the remaining retina is vascularized. In other infants, abnormal blood vessels proliferate from this ridge; and progressive disease can cause exudation, hemorrhage, and fibrosis, with subsequent scarring or retinal detachment (i.e., the retina is pulled off the back of the eye). The presence of plus disease, in which dilated and tortuous blood vessels occur in the posterior pole of the eye, is especially ominous for an adverse visual outcome.

ROP occurs in 16 to 84 percent of infants born with gestational ages of less than 28 weeks, 90 percent of infants with birth weights of less than 500 or 750 grams, and 42 to 47 percent of infants with birth weights of less than 1,000 or 1,500 grams (CRPCG, 1988, 1994; Fledelius and Greisen, 1993; Gibson et al., 1990; Gilbert et al., 1996; Lee et al., 2000; Lefebvre et al., 1996; Lucey et al., 2004; Mikkola et al., 2005; Repka, 2002). Fortunately, severe ROP requiring therapy is less common, occurring in 14 to 40 percent of infants with gestational ages of less than 26 weeks, 10 percent of infants with gestational ages of less than 28 weeks, 16 percent of infants with birth weights of less than 750 grams, and 2 to 11 percent of infants with birth weights of less than 1,000 or 1,500 grams (Coats et al., 2000; Costeloe et al., 2000; Hintz et al., 2005; Ho and Saigal, 2005; Lee et al., 2000; Mikkola et al., 2005; Palmer et al., 1991). ROP resolves without significant visual loss in the majority (80 percent) of infants (CRPCG, 1988; O'Connor et al., 2002). Repka and colleagues (2000) found that involution occurred in 90 percent of infants with ROP by 44 weeks of postmenstrual age.

Treatments have improved the visual outcomes for children with severe ROP (i.e., threshold or plus disease, stages 3 and 4). The ablation of abnormal peripheral vessels with cryotherapy (in earlier studies) and laser therapy (in the last decade) have led to favorable visual outcomes in at least 75 percent of infants with severe ROP (CRPCG, 1988, 1994; Repka, 2002; Shalev et al., 2001; Vander et al., 1997). Continuing improvements in treatments and more timely treatments of severe ROP have served to reduce the proportion of children with severe visual impairment or blindness from 3 to 7 percent down to 1.1 percent in children with birth weights of less than 1,000 or 1,500 grams (Doyle et al., 2005; Hintz et al., 2005; Tudehope et al., 1995; Wilson-Costello et al., 2005) (see Chapter 11). Severe visual impairment or blindness occurs in 0.4 percent of children with gestational ages of 27 to 32 weeks, 1 to 2 percent of children with gestational ages of less than 26 or 27 weeks, 4 percent of children with gestational ages of 24 weeks, and 8 percent of children with gestational ages of less than 24 weeks (Marlow et al., 2005; Vohr et al., 2005).

Timely diagnosis and the prompt treatment of ROP are essential for improving visual outcomes. Screening ophthalmologic examinations require an experienced examiner and careful examination of the retina to the periphery with an indirect ophthalmoscope and lid speculum after dilation of the pupils. Revised guidelines for screening preterm infants for ROP have recently been published, with recommendations for which infants should be screened (infants with birth weights of less than 1,500 grams or gestational ages of less than 32 weeks or selected other preterm infants with an unstable clinical course), the timing and frequency of screening examinations, and the indications for treatment (Section on Ophthalmology, AAP, 2006)

Although visual outcomes have improved, ROP continues to be a major problem, especially in the most immature infants. The primary method of prevention is to prevent preterm births. Prevention of wild swings in blood pressure, blood oxygen and carbon dioxide levels, and acidosis has been recommended (Madan et al., 2005). There is much interest in the role of oxygen in ROP, but the optimal blood oxygen levels and oxygen saturation levels remain controversial (Saugstad, 2005; STOP-ROP, 2000; Tin 2002; Tin and Wariyar, 2002). Although the intravenous administration of high doses of vitamin E appears to reduce the incidence of severe ROP and blindness in infants with birth weights of less than 1,500 grams, it also appears to increase the incidence of sepsis and IVH (Brion et al., 2003).

Other ophthalmologic complications of prematurity include refractive disorders (especially myopia), strabismus (i.e., ocular misalignment), amblyopia (i.e., visual loss associated with reduced development of the visual cortex), optic nerve atrophy, cataracts, and cortical visual impairment (Repka, 2002) (see Chapter 11). Late ophthalmologic problems include angle closure glaucoma (i.e., increased pressure in the eye), retinal detachment, and phthisis (i.e., shrinkage and disorganization of the eye severely affected by ROP); but fortunately, these are rare. Severe threshold ROP is associated with other complications of prematurity, including BPD/CLD and IVH.

Central Nervous System

Neuromaturation is a dynamic process in which the central nervous system (CNS) is formed by a continuous interaction between the programmed genetic processes encoded within the genome and then the intrauterine environment, followed by the extrauterine environment. The successive turning on and then turning off of specific genes propel development forward, whereas surrounding cells, temperature, nutrients, and unknown environmental factors influence cell division, differentiation, function, connections, and migration. At 16 days from conception, the neural plate, which contains the cells that form the brain, is formed. A neural groove then forms and then begins to close to become the neural tube by 3 to 4 weeks from conception. At one end of the neural tube, embryonic brain vesicles form and begin to differentiate into the forebrain, midbrain, and hindbrain (i.e., the prosencephalon, mesencephalon, and rhombencephalon, respectively) (Capone and Accardo, 1996). By the end of the 6th week, the basic subdivisions of the adult brain have formed. Neurons and their glial support cells actively divide during the first trimester, with the peak period of proliferation between the 2nd and 4th months of gestation. Neuronal migration is the mass movement of neurons from where they were formed to an ultimate destination in a specified layer of the brain and occurs between the 3rd and 5th months of gestation.

Fetal movement begins shortly after the brain begins to differentiate and can be detected by prenatal ultrasound as early as 8 to 10 weeks from conception. Fetal and infant activity and sensory input shape the development of the CNS. The fetus moves in response to cutaneous stimulation by 9 to 11 weeks and demonstrates the earliest signs of primitive reflexes (i.e., rooting and grasping) (Hooker, 1952; Hooker and Hare, 1954; Humphrey, 1964). Neurons continue to differentiate, and axons grow out and connect to dendrites to form synapses from the 6 month of gestation to at least 3 years from term. A complex and extensive network of neuronal circuits form; and they are shaped by patterns of electrical activity promoted by sensory input, movement, and responses to the environment. Fetal movements and responses are necessary for the normal development of the limbs and the CNS. Ongoing activity, learning, and sensory input determine which circuits are reinforced, whereas unused circuits are pruned. Myelination covers the neuron with a lipid sheath and reduces conduction times. The myelination process begins as early as 6 months gestation in some regions of the CNS and continues throughout childhood.

Incomplete formation of the CNS makes neonates vulnerable to CNS injury, especially if the infant was born preterm. Injury to the CNS can occur during pregnancy, labor, delivery, the transition to extrauterine life, or a subsequent illness or exposure. Many etiologies of preterm delivery (e.g., infection and maternal illness) contribute to fetal CNS injury. Concerns about the ability of the extremely preterm infants to tolerate the contractions of labor and the trauma of vaginal delivery have raised the question as to whether delivery by cesarean section is neuroprotective (Grant and Glazener, 2001). Trials to evaluate this question have suffered from recruitment problems, and there is not sufficient evidence of improved infant outcomes to balance the increased morbidity for mothers. Infants born preterm also have more difficulties with the transition from placental support to extrauterine life and the many vascular changes that occur.

In preterm infants, the white matter around the ventricles and highly vascular germinal matrix eminence are especially vulnerable to injury (de Vries and Groenendaal, 2002; Gleason and Back, 2005; Madan and Good, 2005). They have difficulties with autoregulation of cerebral blood flow (i.e., maintaining adequate cerebral blood flow, despite changes in blood pressure). Ischemia, hypoxia, and inflammation contribute to CNS injury in the preterm infant, but the relative importance of these factors remains controversial. The most common signs of CNS injury in preterm infants are IVH, intraparenchymal hemorrhage (IPH; bleeding within the substance of the brain), and white matter injury (including periventricular leukomalacia [PVL]). Neuroimaging studies, including ultrasound, computerized tomography, and magnetic resonance imaging (MRI), provide ways to visualize brain injury in infants. Ultrasound has the advantage of being cheaper and easily available (i.e., it can be performed at the bedside), but MRI is increasingly being used for better visualization of the brain parenchyma.

Germinal Matrix Injury, IVH, and IPH

IVH generally begins with bleeding into the germinal matrix just below the lateral ventricles (i.e., a subependymal or germinal matrix hemorrhage). During the late second and early third trimesters, the subependymal germinal matrix supports the development of cortical neuronal and glial cell precursors, which migrate to the cortical layers. The germinal matrix is highly vascularized, with a rich capillary network and a relatively poor supportive matrix. Blood filling the lateral ventricles may dilate the ventricles. The incidence and severity of IVH increase with decreasing gestational age and birth weight. Factors that contribute to IVH include hypotension, hypertension, fluctuating blood pressures, poor autoregulation of cerebral blood flow, disturbances in coagulation, hyperosmolarity, and injury to the vascular endothelium by oxygen free radicals. In 10 to 15 percent of infants a germinal matrix hemorrhage will obstruct venous return and lead to venous infarction of brain tissue (called IPH) (de Vries and Groenendaal, 2002).

Severe IVH can lead to ventricular dilation and posthemorrhagic hydrocephalus if there is an obstruction to the flow of cerebrospinal fluid, with increased intracranial pressure. Intermittent spinal taps or ventricular taps (i.e., drawing off of the cerebrospinal fluid with a needle) can relieve this pressure. This should be done primarily if the infant is symptomatic, as studies have demonstrated no benefits to regular taps of asymptomatic infants (Whitelaw, 2001). Once the blood is mostly cleared from the ventricles, a ventriculoperitoneal (VP) shunt can be surgically placed to drain the cerebrospinal fluid into the abdominal cavity where it is absorbed. De Vries and Groenendaal (2002) found that a third of preterm infants with large IVH required a VP shunt. Neither diuretics nor streptokinase (a clot buster) reduces the need for a shunt, nor do they improve outcomes (and a borderline increase in motor impairment was detected at 1 year of age after the use of diuretics) (Whitelaw, 2001; Whitelaw et al., 2001).

Infants with subependymal or germinal matrix hemorrhage or IVH without ventricular dilation have a good prognosis; but those with IVH with ventricular dilation, posthemorrhagic hydrocephalus or IPH are at an increased risk of neurodevelopmental disability (de Vries and Groenendaal, 2002). As many as 11 percent of infants with birth weights of less than 1,500 grams have IVH with ventricular dilation or IPH (Lee et al., 2000; Lemons et al., 2001). The prevalence of neurodevelopmental disabilities in preterm infants with severe IVH and ventricular dilation or posthemor-rhagic hydrocephalus ranges from 20 to 75 percent (de Vries et al., 2002; Fernell et al., 1994). Although early studies showed a high incidence of neurodevelopmental disabilities with IPH among preterm infants, recent studies have shown that the prevalence of disability varies with the size and the location of the hemorrhage (de Vries and Groenendaal, 2002; de Vries et al., 2002; Guzzetta et al., 1986). A study of infants born between 1979 and 1989 with gestational ages of less than 33 weeks found that the prob-abilities of a major disability at age 8 years were 5 percent for infants with a normal ultrasound, germinal matrix hemorrhage, or small IVH without ventricular dilation and 41 percent for infants with ventricular dilation, hydrocephalus, or cerebral atrophy (Stewart and Pezzani-Goldsmith, 1994).

Antenatal betamethasone (a corticosteroid) reduces the incidence of IVH in preterm infants, but many other treatments have been less successful (Crowley, 1999; NIH, 1994). There is not enough evidence to support the antenatal use of either phenobarbital or vitamin K to prevent IVH (Crowther and Henderson-Smart, 2003; Shankaran et al., 2002). Postnatal phenobarbital did not significantly improve the incidences of IVH, severe IVH, posthemorrhagic ventricular dilation, severe neurodevelopmental dis-ability, or death; and there was a trend toward a longer duration of ventila-tion (Whitelaw, 2001). A meta-analysis of five trials of prolonged neuro-muscular paralysis with pancuronium treatment in preterm infants with asynchronous breathing concluded that although pancuronium did help decrease the incidences of IVH and pneumothorax, concerns about its safety and long-term pulmonary and neurological effects precluded recommenda-tion of its routine use (Cools and Offringa, 2005). Intramuscular doses of vitamin E may have reduced the incidence of IVH in preterm infants, but they were also associated with an increased incidence of sepsis (and high doses may increase the risk of IVH) (Brion et al., 2003). The prophylactic use of indomethacin in the first hours and days after delivery reduced the incidence and severity of IVH, especially in preterm boys, but the use of indomethacin results in many side effects (e.g., renal complications, NEC, and gut perforation) and it has little sustained effect on neurodevelopmental outcomes (although it might improve the verbal abilities of boys) (Fowlie and Davis, 2002; McGuire and Fowlie, 2002; Ment et al., 2004; Schmidt et al., 2004). As with other complications of prematurity, the prevention of preterm birth would be the most effective way to prevent IVH and IPH.

White Matter Injury and Periventricular Leukomalacia

Injury to the periventricular white matter is a sign of CNS injury and is a complication of preterm birth. Its pathogenesis is currently the subject of extensive study (Damman et al., 2002; Wu and Colford, 2000) (see Chapter 6). White matter injury includes a spectrum of CNS injuries, from focal cystic necrotic lesions (also called PVL) to ventricular dilation with irregular ventricular edges or cerebral atrophy (as a result of the resorption of injured brain tissue) and extensive and bilateral white matter lesions. A complex interplay of etiologic factors predisposes the preterm infant's white matter to injury, but the gray matter may be injured as well. Poor blood flow to regions of the brain because of obstruction, low blood pressure or an immature vascular system, poor autoregulation of cerebral blood flow, hypoxia, the vulnerability of preoligodendrocytes (i.e., supporting cells), excitatory neurotransmitters (e.g., glutamate), and harmful inflammatory substances (e.g., cytokines and free radicals) carried by the blood can all contribute brain injury. A meta-analysis found significant relationships between clinical chorioamnionitis, PVL, and cerebral palsy in preterm infants (Wu and Colford, 2000).

Imaging of white matter injury is more difficult than imaging of IVH or IPH (de Vries and Groenendaal, 2002). Ultrasounds should be repeated at 3 to 4 weeks after birth and at 34 to 36 weeks of postmenstrual age to detect signs of white matter injury, which evolve over time. The first sign may be an uneven density of the white matter that resolves (transient echogenicity) or that evolves into cystic lesions. Cystic lesions can collapse, so the timing and the quality of the ultrasound examinations are crucial for the detection of white matter injury. MRI is helpful for the detection of patchy or nonhomogeneous echogenicity.

Children with cystic PVL have a high risk of neurodevelopmental disabilities, and the more extensive that it is, the higher the risk that the children have (e.g., the risk is 100 percent with extensive bilateral cystic PVL) (Holling and Leviton, 1999; Rogers et al., 1994; van den Hout et al., 2000). These children are also at high risk for the development of cerebral palsy, which tends to be more severe with extensive PVL; cognitive impairments; and cortical-visual impairments with visual-perceptual problems. Children with more focal or unilateral cystic PVL also have a high incidence of cerebral palsy (up to 74 percent), but it tends to be a milder motor impairment (Pierrat et al., 2001). Approximately 10 percent of children with periventricular echodensities develop cerebral palsy, generally in the form of mild spastic diplegia. MRI studies of infants born at term and older children have detected reduced regional cortical volumes (especially in sensorimotor regions and in both white and gray matter) that correlate with cognitive or neuromotor impairments (Inder, 2005; Peterson et al., 2000). There has been a paucity of studies of strategies for the prevention of white matter injury and the amelioration of the effects of white matter injury. The effects of neuroprotective medications for IVH (e.g., indomethacin) on white matter injury are not clear, especially as the definitions of IVH are changing to include not just PVL but also irregular ventricular dilation and cortical atrophy. Some intriguing studies of insufficient naturally occurring developmentally regulated neuroprotective substances (e.g., hydrocortisone, thyroxine, and erythroietin) have suggested that they are associated with increased rates of mortality, BPD/CLD, and possibly, negative neurodevelopmental outcomes (Kok et al., 2001; Osborn, 2000; O'Shea, 2002; Scott and Watterberg, 1995; Sola et al., 2005; van Wassenaer et al., 2002; Watterberg et al., 1999). Many avenues are available for study and exploration, and research into the causes of preterm brain injury and neuroprotective strategies and the NICU interventions that can be undertaken to improve the neurodevelopmental outcomes of preterm infants is very much needed.

Complications for Near-Term or Late-Preterm Infants

For many years, attention has focused on high-risk obstetric and neonatal intensive care for extremely preterm infants and infants born at the lower limit of viability, although very little attention has been paid to the majority of preterm infants who are born near term (also called late-preterm infants). Although many deliveries of near-term infants are spontaneous or are indicated for maternal or fetal circumstances, it is important to keep in mind that these larger preterm infants born near term are more vulnerable to complications and disabilities than full-term infants. Although complications in near-term infants are not as frequent as they are in more-preterm infants, near-term infants have more perinatal and neonatal complications than full-term infants (Allen et al., 2000; Amiel-Tison et al., 2002; Wang ML et al., 2004). One study found that the incidence of RDS was as high as 15 percent among infants born at 34 weeks of gestation, whereas it was 1 percent among infants born at 35 to 36 weeks of gestation (Lewis et al., 1996). In a New England study of infants born at 35 to 36 weeks of gestation, more preterm infants than full-term control infants had evaluations for sepsis (37 and 13 percent, respectively), problems with temperature stability (10 and 0 percent, respectively), hypoglycemia (16 and 5 percent, respectively), respiratory distress (29 and 4 percent, respectively), and jaundice (54 and 38 percent, respectively) (Wang ML et al., 2004). Poor feeding was more likely to delay the discharge of near-term infants than full-term infants (76 and 29 percent, respectively), and their hospital costs were higher (the mean cost difference between near-preterm and full-term infants was $1,596, with a median increase in cost of $221 per preterm infant). Accurate identification of late-preterm infants, even if they have normal birth weights, allows better anticipation and management of the complications associated with preterm birth.

Accurate estimates of gestational age and better measures of fetal and infant maturity would provide important information for clinical decision making. Health care providers and families need to carefully weigh the advantages of earlier delivery against the health, financial, and economic costs of preterm delivery.

NEURODEVELOPMENTAL SUPPORT

Neurodevelopmental care is an approach to the intensive care of preterm and sick full-term infants in an NICU that supports neuromaturation and that also provides care for acute and chronic illnesses. Just as the intrauterine environment influences fetal development, the NICU environment influences the development of infants born preterm. The elements that make up the provision of neurodevelopmental support include NICU design and lighting, nursing routines and care plans, feeding methods, management of pain, attention to sensory input, activity and signs of stress, and the involvement of the parents in the care of their infants (Aucott et al., 2002). Although a number of studies have been conducted to evaluate the efficacies of various aspects of neurodevelopmental support in improving the outcomes for infants born preterm, few have yielded conclusive results. Conducting good randomized, controlled trials has proven to be quite difficult and expensive. Neurodevelopmental support is an important area that requires further study, both for the efficacy of the interventions that are used and for obtaining a better understanding of how NICU interventions support (or interfere with) the neuromaturation of infants born preterm.

The NICU presents preterm infants with an overwhelming amount of stimuli because of the active hospital environment and the infant's exposure to multiple medical procedures (Aucott et al., 2002; Gilkerson et al., 1990). To minimize adverse stimuli and to support neuromaturation, NICUs therefore seek to implement strategies that mimic the intrauterine environment and that provide more appropriate stimuli that are geared to the infant's state of alertness and responses (Aucott et al., 2002; Conde-Agudelo et al., 2005; Phelps and Watts, 2002; Pinelli and Symington, 2006; Stevens et al., 2005; Symington and Pinelli, 2006; Vickers et al., 2004). For example, attention to how infants are positioned and handled can influence the development of their posture and muscle tone. Some NICUs have adopted more comprehensive approaches to developmental care, including kangaroo care and the Neonatal Individualized Developmental Care and Assessment Program (NIDCAP) (Conde-Agudelo et al., 2003; Symington and Pinelli, 2006).

It is not unusual for parents of critically ill neonates to feel overwhelmed by the technology that they encounter in the NICU and to have difficulty connecting with their newborn infant underneath all the NICU equipment. Family-centered NICU care is more of a philosophy than a program (Malusky, 2005) and involves providing families with comfortable seating, rocking chairs, privacy, and liberal visiting hours; encouraging them to bring in family photos or tapes of their voices; and saving bathing and feeding for family visits.

Breast-Feeding

Besides providing milk that is more easily digested by vulnerable preterm infants, breast-feeding facilitates attachment by ensuring that the mother has a primary role in her baby's recovery (Kavanaugh et al., 1997; Meier, 2001). Preterm infants fed breast milk have lower risks of infection and NEC, learn to nipple feed better, have higher cognitive scores, and may have a lower risk of chronic gastrointestinal diseases and allergies (AAP, 2006; Mizuno et al., 2002; Mortensen et al., 2002). Women who breast-feed have less postpartum blood loss, enhanced bone mineralization, and a reduced risk of ovarian and breast cancer (AAP, 2006).

Sensory Input and the NICU Environment

Early attempts to improve an infant's environment focused on providing sensory stimuli, including rocking, stroking, holding, and moving, as well as auditory stimuli (e.g., the mother's recorded voice and music) and visual stimuli, either alone or in combination (Aucott et al., 2002; Barnard and Bee, 1983; Mueller, 1996). Most studies of these interventions were flawed by small sample sizes, inadequate controls, or a failure to mask outcome evaluators. Few studies addressed the difficulty of confining an intervention to the study group without carryover to the control group. Finally, most studies failed to take into account background stimulation or the infant's state of alertness and response to the stimulation.

The ability to control the frequency, duration, and intensity of incoming stimuli is an important aspect of learning. Fetuses and preterm infants respond to sound and light as early as 24 to 26 weeks of gestation (Allen and Capute, 1986; Johansson et al., 1992). Preterm infants can visually fixate and recognize visual patterns as early as 30 to 32 weeks of gestation (Allen and Capute, 1986; Dubowitz et al., 1980; Hack et al., 1976, 1981).

Fragile preterm infants, however, are easily overwhelmed by sensory stimuli and respond by closing their eyes, turning away, or even showing physiological instability (e.g., a drop in oxygen saturation levels). The NICU bombards preterm infants with multiple, invariable stimuli, including bright fluorescent lights, noise, and frequent handling (Aucott et al., 2002; Chang et al., 2001; Robertson et al., 1998). Infants with apnea receive tactile stimulation, and many procedures cause discomfort or pain. The ability to habituate to repeated aversive stimuli can be present as early as 24 to 30 weeks of gestation, but it requires the expenditure of energy, and the ability to respond may be imperfect in preterm infants (Allen and Capute, 1986).

Current NICU efforts focus on modifying the NICU environment, routines, and equipment to reduce noise and bright lights (Ashbaugh et al., 1999; Robertson et al., 1998; Walsh-Sukys et al., 2001). In addition to dimming bright overhead lights, measures can be easily adopted to indirectly shield infants' eyes. Complete eye shielding or ear coverings are not beneficial, but decreases in light and sound stimuli on a circadian rhythm appear to promote weight gain (Brandon et al., 2002; Phelps and Watts, 2002; Zahr and de Traversay, 1995). Coordinating and clustering nursing and physician care avoids waking the infant unnecessarily, but there are concerns that clustered care may be too stressful for infants born before 30 weeks of gestation (Holsti et al., 2005).

Positive interactions and stimulation may be beneficial, as long as the infant's responses are carefully monitored (and are therefore contingency based). Lullabies, parents' voices, and rocking may improve the infant's weight gain and shorten the length of the hospital stay (Gaebler and Hanzlik, 1996; Gatts et al., 1994; Helders et al., 1989). Rhythmic vestibular stimulation may facilitate quiet sleep but does not significantly influence weight gain, the frequency of apnea, feeding, or neurodevelopmental outcomes (Darrah et al., 1994; Osborn and Henderson-Smart, 2006a,b; Saigal et al., 1986; Thoman et al., 1991). Although kinesthetic stimulation may reduce the frequency of apnea, it does not prevent it and is less effective than medication (Henderson-Smart and Osborn, 2002; Osborn and Henderson-Smart, 2006a,b). Nonnutritive sucking (i.e., providing a pacifier for the infant to suck on during tube feeding) is associated with improved feeding and a shorter length of hospitalization (Pinelli and Symington, 2006). Some data suggest that gentle massage of physiologically stable preterm infants improves weight gain and decreases the length of the hospital stay (Vickers et al., 2004). Many believe that the best auditory, visual, kinesthetic, vestibular, and tactile stimulation interventions are positive interactions with the parents, who can easily be taught how to recognize and monitor their infants for signs of discomfort or sensory input overload.

Pain and Discomfort

The relationships between frequent or chronic pain, the stress response, cortisol levels, and the neurodevelopment of the preterm infant are extremely complex (Grunau, 2002; Grunau et al., 2005). The fetus or preterm infant responds to painful stimuli with increases in cortisol and endorphin levels as early as 23 weeks of gestation, but the neurotransmitters that attenuate pain develop later in postnatal life (Anand, 1998; Fitzgerald et al., 1999; Franck et al., 2000).

Preterm infants have an increased sensitivity to pain, and stimuli (such as handling) may be painful. These frequent painful experiences that preterm infants encounter in an NICU could lead to structural and functional alterations of their nervous system and subsequent altered pain responses through childhood (Anand, 1998; Anand et al., 2001; Grunau et al., 1998, 2001).

Guidelines for the management of pain in newborns have been published (Anand et al., 2001). The most widely used medications for the treatment of severe acute pain are morphine and fentanyl. Soothing measures (nonnutritive sucking of oral sucrose on a nipple) are also provided during minor procedures (Stevens and Ohlsson, 2000; Stevens et al., 2004). Studies have not consistently demonstrated the benefits of the routine treatment of mechanically ventilated newborns with narcotics (preemptive analgesia), however (Bellu et al., 2005; Grunau et al., 2005).

Positioning and Handling

Attention to how preterm infants are positioned and handled in the NICU may influence their posture and motor development after their discharge to home (Aucott et al., 2002). Failure to attend to how infants are positioned in an NICU can have adverse consequences, and small modifications in routine care take no additional time, nor do they incur additional cost.

In utero, fetuses are tightly flexed and contained (i.e., they have firm boundaries) and are bathed in amniotic fluid, which decreases the influence of gravity. Normal neuromaturation can therefore be promoted by positioning the infant in a manner that mimics the infant's position in the intrauterine environment with extremity flexion and hip adduction, the avoidance of neck and trunk extension, and the promotion of body symmetry.

Because of their physiological instability, critically ill preterm infants receive minimal handling and stimulation but are repositioned on a regular basis according to nursing protocols (Aucott et al., 2002). Attention to how they are positioned can easily be incorporated into their routine care. More comfortable breathing, better oxygenation, and more time in deep sleep have been noted in preterm and sick infants in the prone position than in infants in the supine position (lying on their side) (Grunau et al., 2004b; Wells et al., 2005).

Infants with narcotic abstinence syndrome have fewer signs of opiate withdrawal and better caloric intake when they are positioned more in the prone position (Maichuk et al., 1999). Although obstructive apnea is often effectively treated by repositioning an infant's head and neck, placement of the infant in the prone position and kinesthetic and vestibular stimulation are not as effective as methylxanthines for the treatment of apnea of prematurity (Henderson-Smart and Osborn, 2002; Keene et al., 2000, Osborn and Henderson-Smart, 2006a,b).

A study of 21 intubated NICU infants on ventilators and in the supine position documented evidence of obstructed cerebral venous drainage when their heads were turned to the side, with resolution when they were positioned with their heads midline (Pellicer et al., 2002). Another series of studies demonstrated that more-preterm infants who were predominantly in the supine position in the NICU had asymmetries, asymmetric flattening of the skull, an early preference for use of the right hand, and an asymmetric gait (Konishi et al., 1986, 1987, 1997). Other neuromotor abnormalities formerly observed during infancy in a large proportion of preterm infants appear to have been influenced by how they were positioned in the NICU (e.g., shortened tibial bands from being in a frog-legged position and shoulder retraction with neck extensor hypertonia) (Amiel-Tison and Grenier, 1986; de Groot et al., 1995; Georgieff and Bernbaum, 1986). Hyperextension and hip contractures can make hand exploration, rolling, and sitting more difficult to achieve.

Although many small randomized controlled trials of NICU interventions have not definitively demonstrated beneficial effects, interventions that focus on mimicking the intrauterine environment appear to have at least some transient positive effects on motor development (Blauw-Hospers and Hadders-Algra, 2005; Goodman et al., 1985; Piper et al., 1986; Symington and Pinelli, 2006). Several small studies have found that stable preterm infants gain more weight and have improved bone mass when they are provided with some controlled physical activity each day (Moyer-Mileur et al., 1995, 2000). Allowing older infants to play in prone on a firm surface ("tummy time") improves their ability to control their heads by strengthening antigravity muscles and improves their balance skills and shoulder stability (but has no effect on cognitive outcomes) (Mildred et al., 1995; Ratliff-Schaub et al., 2001).

Parents can use this approach during their visits, which provides an opportunity for them to be involved in their child's care. Nurses and parents can easily use positioning aids, rolled blankets, or swaddling to position preterm infants symmetrically with their extremities flexed, shoulders placed forward, and hips adducted to promote normal neuromaturation. Modeling of this approach for families in the NICU also enhances carryover to post-NICU care and promotes the parents' interest in providing neurodevelopmental support for their infant.

Neonatal Individualized Developmental Care and Assessment Program

Als devised a highly organized comprehensive system for providing neurodevelopmental support in an NICU (Als, 1998). This system, commonly known as NIDCAP, has generated much interest and is often equated with NICU developmental care (Ashbaugh et al., 1999). Its systematic implementation requires development of NICU developmental care teams with dedicated staff trained and certified in NIDCAP, the systematic observation of the behavior of the infants, the coordination of care, and careful monitoring of the infant's physiological responses. An individual developmental care plan is designed for each infant, with efforts to decrease adverse elements in the NICU environment.

Although some studies, including randomized clinical trials, have demonstrated the beneficial effects of NIDCAP on short-term growth, the duration of ventilation, the need for tube feedings, hospital stays, and cognitive abilities, many of these studies have been criticized for their small sample sizes or because they lacked masked outcome evaluators (Symington and Pinelli, 2006). In addition, for every positive effect reported, other studies have provided conflicting results. Because NIDCAP includes multiple interventions, it has been difficult to determine the efficacy of any single intervention. A recent paper found differences in brain structure and behavior at 8 months of age for infants who were part of NIDCAP, but further research is needed to assess longer-term outcomes (Als et al., 2004).

Cost has been cited as a reason for the lack of full implementation of NIDCAP, but no studies have addressed the economic impact of NIDCAP implementation (Symington and Pinelli, 2006). Only 30 percent of responders to a nursing survey published in 1999 worked in an NICU with a dedicated developmental care team and budget, although most reported the incorporation of aspects of NIDCAP care into their practices. The *Cochrane Review* concludes, "Before a clear direction for practice can be supported, evidence demonstrating more consistent effects of developmental care interventions on important short- and long-term clinical outcomes is needed. The economic impact of the implementation and maintenance of developmental care practices should be considered by individual institutions" (Symington and Pinelli, 2006).

Kangaroo Care

Kangaroo care provides skin-to-skin care by placing the naked preterm infant in an upright position between the mother's breasts and allows unlimited breast-feeding. This concept of caring for preterm infants originated in Bogota, Colombia, as a low-cost way to assist preterm infants with temperature regulation, nutrition, and stimulation (Charpak et al., 1996). Kangaroo care is initiated after a routine period of stabilization after birth. A number of studies from developing countries, including a few randomized controlled trials, suggest that kangaroo care improves weight gain (an additional 3.6 grams per day), reduces the incidence of nosocomial (i.e., hospital-acquired) infections, and reduces the incidences of severe illness and respiratory disease up to 6 months of age (Conde-Agudelo et al., 2003). Mothers who provided kangaroo care were more likely to continue to breast-feed and were more satisfied with the care that their infants received in the NICU.

Finding 10-1: Few postnatal intervention strategies that can be used to improve outcomes for children born preterm have been evaluated, and such intervention strategies are needed, especially for more immature preterm infants.

VARIATIONS IN NEONATAL COMPLICATION RATES

The complications of the newborn period noted in this chapter reflect in part the difficulty of establishing extrauterine life with immature organs. However, some of these complications may also reflect the interventions used in the NICU to sustain life. The question about variations in complication rates as a function of differences in management practices in the NICU was initially raised by a report of the substantial variations in the rate of bronchopumonary dysplasia or chronic lung disease among eight NICUs (Avery et al., 1987). The rates varied from a low of 5 percent in one NICU to almost 40 percent in another and could not be explained by the approaches to the management of respiratory distress syndrome reported by the NICUs, with one exception. The site with the lowest rate of chronic lung disease rarely used mechanical ventilation and tolerated blood gas values out of the physiological normal range. The interpretation of these variations was unclear, however. Even for a given gestational age, the severity of the complications may vary among infants, and without some measure of admission severity or case mix, units with higher rates of complications may simply be admitting sicker infants.

Addressing this issue required the development of admission severity measures, which occurred during the 1990s (Richardson et al., 1998). With the development of two measures that assess the degree to which measures of physiological processes like oxygenation and blood pressure fall outside of the normal range, numerous investigators have documented variations in neonatal outcomes overall (Sankaran et al., 2002) as well as variations in specific complications (Aziz et al., 2005; Darlow et al., 2005; Lee et al., 2000; Olsen et al., 2002; Synnes et al., 2001) that cannot be explained by the severity of the infant's condition on admission. Likewise, after adjusting for the severity of the infants' conditions on admission, substantial differences in management have also been noted (Al-Aweel et al., 2001; Kahn et al., 2003; Lee et al., 2000; Richardson et al., 1999a; Ringer et al., 1998). Although most of this work has primarily been done with infants born before 32 weeks of gestation, data that are emerging indicate that such variations are also encountered in the complication rates and management of late-preterm infants (Blackwell et al., 2005; Eichenwald et al., 2001; Lee et al., 2000; Richardson et al., 2003). Although such variations may have less of an impact on survival and morbidity in the late-preterm infants than in earlier preterm infants, even minor variations among hospitals, such as a week's difference in discharge time between those with the earliest gestational age at discharge compared with those with the latest, may have substantial economic benefits, because these late-preterm infants account for almost half of all NICU stays.

The observation of such variations, some of which appear to be unrelated to the clinical condition of the infant, has prompted efforts to reduce the variation and improve outcomes with existing technologies. As reviewed in a supplement to the journal *Pediatrics*, several groups are implementing quality improvement strategies to reduce the rates of unnecessary adverse outcomes (Horbar et al., 2003; Ohlinger et al., 2003), with some evidence of success (Chow et al., 2003).

Finding 10-2: Substantial interinstitutional variations in the complication rates for infants born preterm have been documented, and some outcomes, like physical growth, remain suboptimal.

CONCLUSIONS

Although the mortality rate for preterm infants and the gestational age-specific mortality rate have dramatically improved over the last 3 to 4 decades, preterm infants remain vulnerable to the many complications of prematurity. Infants born at the lower limit of viability have the highest mortality rates and the highest rates of all complications of prematurity. Few studies have reported mortality and morbidity rates in gestational age-specific categories, which limits the information available for the counseling of the parents before preterm delivery and for decision making on the timing and the mode of delivery of an infant who will be born preterm. Better methods of evaluating fetal and infant maturity may improve the ability to predict the many complications of prematurity.

Although much progress in the treatment of preterm infants has been made, many of the medications and treatment strategies used in the NICU have not been adequately evaluated for their efficacies and safety. Even though progress in neuroimaging of brain structure of preterm infants is being made, research is needed to provide better indicators of CNS function and means for prediction of long-term neurodevelopmental outcomes. The high rates of neurological injury in preterm infants highlight the need for better neuroprotective strategies and postnatal interventions that support the extrauterine neuromaturation and neurodevelopment of preterm infants. Long-term health and neurodevelopmental outcomes should be the focus of new trials of treatments and intervention strategies for neonates born preterm.

11

Neurodevelopmental, Health, and Family Outcomes for Infants Born Preterm

ABSTRACT

Although advances in high-risk obstetric and neonatal care have resulted in improved survival of infants born preterm, many studies have documented the prevalence of a broad range of neurodevelopmental impairments in preterm survivors. The spectrum of neurodevelopmental disabilities includes cerebral palsy, mental retardation, visual and hearing impairments, and more subtle disorders of central nervous system function. These dysfunctions include language disorders, learning disabilities, attention deficit-hyperactivity disorder, minor neuromotor dysfunction or developmental coordination disorders, behavioral problems, and social-emotional difficulties. Preterm infants are more likely to have lower intelligence quotients and academic achievement scores, experience greater difficulties at school, and require significantly more educational assistance than children who were born at term. Preterm infants have an increased risk of rehospitalization during the first few years of life and increased use of outpatient care. Among the conditions leading to poorer health are reactive airway disease or asthma, recurrent infections, and poor growth. The smallest and most immature infants have the highest risk of health problems and neurodevelopmental disabilities. Limited evidence of the impact of prematurity on families suggests that caring for a child born preterm has negative and positive effects that change over time, that these effects extend to adolescence and are influenced by different environmental factors over time, and that many areas of family well-being are affected. The prevalence of neurodevelopmental disabilities and health impairments varies. This is not surprising, in light of the multiple etiologies and complications of preterm birth and the variability of both the intrauterine and the extrauterine environments to which fetuses and children born preterm are exposed. In recognition of the increased developmental and emotional risks of children born preterm, several interventions have focused on the provision of services in the early years of life to prevent subsequent developmental and health problems. Although early interventions have a short-term impact, it has been more difficult to demonstrate more long-term benefits.

At first glance, a wealth of data seems to be available for characterization of the outcomes of infants born preterm; however, as with many other areas addressed in this report, much of this literature uses birth weight as the measure of prematurity (see Chapter 2). The use of birth weight as a selection criterion for studies of the outcomes for infants born preterm introduces a well-recognized bias by including various proportions of more mature infants who experienced intrauterine growth retardation (IUGR). Many infants with IUGR are small for gestational age when they are born full term (i.e., at 37 to 41 weeks of gestation). Most infants with birth weights of less than 1,500 grams are preterm, but those who also have IUGR are vulnerable to the complications of both IUGR and prematurity (Garite et al., 2004). A number of the more recent studies have reported on the outcomes for preterm infants by gestational age category, but as in other parts of this report, this chapter uses birth weight-specific data when information by gestational age is not available.

Finding 11-1: Most studies of the outcomes of preterm birth use birth weight criteria for the selection of study participants. Few studies report on the outcomes for preterm infants by gestational age. In addition to infants born preterm, studies with samples of infants with birth weights less than 2,500 grams include full-term infants who are small for gestational age.

When this literature is examined, it is also well to keep in mind that preterm delivery is not a disease with a fixed set of outcomes. Rather, preterm delivery increases the risk of adverse outcomes that are also seen in term infants. Nevertheless, the more preterm an infant is, the greater the risk of adverse outcomes. Thus, these outcomes are a probability for a group and not a certainty for any given infant. Although the adverse outcomes associated with preterm delivery are discussed individually, readers should be aware that individual children may experience more than one outcome. Thus, it would not be unusual for a child to have some coordination difficulty and a specific health problem like asthma. Indeed, multiple milder problems may create more functional difficulties than a single, more severe one.

Relatively few studies of the outcomes for infants born preterm provide comparison groups, and those that do have almost uniformly selected healthy full-term infants or infants with birth weights above 2,500 grams. Some have used siblings or classmates as comparisons. The study question determines the criteria used to select the comparison group. Some have proposed the use of infants or children who experienced other life-threatening conditions to provide a better sense of the disabilities and outcomes from serious neonatal health problems.

Finally, a number of biological and environmental factors may affect the risk of adverse outcomes independent of gestational age or birth weight. To the extent that such independent risk factors have been identified, including some of those that may ameliorate the risks due to prematurity, they are discussed. Nevertheless, researchers are far from understanding all these factors, and prediction of the outcome for an individual child born preterm with any degree of certainty remains impossible.

This chapter describes the outcomes of preterm birth from a life-span perspective, including the prevalence of neurodevelopmental disabilities, health-related quality of life, and functional outcomes to adolescence and early adulthood. The chapter concludes with a discussion of intervention strategies that can be used for the developmental support of children who were born preterm after discharge from the neonatal intensive care unit (NICU).

NEURODEVELOPMENTAL DISABILITIES

Among the earliest concerns about the health of premature infants was the association between preterm delivery and neurodevelopmental disabilities. Neurodevelopmental disabilities are a group of chronic interrelated disorders of central nervous system function due to malformation of or injury to the developing brain. The spectrum of neurodevelopmental disabilities includes the major disabilities: cerebral palsy (CP) and mental retardation. Sensory impairments include visual impairment and hearing impairment. The more subtle disorders of central nervous system function include language disorders, learning disabilities, attention deficit-hyperactivity disorder (ADHD), minor neuromotor dysfunction or developmental coordination disorders, behavioral problems, and social-emotional difficulties.

Early studies focused primarily on cognitive impairment, as measured by intelligence quotient (IQ) and by the detection of motor abnormalities on standardized neurological examinations. A landmark study, the Collaborative Perinatal Project of the National Institute of Neurological and Communicative Disorders and Stroke, monitored 35,000 children born before neonatal intensive care (i.e., in the late 1950s and early 1960s) for 7 years. Although only 177 children born at less than 34 weeks gestation survived, the study documented the increased risk of cognitive and motor impairment as a function of decreasing gestational age. It highlighted the need for neurodevelopmental follow-up of populations born preterm, especially as the emergence of neonatal intensive care and high-risk obstetric care dramatically reduced gestational age-specific mortality rates but not preterm birth rates (see Chapters 1, 2, and 10). The history of neonatal intensive care is not only one of miracles achieved, but also of therapeutic misadventures (Allen, 2002; Baker, 2000; Silverman, 1980; Silverman, 1998). Iatrogenic complications have contributed to adverse health and neurodevelopmental outcomes in the past, but a shift from a trial and error approach toward evidence-based medicine is establishing a more empiric basis for treating mothers and preterm infants. Although new therapies are generally evaluated in randomized clinical trials, the safety and efficacy of many currently used treatments and medications have not been adequately studied (see Chapter 10).

The resulting literature demonstrates wide variations in the prevalence of neurodevelopmental disabilities (Allen, 2002; Aylward, 2002b; Aylward, 2002a; Aylward, 2005). Much of this variation is due to methodological issues, for example, a lack of uniformity in sample selection criteria, the method and the length of follow-up, follow-up rates, and the outcome measures and the diagnostic criteria used. Variations in outcome frequencies reported also reflect differences in the population base and in clinical practice. Whenever possible, outcomes data are provided by gestational age categories for preterm infants born in the 1990s to the present. However, because the age of evaluation determines which outcomes can be assessed, recent studies of the outcomes for adolescents who were born preterm report on preterm births that occurred in the 1980s. The time lag required for follow-up makes caution necessary in generalizing reported adolescent and adult outcomes to preterm infants who survive with the technology available today. Perinatal and neonatal risk factors do not reliably predict these long-term outcomes. Therefore, research is needed to identify better neonatal predictors of neurodevelopmental disabilities, functional abilities, health and other long-term outcomes.

Motor Impairment

Cerebral Palsy

Cerebral palsy (CP) is a general term to describe a group of chronic conditions that impair control of movement and posture. CP is due to malformation of or damage to motor areas in the brain, which disrupts the brain's ability to control movement and posture. Symptoms of CP may range from mild to severe, change over time and differ from person to person, and include difficulty with balance, walking, and fine motor tasks (such as writing or using scissors) and involuntary movements. Many people with CP also have associated cognitive, sensory, social, and emotional disabilities (NIDS, 2005).

The diagnosis of CP may not become certain until the second year of life. As many as 17 to 48 percent of preterm infants demonstrate neuromotor abnormalities during infancy (e.g., abnormal muscle tone or asymmetries) (Allen and Capute, 1989; Khadilkar et al., 1993; Pallas Alonso et al., 2000; Vohr et al., 2005). Some of these infants go on to develop significant neuromotor abnormalities and motor delays that signify CP, but most do not. Although neuromotor abnormalities tend to resolve or do not interfere with function, transient neuromotor abnormalities are associated with an increased risk of later school and behavioral problems (Drillien et al., 1980; Khadilkar et al., 1993; Sommerfelt et al., 1996; Vohr et al., 2005).

The severity of CP is determined by the type of CP, which limbs are affected, and the degree of functional limitation. Increasingly, investigators are distinguishing between mild CP and moderate to severe (i.e., disabling) CP (Doyle and Anderson, 2005; Grether et al. 2000; Vohr et al., 2005; Wood et al., 2000). Many longitudinal studies of the outcomes for preterm infants show good stability between motor assessments at 18 to 30 months of age and at school age (Hack et al., 2002; Marlow et al., 2005; Wood et al., 2000).

The smallest and most immature infants have the highest risk of CP. In their seventh report of CP in Sweden, Hagberg and associates (1996) reported an almost stepwise increase in the prevalence of CP with gestational age: 1.4 per 1,000 live births for children born at more than 36 weeks gestation, 8 per 1,000 live births for children born between 32 and 36 weeks gestation, 54 per 1,000 live births for children born between 28 and 31 weeks gestation, and 80 per 1,000 live births for children born at less than 28 weeks of gestation. Because they report prevalence as the number who have CP per 1,000 live births, infants who die are included in the denominator.

For the most immature infants, another meaningful statistic is the rate of CP among survivors. On the basis of data for preterm survivors born in the late 1980s through the 1990s, the rate of CP increases with decreasing gestational age or birth weight category (Table 11-1) (Colver et al., 2000; Cooke, 1999; Doyle et al., 1995; Doyle and Anderson, 2005; Elbourne et al., 2001; Emsley et al., 1998; Finnstrom et al., 1998; Grether et al., 2000; Hack et al., 2000, 2005; Hansen and Greisen, 2004; Hintz et al., 2005; Lefebvre et al., 1996; Mikkola et al., 2005; O'Shea et al., 1997; Piecuch et al., 1997a,b; Salokorpi et al., 2001; Sauve et al., 1998; Stanley et al., 2000; Tommiska et al., 2003; Vohr et al., 2000, 2005; Wilson-Costello et al., 2005; Wood et al., 2000). Only 0.1 to 0.2 percent of full-term children develop CP, whereas 11 to 12 percent born at 27 to 32 weeks of gestation and 7 to 17 percent born at less than 27 or 28 weeks of gestation develop CP (Doyle, 2001; Elbourne et al., 2001; Finnstrom et al., 1998; Lefebvre et al., 1996; Vohr et al., 2005). A comprehensive British study of preterm infants born in 1995 with gestational ages of less than 26 weeks diagnosed CP in 20 percent of the survivors at 6 years of age (Marlow et al., 2005). In the few reported survivors with birth weights of less than 500 grams, a quarter to a half developed CP (Sauve et al., 1998; Vohr et al., 2000).

Many more studies have reported on the outcomes of CP in terms of birth weight categories. In a review of 17 studies published from 1988 to 2000, Bracewell and Marlow (2002) estimated that approximately 10 percent of preterm infants with birth weights of less than 1,000 grams developed CP. An older meta-analysis of 85 studies of infants with birth weights of less than 1,500 grams estimated that 7.7 percent of survivors developed CP (Escobar et al., 1991). Studies of 18- to 20-year-olds reported that from 5 to 7 percent of those who were born with birth weights of less than 1,500 grams and up to 13 percent of those born with birth weights of less than 1,000 grams had CP (Ericson and Kallen, 1998; Hack et al., 2002; Lefebvre et al., 2005; Saigal et al., 2006a). A Swedish study of young men born as singletons from 1973 to 1975 with birth weights of less than 1,500 grams estimated an odds ratio for CP of 55 (95 percent confidence interval = 41 to 75) (Ericson and Kallen, 1998).

With continuing improvements in high-risk obstetric and neonatal intensive care over the last several decades, several studies have demonstrated small increases or decreases in the overall prevalence of CP (Colver et al., 2000; Hagberg et al., 1996; Stanley and Watson, 1992; Stanley et al., 2000). However, any improvements in gestational age- or birth weight-specific rates of CP are offset by dramatic decreases in the rates of infant mortality. The net result is that more preterm children survive, but more children have CP as well.

Many regional studies of children with CP find an overrepresentation of preterm children with CP than the number expected for their birth rates (Table 11-1) (Amiel-Tison et al., 2002; Colver et al., 2000; Cummins et al., 1993; Dolk et al., 2001; Hagberg et al., 1996; MacGillivray and Campbell, 1995; Petterson et al., 1993; Stanley and Watson, 1992). Although only 1.4

TABLE 11-1 Rates of Cerebral Palsy in Preterm Children by Gestational Age Category

Study	Year(s) of Birth	Age (yr)	Follow-up Rate (%)	Number of Subjects	Gestational Age (wk)	Rate of Cerebral Palsy (%)
Hintz et al., 2005[a]	1996–1999	1.8	87	467	<25	21
	1993–1996		77	360	<25	23
Vohr et al., 2005[a]	1997–1998	1.8	84	910	<27	18
			82	512	27–32	11
	1995–1996	1.8	84	716	<27	19
			81	538	27–32	11
	1993–1994	1.8	74	665	<27	20
			70	444	27–32	12
Mikkola et al., 2005	1996–1997	5	95	103	<27	19
Tommiska et al., 2003	1996–1997	1.5–2	100	5	22–23	20
				18	24	11
				34	25	12
				47	26	11
Wood et al., 2000	1995	2.5	92	283	<26	18
Emsley et al., 1998	1990–1994	2.2–6.1	100	40	23–25	18
Piecuch et al., 1997b	1990–1994	>1	95	18	24	11
				30	25	20
				38	26	11
				94	24–26	13
Jacobs et al., 2000	1990–1994	1.5–2	90	274	23–26	15
Doyle, 2001	1991–1992	5	98	221	23–27	11
Finnstrom et al., 1998[a]	1990–1992	3	98	362	23–24	14
					25–26	10
					>26	3
Lefebvre et al., 1996	1991–1992	1.5	85	9	24	11
				24	25	25
				40	26	27
				72	27	10
				72	28	17
				217	24–28	17

[a]Birth weight less than 1,000 grams.

percent of infants are born at less than 32 weeks of gestation, they comprise 26 percent of children with CP. Four percent of all live births are born at 32 to 36 weeks of gestation, and they constitute 16 to 37 percent of children with CP. Although less than 10 percent of births are preterm, approximately 40 to 50 percent of children with CP are born preterm.

Although children born preterm are vulnerable to all types of CP, the most common type is spastic diplegia (Hack et al., 2000; Hagberg et al., 1996; Wood et al., 2000). Spasticity is characterized by tight muscle tone, increased reflexes, and limited movement around one or more joints. Spasticity of both lower extremities but no or very little involvement of the arms constitutes spastic diplegia. Although most children with spastic diplegia require physical therapy and medical interventions (e.g., orthopedic surgery, orthoses, or Botulinum Toxicum injections), many children with spastic diplegia are quite functional by school age. In a study of children born at less than 26 weeks gestation, 43 percent with spastic diplegia were unable to walk and 43 percent had an abnormal gait at 6 years of age (Marlow et al., 2005).

A large regional study of Swedish preterm children with CP reported that 66 percent had spastic diplegia, 22 percent had spastic hemiplegia, and 7 percent had spastic quadriplegia (Hagberg et al., 1996). Associated deficits were common: 39 percent had mental retardation, 26 percent had epilepsy, 18 percent had severe visual impairment, and 23 percent had hydrocephalus. The proportion of children with CP who had spastic diplegia decreased with increasing gestational age category: 80 percent for children born at less than 28 weeks of gestation, 66 percent for children born at between 28 and 31 weeks of gestation, 58 percent for children born at between 32 and 36 weeks of gestation, and 29 percent for children born at greater than 36 weeks of gestation. The proportion of children with hemiplegia increased with gestational age: 10 percent for children born at less than 28 weeks gestation, 16 percent for children born at between 28 and 31 weeks gestation, 34 percent for children born at between 32 and 36 weeks gestation, and 44 percent for children born at less than 36 weeks gestation.

Coordination and Motor Planning

Children with incoordination and motor planning problems are less likely to enjoy and participate in many preschool and playground activities. Minor neuromotor dysfunction is a diagnosis used to describe infants and children who have persistent neuromotor abnormalities but minimally to mildly impaired motor function. Children with minor neuromotor dysfunction may have mild motor delay but are able to walk by age 2 years and have good mobility. They have a higher risk of coordination difficulties, motor planning problems, fine motor incoordination, or sensorimotor integration problems (which at preschool and school age may be diagnosed as developmental coordination disorder) (Botting et al., 1998; Hadders-Algra, 2002; Hall et al., 1995; Khadilkar et al., 1993; Mikkola et al., 2005; Pharoah et al., 1994; Vohr and Coll, 1985). In a study of 5-year-olds born between 1996 and 1997 with birth weights of less than 1,000 grams, 51 percent had coordination problems, 18 to 20 percent had abnormal reflexes or abnormal posture, and 17 percent had exceptional involuntary movements (Mikkola et al., 2005). Sensorimotor integration problems can range from inability to tolerate certain textures of food or clothing (e.g., an inability to tolerate lumpy food or the tag on the back of a T-shirt) to difficulty following demonstrated directions (e.g., how to put on a shirt or tie shoelaces) or an inability to tolerate motion (e.g., swinging).

Preterm children, even those with normal intelligence and no CP, have more difficulties than full-term children with fine motor, visual motor, visual perceptual, and visual spatial tasks. These tasks include drawing, cutting with scissors, dressing, writing, copying figures, perceptual mapping, spatial processing, finger tapping, and pegboard performance. In a study of 5-year-old children with birth weights of less than 1,500 grams, 23 percent had impaired fine motor skills and 71 percent scored 1 standard deviation or more below average on tests of fine motor function (Goyen et al., 1998). Below-average performances in visual motor skills and visual perceptual tasks were noted for 17 and 11 percent of the children, respectively. These problems were most common in children born at less than 28 weeks of gestation. Even the more mature preterm children are at risk for these problems; a third of school-age children born at 32 to 36 weeks of gestation had poor fine motor and writing skills (Huddy et al., 2001).

Failures at gross motor, fine motor, sensorimotor, and visual perceptual activities are mild in comparison with the difficulties with mobility and adaptive skills that many children with CP face. Nonetheless, these subtle abnormalities of central nervous system function can, over time, adversely influence the child's self-esteem and peer relationships, which in turn contribute to a cycle of frustration and despair that interferes with academic progress and social relationships. Early recognition of these subtle deficits allows modification of expectations, teaching methods, and the environment to support the development of these children and prevent adverse secondary consequences.

Cognitive Impairment

Cognitive Test Scores and Mental Retardation

Intelligence is not one skill but a composite of multiple cognitive processes, including visual and auditory memory, abstract reasoning, complex language processing, understanding of syntax, visual perception, visual motor integration, and visual spatial processing. A variety of standardized intelligence tests are available for use with children at each age level. Scores across a variety of cognitive tasks are summed to form an IQ or, for younger children, a developmental quotient (DQ) (Lichtenberger, 2005). Cognitive assessments of very young infants are limited in their predictive ability because of their reliance on assessment of visual-motor and perceptual abilities. As children mature, more verbal and abstract cognitive processes can be evaluated, and scores more accurately reflect their abilities. Cognitive tests are standardized for diverse large populations, with an IQ score of 100 considered the population mean.

The IQ score is a global score that does not include information about subtle dysfunctions. The full range of cognitive deficits seen in preterm children is not well described by the IQ score, and further cognitive analyses are necessary. Many preterm children have a wide scatter in their cognitive abilities, with excellent performance in some areas but relative weakness in other areas, and these contribute to difficulties in the classroom and at home.

Calculation of a DQ for preterm infants is complicated by whether their age should be calculated from their birth date (i.e., the chronological age) or from their due date (i.e., age corrected for the degree of prematurity). This issue is more important arithmetically the younger the infant is and the lower the gestational age at birth was. For example, a 6-month-old preterm infant born 3 months early who has skills at the normal level for a 3-month-old would have a normal DQ of 100 if it was corrected for the degree of prematurity but would be considered delayed in skill attainment, with a DQ of 50, if the chronological age was used.

For the most part, neuromaturation of the preterm infant in the NICU proceeds along the same timeline as intrauterine development (Allen, 2005a; Saint-Anne Dargassies, 1977). From biological and maturational perspectives, few environmental influences significantly accelerate neuromaturation, and most agree that one should fully correct for the degree of prematurity when preterm infants are evaluated and that this correction should be incorporated for at least the first 2 years of life (Allen, 2002; Aylward, 2002a). Whether or not one corrects for the degree of prematurity may influence IQ scores for up to 8 years (Rickards et al., 1989).

Mental retardation is a disability that originates in childhood and is characterized by significant limitations both in intellectual functioning and in adaptive behavior, as expressed in conceptual, social, and practical adaptive skills (AAMR, 2005). Intellectual functioning is considered subaverage or significantly limited when an individual's IQ score is 2 or more standard deviations below the mean on a standardized intelligence test (generally an IQ less than 70 or 75, depending on the test). Borderline intelligence is when an individual's IQ score is between 1 and 2 standard deviations below the mean (generally, IQs of 70 to 80 or 85).

In a study of children with mental retardation in Norway, children born at 32 to 36 weeks of gestation had a 1.4 times increased risk of mental retardation than full-term children, and this risk increased to 6.9-fold for children born at less than 32 weeks of gestation (Stromme and Hagberg, 2000). The risks of mental retardation in children born preterm compared with those in children born with normal birth weights increase from 2.3-fold for children with birth weights of 1,500 to 2,499 grams to 12-fold for children with birth weights of less than 1,500 grams, 15-fold for children with birth weights of less than 1,000 grams, and 22-fold for children with birth weights of less than 750 grams (Resnick et al., 1999; Stromme and Hagberg, 2000). Nonetheless, children born at less than 32 weeks of gestation or with birth weights of less than 1,500 grams comprised only 4 percent of children with mental retardation.

On the basis of data for preterm children born in the late 1980s and 1990s, survivors born preterm with the lowest gestational ages and birth weights have the highest risk of mental retardation and borderline intelligence (Tables 11-2 and 11-3). A recent large study of infants born at less than 26 weeks gestation in 1995 in the British Isles and evaluated at age 6 years reported that 21 percent had an IQ 2 or more standard deviations below the test mean and 25 percent had borderline intelligence (i.e., IQs 1 to 2 standard deviations below the test mean), whereas for the controls born full term the rates were 0 and 2 percent, respectively (Marlow et al., 2005).

Studies that compare preterm children's performance on intelligence tests against published test norms may underestimate their cognitive disadvantage. Although cognitive tests are standardized on the basis of a mean IQ of 100 for normal populations, there is a tendency for the mean IQ score in normal or control populations to drift upward over time. Marlow et al. (2005) noted a mean cognitive score of 106 in their full-term classmate controls. With restandardization, the percentage of children born before 26 weeks of gestation who had cognitive scores 2 standard deviations or more below the full-term comparison group's mean score rose from 21 to 41 percent.

Children born full term with normal birth weights and raised in similar environments have generally served as comparison groups in studies of the outcomes of preterm birth. In a 1989 meta-analysis, 4,000 children born with birth weights of less than 2,500 grams had a mean IQ that was 5 to 7 points lower than the mean for 1,568 controls who were born full term (Aylward et al., 1989). In more recent studies of children with birth weights of less than 1,500 or 1,000 grams, the preterm children have mean IQ scores that were 10 to 17 points, or 1 standard deviation, below those for the full-term controls (Breslau et al., 1994; Doyle and Anderson, 2005; Grunau et al., 2002; Halsey et al., 1996; Hansen and Greisen, 2004; Whitfield et al., 1997).

A 2002 meta-analysis of 16 case-control studies of children aged 5 years old or older and born from 1975 to 1988 noted significantly lower cognitive scores for 1,556 children born preterm compared with those for 1,720 controls born full term, with a weighted mean difference of 10.9 (95% CI 9.2–12.5) (Bhutta et al., 2002). When only studies that excluded severely neurologically impaired children born preterm were analyzed, the weighted mean difference was 10.2 (95% CI 9.0–11.5).

Many studies have noted a trend toward lower mean cognitive scores with decreasing gestational age and birth weight categories (Tables 11-2 and 11-3) (Bhutta et al., 2002; Doyle and Anderson, 2005; Hall et al., 1995; Halsey et al., 1996; McCarton et al., 1997; McCormick et al., 1992; Saigal, 2000c; Taylor et al., 2000; Wilson-Costello et al., 2005).

There is some controversy as to the consistency of individual DQ and IQ scores over time. Artifacts of intelligence testing contribute to this confusion. One small study of infants with birth weights of less than 1,000 grams found lower Bayley Scale of Infant Development cognitive scores at 18 to 20 months from term than at 8 months from term, and this was associated with infant behavioral characteristics and family income (Lowe et al., 2005). The Bayley test items are, by necessity, heavily weighted toward visual motor abilities during the first year, but during the second year language concepts can be evaluated. In a study with 200 children with birth weights of less than 1,000 grams, Hack and colleagues (2005a) noted a significant improvement between the Bayley scores at age 20 months and cognitive scores at age 8 years (means, 76 and 88, respectively). The proportion of children with cognitive impairment (i.e., IQ scores 2 or more standard deviations below the test mean) decreased from 39 percent at age 20 months to 16 percent at age 8 years. This difference could be an artifact of the use of different tests at different ages. Ment and colleagues (2003) reported an increase in vocabulary test scores of 10 or more points in 45 percent of children with birth weights of less than 1,500 grams when they were retested at age 96 months after initial testing at age 36 months.

Further complicating the interpretation of these differences is the upward drift of IQ scores as a function of increased time from standardization (Flynn, 1999). Improvement in IQ scores with age is most common in children born preterm who have no neurological injuries or impairment and whose mothers have high levels of educational attainment (Hack et al., 2005; Koller et al., 1997; Ment et al., 2003). Despite improvements in their IQ scores with age, these children had more academic problems than children with stable IQ scores in the average range (Hack et al., 2005).

TABLE 11-2 Mean IQ Scores in Children Born Preterm and Full Term

Study	Year(s) of Birth	Age (yr)	Number of Subjects
Marlow et al., 2005	1995	6	241
Caravale et al., 2005	1998	3-4	30
Mikkola et al., 2005	1996–1997	5	103
		5	172
		2	78
Wilson-Costello et al., 2005	1990–1998	1.8	143
			269
		1.8	412
	1982–1989	1.8	51
			160
			211
Doyle et al., 2005	1991–1992	8	209
	1985–1987		192
	1979–1980		77
Taylor et al., 2000	1982–1986	11	60
			55
Halsey et al., 1996	1984–1986	7	54
			30
McCarton et al., 1997[a]	1984–1985	8	561
			313
Hall et al., 1995	1984	8	44
			255
Lefebvre et al., 2005	1976–1981	18	59
Saigal, 2000c	1977–1982	12–16	40
			110
			150
Hack et al., 2002	1977–1979	20	242
Men			113
Women			123

Rate of Follow-up (%)	Gestational Age (wk)	Birth Weight (g)	Mean IQ Score (Standard Deviation)	
			Preterm Group	Full-Term Control Group
78	<26		82.1 (19.2)	105.7 (11.8)
65	30–34		110.8 (10.4)	121 (10.6)
86	<27		94 (19)	
85		<1,000	96 (19)	
91			95 (13)	106 (10)
91		<750	80.3 (20)	
91		750–999	85.3(19)	
91		<1,000	86.3 (19)	
88		<750	81.4(21)	
88		750–999	87.9 (19)	
88		<1,000	86.4 (20)	
87		<1,000	94.9 (15.8)	104.9 (14.1)
91			94.2 (16.9)	
87			96.3 (15)	
82		<750	78 (17.4)	99.1 (18.1)
85		750–1,499	89.5 (14.4)	
80		<1,000	95.4 (18.7)	112.4 (19.6)
93		1,500–2,500	109.7 (15.1)	
89		<2,001	88.3, 89.5	intervention trial
		2,001–2,500	96.5, 92.1	intervention trial
81		<1,000	90.4 (11.1)	102.5 (12.4)
		1,000–1,499	93.7 (13.6)	101.1 (12.4)
75		<1,000	94 (12)	108 (14)
89		<750	86(20)	102(13)
		750–999	91(18)	
89		<1,000	89(19)	
78		<1,500	87	92
			87.6 (15.1)	94.7 (14.9)
			86.2 (13.4)	89.8 (14.0)

TABLE 11-3 Proportion of Survivors of Preterm Birth With and Without Cognitive Impairment

Study	Year(s) of Birth	Age (yr)	Rate of Follow-up (%)
Hintz et al., 2005	1996–1999	1.8	
			82
	1993–1996		
			74
Vohr et al., 2005	1997–1998	1.8	84
			82
	1993–1996		84
			81
	1993–1994		70
			74
Mikkola et al., 2005	1996–1997	5	85
			89
Marlow et al., 2005[a]	1995	6	78
Wood et al., 2005[a]	1995	2.5	
			92
Piecuch et al., 1997b	1990–1994	0.8–5.5	
			91
Emsley et al., 1998	1990–1994	1.5–6.1	100
	1984–1989	3.3–10.5	100
Jacobs et al., 2000	1992–1994	1–2	90
	1982–1987		
Msall et al., 1993	1983–1986	4	97
Wilson-Costello et al., 2005	1990–1998	1.8	
			90
	1982–1998	1.8	
	1982–1989		87
Hack et al., 2005	1992–1995	8	84
Hack et al., 2000	1992–1994	1.8	92
Doyle et al., 2004a	1991–1992	8	93
	1985–1987		97
	1979–1980		98

Number of Subjects	Gestational Age (wk)	Birth Weight (g)	Percentage of Subjects with Scores:		
			2 SDs below the Mean	1–2 SDs below the Mean	Normal
121	<24		52	26	22
315	24		44	25	31
436	<25		47	24	29
102	<24		38	36	26
239	24		40	28	32
341	<25		40	30	30
910	22–26	<1,000	37		
512	27–32	<1,000	23		
716	22–26	<1,000	39		
538	27–29	<1,000	26		
665	22–26	<1,000	42		
444	27–29	<1,000	30		
102	<28		12		
206		<1,000	9		
241	<26		21	25	54
19	<24		27	31	42
69	24		30	40	30
143	25		30	31	39
231	22–25		30	34	36
18	24		39	33	28
30	24		30	23	47
38	26		11	18	71
86	24–26		23		
40	23–25		15		
24	23–25		13		
274	23–26		26		
96	239			27	
149	<28		10		
143		500–749	34	18	49
269		750–999	22	19	60
412		500–999	26	18	56
51		500–749	28	28	45
160		750–999	18	24	59
211		500–999	20	25	56
200		<1,000	16	21	63
221		<1,000	42	26	32
224		<1,000	16.5	25	58.5
206			16	27	57
87			16	33	51

continued

TABLE 11-3 Continued

Study	Year(s) of Birth	Age (yr)	Rate of Follow-up (%)
Piecuch et al., 1997a	1989–1991	≥1	88
Taylor et al., 2000	1982–1986	11	82
			85
			80
Saigal et al., 2000c	1977–1982	12–16	89
			89
			86

NOTE: SD = standard deviation.

Adolescents and young adults who were born preterm continue to demonstrate a cognitive disadvantage compared with those who were born fullterm. When young adults who were born with birth weights of less than 1,000 grams were tested at a mean age of 18 years, they were found to have lower verbal, performance, and full-scale IQ scores than fullterm controls: 93 and 106, 97 and 109, and 94 and 108, respectively ($p < 0.0001$) (Lefebvre et al., 2005). Hack and colleagues (2002) evaluated 20-year-olds who were born with birth weights of less than 1,500 grams and found a mean IQ of 87, whereas the mean IQ was 92 for controls who were born with normal birth weights. Only half (51 percent) had an IQ score above 84, whereas 67 percent of adults who were born full term had IQ scores above 84. When Saigal and colleagues (2000c) compared 12- to 16-year-olds who were born with birth weights less than 1,000 grams with controls who had normal birth weights, preterm children had lower mean IQ scores even when children with IQ scores below 85 or neurosensory impairments were excluded (mean IQ scores 99 and 104, respectively, $p < 0.001$; for total sample, mean IQ scores were 89 and 102, respectively; $p < 0.0001$).

Preterm children with no neurological impairments demonstrate not only lower mean cognitive test scores but also more problems with specific cognitive processes than fullterm controls (Anderson and Doyle, 2003; Bhutta et al., 2002; Breslau et al., 1994; Grunau et al., 2002; Hack et al., 1993; Mikkola et al., 2005). One study of preschool children who were born at 30 to 34 weeks of gestation and who had no neurological impairments found lower scores not only on the Stanford-Binet IQ test (111 and 121, respectively; $p < 0.001$) but also on tests of visual perception, visual

Number of Subjects	Gestational Age (wk)	Birth Weight (g)	Percentage of Subjects with Scores:		
			2 SDs below the Mean	1–2 SDs below the Mean	Normal
136		<1,000	10	16	74
60		<750	37		
43		750–1,499	15		
41		>2,500	6		
40		<750	22.5	25	52.5
110		750–1000	12	12	76
124		Fullterm	0	8	92

motor integration, memory for location, sustained attention, and vocabulary, as compared to a matched control group of children born at term (Caravale et al., 2005).

A number of studies have demonstrated that preterm children who were born with birth weights less than 1,000 or 1,500 grams and who had normal IQ scores have more problems with attention, executive function (i.e., organization and planning skills), memory, language, learning disabilities, spatial skills, and fine and gross motor function than controls who were born with normal birth weights (Anderson and Doyle, 2003; Aylwarda, 2002a; Goyen et al., 1998; Grunau et al., 2005; Hack and Taylor, 2000; Halsey et al., 1993; Mikkola et al., 2005; O'Callaghan et al., 1996; Ornstein et al., 1991; Rose et al., 2005; Saigal et al., 1991).

School Problems

Difficulty with cognitive processes contributes to the increased risk of school problems seen in children born preterm (Aylward, 2002a; Grunau et al., 2002). In a study of 153 children born at less than 28 weeks of gestation, only half were ready and able to enter kindergarten with their peers (Msall et al., 1992). Speech and language delays, attention deficits, and learning disabilities were common. Among 8- to 10-year-old children who were born preterm with birth weights of less than 800 or 1,000 grams, 13 to 33 percent repeated a grade, 15 to 47 percent required some special education support, and 2 to 20 percent were in special education placements (Buck et al., 2000; Gross et al., 2001; Whitfield et al., 1997).

In a longitudinal study of 813 Dutch children born at less than 32 weeks gestation or with birth weights less than 1,500 grams, at age 9 years children born preterm had more school-related problems than the general Dutch population: 32 and 14 percent, respectively, functioned below grade level; 38 and 6 percent, respectively, received special education assistance; and 19 and 1 percent, respectively, were in special education classes (Hille et al., 1994). In adolescence (age 14 years), 27 percent received special education services, whereas 7 percent of their peers received special education services (Walther et al., 2000).

By early adolescence, the children who had been born preterm with birth weights of less than 1,000 grams were 3 to 5 times more likely than the controls born fullterm to fail a grade and required 3 to 10 times more special education resources than the controls born fullterm (Klebanov et al., 1994; Saigal et al., 2000c; Taylor et al., 2000). Saigal and colleagues (2005b) found progressive increases in school problems with decreasing birth weight category: 13 percent for fullterm controls, 53 percent for children born with birth weights between 750 and 1,000 grams, and 72 percent for children born with birth weight less than 750 grams. The proportions of children who had been born with birth weights less than 1,000 grams and who were in regular classrooms without grade failures or special education resources were only 42 to 50 percent at 8 to 10 years of age and as low as 36 percent at 18 years of age (Halsey et al., 1996; Klebanov et al., 1994; Lefebvre et al., 2005; Saigal et al., 2000c).

Many difficulties in school reflect the presence of learning disabilities, which become more apparent as children who had been born preterm progress through their education. A specific learning disability is a term that refers to a heterogeneous group of disorders of one or more of the basic psychological processes involved in understanding or in using spoken or written language. These disorders may manifest as significant difficulties with the acquisition and use of listening, speaking, reading, writing, reasoning, or mathematical skills. The diagnosis of a learning disability requires comparisons of performances on tests of academic achievement, cognition, language, visual motor integration, and perceptual abilities. Although the incidence of learning disabilities varies depending on how they are defined, most estimates indicate that 10 percent or less of the general population has evidence of a specific learning disability.

Ample evidence suggests that many more children born preterm have specific learning disabilities than children of normal birth weight born fullterm. By school age, despite normal intelligence, children born with birth weights of less than 1,000 or 800 grams have a 3- to 10-fold increased risk of problems with reading, writing, spelling, or mathematics compared with the risk for their peers who had been born fullterm (Aylward, 2002a; Grunau et al., 2002; Hall et al., 1995; O'Callaghan et al., 1996; Ornstein et al., 1991; Saigal et al., 2000c). The most consistent academic difficulties associated with preterm birth are arithmetic and reading (Anderson and Doyle, 2003; Bhutta et al., 2002; Hack et al., 1994; Klebanov et al., 1994; O'Callaghan et al., 1996; Ornstein et al., 1991; Saigal et al., 2000c). The proportion of children born preterm who experience academic difficulties increases with age as the complexity of the schoolwork increases and efficiency becomes an issue in the higher grade levels (Aylward, 2002a). In a detailed analysis of the nature of the learning disabilities in 8- to 9-year-olds who had been born with birth weights of less than 1,000 grams, Grunau and colleagues (2002) suggested that the children's problems with visual memory, visual motor integration, and verbal intelligence explained many of their difficulties with arithmetic and reading.

As with other neurodevelopmental disabilities and school problems, the prevalence of learning disabilities increases with decreasing gestational age and birth weight: 7 to 18 percent in children born full term, 30 to 38 percent in children born with birth weights 750 to 1,499 grams, 66 percent in children born at less than 28 weeks of gestation, and 50 to 63 percent in children born with birth weights less than 750 grams (Avchen et al., 2001; Aylward, 2002a; Breslau, 1995; Grunau et al., 2002; Hack et al., 1994; Halsey et al., 1996; Hille et al., 1994; Pinto-Martin et al., 2004; Taylor et al., 2000). In a study of 12- to 16-year-olds in three birth weight categories (normal, 750 to 1,000 grams, and less than 750 grams), the proportion with scores 2 or more standard deviations below the mean increased with decreasing birth weight for reading (0, 12, and 23 percent, respectively), spelling (2, 18, and 38 percent, respectively), and arithmetic (5, 32, and 50 percent, respectively) (Saigal et al., 2000c). The parents of more mature preterm children (those with gestational ages 32 to 35 weeks) reported significant problems with mathematics in 29 percent of the children, speaking in 19 percent, reading in 21 percent, and writing in 32 percent (Huddy et al., 2001).

In a study of 20-year-olds, those with birth weights less than 1,500 grams continued to have lower academic achievement scores in mathematics and reading than controls born with normal birth weights (Hack et al., 2002). Fewer of the young adults studied had graduated from high school (74 and 83 percent, respectively). The mean age at graduation was higher for those with lower birth weights (18.2 and 17.9 years, respectively). Fewer men born weighing less than 1,500 grams than men of normal birth weight attended a 4-year college (16 and 44 percent, respectively), but the rates were similar for women (33 and 38 percent, respectively). In a Canadian study of 18-year-olds born with birth weights of less than 1,000 grams, 56 percent obtained a secondary school diploma, whereas 86 percent of the controls who had been born fullterm did so (Lefebvre et al., 2005). In contrast, a recent study of 23-year-old Canadians weighing less than 1,000 grams at birth and controls born with normal birth weights found no differ-ences in the rates of completion of high school, postsecondary education, or university education or the total number of years of education that they had completed (Saigal et al., 2006a).

Visual Impairment

As discussed in Chapter 10, retinopathy of prematurity (ROP) is a com-mon complication of prematurity that increases with decreasing gestational age and birth weight. As a group, preterm children have a higher risk of impaired visual acuity than full-term children (Table 11-4). Myopia (i.e., nearsightedness) is one of the most common visual sequelae, and its inci-dence increases with the severity of ROP and with decreasing gestational age. Myopia occurs in 20 to 22 percent of children born with birth weights of less than 1,251 or 1,751 grams, and 4.6 percent have a high degree of myopia (i.e., ≥ 5 diopters) (O'Connor et al., 2002; Quinn et al., 1998).

Other visual problems include hyperopia and astigmatism (in 12 and 29 percent of children born at less than 29 weeks of gestation, respectively) (Hard et al., 2000). The need for glasses was higher in 7-year-olds born at gestational ages of less than 32 weeks than in controls born fullterm (13 and 4 percent, respectively) (Cooke et al., 2004). At 10 to 14 years of age, visual impairment was more common in children born with birth weights of less than 750 grams than in children born with birth weights of between 750 and 1,499 grams and children born with normal birth weights (31, 13, and 11 percent, respectively), as was the need for glasses (47, 24, and 27 percent, respectively) (Hack et al., 2000). In a British study of children born at less than 26 weeks of gestation, 24 percent of preterm 6-year-olds wore glasses, whereas 4 percent of controls with fullterm gestations did so (Marlow et al., 2005).

Strabismus (i.e., ocular misalignment, or crossed eyes) is also a frequent complication of prematurity. Strabismus has been reported in 3 percent of children born fullterm; 14 to 19 percent of children born with birth weights less than 1,500 grams, birth weights less than 1,750 grams, and gestational ages less than 29 and 32 weeks; and 24 percent of children born at gesta-tional ages less than 26 weeks (Bremer et al., 1998; Hard et al., 2000; Marlow et al., 2005, O'Connor et al., 2002). The risk of strabismus in-creases with intraventricular hemorrhage, periventricular leukomalacia, and the severity of ROP (Bremer et al., 1998; Hard et al., 2000; Hardy et al., 1997; Marlow et al., 2005; O'Connor et al., 2002; O'Keefe et al., 2001). Treatments for strabismus include correction with glasses or surgery, or both. Repka and colleagues (1998) reported that 10 percent of children with severe ROP underwent surgery for strabismus.

The sequelae of strabismus include amblyopia (i.e., suppression of the

TABLE 11-4 Sensory Impairments in Children Born Preterm

Study	Year of Birth	No. of Subjects	Age (yr)	Gestational Age (wk)	Birth Weight (g)	Percentage with Severe Impairment	
						Visual	Hearing
Vohr et al., 2005	1997–1998	910	1.8	22–26		1	1.8
		512		27–32		0.40	1.8
Hintz et al., 2005	1993–1996	355	1.8	<25		2.3	4.3
	1996–1999	467				1.1	2.6
Marlow et al., 2005	1995	241	6	<26		2	6
Jacobs et al., 2000	1990–1994	470	1-2	23–26		2	4
Lefebvre et al., 1996	1987–1992	217	1.5	23–28		0.5	0.5
Wilson-Costello et al., 2005	1990–1998	145	1.8		<750	1	10
		272			750–999	1	6
		682			<1,000	1	7
Mercier et al., 2005	1998–2001	2446	2		<1,000	1.4	2.1
Mikkola et al., 2005	1996–1997	173	5		<1,000	9	4
Hack et al., 2005b[a]	1992–1995	200	8		<1,000	0	2
Hack et al., 2000	1992–1995	221	1.8		<1,000	1	9
Hansen and Greisen, 2004	1994–1995	183	5	<28	<1,000	3.3	0
Doyle et al., 2005	1991–1992	224	8		<1,000	1.3	1.3

[a]Two percent of the subjects required hearing aids and 14 percent had hearing impairments.

visual input to the cortex) and a loss of binocular vision. Amblyopia has been found to occur in 1 to 4 percent of the general population, 2.5 percent of preterm infants without ROP, 12 percent of children with ROP, and 20 percent of children with severe ROP (Cats and Tan, 1989; Repka et al., 1998). The rate of the absence of stereopsis was higher in 7-year-olds born at less than 32 weeks of gestation than in controls born at fullterm (16.5 and 3.8 percent, respectively) (Cooke et al., 2004). Optic nerve atrophy and cortical visual impairment can also influence visual acuity in preterm children (Repka, 2002).

Although late or severe ophthalmic findings, including cataracts, angle closure glaucoma, and retinal detachment, are uncommon in children born preterm, they interfere with function and quality of life in children, adolescents, and adults when they occur (Kaiser et al., 2001; Machemer, 1993; Repka, 2002). Cataracts have been associated with untreated ROP and severe ROP (Kaiser et al., 2001; Repka et al., 1998). Glaucoma presents as an acute illness because of the severely increased pressure within the eye globe. The abnormal neovascular tissue of ROP can progressively and silently fold, exert traction, and tear or even detach the retina, causing a loss of vision (Kaiser et al., 2001; Machemer, 1993). Although most retinal tears or detachments occur in those with severe ROP, some children born preterm had mild or no ROP but a high degree of myopia (Kaiser et al., 2001). Surgical treatments, which include placement of a flexible band (i.e., a scleral buckle) around the eye to reduce tractional forces and vitrectomy (i.e., replacement of the vitreous fluid of the eye with sterile fluid), can restore visual function to some individuals. Severe detachment results in poor vision, with only light perception or, if the detachment is complete, no vision.

Ophthalmic morbidities are common in survivors of preterm birth, and early detection carries the best prognosis. Half of children with birth weights less than 1,751 grams had ophthalmic morbidities when they were evaluated at ages 10 to 12 years, whereas 20 percent of fullterm controls had ophthalmic morbidities (O'Connor et al., 2002). Although the risk was highest in individuals with severe ROP, ophthalmic morbidities were more common in survivors of preterm birth who had no or only very mild ROP than in controls born fullterm. Whether these ophthalmic problems contribute to the higher rate of visual perceptual deficits in the survivors of preterm birth (42 percent of 5- to 9-year-old children born at gestational ages less than 29 weeks compared with 14 percent of controls born fullterm) is not well understood (Hard et al., 2000, see section on Cognition). For some of these children, even if their visual system is intact, dysfunction of visual processing in the occipital cortex impairs their ability to perceive and understand visual patterns (drawings of figures, letters on a page).

Although the causes of ROP, ophthalmic morbidities, and visual perceptual deficits are, for the most part, unknown, identification of these morbidities allows their correction or amelioration, thereby improving functional outcomes. There is not yet adequate recognition of the need for regular ophthalmologic follow-up during the life span of survivors of preterm birth and assessment of their visual perceptual abilities when they are of preschool and school age (Hard et al., 2000; Kaiser et al., 2001; Repka, 2002).

Hearing Impairment

Children born preterm have a higher incidence of hearing loss than the general population. In the majority of studies of children born in the 1990s, severe hearing impairment occurred in 2 to 4 percent of children who had been born at less than 25 weeks gestation and 1.5 to 3 percent of children who had weighed less than 1,000 grams at birth (Doyle and Anderson, 2005; Hansen and Greisen, 2004; Hintz et al., 2005; Vohr et al., 2005). A British study of 6-year-old children born in 1995 at gestational ages of less than 26 weeks reported that 3 percent had profound sensorineural hearing impairment that could not be corrected with hearing aides, 3 percent had sensorineural hearing impairment that could be corrected with hearing aides, and 4 percent had mild hearing impairment (Marlow et al., 2005). Among the comparison group of children who had been born fullterm, 1 percent had hearing impairment that could be corrected with hearing aides and 1 percent had mild hearing impairment. A Swedish study of 18- to 19-year-olds born between 1973 and 1975 with birth weights of less than 1,500 grams found impaired hearing in 7 percent (Ericson and Kallen, 1998). An Australian study of 14-year-olds who had been born with birth weights of less than 1,000 grams reported that 5 percent required hearing aides (Doyle and Casalaz, 2001). When hearing impairment was defined as no perception of sounds at or above 40 dB in the better ear, bilateral hearing impairment occurred in 1.6/1,000 children aged 3 to 10 years, and in 7.5/1,000 of children born before 29 weeks gestation (Chapter 12, Table 12-8).

Some data suggest that preterm infants have difficulty with auditory processing and auditory discrimination, which involve multiple neural pathways to the cortex of the brain. A study of preterm infants born between 24 and 32 weeks of gestation who had normal cranial ultrasounds assessed event-related potentials (neurophysiological recordings) to evaluate learning and memory of patterns of speech sound discrimination (Therien et al., 2004). Unlike the fullterm controls, preterm infants were unable to discriminate between the speech of their mother and a stranger and demonstrated deficits in discriminating simple speech sounds and auditory recognition memory. Because speech discrimination is necessary for speech recognition, these types of deficits compromise the acquisition of language skills.

There is universal agreement regarding the importance of hearing for speech and language acquisition, and of the need to identify hearing impairment as early as possible. For this reason, most states in the United States are implementing plans to screen the hearing of all newborns (White, 2003). Because of their risk of hearing impairment and language processing problems, the hearing of all preterm infants should be screened before they are discharged from the hospital and later at the first sign of language delay or recurrent ear infections. Many infants with hearing impairment respond favorably to hearing aides, and a number of strategies can be used to teach language even when amplification is ineffective (Gabbard and Schryer, 2003; Gravel and O'Gara, 2003; Yoshinaga-Itano, 2000). Recent evidence also suggests that cochlear implants are the most successful when they are implanted early in infancy (Niparko and Blankenhorn, 2003).

Behavioral and Social-Emotional Problems

Behavior and social-emotional problems are more difficult to define clinically, and most of these data are elicited from surveys of parents and teachers. Symptoms suggestive of ADHD occur two to six times more frequently in children born preterm with birth weights of less than 1,000 grams, less than 1,500 grams, and less than 2,000 grams than in controls born fullterm (9 to 15 percent diagnosed with ADHD compared with 2 percent of controls born fullterm) (Aylward, 2002a; Bhutta et al., 2002; Breslau, 1995; Levy, 1994; Pharoah et al., 1994; Saigal et al., 2001; Stjernqvist and Svenningsen, 1995; Szatmari et al., 1990; Taylor et al., 1998). Refinement of descriptions of impairments of attention and behavior provides further insight into the problems children born preterm and their families face. In a study of 8-year-old children born at less than 28 weeks of gestation or with birth weights of less than 1,000 grams, the preterm children had significantly lower scores for processing speed, attention, and working memory and higher scores for hyperactivity than those for children born with normal birth weights (Anderson and Doyle, 2003). Middle-school children who weighed less than 750 grams at birth were found to have a much higher prevalence of symptoms of executive function disorder, including difficulties with planning, problem solving, organizing, and abstracting, which can seriously influence their function and behavior at school and at home (Taylor et al., 2000).

Parents and teachers report that preterm children with birth weights of less than 1,000 or 1,500 grams lag behind their peers in social competence and behavior and that this is unrelated to their IQ scores (Anderson and Doyle, 2003; Breslau et al., 1988). It is especially true for boys. In a large study of 8- to 10-year-old children born between 1978 and 1981, significantly more children with birth weights of less than 2,500 grams than children born with normal birth weights had behavioral problems, but there were no significant differences among the low birth weight categories (i.e., 27 to 29 percent for children with birth weights of less than 1,000, 1,001 to 1,500, and 1,501 to 2,500 grams versus 21 percent for children with birth weights of greater than 2,500 grams) (McCormick et al., 1992, 1996). Specifically, the children born preterm had higher subscores for hyperactivity and whining and were perceived to be less competent in athletics, behavior, and scholastics. Both teachers and parents rated 8- to 10-year-old children born at less than 28 weeks gestation or with birth weights less than 1,000 grams as having more behavioral symptoms (especially more somatic complaints and atypical behaviors), less adaptability, and fewer social and leadership skills than controls born with normal birth weights (Anderson and Doyle, 2003).

The evidence examining the relationship between low birth weight or preterm birth and autism is mixed. While some studies suggest a positive association (Finegan and Quarrington, 1979; Hultman et al., 2002; Indredavik et al., 2004; Larsson et al., 2005; Wilkerson et al., 2002), other studies have concluded that there is not an increased risk of autism in children born low birth weight or preterm (Deykin and MacMahon, 1980; Mason-Brothers et al., 1990; Piven et al., 1993; Williams et al., 2003). One study suggests that perinatal and obstetric factors might interact to impact birth outcomes (Eaton et al., 2001).

Conduct disorders are more common in children born preterm, but so are traits such as shyness, unassertiveness, withdrawn behavior, and social skill deficits (Bhutta et al., 2002; Grunau et al., 2004; Sommerfelt et al., 1996). In a meta-analysis of 16 case-control studies of children 5 years old or older who had been born preterm, 13 (81 percent) of the studies found that children born preterm had more behavioral problems than controls born fullterm (Bhutta et al., 2002). Two-thirds of the studies found a higher prevalence of ADHD, 69 percent found a higher prevalence of externalizing symptoms (e.g., delinquency), and 75 percent found a significantly higher prevalence of internalizing symptoms (e.g., anxiety, depression, and phobias). Many of these children withdraw from challenging tasks. Many preterm children with nonverbal learning disabilities have social skill deficits that seriously influence their social interactions and peer relationships (Aylward, 2002a; Fletcher et al., 1992). At school age, children born at less than 29 weeks of gestation were more often the target of verbal bullying by their peers than fullterm controls (Nadeau et al., 2004).

Adolescents and adults born preterm are less likely to demonstrate risk-taking behaviors than controls who were born fullterm. A recent study of young adults born from 1980 to 1983 in Britain found that fewer of those born with birth weights less than 1,500 grams than controls born fullterm drank alcohol or used illicit drugs, but there were no differences in the rates of smoking or sexual activity (Cooke, 2004). In the United States, young adults with birth weights less than 1,500 grams reported lower rates of alcohol and illicit drug use than controls with normal birth weights, but the two groups showed similar rates of tobacco use (57 and 59 percent of the men, respectively, and 40 and 48 percent of the women, respectively) (Hack et al., 2002). The men in the sample were also less likely to violate the law (37 and 52 percent, respectively), and this was primarily due to the lower rates of illicit drug use and truancy. The women were less likely to have had intercourse by age 20 years (65 and 78 percent, respectively) and to have had children (13 and 24 percent, respectively). These differences in risk-taking behaviors persisted even when the data for young adults with neuro-sensory impairments were excluded from the analysis. Both men and women with birth weights of less than 1,500 grams reported fewer delinquent behaviors, and women reported higher rates of anxiety-depression and withdrawal behaviors, fewer friends, and poorer family relationships than controls born with normal birth weights (Hack et al., 2004). An older study of Danish teenagers found no differences in the rates of alcohol or drug use between those born weighing less than 1,500 grams and controls born with normal birth weights (Bjerager et al., 1995).

Severity of Disability

Many outcomes researchers recognize the limitations of reporting the outcomes for individuals born preterm only in terms of the diagnoses of specific neurodevelopmental disabilities and have defined and reported on the severity of disability as well. For 8-year-olds born in 1991 and 1992 in Australia, severe disability (i.e., severe CP, blindness, or IQ scores 3 or more standard deviations below the mean) occurred in 9 percent of the children with birth weights of less than 1,000 grams and 12 percent of the children with birth weights of less than 750 grams (Doyle and Anderson, 2005). Moderate disability (i.e., moderate CP, deafness requiring hearing aides, or IQ scores 2 to 3 standard deviations below the mean) occurred in 10 percent of those with birth weights less than 1,000 grams and 15 percent of those with birth weights less than 750 grams. Mild disability (i.e., mild CP or IQ scores 1 to 2 standard deviations below the mean) occurred in 25 percent of children weighing less than 1,000 grams at birth and 33 percent of children weighing less than 750 grams at birth. More than half (56 percent) of the children with birth weights of less than 1,000 grams and 40 percent with birth weights of less than 750 grams had no disabilities.

Although a relatively small proportion of children born preterm have multiple disabilities, this group of children faces significant challenges with respect to mobility, academics, and the transition toward independence.

Multiple disabilities were seen in 5 percent of kindergartners born at less than 28 weeks of gestation (Msall et al., 1992). By using the definitions of handicap based on the Education for All Handicapped Children Act (P.L. 94-142), 2.5 percent of the parents of children born with normal birth weights reported that their child had multiple handicaps, whereas 5 percent of the parents of children born with birth weights of between 1,501 and 2,500 grams, 12 percent of the parents of children born with birth weights of between 1,001 and 1,500 grams, and 14 percent of the parents of children born with birth weights of less than 1,000 grams reported that their child had multiple handicaps (Klebanov et al., 1994). In a sample of infants born with birth weights less than 1,000 grams, 14 percent of the infants born at greater than 32 weeks of gestation had a severe disability (Mercier et al., 2005). In contrast, severe disability was reported in 100 percent of the infants born at less than 22 weeks of gestation, 48 percent of those born at 22 to 23 weeks of gestation, 37 percent of those born at 24 to 25 weeks of gestation, and 25 percent of those born at 26 and 27 weeks of gestation.

The presence of any neurosensory and neurodevelopmental impairment has been investigated in a number of studies of preterm infants. These impairments include: moderate to severe CP, cognitive impairment 2 or more standard deviations below the mean, blindness in both eyes, and hearing loss requiring amplification in both ears. For children born preterm in the 1990s, 28 percent born at 27 to 32 weeks gestation, 13 to 25 percent weighing less than 1,000 grams at birth, 45 percent born at less than 27 weeks of gestation, 58 percent born at 24 weeks of gestation, and 61 percent born at less than 24 weeks of gestation had neurosensory or neurodevelopmental impairment, whereas 1 percent of controls born fullterm had such impairments (Hansen and Greisen, 2004; Hintz et al., 2005; Saigal et al., 2000c; Vohr et al., 2005; Wilson-Costello et al., 2005). Hack and colleagues (2002) reported a major neurodevelopmental disability rate of only 10 percent among young adults born with birth weights of less than 1,500 grams.

The probability of survival without a neurosensory impairment or a major disability increases with increasing gestational age. As many as 56 to 77 percent of children born with birth weights less than 1,000 grams and birth weights less than 750 grams survive and are free of major disability (Doyle and Anderson, 2005; Hack and Fanaroff, 1999; Hansen and Greisen, 2004; Piecuch et al., 1997a,b; Saigal et al., 1990; Wilson-Costello et al., 2005). However, among children born at less than 26 weeks gestation, only 20 percent were free of disability at age 6 years, with 34 percent of these children having a mild disability, 24 percent having a moderate disability, and 22 percent having a severe disability (Marlow et al., 2005). This is similar to the 21 percent of survivors born at gestational ages less than 25 weeks who had no impairments reported by Hintz and colleagues (2005).

Some use the term "intact survival," calculated as the number of survivors who are "normal" divided by all live births. Generally, "normal" means no major cerebral palsy, mental retardation, or severe sensory impairment (i.e., no neurosensory impairment). As a concept, intact survival is most useful at the limit of viability, when the mortality rate is so high. Two recent regional studies have reported survival without major disability: 0 to 0.7 percent for those with gestational ages of less than 23 weeks, 6 percent to 35 percent for those with gestational ages of 23 weeks, 13 to 42 percent for those with gestational ages of 24 weeks, and 31 to 56 percent for those with gestational ages of 25 weeks (Doyle, 2001; Wood et al., 2000). This concept of survival without disability may be useful for discussions with prospective parents as they face the impending delivery of their infant at less than 26 weeks gestation (see Appendix C).

Disability in Late Preterm or Near-Term Infants

The rates of mortality (discussed in Chapter 10) and neurodevelopmental disability for moderately preterm infants; that is, those born between 32 and 36 weeks gestation or those weighing 1,500 to 2,499 grams at birth, are higher than those for infants born fullterm (although they are lower than those for infants born more prematurely). Although children born between 32 and 36 weeks of gestation constitute only about 8 to 9 percent of all births, they account for 16 to 20 percent of children with CP (Hagberg et al., 1996; MacGillivray and Campbell, 1995). Children born late preterm (or near term) have also been reported to have more developmental delays of infant milestones (those born at 33 to 36 weeks gestation) and more difficulty with hyperactivity, fine motor skills, mathematics, speaking, reading, and writing (those born at 32 to 35 weeks gestation) (Hediger et al., 2002; Huddy et al., 2001).

Functional Outcomes

Authors of studies of the outcomes for children born preterm have struggled with how to convey the full range of outcomes. Although the majority have focused on cognitive outcomes and clinical diagnoses of neurodevelopmental disabilities, some have taken a more practical approach and have described what survivors of preterm birth have been able to do.

The acquisition of motor and adaptive milestones is a means of conveying the functional abilities of a toddler. Wood and colleagues (2000) found that at 30 months from term 90 percent of preterm infants born at less than 26 weeks gestation could walk, 97 percent could sit, 96 percent could feed themselves with their hands, and 6 percent could speak. In a similar study of children weighing less than 1,000 grams at birth, at 18 months from term 93 percent could sit, 83 percent could walk, and 86 percent could feed themselves (Vohr et al., 2000). A study of developmental data from the National Health and Nutrition Examination Survey found higher frequencies of motor and social developmental delays in children born preterm (at less than 37 weeks gestation), including the children born moderately preterm at 33 to 36 weeks of gestation (Hediger et al., 2002). Based on their rate of attainment of milestones compared with the rate for other children of the same age, for each week of gestation below full term, the developmental scores of boys decreased by 0.1 point.

Several studies have reported on the functional abilities of 5- to 6-year-old children born preterm. In a study of 149 children born at less than 28 weeks gestation who were in kindergarten, 95 percent could walk and perform basic self-care skills and were continent during the daytime (Msall et al., 1992). Most of the children who had neurodevelopmental disabilities were still able to function well: 87 percent could walk one block, 84 percent talked in sentences, and 81 percent could perform self-care tasks. In a study of 5-year-olds weighing less than 1,500 grams at birth, the results were reported in terms of the proportion of children with severe functional limitations (e.g., mobility, self-care, and social communication) (Palta et al., 2000). Severe functional limitations were identified in more children with CP (57 percent for self-care, 89 percent for mobility, and 32 percent for social communication) than in those without CP (5 percent for self-care, 21 percent for mobility, and 8 percent for social communication). Marlow and colleagues (2005) reported on the motor functions of 6-year-olds born at less than 26 weeks gestation: 6 percent could not walk, 6 percent walked independently but with an abnormal gait, and the remainder were functional with respect to walking and hand use.

A study of 5.5-year-old children born with birth weights of less than 1,250 grams found an increase in the proportions of children with severe functional limitations with an increasing severity of ROP: 4 percent with no ROP, 11 percent with prethreshold ROP, and 26 percent with severe threshold ROP (Msall et al., 2000). Severe functional limitations were common in children with severe ROP and poor vision (77 percent for self-care, 43 percent for mobility, 50 percent for continence, and 66 percent for social communication). Children who were born preterm and who had good vision fared better: 25 percent had self-care limitations, 5 percent had mobility limitations, 4.5 percent were not continent, and 22 percent had limitations in social communication skills.

Hack and Taylor (2000) found that 14-year-old children with weights of less than 750 grams at birth had significantly higher prevalences of functional limitations and a greater need for special services than children who weighed 750 to 1,499 grams at birth and controls born fullterm. Only 3 percent of those born weighing less than 750 grams and 2 percent of those born weighing 750 to 1,499 grams (and no controls) had severe functional impairments that interfered with feeding, dressing, washing, or toileting themselves. Compared with control children born fullterm, children with birth weights less than 750 grams were more likely to have mental or emotional delays, restrictions in activity, and visual difficulties (odds ratios = 4.7, 5.1, and 3.9, respectively). They were more likely to need special education, counseling, and special arrangements at school (odds ratios = 5.0, 4.8, and 9.5, respectively).

Later functional outcomes can be expressed in terms of the highest educational level achieved and the transition to adulthood. A study that linked data from the Swedish Medical Birth Registry with the National Service Enrollment Register found that not only did 18- to 19-year-olds born from 1973 to 1975 with birth weights of less than 1,500 grams have higher rates of CP (odds ratio = 55.4), mental retardation (odds ratio = 1.7), myopia (odds ratio = 3.3), and severe hearing impairment (odds ratio = 2.5); but they also tended to leave the school system early (odds ratio = 1.6) (Ericson and Kallen, 1998). Hack and colleagues (2002) found that fewer 20-year-olds born from 1977 to 1979 with birthweights less than 1,500 grams than controls who had normal birth weights graduated from high school or earned general equivalency diplomas (74 and 83 percent, respectively) and that fewer men attended 4-year colleges (16 and 44 percent, respectively). These differences persisted even when the data for those with any neurosensory impairment were excluded from the analyses.

Other investigators have found lower rates of graduation from high school among young adults born weighing less than 1,000 or 1,500 grams compared with the rates for controls with normal birth weights (Cooke et al., 2004; Lefebvre et al., 2005). In a comparison of performance on exams at the end of secondary school in Great Britain (i.e., the General Certificate of Secondary Education), matched control graduates born fullterm scored more points per test and more total points than graduates born with birth weights less than 1,500 grams (Pharoah et al., 2003). On the other hand, among a fairly privileged group of young adults born from 1977 to 1982 with birth weights less than 1,000 grams, Saigal and colleagues found no significant differences in the levels of educational attainment or the rates of continuing with higher education compared with those for the controls born with normal birth weights (Saigal et al., 2006a).

Tideman and colleagues (2001) reported that 19-year-olds born at less than 35 weeks gestation gave similar reports of self-esteem as controls born fullterm. Sixteen- to 19-year-olds born from 1981 to 1986 with birth weights of less than 800 grams reported less self-confidence with athletics, school achievement, job confidence, and romance than controls born fullterm (Grunau et al., 2004). Despite feeling less attractive than their peers who had been born with normal birth weights, young adults born from

1980 to 1983 with birth weights of less than 1,500 grams had similar social activities and similar experiences with sex (Cooke et al., 2004). More young adults who had been born preterm were parents, but they had lower rates of participation in higher education and paid employment.

Saigal and colleagues (2006a) found no significant differences in high school graduation rates, the level of education attained, rates of employment, rates of independent living, marriage or cohabitation status, or rates of parenthood between 22- and 25-year-olds born weighing between 501 and 1,000 grams and those born with normal birth weights. Subanalyses, however, revealed that more participants born with extremely low birth weights reported that they were neither in school nor employed, although these differences disappeared when those with disabilities were excluded. These results suggest that individuals born preterm can make a successful transition into adulthood. It is noted, however, that the participants in this sample were predominantly white, were from relatively advantaged homes, and had access to universal health care.

Summary

The spectrum of neurodevelopmental disabilities and functional outcomes in children, adolescents, and young adults born preterm is wide. Likewise, the prevalences of neurodevelopmental disabilities and neurosensory impairments in people born preterm are quite variable. This is not surprising, in light of the multiple etiologies and complications of preterm birth, the variability of both the intrauterine and the extrauterine environments to which they are exposed, and the infinite genetic variations of humans.

Finding 11-2: There is tremendous variation in the outcomes reported for individuals born preterm. Much of this variation is due to a lack of uniformity in study sample selection criteria, the study methodologies used, the age of evaluation, and the measurement tools and cutoffs used.

Finding 11-3: Few long-term studies of adolescents and adults born preterm have been conducted. Good indicators of the functional development of the central nervous system of preterm infants in neonatal intensive care units are lacking, and predictors of long-term neurodevelopmental and health outcomes are inadequate.

FACTORS THAT INFLUENCE
NEURODEVELOPMENTAL OUTCOMES

Many factors influence the outcomes for infants born preterm, including gestational age at birth, complications that injure the brain, variations in the clinical management of infants at various health care institutions, the family's socioeconomic condition, and the mother's mental health. As discussed above, children who were born more prematurely and who were sicker tend to have more health and developmental problems. The marked variations in neurodevelopmental and health outcomes for preterm infants is the result of variations in the etiologies of preterm birth, intrauterine environments, complications of prematurity, NICU management and treatments, and home environments. Although many factors influence the outcomes for individuals born preterm, the many studies that have evaluated demographic, prenatal, perinatal, and neonatal predictors have not been able to devise a method of determining the outcome for an individual infant. Predictors of outcomes can identify groups of infants with a high risk of disability who may benefit from intensive developmental support and community services. Further research to refine the predictors may also provide insights into the etiologies and the mechanisms of organ injury and recovery in preterm infants.

The processes that lead to preterm birth and the subsequent treatments necessary to support life (i.e., neonatal intensive care) can injure immature organ systems that are not ready to support life in the extrauterine environment. Maternal illness can influence fetal growth, fetal organ development, preterm delivery, and infant health and neurodevelopmental outcomes. A growing concern is the impact of infection and inflammation on the mother and the fetus: inflammatory mediators have been implicated in proposed mechanisms of preterm delivery and fetal brain injury leading to CP and cognitive impairments (Andrews et al., 2000; Dammann et al., 2002, 2005; Goldenberg et al., 2005; Gravett and Novy, 1997; Hagberg et al., 2005; Holling and Leviton, 1999; Wu and Colford, 2000) (see Chapters 6 and 10). Research is needed to understand the relationships between the genome, factors that control inflammation, and development of the brain, the neurotransmitter system within the brain, and immune system (Raju et al., 2005).

Although prenatal and intrapartum factors can adversely influence the outcomes for infants born preterm, many neonatal factors are stronger predictors (Allen, 2005b). The strongest neonatal predictors are the severity of the acute illness, measures of bronchopulmonary dysplasia/chronic lung disease (BPD/CLD), severe ROP, and signs of brain injury (Allen, 2005b; Doyle, 2001; Emsley et al., 1998; Hack et al., 2000; Hintz et al., 2005; Piecuch et al., 1997a,b; Schmidt et al., 2003; Vohr et al., 2005). The effect of BPD/CLD on neurodevelopment may be due to difficulties with nutrition and growth, management of ventilators and oxygen supplementation, or the use of postnatal steroids or other medications (Bhutta and Ohlsson, 1998; Halliday and Ehrenkranz, 2001a,b,c; Kaiser et al., 2005; Saugstad, 2005; Thomas et al., 2003; Tin, 2002; Tin and Wariyar, 2002; Wood et al., 2005). Because various management strategies influence outcomes, one factor that would be expected to influence outcomes is the institution(s) at which the infant was managed clinically (Vohr et al., 2004).

Signs of brain injury on neuroimaging studies (e.g., ultrasound or magnetic resonance imaging), neurodevelopmental examination, and analysis of infant movements are some of the strongest neonatal predictors of preterm motor and cognitive outcomes. Predictive neuroimaging findings include severe intraventricular hemorrhage, intraparenchymal hemorrhage, hydrocephalus, porencephaly, periventricular leukomalacia, and other signs of white matter injury (Doyle, 2001; Hack et al., 2000; Hintz et al., 2005; Ment et al., 2003; Piecuch et al., 1997a,b; Pinto-Martin et al., 1995; Rogers et al., 1994; Tudehope et al., 1995). Measures of infant neurological function, including neurodevelopmental examination and assessment of general movements, are independently predictive and enhance the predictive capability when they are used in combination with neuroimaging (Allen and Capute, 1989; Einspieler and Prechtl, 2005; Gosselin et al., 2005; Mercuri et al., 2005). Neuroimaging technologies have begun to demonstrate reduced brain volumes, involving the cortex (especially parietal and sensorimotor areas) and deep nuclear structures, in infants and children born preterm as compared with fullterm control children (Peterson et al., 2000; Peterson, 2003). Reduction in brain volume has been associated with white matter injury and cognitive deficits. Research into the nature of brain-behavior relationships, including relationships between brain structural and functional development, areas of the brain typically affected by brain insult and their corresponding neurodevelopmental and behavioral deficits, and how plasticity is manifested as recovery from brain injury could provide insight into better predictors of neurodevelopmental outcomes as well as neuroprotective strategies (Peterson, 2003; Raju et al., 2005).

The developing preterm infant is not immune to environmental factors, and preterm birth may interact with poverty toward further disadvantage. There is a wealth of information on how a child's low socioeconomic status adversely affects the outcomes for the child in general (Brooks-Gunn and Duncan, 1997). It is also well documented that preterm infants are disproportionately poor (see Chapter 4). Not only does poverty increase the risk of being born preterm but it also independently increases the risk of adverse outcomes. The effect of poverty directly relates to the design of postdischarge interventions. Even controlling for birth weight or prematurity, poverty worsens the outcomes for preterm infant, particularly cognitive outcomes (McGauhey, 1991).

There is some evidence that maternal mental health influences the outcomes for children born preterm. In general, children of depressed mothers do not fare well (independently of poverty, which increases the risk of depression) (Downey and Coyne, 1990; Zuckerman and Beardslee, 1987). As discussed above, the mothers of preterm infants experience more depression, and that affects their parenting abilities (Singer et al., 1999, 2003). Maternal mental distress early in a child's life has long-term effects on child behavior (Gray et al., 2004).

Evidence suggests that educational and other programs may improve outcomes and have especially been shown to mitigate the effects of poverty (Barnett, 1995; Devaney et al., 1997; Yoshikawa, 1995). Potentially beneficial effects from developmental support in the NICU are discussed in Chapter 10. Early intervention programs that may affect the outcomes of premature infants after discharge from the NICU are discussed below. Research into preterm health and neurodevelopmental outcomes should address the complex and intricate relationships between biomedical, proximal, and distal environmental and behavioral influences. Consideration should be given to specific and discrete outcomes, ages at time of exposure to environmental variables, mediators and moderators of environmental influences, and use of multivariate modeling.

HEALTH AND GROWTH

Health

As with much of the literature reviewed in this volume, studies of the health of premature infants after discharge from the hospital have been characterized largely in terms of birth weight (Doyle et al., 2003b). The most frequently cited evidence of a higher risk for adverse health status among low birthweight and preterm infants is an increased risk of rehospitalization during the first few years of life. Infants born weighing 1,500 grams or less are four times more likely than normal birth weight infants to be hospitalized in the first year of life (McCormick et al., 1980) and are more likely to have a disproportionate duration of stay for these hospitalizations (Cavalier et al., 1996). Among infants born with birth weights of 2,500 grams or less, the relative risk of rehospitalization in one study was about twice that of heavier infants, and again, these infants had longer lengths of stay in the hospital (Cavalier et al., 1996).

More recently, attention has been shifted to the risk of rehospitalization associated with prematurity. Although the findings of these studies are difficult to compare with those from the older literature based on birth weight, these studies suggest that preterm infants are also more likely to be rehospitalized (Escobar et al., 1999; Martens et al., 2004). For example, among infants born preterm, those born at earlier gestations compared to those born moderately preterm were at greater risk of rehospitalization (Joffe et al., 1999). Children born with birth weights below 2,500 grams also make more use of outpatient health care (Jackson et al., 2001) and incur significantly higher medical and nonmedical costs (McCormick et al, 1991) compared to children born with normal birth weights. Furthermore, as with other measures of health care utilization, the rates of rehospitalization vary among institutions (Escobar et al., 2005; Martens et al., 2004).

The increased risk of rehospitalization for preterm and low birth weight infants is likely a reflection of their compromised health status. Children born with birth weights below 1,500 grams suffer increased morbidity (McCormick et al., 1992) compared to children with normal birth weights. The psychosocial environment is also important for children born with birth weights below 2,500 grams, as those with high psychosocial risk have worse health status than children in low and moderate risk categories (McGauhey et al., 1991). Furthermore, in comparison to children with normal birth weights, chronic health conditions have a stronger impact on the school achievement and participation, and behavior problems of children with birth weights below 2,500 grams (McGauhey et al., 1991). The impact of LBW extends into adolescence. Adolescents with birth weights below 1,500 grams have higher blood pressure than those with normal birth weights (Doyle et al., 2003a).

Growth

Besides acute and chronic conditions, infants born preterm or with birth weights below 2,500 grams also experience poorer growth. The first 3 years of life evidence a discrepancy in the growth patterns of children with birth weights below 2,500 grams, compared to those with normal birth weights (Binkin et al., 1988; Casey et al., 1991). Poor growth resulting from intrauterine, neonatal, or postnatal growth failure has been documented widely among children with birth weights below 1,500 grams (Binkin et al., 1988; Casey et al., 1991). Studies performed with adolescents who with birth weights less than 2,500 grams suggest that their anthropometric measurements are lower than those of adolescents with normal birth weights. Similarly, a study by Peralta-Carcelen and colleagues (2000) showed lower growth measures for adolescents born at birth weights less than 1,000 grams who survived without a major neurodevelopmental disability, compared to those with normal birth weights.

However, other studies suggest that there is catch-up growth. Hack and colleagues (1984) found that catch-up growth occurs during the first 2 to 3 years of life. A more recent study of children with birth weights less than 1,500 grams documented catch-up growth during the first 8 years of life, with poorer growth attainment among those who were small for gestational age (SGA) (Hack et al., 1996). Ford et al. (2000) also documented catch-up growth among children with birth weight less than 1,500 grams although they are still smaller than those born with normal birth weights. Another study also found that 18–19 year old boys with birth weights less than 1,500 grams were shorter and lighter than their counterparts with normal birth weights (Ericson and Kallen, 1998). Finally, Saigal and colleagues (2001) found that adolescents with birth weights less than 1,000 grams demonstrated patterns of catch-up growth between age 8 and adolescence.

Studies on the ultimate growth attainment or growth during the adolescent years and into early adulthood for individuals born preterm are only recently appearing in the literature. Doyle and colleagues (2004b) found compromised growth among survivors up to age 8 who were born with birth weights less than 1,000 grams, but by age 14 and up to age 20 they had reached average height and weight. Despite the persistence of lower height among survivors with birth weights less than 1,000 grams, Saigal and colleagues (2001) showed that most of their adolescents were within 2 standard deviations of the mean. Furthermore, Hack and colleagues (2003) documented gender differences. In childhood (8 years), males with birth weights less than 1,500 grams were shorter and lighter than counterparts with normal birth weight, whereas females were lighter but not significantly shorter than their counterparts with normal birth weights (Hack et al., 2003). The discrepancy for males persisted at 20 years, but females did not demonstrate subaverage height and weight at early adulthood (Hack et al., 2003). The predictors of height and weight also differed for males and females. For females, black race and chronic illness predicted weight, and maternal height and birthweight standardized score predicted height at 20 years of age (Hack et al., 2003). The predictors of height for males were the same as the females' with duration of neonatal hospital stay and SGA birth as additional predictors of height (Hack et al., 2003).

Many of these findings suggest that by adolescence children born preterm experience catch-up growth. Since sexual maturation is an important aspect of adolescent development, studies on growth attainment for preterm infants during the adolescent years should evaluate sexual maturity. Another area for further research to elucidate the factors involved in catch-up growth among LBW survivors is nutrition. Weiler and colleagues (2002) found that despite the impact of preterm birth on attainment of normal height in young adulthood, bone mass is appropriate.

Health-Related Quality of Life

Health, as formulated by the World Health Organization (WHO, 1958) is a "state" of complete physical, mental, and social well-being and not merely the absence of disease or infirmity. Health-related quality of life (HRQL) is a narrower concept that considers the net impact or consequence of a disease or impairment and implicitly reflects the personal values of the individual (Gill and Feinstein, 1994). Measurement of HRQL can be used for comparisons with different disease conditions, as well as for cost-effectiveness and cost-utility analyses.

The challenge in pediatrics is that children are constantly developing and changing; and their personal values may also evolve over time (Rosenbaum and Saigal, 1996). Traditionally, parents or caregivers have been accepted as reliable proxy respondents on behalf of younger children or those with severe disabilities. However, there is evidence that proxy responses by parents correlate poorly with the perceptions of children. Parents have more consistent agreement with children for observable functioning (physical health), than for emotional and social functioning. Overall, parents are generally more negative, and their responses may be influenced by the burden of caregiving (Eiser and Morse, 2001). Also, health professionals have limited abilities to judge patients' HRQL, and their values may differ from those of children and their parents (Saigal et al., 1999). Further work is required to understand how the characteristics of patient proxy responses influence agreement. However, it is acknowledged that although children's perspectives may differ from that of parents or health professionals, they are valid, and should be accepted. There are strong arguments for obtaining HRQL perspectives from multiple respondents (Eiser and Morse, 2001). Recently a few "generic" and "disease-specific" HRQL instruments been developed to measure the physical, psychological, and social domains of health in young children from their own perspective. To date, there are limited studies on Quality of Life (QL) in children, and even fewer in children born preterm. In this section a few such studies conducted at various ages are described.

On a preschool quality of life questionnaire (TAPQOL) (Fekkes et al., 2000) administered to parents and neonatologists in the Netherlands, 1- to 4-year-old children born before 32 weeks gestation were reported to have significantly lower HRQL than the reference group (Theunissen et al., 2001). However, the study found differences between the neonatologists' and parents' perceptions of HRQL in terms of what conditions needed treatment. A Canadian study from British Columbia (Klassen et al., 2004) used both the Infant Toddler Quality of Life Questionnaire (ITQOL) (Landgraf et al., 1999) and the Health Status Classification System for Preschool children (Saigal et al., 2005a) and found that the 1,140 children who required

NICU care at birth had poorer health status and HRQL on a range of domains compared with the findings for 393 children who had been born fullterm.

A series of studies on the HRQL of children born in Ontario Canada between 1977 and 1982 weighing less than 1,000 grams were conducted by Saigal and colleagues. In the initial study of 156 8-year-old children who weighed less than 1,000 grams at birth and 145 fullterm controls (Saigal et al., 1994b), health status was determined by health professionals using a multiattribute classification system, which also provided the levels of functional limitations (Feeny et al., 1992). This descriptive information was used to map HRQL scores using a utility function formula (HUI2), based on preferences about hypothetical health states expressed by the general public (Torrance, 1995). The children with birth weights less than 1,000 grams had functional limitations in several attributes, and mean HRQL scores were significantly lower than in controls (Saigal et al., 1994b). In a subsequent study of the same cohort (Saigal et al., 1996), directly measured preferences were elicited for the first time at adolescence using the standard gamble technique (method for eliciting patient preferences when there is uncertainty about the outcome). The teenagers born weighing less than 1,000 grams reported a higher frequency and more severe functional limitations in their health status in several domains as compared to fullterm controls. Although their overall mean HRQL scores were significantly lower, the majority of adolescents with birth weight less than 1,000 grams viewed their HRQL to be similar to normal birth weight controls (71% vs 73%). Parents of both groups rated their adolescent children's HRQL higher than the children's self-ratings (Saigal et al., 2000b).

In a further study to determine whether the preferences of health professionals differed systematically from those of the Ontario teenagers and their parents, hypothetical health scenarios were employed, and preferences were elicited by standard gamble technique (Saigal et al., 1999). Although there was a fair degree of agreement between the groups for milder disabilities, parents and teenagers appeared to be more "accepting" of the more severely disabling health states than health professionals. These findings have clinical implications for medical decision making around the birth of a very preterm infant.

Other investigators have measured parental perspectives of HRQL in 244 10-year-old children who weighed less than 1,250 grams at birth. These children participated in the landmark CRYO trial for retinopathy of prematurity (ROP) (CRPCG, 1988). Using the HUI2 system (Feeny et al., 1992), threshold ROP was associated with functional limitations in health and reduction in HRQL scores and, as expected, children with poorer visual outcomes had lower HRQL scores (Quinn et al., 2004). HRQL in relation to the severity of abnormality on brain ultrasounds was measured in a cohort of adolescents born preterm (Feingold et al., 2002). Paradoxically, the overall self-perceived HRQL of adolescents with a higher degree of severity of intraventricular hemorrhage was better than that of adolescents with mild (i.e., grade 0 to 2) intraventricular hemorrhage.

Recently, several studies have reported the HRQL in young adults born preterm. In a telephone survey, the quality of life of 85 Danish young adults born between 1971 and 1974 in Denmark with birth weights less than 1,500 grams was compared with that of subjects with normal birth weights by using both objective and subjective measures (Bjerager et al., 1995). Although the self-reported quality of life scores for those with physical and mental handicaps were significantly lower, the scores of nondisabled subjects were comparable to those of the group with normal birth weights. In a subsequent study in Denmark, a cohort of young adults born from 1980 to 1982 with birth weights less than 1,500 grams had similar subjective quality-of-life scores but lower objective quality-of-life scores compared to the reference group (Dinesen and Greisen, 2001). Tideman and colleagues (2001) found that on the visual analogue scale, the HRQL of 19-year-olds born at less than 35 weeks gestation was similar to the HRQL of the normal birth weight group. The quality of life of a British cohort of young adults with birth weights less than 1,500 grams assessed by SF-36 (Short Form 36 Health Survey) was found to be similar to that of normal birth weight group (Cooke 2004). Similarly, at a mean age of 23 years, Saigal and colleagues (2006b) found no differences in the self-reported mean HRQL scores in the Ontario young adults weighing less than 1,000 grams compared to normal birth weight controls.

Although measurement of quality of life appears to be popular, a well-defined theoretical framework for the accurate assessment of the child's conceptual and developmental viewpoint is not yet available (Jenney and Campbell, 1997). Furthermore, most of the currently available quality-of-life measures focus to a large extent on how children are functioning in different domains as determined by age-appropriate roles. Although functional measures provide considerable valuable information, they are considered to be tapping health profiles and not the values of individual subjects (Gill and Feinstein, 1994). Such health profiles generally paint a picture more negative than that obtained when personal valuation is sought (Guyatt and Cook, 1994). However, in-person interviews are time consuming and expensive and impose considerable cognitive demands on respondents. Feeny et al. (2004) compared directly measured standard gamble utility scores of the Ontario cohort at adolescence with indirectly measured scores from the HUI, based on self-assessed health status but valued using community preferences. Although HUI scores matched directly measured utility scores reasonably well at the group level, at the individual level they were poor substitutes for directly measured preferences.

Finally, despite the growing literature, measurement of self-reported quality of life continues to be viewed with skepticism by the medical community and even by some parents (Hack, 1999; Harrison, 2001). Although a considerable challenges the view that the quality of life of people with disabilities is inevitably compromised, the prevailing perception appears to be largely negative.

Fetal Origins of Adult Disease

The "fetal origins" hypothesis proposes that undernutrition in utero at critical periods of development, programs or permanently alters fetal metabolism and renders the individual susceptible to future cardiovascular disease (CVD) and metabolic derangements of glucose metabolism (Barker et al., 1989a). This hypothesis originated in a retrospective study in which it was noted that men whose birth weights were below the 5th percentile had a higher risk of dying from coronary artery disease than men with a higher birth weight. Subsequent investigations with other populations have confirmed this relationship (Barker et al., 1993a; Martyn et al., 1998) and noted that it also exists in women (Osmond et al., 1993; Osmond et al., 2000; Rich-Edwards et al., 1997).

Low birth weight is reported to be associated with established cardiovascular risk factors, including dysglycemia, dyslipidemia, and hypertension (Barker et al., 1993b; Lithell et al., 1996). Upon meta-analysis, however, the association between birth weight and blood pressure or dyslipidemia is weaker than initially thought, with the larger studies showing the smallest relationship (Huxley et al., 2002). In a recent meta-analysis, the pooled relative risk for coronary artery disease among the 6,056 subjects who weighed 5.5 pounds or less at birth was 1.26 (95% CI 1.11–1.44) compared with the risk for the 80,802 subjects who weighed more than 5.5 pounds at birth (Raju, 1995). Animal studies have provided supportive evidence in favor of this programming hypothesis, although often after the use of extreme nutritional insults during fetal life (Coates et al., 1983).

Despite the growing number of reports on an association between low birth weight, cardiovascular risk factors and surrogate markers of CVD, most studies investigating the fetal origins of adult disease have used a retrospective design for data collection (Barker et al., 1989a,b, 1993a,b,c; Leeson et al., 2001). Furthermore, many of these studies were conducted with highly selected subgroups of people for whom very little information on pregnancy and perinatal events was available. In addition, most investigators did not differentiate low birth weight from small for gestational age or prematurity, and did not measure postnatal growth. Thus, birth weight and early growth were used as surrogates for overall somatic growth, without data on the presence or the absence of interim growth decelerations or subsequent catch-up growth. Furthermore, social class (paternal occupation) was based on recall by adult subjects 50 to 70 years later and the studies did not control for postnatal modifiers, such as socioeconomic, environmental or behavioral factors, or social deprivation in the early critical period of life (Joseph and Kramer, 1996; Paneth, 1994; Paneth and Susser, 1995; Paneth et al., 1996). In addition, retention rates in most study cohorts were extremely poor with only between 19 and 60 percent of the subjects available for further follow-up (Bhargava et al., 2004; Cooke, 2004; Strauss, 2000).

Only a paucity of studies have been designed to investigate specifically whether the fetal origins hypothesis is also applicable to preterm infants and not just to those who are small for gestational age. Fewtrell and colleagues (2000) examined the relationship between gestational age and size for gestational age on glucose and insulin concentrations at ages 9 to12 years in 385 children who had been born preterm with birth weights less than 1,850 grams. Low birth weight, whether it was due to being born preterm or intrauterine growth restriction, was associated with higher plasma glucose levels 30 minutes after administration of a glucose load. Recently, Hofman and colleagues (2004a) have demonstrated that 4- to 10-year- olds born preterm have metabolic abnormalities similar to those observed in infants born fullterm but small for gestational age and that these occur irrespective of whether the preterm infants are small or appropriate for gestational age. In fact, there did not seem to be an additive effect on reduced sensitivity from being born both preterm and small for gestational age. A subsequent study by the same investigators confirms the reduction in insulin sensitivity, which may be a risk factor for Type II diabetes mellitus (Hofman et al., 2004b). This reduction was similar in infants born between 24 and 32 weeks gestation, suggesting that a critical window exists in the third trimester in which insulin activity is altered. In another study by Hovi et al. (2005), young adults born with birth weights less than 1,500 grams had fasting insulin levels that were 34 percent higher than those for controls, and their mean fasting serum glucose level was also higher (but an oral glucose tolerance test was not done). Unfortunately, these studies examined only 50 percent of the cohort.

Childhood weight gain has also been shown to be an important predictor of measures of insulin secretion and resistance in some studies (Fewtrell et al., 2000). Singhal and colleagues (2003a) have shown that preterm infants with birth weight less than 1,850 grams who received nutrient-enriched formula had higher fasting 32–33 split pro-insulin levels (a marker of insulin resistance) at adolescence. This effect of postnatal diet was a proxy for greater weight gain in infants in the first 2 weeks of life, independently of birth weight, gestational age, and other sociodemographic factors.

The authors propose that relative undernutrition in preterm infants early in life may actually have beneficial long-term effects on insulin resistance. Similar beneficial effects on vascular structure and endothelial function were also observed (Singhal et al., 2004). These studies have raised further controversy regarding the nutritional management of very preterm infants and what should be considered "optimal" catch-up growth.

Other studies have also shown high rates of type II diabetes in individuals who were small for gestational age at birth and who later became overweight as adults (Bavdekar et al., 1999; Eriksson et al., 1999; Newsome et al., 2003). In a recent prospective longitudinal study of 1,492 Indian subjects 26 to 32 years of age, the growth of children in whom impaired glucose tolerance or diabetes later developed was characterized by a low body mass index between birth and 2 years of age, followed by an early adiposity rebound and a sustained and accelerated increase in body mass index until adulthood (Bhargava et al., 2004). In two other studies with young adults, individuals who experienced the largest increase in body mass index and those who remained overweight over time had evidence of vascular change manifest by increased common carotid intima-media thickness (CIMT) (to estimate cardiovascular risk) (Eriksson et al., 2001; Oren et al., 2003). Thus the association of low birth weight and later CVD and metabolic factors is very likely modified by postnatal factors, although this has not been adequately studied.

Body composition, specifically the distribution of the fat and lean bone mass compartments, may also be important predictors of risk of CVD, hypertension and diabetes in adult life. Fat mass and fat-free mass were lower in 8- to 12-year-old children born with birth weights less than 1,850 grams than in children born with normal birth weights (Fewtrell et al., 2004). Such findings may reflect programming of body composition by early growth and nutrition. Indeed, a higher birth weight was associated with a greater fat free mass in adolescents (Singhal et al., 2003b). The authors suggest that an association of low birth weight and lower lean mass may be the underpinnings of programming for suboptimal insulin sensitivity, lower metabolic activity, and a subsequent propensity to greater adiposity and risk of CVD (Singhal et al., 2003b).

Using whole-body magnetic resonance, Uthaya and colleagues (2005) have recently shown that by the time that infants born preterm reached their term age, they had a highly significant decrease in subcutaneous adipose tissue and significantly increased levels of intra-abdominal adipose tissue. They caution that preterm infants may be at risk of metabolic complications later in life through this increased and aberrant adiposity. In a cohort of 132 20-year-old individuals who had been born small for gestational age and average for gestational age and who were born fullterm (Levitt et al., 2005), the association between low birth weight and expression of adult chronic cardiometabolic disease was not dependent on birth weight alone, but was also dependent on its interaction with subsequent fat accumulation (either generally or abdominally) (Levitt et al., 2005).

Fewer studies have explored the association of preterm birth and CVD in adulthood. Irving and colleagues (2000) investigated 61 young adults who had been born with low birth weights less than 2,000 grams at a mean age of 24 years and showed that those who were small because of prematurity were also at risk of hypertension, an adverse metabolic profile (higher plasma insulin triglyceride and total cholesterol levels and lower high-density lipoprotein cholesterol levels) and hyperglycemia as adults. Among the preterm cohort, those who were small for gestational age were not measurably more disadvantaged than those who were average for gestational age. CIMT studies, however, were not performed. A study conducted in the Netherlands attempted to elucidate the effects of prenatal and infancy growth on the lipid and CIMT measures in a very preterm cohort at age 19 years (Martin et al., 2006). Their findings support an effect of current body composition rather than early growth on CVD risk. Two recent studies (Doyle et al., 2003; Hack et al., 2005a) have shown higher systolic blood pressure among very low birth weight infants in late adolescence and young adulthood. However, no relationship was found between intrauterine growth and blood pressure. Not all studies have found higher blood pressure in preterm subjects in childhood (Morley et al., 1994) or at young adulthood (Saigal et al., 2005). Further prospective, long-term studies of preterm infants monitored to adulthood are warranted to confirm whether preterm infants are at increased risk for CVD and metabolic problems as adults.

IMPACT OF PRETERM BIRTH ON FAMILIES

Families caring for a child born preterm face long-term and multilayered challenges. The limited research on this topic suggests that this impact is largely negative (Beckman and Pokorni, 1988; Cronin et al., 1995; Davis et al., 2003; Eisengart et al., 2003; Lee et al., 1991; Macey et al., 1987; McCain, 1990; McCormick et al., 1986; Singer et al., 1999; Stjernqvist and Svenningsen, 1995; Taylor et al., 2001; Veddovi et al., 2001), although some studies found positive outcomes (Macey et al., 1987; Saigal et al., 2000a; Singer et al., 1999). Furthermore, the impact varies according to sociodemographic risk factors as well as the severity of the child's health condition (Beckman and Pokorni, 1988; Cronin et al., 1995; Davis et al., 2003; Eisengart et al., 2003; Lee et al., 1991; McCormick et al., 1986; Rivers et al., 1987; Saigal et al., 2000a; Singer et al., 1999; Taylor et al., 2001; Veddovi et al., 2001).

Most studies on the impact of caring for a preterm infant have focused on those born at less than 32 weeks gestation (Davis et al., 2003) and less than 35 weeks of gestation (Veddovi et al., 2001), although others studied infants with birth weights less than 1,500 grams or less than 1,750 grams (Eisengart et al., 2003; Macey et al., 1987; Singer et al., 1999). Others have used prematurity and low birth weight as a continuous variable (Beckman and Pokorni, 1988). The assessment of outcomes has centered on the mother's psychological well-being in the postpartum period and suggests that the mothers of infants born preterm are at risk of experiencing depressive symptoms (Davis et al., 2003; Singer et al., 1999; Veddovi et al., 2001). Longitudinal studies of children born preterm and with low birth weights in the first 2 to 3 years of life suggest that the levels of maternal depression and psychological distress (Singer et al., 1999), as well as problems related to the child, decreased over time (Beckman and Pokorni, 1988) except among high-risk (defined as having bronchopulmonary dysplasia) infants (Singer et al., 1999). Furthermore, specific factors that may contribute to depressive symptoms include a higher medical risk for the infants, the less frequent use of informal networks to obtain information about their infants, increased use of escape-avoidance coping strategies, and less knowledge of infant development (Eisengart et al., 2003; Veddovi et al., 2001). On the other hand, factors that might buffer these mothers from depressive symptoms include a higher level of educational attainment and support from nurses (Davis et al., 2003).

Families caring for a child who was born preterm continue to manage the effects of prematurity when the children are toddlers (Lee et al., 1991; McCormick et al., 1986; Singer et al., 1999), school age (Cronin et al., 1995; Lee et al., 1991; McCain, 1990; Rivers et al., 1987; Taylor et al., 2001), and adolescents (Saigal et al., 2000a). Studies focusing on these children have mainly included children who were born weighing less than 2,500 grams (Cronin et al., 1995; Lee et al., 1991; McCormick et al., 1986; Rivers et al., 1987; Singer et al., 1999; Taylor et al., 2001); and only one focused on children born weighing less than 1,000 grams (Saigal et al., 2000a). Their findings suggest that the impact on families is long term and that the parents, siblings, finances, and family functioning are all affected (Cronin et al., 1995; Saigal et al., 2000a; Singer et al., 1999; Taylor et al., 2001). Furthermore, the families of children with more severe levels of impairment are the most affected (Cronin et al., 1995; Rivers et al., 1987; Saigal et al., 2000a; Singer et al., 1999; Taylor, 2001).

At the individual level of the impact of a preterm birth on the family, the parents of children born preterm report higher levels of emotional distress (Saigal et al., 2000a; Singer et al., 1999; Taylor et al., 2001) and strain and a compromised sense of mastery (Cronin et al., 1995). One study suggests that some of the factors that parents associate with higher stress levels might include supervision of the child, the child's peer relationships and self-esteem, the impact of the child's difficulties on family routines, and worrying about the child's future (Taylor et al., 2001). The length of time that the newborn preterm infant must stay in the hospital also affects the ability of the mother to fulfill her role in the family (McCain, 1990).

Other studies suggest that there might be gender role differences in parents' perception of problems. Mothers perceived that the preterm birth of a child had a greater impact on their sense of mastery, finances, and employment (Cronin et al., 1995). They also perceived greater satisfaction in caring for their child (Cronin et al., 1995). The mothers also perceived a greater impact when the child was born at a younger gestational age (Lee et al., 1991), experienced more physical symptoms during the pregnancy, and were more likely than the fathers to experience crisis reactions (Stjernqvist, 1992). On the other hand, fathers perceived greater uncertainty, less individual strain (Cronin et al., 1995), and greater effects at lower levels of progression of the infant's development (Lee et al., 1991).

Beyond the impact on each of the parents individually, caring for children born preterm affects other units within the family, including the couple, the siblings, and the family as a whole (Beckman and Pokorni, 1988; Cronin et al., 1995; Macey et al., 1987; McCormick et al., 1986; Saigal et al., 2000a; Singer et al., 1999; Stjernqvist, 1992; Taylor et al., 2001). Specifically, the parent's marital relationship is stressed (Macey et al., 1987; Stjernqvist, 1992), at times leading to divorce (Saigal et al., 2000a), and parenting difficulties emerge (Taylor et al., 2001). Siblings are affected because of the decreased attention that they receive from their parents (Saigal et al., 2000a). The family as a unit is affected by the greater likelihood of not having additional children (Cronin et al., 1995; Saigal et al., 2000a), the financial burden (Cronin et al., 1995; Macey et al., 1987; McCormick et al., 1986; Rivers et al., 1987), limits on family social life (Cronin et al., 1995; McCormick et al., 1986), high levels of adverse family outcomes (family stress and dysfunction) (Beckman and Pokorni, 1988; Singer et al., 1999; Taylor et al., 2001), and parents' difficulty maintaining employment (Macey et al., 1987; Saigal et al., 2000a). Lower income and education place an additional burden on families caring for children born preterm (Cronin et al., 1995; McCormick et al., 1986; Taylor et al., 2001), although one study found that the higher medical risks faced by neonates had more significant impacts on socioeconomically advantaged families (Taylor et al., 2001).

Furthermore, different factors predict family stress at different ages (Beckman and Pokorni, 1988). When the neonate born preterm was 3 months of age, it was found that informal support, the number of siblings, and the family's socioeconomic condition were the most important factors; at 6 months of age, gestational age at birth, home environment, caregiving demands, and the number of parents in the home were the most important;

at 12 months of age, race, home environment, and scores on the Bayley scales of infant development were the most important; and at 24 months of age, birth weight at birth, informal social support, temperament, caregiving demands, and race were the most important (Beckman and Pokorni, 1988).

Families and parents also have positive experiences and demonstrate resilience in caring for a child with impairments related to preterm birth. A study by Saigal and colleagues (2000a) found that parents perceived positive interactions with friends and within the family stemming from their efforts to care for their child born with birth weight less than 1,000 grams. The parents also reported enhanced personal feelings and improved marital closeness (Saigal et al., 2000a). Macey and colleagues (1987) found that at 12 months (corrected for prematurity), 50 percent of the infants' mothers perceived their marriage to be more cohesive. Other studies suggest that these parents perceive their children to be acceptable, attached, and reinforcing (Singer et al., 1999) and to have a greater appreciation for their child than was the case when the child was an infant (Rivers et al., 1987). Thus, the impact of caring for a child born preterm may also contribute to the growth of the family as well as its members.

In summary, the limited evidence presented here suggests that caring for a child born preterm has negative and positive impacts on the family that change over time, that these impacts extend to adolescence and are influenced by different environmental factors across time, and that many areas of family well-being are affected. However, because of the limitations of these studies, further research is needed. First, these findings are limited in their generalizability because of a lack of ethnic and socioeconomic diversity in the samples and because a higher proportion of mothers than fathers were surveyed. Research should strive to balance these sociodemographic factors in the samples used. Second, the measures used to determine the effects of a child born preterm on the family and the child's functional health were not uniform across studies. For example, the effects on the family were measured as the economic burden, parental symptomatology, and parenting stress, among others. Similarly, the child's health and functional health status were assessed on the basis of the presence of serious health conditions in one study, whereas other studies formally assessed functional health status by the use of validated measures.

Future studies could advance knowledge in this area by developing a measure that would capture the particular health and functional health challenges that these families and the children born preterm face. In a recent review of functional health outcomes of preterm children, Donohue (2002) suggested that measures that are sensitive to the child's developmental stage should be developed for children and that the measures for parents should focus on the peculiarities of their role as caregivers for these children.

Third, the few longitudinal studies reviewed in this section suggest that future research is needed to study changes in the impact of a child born preterm on the family over time. The fourth limitation noted in the studies reviewed were the variations in the gestational ages and the birth weights of the infants. Researchers should be encouraged to focus on prematurity by gestational age in addition to birth weight, so that the variations in the impacts on families can be ascertained by gestational age. Finally, studies of the impacts of an infant born preterm on families during the child's infancy should assess outcomes beyond maternal depressive symptoms in the postpartum period.

POST-NICU DISCHARGE INTERVENTIONS

In recognition of the increased developmental and emotional risks for children born preterm, several interventions have focused on the provision of services in the early years of life to prevent subsequent developmental and health problems. Coordinated, community-based, multidisciplinary programs for early intervention, based on the findings of some seminal studies, have been established for children and their families. The types and severities of the conditions affecting children with disabilities are varied, and so are the intensity and the extent of the services provided. Research suggests that these programs may be effective in improving some cognitive outcomes in individual children and can also lead to important improvements in family function (Berlin et al., 1998; Majnemer, 1998; McCormick et al., 1998; Ramey et al., 1992; Ramey and Ramey, 1999). However, long-term follow-up of the children in some of these studies has shown mixed results, with some evidence that differences apparent within 3 years of an intervention all but disappear after time.

Early Infant and Childhood Interventions

Several longitudinal studies have attempted to ascertain the effects of early intervention on the emotional, physical, and developmental outcomes in children born preterm or with disabilities. The Infant Health and Development Program (IHDP) is a multicentered, randomized, controlled, U.S. nationwide study of preterm infants born in 1985 at gestational ages of less than 37 weeks and with birth weights of less than 2,500 grams and their families. Infants and their families were randomly assigned to either the intervention group (n = 377) or the follow-up-only (FUO) group (n = 608) within two birth weight strata: less than 2,000 grams and 2,000 to 2,499 grams. For their first 3 years, both groups received medical, developmental, and social assessments, as well as referrals for services such as health care. An educational intervention for infants and families in the intervention group consisted of home visits (weekly during the first year and every other week thereafter), enrollment in a child development center at 12 months from the due date, and parent group meetings (Ramey et al., 1992). The educational sessions at home and the center encouraged parents to use games and activities to promote their child's cognitive, language, and social skills development; and parents were provided with information on health, safety, and child-rearing topics.

At the outcome evaluation at 36 months from the due date, the children in the intervention group had higher cognitive scores (14 points higher for those with birth weights of 2,000 to 2,499 grams and 7 points higher for those with birth weights of less than 2,000 grams) and fewer behavioral problems than the children in the FUO group (Brooks-Gunn et al., 1992b; McCormick et al., 1993). Receptive language, visual motor, and spatial skills were also improved for those in the intervention group. Even among the smallest infants; that is, those with birth weights of less than 1,500 grams and less than 1,000 grams, IQ scores were higher and behavior was better with the early intervention. The effects were the greatest for the highest-risk children, whose parents had no more than a high school education or were of an ethnic-racial minority status (Brooks-Gunn, 1992a,b). The effects were long lasting for children with birth weights of 2,000 to 2,499 grams. The children of well-educated mothers did not benefit from the intervention (McCormick et al., 1998). Mothers who had less than a high school education reported less emotional distress as a result of the intervention (Klebanov et al., 2001). These findings suggest that early intervention programs should especially target children and families at risk for poor outcomes.

The cohort in the IHDP study was again evaluated at 5, 8, and 18 years of age (Brooks-Gunn, 1992a,b; McCarton et al., 1997; McCormick et al., 2006). Among children with birth weights of 2,000 to 2,499 grams, the differences in IQ scores, behavior, and math and reading achievement persisted, although for the IQ scores the difference decreased to 4 points. In adolescence, the intervention group reported lower rates of engagement in risky behavior (e.g., substance use or delinquency). These findings are consistent with those of other long-term studies of single-site educational interventions for poor healthy children (Campbell et al., 2002; Reynolds et al., 2001; Belfield et al., 2006). The lack of a persistent difference in those with birth weights of less than 2,000 grams raises questions about their subsequent experiences and the need for more sustained support for neurologically vulnerable children.

Avon Premature Infant Project

The United Kingdom Avon Premature Infant Project was a randomized controlled trial in which the parents of 284 infants born at less than 33 weeks gestation received a home-based developmental education program, a social support intervention, or standard care (Johnson et al., 2005). A fullterm reference population served as a control group. Although there were some differences in cognitive, motor, and behavioral outcomes at 2 years of age, there were no differences at 5 years of age (mean age, 58 months and 15 days) among the intervention groups. The children born preterm had poorer cognitive performance than their peers born fullterm. Further analyses, in which the outcomes data were adjusted for social factors, did not reveal any differences between the intervention groups or between subgroups classified by a range of perinatal variables. The authors concluded that the small advantage shown at 2 years of age is no longer detectable at 5 years of age and questioned the effectiveness of early intervention in sustained cognitive, behavioral, and motor functions.

National Early Intervention Longitudinal Study

The National Early Intervention Longitudinal Study (NEILS), sponsored by the Office of Special Education Programs of the U.S. Department of Education, is monitoring more than 3,338 children who have disabilities or who are at risk for disabilities and their families through their experiences in early intervention and into early elementary school. Information about the characteristics of the children and their families, the services that they receive, and the outcomes that they experience is being collected. A nationally representative sample of children between birth and 31 months of age and their families who began early intervention services for the first time between September 1997 and November 1998 has been recruited for the study. NEILS is focusing on, among other issues, the early intervention services that participating children and families receive and the outcomes that participating children and families experience. Because this study will also assess how outcomes relate to variations in child and family characteristics and the services that they received, it has particular relevance for infants born preterm and their families.

A three-stage stratified sampling procedure was used to identify the original sample for the study. Twenty states were selected on the basis of the number of children served in early intervention and the region of the country. These states represented considerable variation with regard to the lead agency and whether or not the agencies served children at risk. The second stage involved the selection of counties on the basis of the estimated number of children served in Part C programs.[1] Three to seven counties

---

[1]Part C of the Individuals with Disabilities Education Act elevated the family component of early intervention to a new level. This legislation replaced the Individualized Education Program for children ages 3 to 21 years with the Individualized Family Service Plan for infants and toddlers with disabilities.

were selected within each state, for a total of 93 counties. The children ranged in age from birth to 30 months when they began receiving early intervention services (between 1997 and 1998).

The initial results from this study have been favorable. In a 2004 report by Bailey et al., it was found that most parents considered early intervention to have had a significant impact on their families, reporting that their families were much better off (59 percent) or somewhat better off (23 percent) as a result of the help and information that the early intervention program provided. Most parents (96 percent) also believed that they were able to help their children learn and develop, although in comparison, when they were asked about their perceived competence in caring for their child's basic needs, fewer (64 percent) reported strong agreement and more (32 percent) reported simple agreement.

A separate assessment of functional status over the time of the intervention showed that the proportion of children with vision, hearing, or motor skills problems stayed constant over the period of the intervention. However, some children who had problems with communication when the services began showed improvement over time (Markowitz, 2004). The assessment also found that 96 percent of the families reported that the intervention helped them become more proficient in working with professionals and advocating for their child's needs.

Summary

Although the short-term impact of early interventions has been well demonstrated, the findings of evaluations of the long-term impact of early interventions for preterm infants have been ambiguous. Long-term prenatal and perinatal cohort studies conducted before the introduction of neonatal intensive care concluded that social factors and the quality of the home environment can compensate for the disadvantages encountered perinatally and neonatally (Wolke, 1998). Recent evidence shows that intervention providing social and environmental enhancement through home visits and child development programs, is associated with catch-up in cognitive and behavioral development in large preterm infants, especially those from socieconomically disadvantaged backgrounds (Brooks-Gunn et al., 1994; Olds and Kitzman, 1993; Ramey and Ramey, 1999). This suggests that these larger preterm infants may not have persistent central nervous system insults. In contrast, although early interventions may have an impact on the outcomes for smaller preterm infants, biological factors may be the best predictors of cognitive and behavioral outcomes at school age.

However, McCormick (1997) and others have argued that the lack of comparability across studies that use such a broad categorization of morbidity is but one methodological flaw recurring in the follow-up literature. Other methodological problems include the failure to characterize the study samples by the eligibility for the study and the number of losses in the cohort, the failure to provide sufficient information with which the representativeness of the sample can be assessed, and the failure to use appropriate controls (McCormick, 1997). In addition, the outcomes being assessed may be too limited. Finally, even for the outcomes selected, many studies fail to incorporate a specific underlying pathogenic or conceptual model to identify potential factors influencing the relationship between the initial state (i.e., prematurity or low birth weight) and the outcomes observed (McCormick, 1997).

Finding 11-4: Early childhood educational and other therapeutic research interventions have been demonstrated to improve outcomes for some infants born preterm; however, it is critical to determine the appropriate intensity, type of service, personnel, and curricula to achieve improvement in interventions.

CONCLUSION

There is a wide range of health and neurodevelopmental outcomes for infants born preterm, and many resources are required to provide the necessary medical, neurodevelopmental and educational support for the children and support for their families. More outcomes data are reported by birth weight categories than by gestational age categories, but until better measures of organ maturation are available, information regarding gestational age is necessary for medical decision making and parent counseling when a preterm delivery is anticipated. Because of their long-term impact, health care providers should focus not on preterm birth but on degree of organ maturity at birth and on short and long-term neurodevelopmental, functional, and health outcomes. Just as the etiologies of preterm birth are multifactorial, the neurodevelopmental, functional, and health outcomes of infants born preterm are determined by interactions among the genome, intrauterine environment, high-risk obstetric and neonatal intensive care provided, the home environment, and available community resources. Future research to develop better predictors of outcomes should focus on the relationships between brain structural and functional development, areas of the brain typically affected by brain insult and corresponding neurodevelopmental and behavioral deficits, and how organ recovery and plasticity occur. Better predictors of outcomes will allow for improved parent counseling, enhance safety of trials of maternal and infant interventions by providing more immediate feedback, and facilitate planning for use of comprehensive follow-up and early intervention resources. Until preterm birth can be prevented, much work also needs to be done to develop treatment strategies that prevent injury to the brain and other organs and support the infant's ongoing development.

12

Societal Costs of Preterm Birth

ABSTRACT

Based on new estimates provided in this chapter, the annual societal economic burden associated with preterm birth in the United States was at least $26.2 billion in 2005, or $51,600 per infant born preterm. Medical care services contributed $16.9 billion to the total cost and maternal delivery costs contributed another $1.9 billion. In terms of longer-term expenditures, early intervention services cost an estimated $611 million, whereas special education services associated with a higher prevalence of four disabling conditions among premature infants added $1.1 billion. Finally, the committee estimates that lost household and labor market productivity associated with those disabilities contributed $5.7 billion.

While more comprehensive than any previous estimate of the cost of preterm birth in the United States, this $26.2 billion estimate is a floor, or minimum. Except for lifetime medical care costs associated with four major disabling conditions, it does not include the cost of medical care beyond early childhood. It includes special educational services and lost productivity costs only for those four conditions, and it includes no caretaker costs. It includes only maternal medical care costs associated with delivery. More comprehensive and refined estimates therefore need to be generated so that policies can be crafted and resources can be directed to obtaining a *better understanding of the full scope of the growing economic burden of preterm birth in the United States.*

The proportions of the total cost accounted for by each cost category mentioned above should be considered with caution, as the estimates reflect a higher degree of precision with respect to what can be most readily assessed for categories of cost that have drawn more extensive resources for their determination, such as early inpatient care, than for cost categories that pose greater methodological challenges for determination and that have received less attention, such as caregiver and maternal costs other than those involved with delivery.

While previous chapters in this report summarize and assess the literature on the causes and consequences of preterm birth, this chapter presents the results of new research undertaken by the Committee on the economic consequences of preterm birth, and places this research within the context of a select literature on the topic. A more systematic review of the literature on the cost of preterm birth can be found in Appendix D (Zupancic, 2006). Medical care costs in infancy for children born preterm, particularly those related to initial hospitalization, have received relatively extensive attention in the published literature compared with the amount of attention given to noninpatient and postinfancy medical care costs (Zupancic, 2006).

Based on the Committee's estimates, the annual societal economic burden associated with preterm birth in the United States was at least $26.2 billion in 2005, or $51,600 per infant born preterm (Table 12-1). The referent for these estimates was the resources expended on full-term infants; that is, these costs are above and beyond what would have been expended had these infants been born at term. Nearly two-thirds of the societal cost was accounted for by medical care. The share that medical care services contributed to the total cost was $16.9 billion ($33,200 per preterm infant), with more than 85 percent of those medical care services delivered in infancy. Maternal delivery costs contributed another $1.9 billion ($3,800 per preterm infant). Early intervention services cost an estimated $611 million ($1,200 per preterm infant), whereas special education services associated with a higher prevalence of four disabling conditions including cerebral palsy (CP), mental retardation (MR), vision impairment (VI), and hearing loss (HL) among premature infants added $1.1 billion ($2,200 per preterm infant). Lost household and labor market productivity associated with those disabilities contributed $5.7 billion ($11,200 per preterm infant).

These new cost estimates for medical care received beyond infancy for those born preterm are among the first ever such estimates obtained in the

TABLE 12-1 Estimated Cost of Preterm Birth, United States, Aggregate and Cost per Case

| Cost | Medical Care Costs | | | Early Intervention Costs | Special Education Costs (4 DDs) | Lost Productivity Costs (4 DDs) | Maternal Delivery Costs | Total Costs |
	Birth to Age 5 Years	6 years & older (4 DDs)	Total					
Aggregate (millions)	15,887	976	16,863	611	1,094	5,694	1,935	26,197
Per case	31,290	1,920	33,210	1,203	2,150	11,214	3,812	51,589

NOTE: All amounts are in 2005 dollars. 4 DD = the four developmental disabilities.

United States. Nevertheless, the estimates beyond early childhood include the costs for only a subset of those with the four disabling conditions associated with preterm birth which, in and of themselves, are likely conservative because of the limitations of the data on the level of certain rehabilitation and therapy services provided as well as the costs for long-term care. Of even greater significance, perhaps, is the paucity of evidence regarding certain entire categories of costs. The costs of the caregivers of individuals with disabling conditions, for example, can exceed medical care costs, but insufficient data were available to make reliable national estimates of such costs. Estimates of the costs of special education services were also limited by the inclusion of data for special education services for only a subset of the disabling conditions associated with preterm birth. With the exception of the incremental services associated with delivery, maternal care costs were not tabulated.

The relative concentration of medical care costs among extremely preterm infants (less than 28 weeks of gestation) is noteworthy. Although extremely preterm births represent just 6 percent of all preterm births, extremely preterm infants accounted for more than one-third of the total medical costs associated with preterm birth through 7 years of age. On the other hand, because of the much higher proportion of preterm infants born at 28 to 36 weeks of gestation, very preterm infants (those born at 28 to 31 weeks of gestation) and moderately preterm infants (those born at 32 to 36 weeks of gestation) together accounted for the large majority of the total societal costs of preterm birth. The concentration of costs, however, may provide insight into directing specific sets of resources toward the prevention and treatment of preterm birth in a cost-effective manner.

Also of note is the high level of variation and skew underlying several of the cost estimates, even within gestational age categories. Although high rates of mortality among extremely preterm infants, in particular, affect the variance of the costs, it is not the primary driver of the variance. The upper tail of the distribution of costs for medical care—in some cases, the upper 5 percent—is primarily responsible for the higher average medical care costs for young children born preterm and becomes more dominant as they age. This likely reflects the higher average costs associated with disabling conditions among the minority of individuals with such conditions born preterm. Future research on the societal costs of preterm birth should be designed to permit more detailed investigations of the variance and tails of the cost distribution.

All estimates provided here are lifetime estimates of cost, in 2005 constant dollars, associated with the cohort born preterm in the United States in 2003, the last year for which final estimates on birth by gestational age were available from the National Center on Health Statistics. Costs beyond the first year of life were discounted at a 3 percent rate back to the year of birth, in accordance with the economic principle that current consumption is valued over future consumption and with the accepted methodologies used to determine the cost of illness (Gold et al., 1996). The remainder of this chapter provides greater detail on the methodology used to make national estimates of the cost of preterm birth as well as a more detailed breakdown of the summary costs provided above by cost category. Part of the literature on cost-effectiveness with respect to preterm birth is also addressed.

COST-OF-ILLNESS METHODOLOGY
APPLIED TO PRETERM BIRTH

The societal costs associated with illness are conventionally broken down into direct and indirect costs. Direct costs include the value of the resources used to treat the condition, such as medical care, special education, and developmental services. Indirect costs include the value of resources lost to society, such as the reduced labor market productivity or the reduced level of household productivity due to heightened morbidity or premature mortality. Costs are incremental relative to referent or counterfactual assumptions. Except where otherwise stated, the estimates of the societal costs of preterm birth provided here use term birth (37 weeks of gestation or greater) as the referent.

The relevant costs included are not conceptually restricted to those associated with the affected individual. Maternal, caregiver, and family costs are also relevant. Maternal costs include the incremental costs of prenatal care and delivery services, the costs of any extended care associated with maternal morbidity arising from the pregnancy, and the costs of added precautionary care in subsequent pregnancies, even if the subsequent birth goes to term. Caregiver costs appropriately include travel expenses for extended care of the preterm infant, in addition to the incremental value of time devoted to caring for the infant or child born preterm.

Insufficient information was available to estimate reliably the national burden for all of the cost categories listed above. However, estimates were made for a portion of the lifetime costs for medical care, special education services, and household and work productivity losses for the affected individual. A national estimate of early intervention services was also made, based on the extent and cost of such services provided in Massachusetts. Among the family costs, only an estimate of maternal delivery costs was included.

New estimates of the inpatient and outpatient medical care costs associated with preterm birth through 7 years of age are provided on the basis of the medical care services provided to a cohort of 23,631 individuals born in Utah from 1998 to 2000 and covered under a major integrated health care system. These data also served as the basis for making maternal delivery cost estimates. Additional estimates on the incremental lifetime medical care costs beyond age 5 years are provided for four disabling conditions associated with preterm birth: CP, MR, VI, and HL. Estimates of incremental special education costs and lost household and labor market productivity were also tabulated for these conditions. All estimates of preterm birth associated with these conditions drew upon published analyses and unpublished tabulations from the Metropolitan Atlanta Developmental Disability Surveillance Program (MADDSP).

The cost estimates presented capture the annual discounted present value of the resources projected to be used or lost by the cohort born preterm in a single year rather than the costs incurred annually by the prevalent population in the nation that was born preterm. This cohort, or "incidence," approach essentially involves the construction of a synthetic cohort on the basis of current patterns of resource utilization by age or age category. The cost estimates obtained by this approach lend themselves particularly well to the evaluation of programs aimed at prevention.

MEDICAL CARE COSTS DUE TO PRETERM BIRTH

Birth to Early Childhood

To date, research on the medical care costs of preterm birth has focused nearly exclusively on inpatient care, primarily on the initial hospitalization of the infant (Zupancic, 2006). Certain studies have provided estimates of inpatient hospitalization costs exclusively for infants born with extremely low birth weights (The Victorian Infant Collaborative Study Group, 1997) or very low birth weights (VLBWs) (Rogowski, 2003), others have provided estimates exclusively by gestational age (Phibbs and Schmitt, 2006), and still others have provided estimates by both gestational age and birth weight (BW) (Gilbert et al., 2003; Schmitt et al., 2006). This literature has drawn specific attention to the high costs associated with neonatal intensive care for preterm infants. More than two-thirds of infants born extremely premature (at less than 28 weeks of gestation) and more than one-third of infants born very premature (at 28 to 31 weeks of gestation) in California who survived infancy in 1996 had respiratory distress syndrome and received mechanical ventilation in their initial hospitalization. In comparison, less than 1 percent of infants born at term received mechanical ventilation in their initial hospitalization (Gilbert et al., 2003). Ancillary costs, including respiratory care, laboratory, radiology, and pharmacy costs, contribute heavily to the costs of intensive care for low birth weight (LBW) infants. They represented over 25 percent of the median $53,316 in initial hospitalization costs for those born with VLBWs (<1,500 grams) in a group of hospitals belonging to the Vermont Oxford Network in 1997 and 1998 (Rogowski, 2003).

Less research has been conducted on the medical care expenses of preterm birth beyond early hospitalization. Comprehensive data on medical care delivery and cost for the cohort of infants born between 1998 and 2000 who were covered by Intermountain Healthcare (IHC) Health Plans and who were monitored from birth through 2004 afforded the opportunity to analyze inpatient and outpatient medical care costs associated with preterm birth from birth to age 7 years, well beyond the term covered by any previous study in the United States. In making national estimates, it would have been preferable to have data from several rather than from a single health plan. Resource constraints faced by the committee precluded the incorporation of data from additional plans. As noted below, however, substantial effort was undertaken to stratify the sample and adjust estimates so as to make valid approximation of costs for the nation as a whole.

IHC is a large, nonprofit, fully integrated health care organization headquartered in Utah. In addition to providing a comprehensive set of medical care services under its Health Plans, it also provides services to patients under contract with Medicaid and Medicare, patients covered under non-IHC commercial insurance, and privately paying patients, as well as those receiving charitable care.

Of the 139,517 estimated live births in Utah between 1998 and 2000 (NCHS, 2004b), 81,931, or 59 percent of the total, were born within the IHC network of facilities. One-third of those births were covered under IHC Health Plans, 38 percent were covered by other commercial insurance, 22 percent were covered by Medicaid, and 7 percent were covered through other sources of private payment or by charity.

Finding 12-1: The medical costs of preterm birth during infancy, particularly during the neonatal period, are high and the medical needs are relatively well understood. The long-term medical, educational, productivity, and productivity costs borne by the individual, as well as by the family and society, are not well understood.

The detailed estimates of costs presented here were based strictly on the cohort covered under IHC Health Plans, as records of service utilization and cost were comprehensive for that cohort. The application of exclusion criteria based on clear coding errors for gestational age (less than 22 weeks or more than 43 weeks of gestation) or BW (<450 or >5,000 grams) or the presence of missing fields in certain instances resulted in 23,631 Health Plan infants in the cohort as of birth; 1,902 of these infants were born preterm. By the end of the 48th month of follow-up, the last possible month for all surviving infants in the cohort to be monitored, given the 2004 cut-off, 11,357 subjects (48 percent of the total) remained. The corresponding numbers (percentages) remaining at 48 months by gestational age were 36 (40 percent) among those born at less than 28 weeks of gestation, 73 (42 percent) among those born at 28 to 31 weeks of gestation, 754 (46 percent) among those born at 32 to 36 weeks of gestation, and 10,494 (48 percent) among those born at 37 weeks of gestation or later. To maintain robustness, resource utilization and cost estimates were pooled for the cohort over years 3 and 4 and for years 5 through 7.[1]

Extrapolation of health care utilization and costs across organizations and across geographic areas is potentially confounded by differences in demographics, including the underlying health status of populations, as well as by differences in the health care delivery conventions by provider. For that reason, adjustments of charges to costs and adjustments of costs for differences across geographic areas may not be sufficient to project cost estimates from one region to the nation as a whole. Risk adjustment based on differences in population characteristics and further adjustment for organizational differences in the delivery of care may also be required (Rogowski, 1999).

A comparison of demographic and vital statistics, as well as of health care utilization and costs, between the IHC Health Plans cohort and those served outside of the plan but within the IHC network of facilities, was therefore made. A further comparison of the results with published results from other studies on initial hospitalization costs and costs outside of Utah was also performed. The comparison of demographic characteristics and vital statistics of the Health Plans cohort of births with other births in IHC facilities between 1998 and 2000 revealed—as one might expect, given the well-established inverse socioeconomic gradients in the rates of preterm birth and LBW—that those covered by IHC Health Plans were less likely to be born preterm (8.5 percent) and of LBW (6 percent) than those born in IHC facilities and covered by Medicaid (11.2 and 8.7 percent, respectively).

---

[1]These estimates of those remaining in the cohort include all those still enrolled in Health Plans, even if they did not receive medical care services during a specific period. With an additional mortality adjustment, these essentially served as denominators for calculating average cost. Attrition occurred either because of mortality or because of loss of eligibility for coverage. Estimates were adjusted for mortality based on national figures, as discussed below. As long as resource utilization for those otherwise dropping coverage were similar to those remaining in the health plan, such attrition would not affect the estimates. Some attrition, however, particularly among those born extremely premature, was likely due to infants reaching a $1 million lifetime limit. While not common, the selection out of such infants introduced a downward bias into the estimates.

The rates of preterm birth and LBW among births covered by other commercial insurance were nearly identical to those in the IHC Health Plan cohort. The overall rate of preterm birth in the United States in 1999–2000 was 11.6 percent (MacDorman et al., 2005). The rate of infant mortality for those born extremely prematurely and for those born with VLBWs was lower in the IHC Health Plans cohort than in the cohort cared for in IHC facilities not covered by Health Plans; but summary statistics (mean, median, interquartile ranges, and box plots) revealed that the rate of neonatal intensive care unit utilization, the average length of stay, and the average cost of treatment for the initial hospitalization by gestational age were not significantly different between those who were covered by IHC Health Plans and those who were covered by Medicaid or other commercial insurance in IHC facilities. With the incorporation of adjustments for mortality, in other words, the IHC Health Plan cohort yielded reliable estimates of average service utilization across plans by gestational age and BW.

The levels of health care provision under the umbrella of a single organization and for a population with demographics different from those for the nation as a whole (in Utah, the population is younger and has lower proportions of ethnic and racial minorities than the population of the nation as a whole) could still deviate from those for the general population. Because studies of resource utilization associated with preterm birth have been specific to particular organizations or geographic regions, there is no "gold standard" against which a definitive assessment can be made. Table 12-2 provides a summary of the results of several recent studies, including the results for the IHC Health Plans cohort, on the length of stay for initial or early hospitalizations by gestational age and BW. Data from those studies were reconfigured to make more direct comparisons with the IHC Health Plans cohort by gestational age and BW.

The first three columns of Table 12-2 summarize the length-of-stay data for recent population-based studies in the state of California. The samples in each of those studies essentially drew from the same statewide database on hospital discharges linked to vital records. Because of the absence of reporting of charges by the Kaiser Permanente Medical Care System, the lengths of stay for hospitalizations under that system were largely excluded from the statistics in the CA1 and CA2 columns of Table 12-2. The major difference between the hospital stay figures from the study of Gilbert et al. (2003) reported in column CA1 and those from the study of Phibbs and Schmitt (2006) reported in column CA2 is that the former included only survivors of infancy, whereas the latter included all infants. Given that the length of stay for survivors is longer than that for nonsurvivors, it is counterintuitive for the average length of stay reported in the study of Phibbs and Schmitt (2006) to be uniformly longer by gestational age than that reported in the study by Gilbert et al. (2003). Nevertheless, the gradients in the lengths of stay by gestational age are quite similar

TABLE 12-2 Mean Length of Stay for Initial or Early Hospitalizations, by Gestational Age and Birth Weight and by Study

Birth Parameter	Mean Length of Stay (days)							
	CA1	CA2	CA3	NIC/Q	STAT	UK	IHC	(SD)
Gestational age (wk)								
<28	76.0	79.4	NA	NA	NA	24.1	67.4	(41.6)
28–31	31.6	49.8	NA	NA	NA	23.9	44.4	(24.2)
32–36	4.7	5.9	NA	NA	NA	7.2	6.7	(9.3)
All <37	8.0	10.5	NA	NA	16.8[a]	9.3	13.0	16.6[a]
≥37 (term)	1.9[b]	2.6[c]	NA	NA	2.73[a]	3.4	1.5	(1.7)
Birth weight (g)								
<1,500	57.5	NA	47.9	47[d]	NA	NA	53.5	(34.5), 51[d]
1,500–2,500	8.1	NA	9.4	NA	NA	NA	8.4	(11.3)
All <2,500	14.4	NA	16.4	NA	NA	NA	15.9	
≥2,500	1.8	NA	2.3	NA	NA	NA	1.6	(2.1)

NOTE: NA = not available. SD = standard deviation. CA1 = derived from Gilbert et al. (2003) for the cohort of singleton live births in California in 1996 that survived infancy. The length of stay for the initial hospitalization includes interhospital transfers. The estimates largely exclude those for Kaiser Permanente Medical Care Program hospitalizations. CA2 = 1998 to 2000 California birth cohort (Phibbs and Schmitt, 2006). The length of stay is for the initial hospitalization, including interhospital transfers. The estimates largely exclude those for Kaiser Permanente Medical Care Program hospitalizations. CA3 = 2000 California birth cohort (Schmitt et al., 2006). The length of stay is for the initial hospitalization, including interhospital transfers, as well as most Kaiser Permanente Medical Care Program hospitalizations. NIC/Q = Median length of stay for 6,797 VLBW infants born in 1997 and 1998 in 29 of 34 hospitals throughout the United States belonging to the Vermont Oxford Network that participated in the Neonatal Intensive Care Quality Improvement Collaborative in 2000 (Horbar et al., 2003; Rogowski, 2003). The data are strictly the portion of initial hospitalizations within a participating center and therefore exclude that portion of the initial length of stay for 1,364 infants before transfer to a participating center, as well as that portion of the initial stay after transfer out of a participating center (n = 1,264). All data are for before the initiation of the quality improvement initiative. STAT = Medstat (2004). The length of stay is for all hospitalizations in the first year of life, based on 2001 and 2002 claims records for 3,214 premature infants who survived infancy and who were covered as dependents under commercial plans for select large employers in the United States; the selection of premature infants was based on select International Classification of Diseases (Ninth Revision) and diagnosis-related group codes. UK = based on the data of Petrou et al. (2003), covering 239,649 births in southern United Kingdom (Oxfordshire and West Berkshire) from 1970 to 1993. The reported data on initial hospitalizations were based on unpublished tabulations provided to the committee by the authors. IHC = 1998 to 2000 birth cohort (n = 23,631) covered by IHC Health Plans. The data summarize the length of stay for any admissions in the first month, including any readmissions after initial discharge. They exclude transfers associated with the initial hospitalization that took place after the first month of life.

[a]Data are for the entire first year of life.
[b]Data are only for those born at 37 to 38 weeks of gestation.
[c]Data are only for those born at 37 weeks of gestation.
[d]Median length of stay.

between the two studies, and the difference was not statistically significant. The average length of stay and the gradients exhibited by gestational age and BW from the IHC Health Plan cohort reported in the final column are very similar, in this context, to those reported for the California population-based data in columns CA1 to CA3 of Table 12-2.

It should be noted that the IHC data provided in the table summarize the inpatient lengths of stay for all admissions in the first month after birth and therefore exclude transfers from initial hospitalizations that transpire after the first month. The California studies included only the lengths of stay for initial hospitalizations but included all transfers connected to that hospitalization, even if they occurred after the first month. Therefore, among the extremely premature and very premature infants, who have the longest initial hospitalizations and who have the highest rates of transfer after the first month, the California data would be expected to exhibit longer average lengths of stay than the IHC data. Among those born moderately preterm (32 to 36 weeks of gestation), who are more likely to be discharged from their initial hospitalization but then readmitted for other problems within the first month after birth, the IHC data would be expected to reveal relatively longer average lengths of stay. These are the precise patterns exhibited in Table 12-2.

Table 12-2 also reports the median lengths of stay for 6,797 VLBW infants who were born in 1997 and 1998 and who received intensive care in 29 of 34 hospitals located in several states across the United States belonging to the Vermont Oxford Network (Horbar et al., 2003; Rogowski, 2003). Estimates were made before the participation by these hospitals in a neonatal intensive care quality improvement initiative (NIC/Q) beginning in 2000. The 47-day estimate reflects only the portion of initial hospitalizations that transpired within a participating hospital and therefore excludes that portion of the initial length of stay for 1,364 infants before transfer into a study hospital as well as that portion of the initial stay after 1,264 infants transferred out of participating hospitals. Given these exclusion criteria, which generated slightly shorter stays relative to those for the IHC cohort, the median length of stay of 51 days for the IHC cohort is very similar to that of the NIC/Q hospitals.

The STAT column of Table 12-2 is taken from a study of infants who survived their first year of life and provides the average length of stay over that entire year (Medstat, 2004). The sample included infants born between 2000 and 2002 covered under the health plans of certain large employers in the United States. The selection of infants was made on the basis of specific International Classification of Diseases (Ninth Revision) and diagnosis-related group codes and not on the basis of a reported gestational age or BW. Despite such differences, the average length of stay for the IHC cohort, when the length of stay was recalculated for survivors in the entire first year, was 16.6 days, which is nearly identical to the 16.8 days from the Medstat analysis.

Table 12-2 also summarizes data on the length of stay for the initial hospitalization from a population-based cohort study conducted in the United Kingdom (Petrou et al., 2003). The infants in the sample were born between 1970 and 1993 and were monitored for 5 years. Given the vast improvements in neonatal intensive care technology that have taken place since 1970 and that have resulted in dramatic increases in the rates of infant survival, it is not surprising that the average length of stay for the most premature infants in this sample was substantially less than that for the more recent periods in the United States reported in the other columns of Table 12-2. The longer average length of stay among those born at 32 to 36 weeks of gestation and among normal-term infants in the United Kingdom than in the United States reflect the well-established differences in practice patterns between the two countries (Profit et al., 2006).

The comparative data on the length of stay for initial or early hospitalization provided in Table 12-2 suggest that the IHC Health Plans cohort data on health care utilization associated with preterm birth, when adjusted for gestational age and mortality, is reflective of that in other large population-based samples in the United States. When the data are also adjusted for geographic differences in prices, the IHC data were considered sufficiently reliable for the approximation of the rates of medical care utilization and the costs associated with preterm birth for the United States as a whole. Although the intensity and the quality of care per inpatient stay or physician visit cannot be directly observed from the data, they could still create differences in costs between the IHC cohort and the national population. Price-adjusted cost comparisons of initial and early hospital stays by BW between the IHC cohort and those reported in other analyses, however, provided additional support for the conclusion that such differences may not be consequential. An analysis of VLBW infants (birth weights of <1,500 grams) receiving neonatal intensive care in 1997 and 1998 in 29 hospitals belonging to the Vermont Oxford Network, for example, estimated the median cost of the initial hospitalization to be $53,316 in constant 1998 dollars (Rogowski, 2003). Although that study did not include the costs associated with the care received before some transfers to or after some transfers out of the sample hospitals, the comparative figure for first-month hospitalizations among such infants in the IHC cohort was $56,433, which is remarkably similar to that for the Vermont Oxford Network, given the geographic differences and the differences in the costing methodologies applied in the two studies. Geographic and inflation adjustments applied to initial hospitalization costs reported in one California study (Schmitt et al., 2006) demonstrated patterns similar to those reported in Table 12-2 (column CA3) for length of stay.

The algorithm developed by IHC Health Plans for the computation of cost is constructed such that allowed charges are reflective of cost at a detailed level of service provision. Allowed charges for services provided to the IHC cohort between 1998 and 2004 were tabulated and adjusted to 1998 constant dollars on the basis of a separate inflation algorithm developed within IHC. Adjustment of IHC costs to the United States as a whole was based on geographic adjustment factors that were separately constructed for inpatient and outpatient care. The geographic adjustment factor for inpatient care was based on the 1998 Medicare Prospective Payment System wage and capital indices for each metropolitan statistical area (MSA) and for rural Utah. To yield a single inpatient geographic adjustment factor, these area indices were weighted by the population distribution in each Utah MSA and rural Utah, according to intercensus population estimates for 1998; and the capital and wage components were weighted according to their relative contributions to hospital care costs. A parallel method was applied by using Medicare geographic adjustment factors for physician work, practice, and malpractice expenses in Utah to generate an outpatient geographic adjustment factor. An adjustment for national cost inflation between 1998 and 2005 was then made separately for inpatient care and outpatient care on the basis of Medicare Prospective Payment System price adjustments and physician practice expense price adjustments, respectively.

The results for the average medical care cost by gestational age and by year of life are presented in Tables 12-3 through 12-5 separately for inpatient care (Table 12-3), outpatient care (Table 12-4), and total care (Table 12-5). Birth-year inpatient costs constitute the large majority of incremen-

TABLE 12-3 Average Annual Inpatient Costs by Gestational Age and Year of Life, United States, 2005

	Average Annual Inpatient Costs (dollars)			
Gestational Age (wk)	Birth Year	Year 2	Years 3–4	Years 5–7
<28	181,111	2,893	691	123
28–31	85,171	3,519	766	76
32–36	10,855	344	123	66
37–40 (term)	1,895	266	129	64

NOTE: The data are based on the 1998 to 2000 birth cohort covered under IHC Health Plans. The birth-year cost is adjusted for national rates of infant mortality by gestational age (infant deaths were assigned to the first month of life for those born at less than 28 weeks of gestation and to the end of the neonatal period for those born at 28 to 36 weeks of gestation). Normal survival was assumed after infancy. Costs were adjusted geographically to the nation by using Medicare inpatient adjustment factors and were adjusted for inflation between 1998 and 2005 on the basis of the Medicare Prospective Payment System hospital cost index.

TABLE 12-4 Average Annual Outpatient Costs by Gestational Age and
Year of Life, United States, 2005

Gestational Age (wk)	Average Annual Outpatient Costs (dollars)			
	Birth Year	Year 2	Years 3–4	Years 5–7
<28	9,356	9,279	4,254	995
28–31	9,614	4,196	1,767	414
32–36	2,766	1,392	690	557
37–40 (term)	1,430	1,062	532	407

NOTE: The data are based on the 1998 to 2000 birth cohort covered under IHC Health Plans.
The birth-year cost was adjusted for national rates of infant mortality by gestational age (infant deaths were assigned to the first month of life for those born at less than 28 weeks of gestation and to the end of the neonatal period for those born at 28 to 36 weeks of gestation). Normal survival was assumed after infancy. Costs were adjusted to the nation geographically by using Medicare physician practice expense adjustment factors and were adjusted for inflation on the basis of Medicare practice expense inflation between 1998 and 2005.

TABLE 12-5 Average Annual Total Medical Care Costs by Gestational
Age and Year of Life, United States, 2005

Gestational Age (wk)	Average Annual Total Medical Costs (dollars)			
	Birth Year	Year 2	Year 3–4	Years 5–7
<28	190,467	12,172	4,944	1,119
28–31	94,785	7,715	2,534	490
32–36	13,621	1,736	814	643
37–40 (term)	3,325	1,328	661	471

tal medical care costs associated with preterm birth, and the familiar steep
inverse gradient for first-year inpatient medical care costs is evident in the
first column of Table 12-3. Higher incremental inpatient costs are evident
beyond birth through age 4 years for those born at less than 32 weeks of
gestation and through age 7 years for those born at less than 28 weeks
of gestation. Although early inpatient costs are disproportionate relative to
subsequent costs, postinfancy medical care costs associated with preterm
birth are not insignificant. Incremental costs for outpatient care exceed
those for inpatient care beginning in the second year of life, and incremental outpatient care costs continue for children born preterm through age 4
years, regardless of gestational age.

The differences in mean outpatient costs exhibited in Table 12-4 appear to be driven largely by differences in the upper tails of the cost distribution rather than by the median by age 2 (Table 12-6). This upper tail dominance appears to continue with age, particularly for those under 32 weeks of gestation, but sample size limitations because of restriction of the analysis to the upper 5 percent of the sample, coupled with attrition in the later years of the IHC cohort database, precluded a definitive assessment.

The average cost estimates in Tables 12-3 through 12-5 were multiplied by national cohort estimates at each age to make national cost estimates. The size of the birth cohort by gestational age was based on vital statistics for the 2003 birth cohort (Martin et al., 2005), and infant mortality was based on linked birth-death records from 2001 and 2002 (MacDorman et al., 2005). These data indicated that 91, 71, and 56 percent of the cases of infant morality occur in the neonatal period for those born at less than 28, 28 to 31, and 32 to 36 weeks of gestation, respectively. Adjustments were therefore made for average costs in the first year of life for infant mortality, such that all cases of infant mortality were assumed to take place at the end of the first month of life for those born at less than 28 weeks of gestation and at the end of the neonatal period for those born at 28 to 31 and 32 to 36 weeks of gestation. Normal survival was assumed beyond infancy. Costs beyond the first year of life were discounted back to the year of birth at a 3 percent rate. The results for aggregate national costs and the cost per case by gestational age and care category are provided in Table 12-7.

Although the literature on initial hospitalization has often suggested a roughly equal distribution of total inpatient costs between the three groups of infants born preterm—that is, those born extremely preterm (less than 28 weeks of gestation), those born very preterm (28 to 31 weeks of gestation), and those born moderately preterm (32 to 36 weeks of gestation)— the inclusion of a longer period of follow-up in this analysis demonstrates that the overall contribution to inpatient costs among those born extremely preterm is even larger. Given the relatively small numbers of infants born at less than 28 weeks of gestation, this translates into an even steeper cost-concentration curve, with the 6 percent of infants born at less than 28 weeks of gestation accounting for nearly 38 percent of total medical costs (Table 12-7). The cost per preterm infant increases nearly exponentially with each categorical decrease in gestational age. The concentration of neonatal intensive care among those born at the lowest gestational ages, coupled with its very high cost, is a primary driver behind this gradient.

Although the average cost reflects the generally higher cost of preterm birth with progressive decreases in gestational age, the variance of the cost is substantially higher among preterm infants than among term infants. The ratio of the 75th cost percentile to the 25th cost percentile for early inpatient care, for example, is about 3 to 1 for each of the gestational age categories, similar to that found by Phibbs and Schmitt (2006). Although the

TABLE 12-6 Outpatient Medical Care Cost per Case in the Upper Tail of the Cost Distribution by Gestational Age

	Medical Care Cost (dollars)					
	Year 2			Years 3–7		
Gestational Age (wk)	Median	Upper 25%	Upper 5%	Median	Upper 25%	Upper 5%
<28	3,305	7,905	21,117	1,106	3,510	20,127
28–31	785	2,083	12,055	866	1,664	4,432
32–36	533	915	2,658	672	1,545	3,928
37–40 (term)	475	770	1,966	575	1,238	3,149

NOTE: Data are in 1998 dollars.

TABLE 12-7 Total Medical Care Costs of Premature Births by Gestational Age and Category of Service, United States, 2005

Gestational Age (wk)	Aggregate Costs (millions of dollars)			Cost per Case (dollars)		
	Inpatient	Outpatient	Total	Inpatient	Outpatient	Total
<28	5,546	536	6,082	181,409	17,536	198,945
28–31	4,406	669	5,075	87,440	13,285	100,725
32–36	3,855	1,016	4,871	9,034	2,381	11,415
All <37	13,808	2,222	16,030	27,195	4,376	31,571

NOTE: The data are based on the 1998 to 2000 birth cohort covered under IHC Health Plans. The birth-year cost was adjusted for national rates of infant mortality by gestational age (infant deaths were assigned to the first month of life for those born at less than 28 weeks of gestation and to the end of the neonatal period for those born at 28 to 36 weeks of gestation). Normal survival was assumed after infancy. Costs were adjusted geographically to the nation by using Medicare geographic adjustment factors and were adjusted for inflation between 1998 and 2005 on the basis of Medicare cost indices. Costs are incremental, above those of term birth, through age 7 years, with costs beyond infancy discounted to the year of birth at a 3 percent rate. Outpatient care included prescription medications.

distribution of cost is affected by mortality, particularly among those born extremely preterm, the high variance in cost is not driven by mortality (Phibbs and Schmitt, 2006). The association of birth defects with preterm birth (Rasmussen et al., 2001), coupled with the high cost of repair of several of those defects in infancy (Waitzman et al., 1996), may explain part of the variance in cost. More research that formally accounts for comorbidities to explain the variance in cost associated with preterm birth is required.

Finding 12-2: The variance in the costs associated with preterm birth is large, even within gestational age groups. Sufficient knowledge about the factors that explain this variance is not available.

Disability-Specific Costs Beyond Early Childhood

Although few studies have tabulated the medical care costs of preterm birth in early childhood, fewer still have analyzed the medical costs beyond early childhood for those born prematurely. Lifetime estimates of cost, however, have been made for individuals with certain conditions and developmental disabilities associated with preterm birth and LBW, such as specific birth defects (Waitzman et al., 1996), CP (CDC, 2004c; Honeycutt et al., 2003; Waitzman et al., 1996) and MR, HL, and VI (CDC, 2004c; Honeycutt et al., 2003). Prevalence estimates of developmental disabilities in a Centers for Disease Control and Prevention (CDC) study (CDC, 2004c) were drawn from MADDSP, which CDC established in 1991 to identify children with these developmental disabilities (Yeargin-Allsopp et al., 1992). The CDC study, together with unpublished tabulations of differences in the prevalence of each developmental disability by gestational age from MADDSP (see Table 12-8), permitted the assessment of the incremental lifetime direct medical and special education costs as well as the indirect costs of lost household and labor market productivity for those born preterm with the four developmental disabilities presented here.

Cost estimates from the CDC study that served as the basis for cost estimates provided here were based on cross-sectional data on age-specific average service utilization multiplied by average cost or on labor market productivity multiplied by average compensation for those with these developmental disabilities relative to the population as a whole. These cross-sectional data were then applied to a synthetic cohort, based on prevalence data from the MADDSP and on survival estimates from the literature. Costs were discounted back to birth at a 3% rate.

Service utilization, labor market participation rates, and cost estimates were made from national databases. The primary sources for disability-specific service utilization were the 1994 and 1995 National Health Interview Survey-Disability Supplement (NHIS-D) (inpatient, prescription medi-

TABLE 12-8 Cases and Prevalence of Developmental Disabilities by Gestational Age Among Survivors to Age 3 Years, MADDSP

Developmental Disability and Statistic	Gestational Age					Total	Born Preterm	Risk Ratio	Risk Difference
	20–23 wk	24–28 wk	29–32 wk	33–36 wk	>37 wk				
No. of 3-Year Survivors: 1981–1991 births[a]	421	2,364	6,281	31,568	293,949	334,583	40,634		
Cerebral palsy									
No. of cases	21	118	105	100	383	727	344		
Prevalence[b]	49.9	49.9	16.7	3.2	1.3	2.2	8.5	6.5	7.2
(95% CI)[c]	(31.1–75.2)	(41.5–59.5)	(13.7–20.2)	(2.6–3.9)	(1.2–1.4)	(2.0–2.3)			
Mental retardation									
No. of cases	32	144	171	407	1,988	2,742	754		
Prevalence[b]	76.0	60.9	27.2	12.9	6.8	8.2	18.6	2.7	11.8
(95% CI)	(52.6–105.6)	(51.6–71.3)	(23.3–31.6)	(11.7–14.2)	(6.5–7.1)	(7.9–8.5)			
Hearing loss									
No. of cases	6	15	12	30	214	277	63		
Prevalence[b]	14.3	6.3	1.9	1.0	0.7	0.8	1.6	2.1	0.8
(95% CI)	(5.2–30.8)	(3.6–10.4)	(1.0–3.3)	(0.6–1.4)	(0.6–0.8)	(0.7–0.9)			
Vision impairment									
No. of cases	5	38	18	31	154	246	92		
Prevalence[b]	11.9	16.1	2.9	1.0	0.5	0.7	2.3	4.3	1.7
(95% CI)	(3.9–27.5)	(11.4–22.0)	(1.7–4.5)	(0.7–1.4)	(0.4–0.6)	(0.6–0.8)			

[a]Birth cohort of 3-year-old survivors for children with cerebral palsy, mental retardation, hearing loss, or vision impairment.
[b]Per 1,000 children.

cations, therapy and rehabilitation, long-term care and the 1994 and 1995 National Health Interview Survey (NHIS) (physician visits). Pricing of out-patient medical care services relied primarily on the 1987 National Medical Expenditure Survey (NMES), whereas inpatient service cost was based on charge data from the 1995 Healthcare Cost and Utilization Project adjusted to costs using Medicare cost-to charge ratios. The receipt of special education services by developmental disability was based on the MADDSP, whereas special education placement category for those receiving services by disability was taken from the NHIS-D. Average special education costs were then estimated based on the incremental price of placements from Moore et al. (1988b). Disability-specific work limitation estimates were based on the NHIS-D, while earnings losses associated with such limitations were based on the Survey of Income and Program Participation (SIPP) (Honeycutt et al., 2003). Costs taken from that study for this report were inflated to 2005 based on Medicare reimbursement indices for medical care, weighted by type of service, and on the employee compensation index for public education (special education services costs) and the general employee compensation index (lost productivity estimates).

Estimates of lifetime medical care costs per individual with one or more of the four developmental disabilities, regardless of gestational age, ranged from $23,209 for those with HL to $123,205 for those with MR, expressed in 2000 dollars (Honeycutt et al., 2003) (Table 12-9). Although long-term care constitutes a large proportion of medical costs for those with developmental disabilities, inpatient hospitalization and physician visits also contribute significant costs. Long-term care costs represented about 44 percent of the medical care costs for individuals with MR, but physician visits and inpatient hospitalization accounted for more than 40 percent of the costs (Table 12-9). For those with CP, HL, and VI, physician visits and inpatient hospitalization accounted for more than two-thirds of the medical care costs (Honeycutt et al., 2003). These estimates of long-term care costs are particularly conservative, as such care for children under age 18 years and for those in institutionalized settings was not included. Long-term care costs for those with CP, for example, were found to be more than 63 percent of the lifetime medical care costs in earlier work, based on a cohort of individuals with CP born in California, which included estimates for those institutionalized in that state's developmental centers (Waitzman et al., 1996).

Excess cases of the four developmental disabilities associated with preterm birth were based on unpublished tabulations from MADDSP on the prevalence of the four developmental disabilities by gestational age for the cohort born from 1981 to 1991 surviving to age 3 years. With the exception of HL among infants born at 33 to 36 weeks of gestation, among whom the difference in prevalence of HL relative to that among infants born at term was of only marginal significance, the prevalence of all four

TABLE 12-9 Estimates of Per-Person Lifetime Incremental Direct Medical Costs by Developmental Disability

Developmental Disability	Direct Cost (dollars)						
	Physician Visits	Prescription Medications	Inpatient Stays	Assistive Devices	Therapy and Rehabilitation[a]	Long-Term Care[b]	Total Medical Costs
Mental retardation	19,133	3,513	30,151	3,078	13,181	54,185	123,205
Cerebral palsy	37,136	4,035	19,636	3,053	16,365	2,944	83,169
Hearing loss	8,129	106	8,683	5,438	735	0	23,209
Vision impairment	4,538	24	20,310	1,330	5,024	832	32,058

NOTE: Data are in 2000 dollars and assume a 3 percent discount rate.

[a]Assumes that therapy and rehabilitation services are used by children only.
[b]Assumes that long-term care services are used by adults only; these data are only for the noninstitutionalized population.

SOURCE: Honeycutt et al. (2003). Reprinted from *Using Survey Data to Study Disability: Results from the National Health Interview Survey on Disability*, Honeycutt et al., Economic costs of mental retardation, cerebral palsy, hearing loss, and vision impairment, Pg. 217, © 2003, with permission from Elsevier.

developmental disabilities was significantly higher among preterm infants than among term infants. The prevalence exhibited a distinct inverse gradient by gestational age (Table 12-8). Although births at less than 28 weeks of gestation constituted 0.8 percent of all births, for example, extreme prematurity accounted for 19, 6, 7.5, and 17.4 percent of all cases of CP, MR, HL, and VI, respectively (Table 12-8). In addition, although extremely preterm births represented just 6.9 percent of all preterm births in the MADDSP sample of survivors to age 3 years, children born extremely preterm accounted for more than 40, 23, 23, and 47 percent of all individuals born preterm with CP, MR, HL, and VI, respectively. The ratios of the rates of CP, MR, VI, and HL among preterm infants to those among term infants surviving to age 3 years were 6.5, 2.1, 2.1, and 4.3, respectively. Prevalence differences, given in the final column of Table 12-8, were used to estimate the excess number of cases of each developmental disability among survivors born preterm. Prevalence by birth weight category demonstrated similarly sharp gradients (Table 12-10).

Several of the infants displaying one of the four index developmental disabling conditions had multiple index disabling conditions, and aggregation of the costs for all these disabling conditions therefore required that such cooccurrences be taken into account to avoid double counting. The cooccurrence rates generated from MADDSP permitted such aggregation (Yeargin-Allsopp et al., 1992). Because per-case costs were not estimated separately for each permutation of multiple conditions, an algorithm was established to assign cases to conditions. The algorithm was adopted by assigning cases hierarchically to the condition with the highest cost among each case with multiple conditions. The implicit assumption was that a case with multiple disabling conditions costs, on average, at least as much as the mean cost of its highest-cost disabling condition. The resulting hierarchical order of conditions, from highest to lowest cost, was MR, CP, VI, and HL. An individual born with both MR and HL, for example, was assigned the average cost of all individuals with MR. On the basis of the data reported by MADDSP, 64 percent of survivors to age 3 years with CP had MR, 73 percent of those with VI had either MR or CP, and 23 percent of those with HL had MR, CP, or VI. Medical care costs were adjusted for inflation to 2005 dollars by using a price index weighted by Medicare medical price and employment cost indices, based on the percentage contributions of inpatient services; outpatient services; and therapy, rehabilitation, and long-term care to the overall treatment of these developmental disabilities.

Because medical care costs for all premature infants were reported above for those through age 7 years, medical care cost estimates for these four developmental disabilities through age 5 years were subtracted from the total medical care costs in the disability cost study to avoid double counting. The net effect was to reduce the total lifetime medical costs asso-

TABLE 12-10 Cases and Prevalence of Developmental Disabilities by Birth Weight Among Survivors to Age 3 Years, MADDSP

Developmental Disability and Statistic	Birth Weight			
	<1,000 g	1,000–1,499 g	1,500–2,499 g	2,500–2,999 g
No. of 3-year survivors: 1981–1991 births[a]				
	1,147	2,648	23,117	62,451
Cerebral palsy				
No. of cases	101	130	166	107
Prevalence[b]	88.1	49.1	7.2	1.7
(95% CI[c])	(72.3–106.0)	(41.2–58.0)	(6.1–8.4)	(1.4–2.1)
Mental retardation				
No. of cases	151	156	464	667
Prevalence[b]	131.6	58.9	20.1	10.7
(95% CI)	(112.6–152.6)		(50.2–68.6)	(18.3–22.0)
Hearing loss				
No. of cases	16	13	41	72
Prevalence[b]	13.9	4.9	1.8	1.2
(95% CI)	(8.0–22.6)	(2.6–8.4)	(1.3–2.4)	(0.9–1.5)
Vision impairment				
No. of cases	44	20	35	50
Prevalence[b]	38.4	7.6	1.5	0.8
(95% CI)	(28.0–51.2)	(4.6–11.6)	(1.1–2.1)	(0.6–1.1)
No. of 3-year survivors: 1986–1993 births[d]				
	1,179	2,231	19,112	50,960

NOTE: The data represent the birth weight-specific prevalence of select developmental disabilities among 3- to 10-year-old children who were born in Atlanta, Georgia, from 1981 to 1993 and who survived to 3 years of age.

ciated with these conditions by less than 5 percent. Because the age categories used in the developmental disability cost study made it difficult to accurately carve out medical care costs for 6- and 7-year-olds separately, cost estimates for those 6- and 7-year-olds were subtracted from the overall medical care costs for preterm birth provided above to avoid double counting. Estimates of the costs at each age were discounted at a rate of 3 percent to the year of birth. Adjustment for the prevalence differences between term and preterm birth by condition and application of the algorithm for mul-

3,000–3,999 g	≥4,000 g	Total	Low Birth Weight	Normal Birth Weight	Risk Ratio	Risk Difference
231,613	35,780	356,756	26,912	329,844		
254	37	795	397	398		
1.1	1	2.2	14.8	1.2	12.2	13.5
(1.0–1.2)	(0.1–1.4)	(2.1–2.4)				
1,402	189	3029	771	2,258		
6.1	5.3	8.5	28.6	6.8	4.2	21.8
(9.9–11.5)	(5.7–6.4)	(4.6–6.1)	(8.2–8.8)			
131	23	296	70	226		
0.6	0.6	0.8	2.6	0.7	3.8	1.9
(0.5–0.7)	(0.4–1.0)	(0.7–0.9)				
106	19	274	99	175		
0.5	0.5	0.8	3.7	0.5	6.9	3.2
(0.4–0.6)	(0.3–0.8)	(0.7–0.9)				
189,441	29,656	292,579				

[a]Birth cohort of 3-year-old survivors for children with cerebral palsy, mental retardation, hearing loss, or vision impairment.
[b]Per 1,000 children.
[c]CI = confidence interval.
[d]Birth cohort of 3-year-old survivors for children with autism.

tiple disabilities discussed above yielded a total of $976 million in lifetime incremental medical care costs associated with preterm birth after age 5 years, or nearly $2,000 per preterm birth. The addition of these costs to the national costs of preterm birth from birth to age 5 years yielded a total national cost of medical care for preterm birth of $16.86 billion in 2005.

The estimate of national medical care cost associated with preterm birth is conservative, in the sense that it includes the costs associated with all premature infants only through the first 5 years of life. The costs beyond age 5 years, as demonstrated by these cost estimates for the four developmental disabilities associated with preterm birth, are quite substantial. Although these conditions associated with preterm birth are among the most disabling, there are several others, including autism and certain birth defects (Rasmussen et al., 2001). Furthermore, the medical care cost estimates for even these four developmental disabilities are conservative, because long-term care provided for the small subset of the population who required institutionalized settings and therapy and rehabilitation services provided for adults were not included.

In summary, extremely preterm birth contributes disproportionately to the medical care costs of prematurity, not only because early medical care for such infants is so expensive but also because survivors have disproportionately high rates of disabling conditions that generate high lifetime medical care costs. Very preterm and moderately preterm infants, however, also have significantly elevated rates of developmental disabilities relative to those for term infants. Although the prevalence of disabilities is lower among this group than among extremely preterm infants, the disproportionate number of births in this category yields a significant contribution to the national cost. Moderately preterm infants, for example, represent over 50 percent of preterm cases with MR.

Treatment for reactive airway disease, for which all premature infants are at risk, and treatment of infection may contribute to higher average outpatient costs among those born preterm. The relatively high outpatient medical care costs in the upper tail of the medical care cost distribution for those born at 32 to 36 weeks of gestation noted earlier is likely explained, in part, by the costs incurred by individuals with developmental disabilities. LBW is clearly a risk factor for developmental disabilities and their associated costs and one that is correlated with gestational age. The extent to which these risk factors contribute independently to these developmental disability costs is not fully understood. Future studies should investigate costs for other disabling conditions, which were not available for these analyses but are prevalent among preterm infants such as asthma and attention deficit hyperactivity disorder.

EARLY INTERVENTION SERVICES

Evidence from Massachusetts on early intervention (EI) services delivered between the first through third years of life suggests that the rate of provision of such services for preterm infants is significantly higher on a per-case basis than that for term infants. Mean expenditures for such services per case displayed an inverse gradient by gestational age: less than 28 weeks, $7,182; 28 to 30 weeks, $5,254; 31 to 33 weeks, $2,654; 34 to 36 weeks, $1,321; and 37 to 39 weeks, $697 (Clements et al., 2007).

The services that Massachusetts mandates for EI services are more generous, on average, than those mandated by the nation as a whole (personal communication, W. Barfield, 2006). It is unclear, however, whether the level of incremental EI services delivered to children born preterm relative to those delivered to those born term in that state are above the national average. If incremental EI services were delivered in the rest of the country at the same level that they are delivered in Massachusetts, the incremental cost of such services would be an estimated $1,200 per preterm child, or a total of $611 million in 2005 dollars.[2]

SPECIAL EDUCATION COSTS

Much of the literature on the rates of receipt of special education by newborn status has focused on LBW infants, particularly VLBW and extremely low birth weight infants, and has not been estimated from population-based samples (Pinto-Martin et al., 2004). In a 9-year follow-up of a cohort of 1,105 infants born between September 1984 and June 1987 in central New Jersey, both VLBW and birth at a gestational age of less than 28 weeks were found to be significantly associated with the receipt of special educational services, with the odds ratio for those born extremely preterm relative to those born term being higher than the odds ratio for those born VLBW relative to those born with normal BWs (Pinto-Martin et al., 2004). Although a review of the literature revealed a few studies that have made estimates of the costs of special education associated with LBW (Zupancic, 2006), little research on the special education costs specifically associated with preterm birth has been conducted to date. One multivariate study found that LBW added $1,240 (1989–1990 dollars) per child to the annual cost of schooling for children ages 6 through 15 years born with birth weights of less than 2,500 grams (Chaikand and Corman, 1991). This translates into $2,009 in 2005 per LBW child when the employee compensation index for primary and secondary school employees is applied to adjust for inflation between 1989–1990 and 2005.

As with the cost of medical care beyond age 5 years, an estimate of the special education costs due to premature birth was made on the basis of the incremental special education costs specific to four developmental disabili-

---

[2]This calculation assumed the same percentage distribution of services across the first 3 years of life for children born preterm as the distribution of mean costs of EI services for all children. All costs beyond the first year of life were discounted at a 3 percent rate back to the year of birth. Costs were adjusted for the difference in the cost of living between Massachusetts and the nation as a whole and for inflation, gauged by the Employment Cost Index, between 2003 and 2005. Only preterm children surviving infancy were assumed to receive EI services.

ties that have a higher prevalence among those born preterm: MR, CP, VI, and HL. It is noted that the increased use of infertility treatment may lead to special education costs due to its effect on preterm birth via multiple gestations. To the extent that preterm birth associated with multiple gestations leads to the four disabilities that are included in these estimates, such costs are included. The estimates reflect the receipt of services from ages 3 to 18 years, discounted back to the year of birth at a 3 percent rate. The estimates were based on data from CDC (2004c) and unpublished tabulations from MADDSP, as described above. The rate of receipt of special education services by developmental disability was based on the distribution from MADDSP. Allocation among federal special education handicap categories was based on the primary disability for those with MR, VI, and HL and was based on estimates from Waitzman et al. (1996) for CP. Costs for special education were taken from the Special Education Expenditure Project (Chambers et al., 2003). Estimates were incremental; that is, costs above and beyond what would have been spent on regular education. For each case associated with preterm birth, estimated lifetime special education costs were $102,410, $81,655, $125,811, and $92,020 for those with MR, CP, VI, and HL, respectively. In terms of cohort results, updated to 2005 costs, special education for individuals with these four developmental disabilities added an estimated $2,237 per preterm survivor to the overall lifetime cost associated with preterm birth. This translates into a societal cost of $1.1 billion for special education in association with preterm birth.

There is only about a 10 percent difference between the inflation-adjusted estimate per LBW infant from an earlier study (Chaikand and Corman, 1991) and the $2,237 per infant estimate for preterm birth provided here. Although the similarity is intriguing, there were distinct differences in the methodologies and populations underlying the methods used to obtain these estimates. The estimate was for services provided to children who had been born with LBWs from ages 6 to 15 years, whereas the current estimate was for special education services provided to children who had been born with LBWs from ages 3 to 18 years. The estimate provided here, more importantly, is based only on a subset of disabling conditions among children born preterm for whom special education is provided. In that respect, these special education cost estimates are conservative proxies of the full cost of special education services provided to those born preterm. As discussed in Chapter 11, the receipt of special education services is quite prevalent among children born preterm, beyond those with the specific disabilities. However, these costs could not be tabulated.

INDIRECT COSTS:
HOUSEHOLD AND LABOR MARKET PRODUCTIVITY

Lost labor market and household productivity for individuals born preterm may result from disabling conditions, from the more subtle effects of cognitive or behavioral deficits, or from lower intelligence quotients. Lost productivity can result from either premature mortality or heightened morbidity, in which the ability to work or the amount of work, or both, could be affected. One complication for the calculation of indirect mortality and morbidity costs that is generally ignored when infant mortality is considered is the rate of "replacement"; that is, the extent to which a subsequent pregnancy is tied to the first by virtue of the loss. Treatment of this issue is complicated by philosophical as well as economic issues, as each birth is typically treated as an independent event. The effect of replacement on cost, from a societal perspective, might translate into a net reduction in indirect mortality costs associated with the preterm infant, for example, but the amount of reduction would depend on the rate and timing of the replacement as well as on the overall health status of the replacement child. Another potential complication arises with the treatment of multiple gestations associated with preterm birth and the extent to which productivity associated with the multiple gestations should be considered jointly in the analysis of the costs of preterm birth. Although these are legitimate and potentially mitigating factors, they pose significant hurdles for estimation of the costs associated with preterm birth. They are ignored in the estimates provided below, although infant mortality was excluded in the estimates of indirect costs, which could be interpreted as an implicit assumption of 100 percent replacement of such infants with infants that are born at term.

As with the estimates of medical care costs beyond 5 years of age and special education costs, the CDC analysis (CDC, 2004c), together with unpublished tabulations from MADDSP, permitted estimates of the lifetime incremental indirect costs associated with excess cases of MR, CP, VI, and HL associated with preterm birth. Work limitations for each disabling condition were estimated from the NHIS-D, earnings reduction was drawn from the Survey of Income and Program Participation, and age-sex earnings and household productivity values were taken from the work of Grosse (2003). After multiple index conditions were accounted for and after adjustment of the costs to 2005 dollars by use of the employment compensation index, the results indicate that excess cases of these conditions associated with preterm birth contributed $11,214 in indirect productivity costs per case, or $5.7 billion to the overall national cost of preterm birth in 2005.

FAMILY COSTS

Maternal Costs

Several studies have estimated the excess maternal costs associated with the birth of an LBW infant and with preterm birth (Zupancic, 2006). Most such studies focused strictly on elevated delivery costs, although two recent U.S. studies incorporated prenatal hospital admissions as well (Gilbert et al., 2003, Schmitt et al., 2006). One study included any subsequent transfers until the mother was ultimately discharged (Gilbert et al., 2003).

Use of the estimates from the IHC cohort data used above to estimate medical costs for infants and children reveal, in line with much of the findings in the literature, that maternal delivery costs are significantly higher for preterm deliveries than for term deliveries and that there is a distinct inverse gradient by gestational age and BW. On the basis of those data, with adjustments for geographic differences in cost and for inflation, the incremental delivery costs by gestational age were $11,737, $9,153, and $2,613 for infants born at less than 28, 28 to 31, and 32 to 36 weeks of gestation, respectively. These excess maternal delivery costs associated with preterm birth translated into $1.9 billion in total costs in 2005. This cost does not include the excess costs associated with prenatal care, including prenatal inpatient admissions, nor does it include postnatal costs associated with the provision of services for maternal morbidity or for services undertaken to reduce the risk in subsequent pregnancies, in the event that such pregnancies go to term.

Caregiver Costs

Outside of the initial hospitalization, there has been a paucity of research on the out-of-pocket travel costs for caregivers associated with the incremental medical services provided to preterm infants. Productivity losses have also received scant attention (Zupancic, 2006), although such caregiver costs for disabling conditions can exceed the costs of care for the affected individuals themselves (Tilford et al., 2001). One recent study among large employers, in which mothers were both employed and the primary beneficiary on the company's health plan, found that mothers lost an estimated $1,513 in annual wages and benefits more in short-term disability following a preterm birth than after a term birth. The estimate was $2,766 when the synergies that are lost with coworkers when a worker needs to be replaced on short notice are modeled (Medstat, 2004). Although these estimates are suggestive of the loss of significant numbers of hours at work by the mother because of a preterm birth, the sample was too restricted and the identification of premature birth too broad to be able to make generalizations to the national population. More research on the family costs associated with preterm birth needs to be conducted to more fully understand its societal burden.

ECONOMIC EVALUATION OF INTERVENTIONS TO REDUCE PRETERM BIRTH AND ITS CONSEQUENCES

Economic evaluation of interventions that can be used to reduce the rates of preterm birth and its adverse consequences can aid in decision making regarding the development and integration of new technologies and programs. The techniques for such an evaluation take on several different forms. Cost identification assesses the burden of illness and the features of its distribution in economic terms, as with the estimates provided above. Such estimates can form part of the foundation for the comparison of the cost with the outcome. Identified costs that are averted from primary or secondary prevention of preterm birth, for example, can be treated as benefits in benefit-cost or cost-reduction analysis.

Cost-effectiveness analysis is distinct from benefit-cost analysis, in that outcomes are expressed in some unit of health improvement, such as a reduction in the numbers of cases of a health-limiting condition or the numbers of lives or years of life saved rather than in strict monetary terms. The cost per unit of gain, or effectiveness, among interventions can be compared, as long as the health improvements are expressed in a single metric. The fact that most interventions have diverse health consequences means that such comparisons are often limited. Cost-utility analysis is a form of cost-effectiveness analysis in which health outcomes are expressed in a single metric, such as quality-adjusted life years (QALYs), to afford the assessment of the relative effectiveness of programs with diverse health consequences (Drummond et al., 2003; Gold et al., 1996). The conversion of QALYs into monetary units permits the translation of cost-effectiveness into a cost-benefit, but such a conversion is controversial largely because the tradeoffs that are used to elicit preferences over health states in developing QALYs, as opposed to so-called willingness-to-pay preference measures, are too constrained to comport with the theoretical foundations of valuation in welfare economics. A recent expert panel therefore recommended against the use of this practice (IOM, 2006).

It should be emphasized, as well, that although the average performance of an intervention or program may prove to be of net benefit, the incremental expansion of such efforts may not prove to be of net benefit. Appropriate economic evaluation in decision making often requires the assessment of a marginal net benefit rather than an average net benefit.

To date, there have been limited analyses of the cost-benefit or the cost-effectiveness associated with interventions for preterm birth. One global cost-benefit analysis of the reduction in mortality and morbidity associated with LBW due to advances in neonatal intensive care technology between 1950 and 1990 found that the net societal return was not only high but also outweighed that of several other widely used technologies in health care (Cutler and Meara, 2000). Although the historical advances in neonatal intensive care technology have been vast, as have the increases in the associated costs, the analysis was based on limited available data on the extent of and the quality of life associated with the developmental disabilities associated with LBW. It also ignored the effects of LBW on the quality of life of the family and caregivers and implicitly assumed a zero replacement rate; that is, that no subsequent births were tied to infant deaths associated with LBW. It also converted QALYs to dollars, which, as noted above, runs contrary to the recommendations of a recent expert panel on health valuation (IOM, 2006). Notwithstanding these limitations, the analysis provides a provocative case for the fact that cost-increasing neonatal technologies generate a net societal value. Because the results are tabulated as an average return over a historical period, however, they could not serve as the basis for the incremental evaluation of new technologies or programs for the prevention or treatment of LBW, as the authors noted (Cutler and Meara, 2000).

One recent study of the initial hospitalization cost by week of gestational age for the cohort born in California between 1998 and 2000 demonstrated that substantial reductions in such costs, on average, could be garnered by extending gestation by an additional week, particularly among those infants born at less than 32 weeks of gestation (Phibbs and Schmitt, 2006). The large interquartile variance in cost among those born at each week of gestational age, however, even after accounting for infant mortality, reinforced the high degree of uncertainty over the extent of the savings that would actually be reaped through selective extensions of gestation rather than through general extensions of gestation. In a similar approach applied to LBW, another study found that even small increases in BW could generate significant savings in medical care costs in the first year of life, although such an incremental weight gain among those infants born with a birth weight below a threshold of 750 grams might generate increases in medical costs (Rogowski, 1998). These analyses represent a solid methodological foundation for a more refined economic evaluation of the interventions and programs aimed at the prevention of preterm birth that include longer-term and broader categories of outcomes and associated costs.

CONCLUSIONS

The cost of preterm birth to the nation exceeds $26.2 billion annually and $51,500 per infant born preterm. Although a disproportionate share of these costs is incurred in the form of neonatal intensive medical care services and among those born extremely preterm, the estimates provided in this chapter demonstrate that substantial incremental costs associated with preterm birth extend after the initial hospitalization and among the majority of infants born even just a few weeks preterm. Furthermore, the costs are not limited to medical care services. Substantial costs associated with preterm birth are due to early intervention and special education services associated with elevated rates of disabling conditions, and to lost household and labor market productivity over the life span.

Although relatively little research has been devoted to the maternal and caregiver costs associated with preterm birth, such costs are likely quite substantial. More research on the long-term and nonmedical care costs associated with preterm birth, including maternal and caregiver costs, needs to be conducted to have a more comprehensive understanding of its societal burden. Such research should also address the distribution of cost by gestational age and across public and private payers. Other areas that will be important to investigate include the ways in which reimbursement for obstetrical services may affect the costs of preterm birth. For example, do low reimbursement and high malpractice costs in certain regions of the country affect care? Given that preterm births generate revenue for hospitals through NICU charges, how might this affect health systems' incentive to reduce preterm births? How this transpires may vary depending on the degree of integration of the health care system, and the specific mechanisms for reimbursement. Examining potential incentives to encourage health care providers and systems to reduce preterm births should be considered. This, of course, will require advances in the field to better understand causes of preterm birth and effective interventions to prevent its occurrence. The reader is referred to Chapter 14 for further discussion of the financing of health care and the organization and quality of perinatal and neonatal care. The results of these additional investigations will form the basis for more refined economic evaluations of interventions that may reduce the associated societal burden of preterm birth.

Section IV

Consequences of Preterm Birth

RECOMMENDATIONS

Recommendation IV-1: *Develop guidelines for the reporting of infant outcomes. The National Institutes of Health, the U.S. Department of Education, other funding agencies, and investigators should develop guidelines for determining and reporting outcomes for infants born preterm that better reflect their health, neurodevelopmental, educational, social, and emotional outcomes across the life span and conduct research to determine methods that can be used to optimize these outcomes.*

Specifically,

• Outcomes should be reported by gestational age categories, in addition to birth weight categories; and better methods of measuring fetal and infant maturity should be devised.
• Obstetrics-perinatology departments and pediatrics-neonatology departments should work together to establish guidelines to achieve a more uniform approach to evaluating and reporting outcomes, including ages of evaluation, measurement tools, and the minimum duration of follow-up. The measurement tools should cover a broad range of outcomes and should include quality of life and the elicitation of outcome preferences from adolescents and adults born preterm and their families.
• Long-term outcome studies should be conducted into adolescence

and adulthood to determine the extent of recovery, if any, and to monitor individuals who were born preterm for the onset of disease during adulthood as a result of being born preterm.

• Research should identify better neonatal predictors of neurodevelopmental disabilities, functional outcomes, and other long-term outcomes. These will allow improved counseling of the parents, enhance the safety of trials of interventions for mothers and their infants by providing more immediate feedback on infant development, and facilitate planning for the use of comprehensive follow-up and early intervention services.

• Follow-up and outcome evaluations for infants involved in maternal trials of prenatal means of prevention or treatment of threatened preterm delivery and infant trials of means of prevention and treatment of organ injury not only should report the infant's gestational age at delivery and any neonatal morbidity but also should include neurological and cognitive outcomes. Specific outcomes should be tailored to answer the study questions.

• Research should identify and evaluate the efficacies of postnatal interventions that improve outcomes.

Recommendation IV-2: *Investigate the economic consequences of preterm birth. Researchers should investigate the gaps in understanding of the economic consequences of preterm birth to establish the foundation for accurate economic evaluation of the relative value of policies directed at prevention and guidelines for treatment.*

This research should

• assess the long-term educational, social, productivity, and medical costs associated with preterm birth, as well as the distributions of such costs;

• undertake multivariate modeling to refine the understanding of what drives the large variance of the economic burden, even by gestational age at birth;

• be ongoing to provide the basis for ongoing assessments; and

• establish the basis for refined economic assessment of policies and interventions that would reduce the economic burden.

SECTION V

RESEARCH AND POLICY

13

Barriers to Clinical Research on Preterm Birth and Outcomes for Preterm Infants

ABSTRACT

The complex of interrelated biological, psychological, and social factors involved in preterm birth necessitate a multidisciplinary approach to research directed at understanding its etiologies, pathophysiology, diagnosis, and treatment. This research must be conducted over a sustained period of time and requires stable funding. In addition to the scientific and clinical challenges of preterm birth, other important barriers must also be addressed. Although some of these barriers are common to all clinical disciplines, others are unique to physician scientists trained in obstetrics and gynecology. Of primary importance are the recruitment and participation of scientists in the type of investigation that must be pursued to address prematurity. Other barriers include issues related to career choices and training; the difficulties of conducting clinical investigations, particularly drug studies, during pregnancy; the relatively low levels of research funding, given the size of the problem; ethical and liability issues; and the need for coordinated scientific leadership in the field.

The barriers to conducting research faced by physician scientists trained in obstetrics and gynecology were the subject of a workshop hosted by the Institute of Medicine (IOM) Committee on Understanding Premature Birth and Assuring Healthy Outcomes on August 10, 2005. Although some of these barriers are common to all clinical disciplines, others are unique to obstetricians and gynecologists. Workshop speakers addressed issues related to the workforce available to conduct research, career development, funding available for research, ethical and liability issues in reproductive research, training required for conducting reproductive research, and academic leadership challenges (see Appendix A for the agenda and participants). This chapter presents a summary of presentations on these topics.

CAREER DEVELOPMENT

In general, there has been a significant shortfall over time in the resources needed to train clinical investigators and to support clinical research. Numerous reports produced over the past decade have focused on the need to (1) increase the number of physician scientists (IOM 1992; IOM, 1994; Nathan and Wilson, 2003; NIH, 1997), (2) increase interdisciplinary efforts among the clinical and basic sciences (Nathan, 2002; NRC, 2004), (3) promote multidisciplinary and translational research as a means of solving complex health problems (Nathan, 2002), and (4) foster the independence of young investigators (NRC, 1994, 2000, 2005). All of these issues are relevant to fostering careers and promoting research in preterm birth. Thus, as clinical research needs are addressed more broadly, research on preterm birth—which is inherently interdisciplinary, multidisciplinary, and translational—will benefit. This section focuses on issues specific to promoting careers in clinical research on preterm birth.

Training Scientists for Future Reproductive Research

A major roadblock to advancing research on preterm birth and its consequences is the lack of experienced clinician scientists to conduct research and serve as mentors in obstetrics and gynecology departments as well as in pediatrics departments. Experienced mentors are needed to help research trainees plan their careers and support their development. Particularly needed are investigators who are successful with receiving funding from the federal research funding system. However, it is not clear that a significant pool of R01[1] grant-funded investigators is available to take on the task of mentorship in research on preterm birth.

---

[1]R01 grants provide support for health-related research and development based on the mission of the NIH.

Resources for Training

Despite the continuing shortage of clinical scientists, the National Institutes of Health (NIH) has made substantial investments in the training of biomedical scientists, particularly physician scientists. Some programs have been specific to reproductive health; for example, the Reproductive Scientist Development Program. This is an obstetrics and gynecology-focused research training program for those who have completed a residency. It has had excellent success in preparing investigators who have gone on to obtain individual, extramural support, primarily from NIH. In addition, NIH's Women's Reproductive Health Research program and the Building Interdisciplinary Research Careers in Women's Health program are contributing to increasing the pool of physician scientists working in areas relevant to women's health.

NIH has also instituted a program of K02 (career development) grants. Those who have achieved an R01 grant can apply for these K02 grants to gain extra protected time to pursue research. K23 awards are available for more advanced clinical research, as are the smaller research grants, R03 and R21 grants. These grants cover the complete cost of training individuals for careers in biomedical science, both doctoral scientists and physician scientists (see below).

In the private sector, the American Association of Gynecology and Obstetrics Foundation (AAOGF) has partnered with the Society for Maternal-Fetal Medicine to provide 3 years of research support designed to supplement the standard 3-year clinical fellowships in maternal- fetal medicine. Each organization contributes $150,000 annually so that each fellow receives $100,000 per year for 3 years. Many, but not all, fellows study prematurity-related topics. AAOGF also has a similar partnership with the American Board of Obstetrics and Gynecology to provide research support for beginning investigators in obstetrics and gynecology. In the area of pediatrics, a 3- to 4-year postresidency physician scientist program has been established and funded by the Association of Pediatric Department Chairs, the National Institute of Child Health and Human Development, and various foundations.

Despite these efforts, a shortage of clinical researchers in the areas of perinatology, neonatology, developmental disabilities, and health services remains. Knowledge in all these areas is critical to achieving a better understanding of preterm birth and its consequences for individuals who survive after they are born preterm. Importantly, few opportunities exist for pediatricians and for obstetricians and gynecologists to train and work together in active association with investigators in epidemiology and the biological, behavioral, and social sciences.

Costs

Cost is a significant barrier to the training of clinical scientists. The cost of training a doctoral student is about $200,000 over the course of 4 years of medical school, including a stipend and tuition.[2] Graduate medical education funds for a residency position total at least $200,000, and then a 3-year fellowship in maternal-fetal medicine or neonatology costs another $200,000. A postdoctoral fellowship of 3 to 4 years to train a biomedical scientist costs another $300,000 to 400,000. Start-up expenses for a new faculty member are about $750,000.[3] The Burroughs-Wellcome Fund has generated excellent data on the start-up packages that individuals receive when they take on their first independent academic position as an investigator (see below). In general, these funds do not come from NIH but, rather, are provided by research institutions. In total, it costs more than $1 million to train a physician scientist.

Length of Training

The research careers of both M.D. and Ph.D. investigators progress slowly. The median age at the time of the first independent appointment to a faculty position was 38 years, and progressively declining numbers of investigators under the age of 35 years are receiving research grants (data from the Association of American Medical Colleges [AAMC] faculty roster as of March 31, 2004 [NRC, 2005]). The median age at which a person receives his or her first R01 grant award is 42 years, and some investigators never receive a second R01 award (NRC, 2005). This has several implications. First, somewhere between the postdoctoral training period and the time of receipt of the first award, individuals are often unable to obtain independently the funds that they need to establish a laboratory and conduct research. In the interim, Ph.D. researchers and their departments must find alternative means of financial support. Second, for M.D. researchers, participation in clinical practice generates income and provides important clinical correlations that inform their research. However, a commitment to clinical practice that takes up more than 10 to 15 percent of their time quickly creates demands that disrupt their focus on research. Moreover, because liability insurance costs for obstetricians are high and are not related to practice volume, physician scientists conducting research related to preterm birth must pay the same malpractice insurance premiums as those

---

[2]Data presented by Jerome Strauss, University of Pennsylvania Medical Center, at the August 2005 IOM workshop.

[3]Data presented by Enriqueta Bond, Burroughs-Wellcome Fund, at the August 2005 IOM workshop.

paid by an obstetrician in full-time practice. This confluence of stresses increasingly forces academic obstetrics and gynecology departments to depend on clinical revenues to pay the costs of academic programs.

All of these factors discourage younger trainees who may want to pursue a career in science. Major structural changes are needed to address this issue. Without such changes, fewer individuals, particularly those in undergraduate medical education, will be willing to consider a research career. This dilemma has been the subject of a previous report of the National Academies, *Bridges to Independence: Fostering the Independence of New Investigators in the Life Sciences* (NRC, 2005).

Need for Change

The committee discussed various options for addressing this complex set of challenges to developing a critical mass of scientists from various disciplines focused on research on preterm birth. The committee determined that a systematic evaluation of the entire process of medical education as a continuum is needed. Ways to streamline postgraduate medical education for those obstetricians and gynecologists who are clearly tracking into an academic path should include some combination of residency, clinical fellowship, and research training that decreases the total postdoctoral education period—a strategy that the disciplines of internal medicine and pediatrics have used successfully—as the time that it takes to prepare a physician with no research experience for a competitive career in investigation has been underestimated. The American Board of Pediatrics, for example, has instituted several special pathways to board certification for those committed to careers as physician scientists. Special pathways should also be considered in obstetrics and gynecology.

In addition, chairs in obstetrics and gynecology departments should encourage and facilitate research activities, provide appropriate start-up funding and laboratory space, and create opportunities for clinicians to conduct research on a part-time basis. Mentors—and young mentors in particular—should be recognized and compensated for their time. Despite the challenges to establishing research careers, the excitement and rewards of research should be showcased for medical students, perhaps by highlighting the success stories of some physician investigators.

Finally, the changing gender demography of academicians must be addressed. Structural issues that impede the progress of women in the academic ranks need to be addressed. Family-friendly policies can facilitate the process of appointments and promotions without compromising the quality and quantity of scholarship. Furthermore, mentorship support that is gender specific and that provides guidance on how female physician scientists can manage career, family, and time should be provided. Having successful role models is also essential. These research training and faculty issues are not specific to obstetrics and gynecology, neonatology, or maternal-fetal medicine.

Who Is Selecting Obstetrics and Gynecology as a Career Path?

A review of those who participate in NIH's Medical Scientist Training Program reveals that few of the talented people who are committing themselves to careers in biomedical research have selected obstetrics and gynecology as their career choice. In addition, Gariti et al. (2005) found that students considering obstetrics and gynecology as a specialty are dissuaded by lifestyle concerns (i.e., a lack of control in scheduling) and liability issues (see Box 13-1). The available data show that obstetrics and gynecology is often at the bottom of the list of the specialty choices of new physicians. Specific to research needs, too few doctors in training consider women's health and the health of mothers as key research areas in which to pursue their scholarly work.

The demographics of those entering obstetrics and gynecology are changing as well, and it is important to be sensitive to these changing demographics in terms of how individuals are prepared to pursue careers in biomedical science and clinical research. There has been a progressive increase in the number of female graduate students in the biomedical sciences and medicine. However, the record for advancement opportunities for women in obstetrics and gynecology is discouraging, even though 70 to 80 percent of those in the residency pool are women. The percentage of female full professors did not change between 1999 and 2003: it remained at 14 percent. This does not compare well with the proportions of female full professors in other areas of medicine or law (see the further discussion below).[4]

Career Development for Women

In the 1970s, women began to see more opportunities and were prepared with the science backgrounds needed to attend medical school. At the time, more than 20 new medical schools opened in a very short period. Approximately 7 years after this increase in the numbers of female students in the early 1970s, the percentage of women faculty started to increase. During the 1970s, the percentage of men who chose the obstetrics and gynecology specialty also began to decrease. About 20 years ago, approximately 11 percent of both men and women in every medical school class

---

[4]These data were presented by AAMC at the August 2005 IOM workshop.

BOX 13-1
Obstetrics and Gynecology Workforce Data

The American College of Obstetricians and Gynecologists (ACOG) has slightly more than 49,000 members, of whom more than 31,000 are practicing in the United States (personal communication, R. Hale, 2005). Of that number, 44 percent are women. An additional 1,500 osteopathic obstetricians and gynecologists practice obstetrics. Urban and suburban areas tend to have the highest concentrations of obstetricians and gynecologists; it is rare for areas with populations of less than 10,000 to have an obstetrician-gynecologist. In those areas family physicians tend to be the obstetricians, although their numbers are dropping rapidly because of the cost of liability Insurance. Approximately 1,100 residents in obstetrics and gynecology complete their training each year. Of this number slightly more than 10 percent go into subspecialty training. Of those who pursue subspecialty training, approximately 30 percent choose maternal-fetal medicine, 25 percent select oncology, 30 percent enter reproductive medicine, and 20 percent select urology-gynecology. The actual numbers vary from year to year, depending on position availability (personal communication, R. Hale, 2005). As of September 2005, there were 1,165 fourth-year residents in obstetrics and gynecology. Seventy-six percent of these fourth-year residents were female (personal communication, A. Strunk, January 10 and January 12, 2006).

Data from ACOG professional liability surveys indicate that in 2003, 22 percent of ACOG members decreased the amount of high-risk obstetric care that they offer, 9.2 percent decreased the number of deliveries, and 14 percent stopped practicing obstetrics altogether because of liability claims or litigation. This compares to respective proportions of 18.7, 6.3, and 8.9 percent of physicians providing affirmative responses to these questions in 1996. Because of the reduced affordability and the lack of availability of liability insurance, in 2003 25.2 percent of ACOG members reported that they decreased the amount of high-risk obstetric care that they provided, 12.2 percent reported that they decreased the number of deliveries, and 9.2 percent reported that they stopped practicing obstetrics altogether. The national response rates for the survey were 44 percent in 1996 and 45.45 percent in 2003 (personal communication, A. Strunk, January 10 and January 12, 2006).

---

selected obstetrics and gynecology. The numbers have decreased some for women but have decreased more dramatically for men. In 2004, 8.5 percent of women and 2.1 percent of men in medical school selected obstetrics and gynecology (AAMC, 2005a).

Data from the faculty roster at AAMC on individuals who pursue careers in obstetrics and gynecology show that in 2004, 74.7 percent of residents in obstetrics and gynecology were women. (In 2004, 98,000 residents and fellows were training in medical schools and teaching hospitals in the United States, of whom 40,000 were women.) About 3,500 women obstetricians and gynecologists (of a total of 4,681 available positions) were in training in the United States in 2004 (AAMC, 2005a).

Today in the United States women represent 51 percent of all applicants to medical school, and that figure is not increasing. In 2004, women represented 50 percent of all first-year medical students, 48 percent of all medical students, 46 percent of all graduates of medical schools, 41 percent of all residents, 30 percent of all faculty, 26 percent of all associate professors, 14 percent of full professors, and 10 percent of all department chairs. In 2004, 10 percent of all medical school deans were women. This proportion represents a doubling of the number of women deans over the last 5 years (AAMC, 2005a).

Faculty Vitality

As mentioned above, fewer medical students are choosing obstetrics and gynecology as their specialty, and research indicates that medical students who had inspiring teachers or a great clerkship experience are more likely to enter a specialty. A snapshot of the 2004 data that are derived annually from the Women in Medicine section of the Office for Faculty Development and Leadership of AAMC provides a framework for a discussion of what is called *faculty vitality*. Faculty vitality is the result of the mutual contribution of institutions and individuals to the achievement of shared goals and is a concept that can help provide a context for ways in which the career development of reproductive scientists might be considered.

Faculty vitality can be thought of in terms of what needs to be offered to boost professional development and provide support. It is organized around the concepts of responsibility, capability, and community for institutions and individuals. From an institutional perspective, the policies for advancement and tenure common in the 19th century were designed to support the academic freedom of those who joined faculties at a young age, but the world has changed significantly since then and the policies have changed little. Employment policies are needed that keep faculty on track for the duration of their careers.

An academic institution enhances its faculty by providing coaching, mentoring, and the other resources needed to facilitate learning. The clinical research community builds its expertise in a variety of conference settings and with funding that extends social and professional networking outside of the laboratory and that develops largely through peer-to-peer problem solving. Clinical researchers also build their professional networks through attendance at meetings. Thus, vitality for clinical researchers could be supported by considering the joint products of clinical care and research, linking collaborative research to career development. Some programs, some of which are described below, accomplish this; but not all young faculty members are aware of them.

Although for both clinician scientists and Ph.D. scientists, the research is the heart of the effort on an individual level, the institution expects a contribution as well. For clinicians, that means clinical practice and grant support for research; for Ph.D. scientists it means grant support. There are several ways to help scientists in these efforts, including the documentation of activities that move researchers forward and the development of management skills related to the researcher's career, office, and laboratory. In addition, leadership by example is needed, as is the ability to share a passion for professional activities.

The following are some of the activities and programs offered nationally through AAMC that may help scientists stay engaged in academic life:

- The Early Career Women in Medicine Program focuses on the issues of orientation to faculty life, including determining the focus of research and how to identify the mentors, grant opportunities, and professional networks necessary to sustain a career.
- The Mid-Career Women in Medicine Program is for associate professors and early full professors, with a focus on how women professors may extend their professional networks and mentor others as a form of leadership.
- The Women Liaison Officers updates are for the women liaison officers at every medical school in the country.
- Faculty Vitae is a new online resource for professional development. Its features include news, resources, and lessons in leadership and management to support U.S. medical schools and teaching hospitals.
- The 80-hour work week was implemented to improve balance between personal and professional lives for all residents.

RESEARCH FOR DRUG DEVELOPMENT

The development of drugs to preterm labor encounters the same challenges encountered during the development of all drugs, as well as the additional challenges of careful adherence to human subject research guidelines when they involve pregnant women and infants. Relevant and tractable targets must be identified, followed by the development of compounds with appropriate affinities, specificities, pharmacokinetic characteristics, cytochrome P450 characteristics, safety profiles, and efficacies. Thus, the characteristics of the drug related to absorption, elimination, and metabolism must be evaluated.

Typically, early drug development studies are conducted as Phase I trials with adult men. In the testing of drugs for the prevention of preterm labor, safety studies must be conducted early and before Phase I studies are conducted with pregnant women. In addition, studies must be able to determine the potential effect on the fetus. This slows the development of new drugs.

The typical practice in the development of drugs for the prevention of preterm labor is to conduct Phase I studies with healthy nonpregnant volunteers, assess the pharmacokinetics of the drug, and then extrapolate the findings to the target population. However, pregnant women have unique physiological characteristics, including changes in the glomerular filtration rate and the up-regulation of cytochrome P450 and PGP. This means that data from Phase I studies cannot be extrapolated perfectly into this patient population, which creates more uncertainty when the drug enters Phase II studies and requires more pharmacokinetic analyses in studies with the target population. Studies of the safety of the drug are also important and must be based on sufficient studies with animals and other preclinical research.

Another challenge in drug development is evaluation of the benefit of a drug. Will a delay in delivery benefit the fetus? Will chronic tocolysis be beneficial? Some preliminary evidence shows that a newborn infant who was born preterm may have a shortened stay in the neonatal intensive care unit (NICU) if the pregnancy can be prolonged. Although the shortened NICU stay might have an economic benefit, it does not necessarily translate into an overall improved clinical outcome (see Chapter 9 subsection on Information Informing Decisions Surrounding Perinatal Interventions for discussion). A delay of preterm labor at later times in gestation (for fetuses at greater than 32 weeks of gestation) may not demonstrate a significant health benefit for the infant, and the benefits of delaying preterm labor are greater at earlier gestational ages, but fewer of these pregnancies are available for study. In addition, it is ethically problematic to use a placebo control group in studies with pregnant women.

Studies of new drugs are further complicated by the fact that the standard for the use of tocolytic agents varies within and among countries. No tocolytic agent has been approved for use by the Food and Drug Administration, although many agents for tocolysis are used off label (that is, for an indication other than that for which they have been approved); for example, magnesium, β_2-antagonists, indomethacin, and nifedipine. Robust data for efficacy, defined as neonatal benefit, are not available for any of these therapies, however (see Chapter 9). Atosiban has been approved for use in Europe as a means of delaying delivery, but it is not approved for use in the

United States because the sponsor was unable to show a significant benefit to the fetus. The lack of data on these agents makes it difficult to design ethical studies. A particularly troublesome concern is whether a reduction in mortality will result in increased morbidity, such as ventricular hemorrhage and respiratory distress. Longer-term follow-up must be performed to evaluate the effects of new drugs on certain end points, such as quality of life, quality of function, or degree of disability.

Biomarkers of preterm labor are also needed to assist with determination of threatened versus actual preterm labor. The identification of biomarkers of preterm labor could refine and reduce the population to be studied and allow treatment only of those patients who are more likely to benefit. For example, one drug being pursued by pharmaceutical developers involves the oxytocin receptor. Data from in vitro and in vivo studies suggest that blockade of the oxytocin receptor is effective in delaying preterm labor. The compound being studied, 221149, is a small nonpeptide molecule that is a selective oxytocin antagonist. Any such molecule, however, must have specificity for the oxytocin receptor to avoid effects on, for example, the hemodynamics of fetal tolerance to physiological stress. The effects of the agent must also be reversible or capable of being slowed.

The pharmaceutical industry is working on drugs in several areas of potential application to preterm labor and relies on teams of investigators to translate the findings from early laboratory studies—that is, Phase I and Phase IIa studies, which test the proof of concept—to clinical use. Other physician scientists are responsible for studying the drug in the later phases. Most of these studies rely heavily on the skills acquired by investigators through such programs as the Medical Scientist Training Program. To succeed in developing drugs for the prevention of preterm labor, the industry must actively recruit people who understand both the basic science and clinical medicine. In collaborating with academic scientists, industry frequently finds the policies of academic institutions regarding intellectual property and conflicts of interest to be complex obstacles, though sometimes necessary safeguards, in research.

Developing drugs to prevent preterm labor is an important research area, for which many barriers exist. Study design for trials of agents is a critical problem for the pharmaceutical industry. A mechanism to facilitate product development would be to establish optimal designs through partnerships between industry, academic researchers, and the FDA.

In addition, moving drug development to prevent preterm birth under the protection of public health drug law might encourage industry interest. Unfortunately, this has been proposed for other "public health" drugs such as contraceptives, but there has been little traction. As noted, family planning and access to contraception could have a significant impact on reducing prematurity. Omnibus legislation that would encourage drug development to improve all aspects of reproductive health would be a welcome advance.

FUNDING FOR RESEARCH ON PRETERM BIRTH

The primary sources of funding for research on premature birth and individuals who survived preterm birth are NIH, the Centers for Disease Control and Prevention (CDC), and nonprofit voluntary health or philanthropic organizations, such as the March of Dimes and the Burroughs-Wellcome Fund. These agencies and organizations support research related to the basic science of the events that lead to preterm labor, interventions that can be taken to prevent preterm labor, treatments for infants who are born preterm, and assessment of the developmental and cognitive outcomes of children who were born preterm. Detailed descriptions of the programs and funding as they were described to the committee at the workshop are provided in Appendix E.

Because of the many scientific perspectives involved in understanding preterm birth, it is difficult to ascertain the total amount of funding available for research on preterm birth specifically. In particular, pinpointing the amount of funding that NIH spends on research on preterm birth is difficult because the funding is codified under a broad general category called *prenatal birth-preterm low birth weight*, which encompasses all research on low birth weight infants, including but not limited to those born preterm, as well as all research concerned with normal and preterm labor and fetal physiology, nutrition, and status. The separation of funding for preterm birth in particular from funding for the general category of prenatal birth-preterm low birth weight is not possible with the information on NIH funding currently available.

Although NIH and CDC provide much of the federal support for research on preterm birth, other federal agencies also contribute to this effort. In addition to the information presented at the IOM committee's workshop, additional information regarding research pertaining to preterm birth has been made available. In 2004, the Interagency Coordinating Council on Low Birth Weight and Preterm Birth of the U.S. Department of Health and Human Services (DHHS) prepared the report *Inventory of Research and Databases Pertaining to Low Birth Weight, Preterm Birth, and Sudden Infant Death Syndrome* (DHHS, 2004). The council compiled the inventory as a first step in stimulating multidisciplinary research, policy initiatives, and collaborations among DHHS agencies to achieve the goal of reducing infant mortality. Secretary Tommy Thompson had requested a department-wide research agenda on low birth weight and preterm birth, which, as discussed in this report, are major contributors to infant mortality. Agencies with research activities related to preterm birth prevention and infants born preterm or with low birth weights and their sequelae include the following:

- Administration for Children and Families
- Agency for Healthcare Research and Quality
  —Centers for Disease Control and Prevention
  —National Center for Birth Defects and Developmental Disabilities
  —National Center for Chronic Disease Prevention and Health Promotion
- National Center for Health Statistics
- Centers for Medicare and Medicaid Services
- Food and Drug Administration
- Health Resources and Services Administration
  —Bureau of Primary Health Care
  —Maternal and Child Health Bureau
- Indian Health Service
- National Institutes of Health
  —National Center for Complementary and Alternative Medicine
  —National Center on Minority Health and Health Disparities
  —National Heart, Lung, and Blood Institute
  —National Institute on Alcohol Abuse and Alcoholism
  —National Institute of Allergy and Infectious Disease
  —National Institute of Child Health and Human Development
  —National Institute on Deafness and Other Communication Disorders
  —National Institute of Dental and Craniofacial Research
  —National Institute of Diabetes and Digestive and Kidney Diseases
  —National Institute on Drug Abuse
  —National Institute of Environmental Health Sciences
  —National Institute of Mental Health
  —National Institute of Nursing Research
- Substance Abuse and Mental Health Services Administration

ETHICAL AND LIABILITY ISSUES IN REPRODUCTION RESEARCH

Many ethical issues involved in reproduction research are being discussed and debated at this time, and some may be obstacles to this research. One issue involves whether there is a benefit to the mother and her fetus of inclusion in reproduction research and whether those who are enrolled in research are better off than those who are not. Another challenge involves the documented prevalence of off-label medication use and the professional obligation to study off-label medication use. For neonates, there has been a discussion of the need for alternative approaches to obtaining informed consent, such as a process that would facilitate research during various clinical emergencies when informed consent cannot be obtained. Other challenges include

- the requirement expressed in 45 CFR 46, Subpart B,[5] that sufficient data from preclinical studies and clinical studies of nonpregnant women and adults are needed to assess the potential risk of an agent or treatment to pregnant women and fetuses before research can proceed;
- conflicts of interest of clinical investigators regarding the termination of pregnancy and the determination of viability;
- innovative practices, such as maternal-fetal surgery; and
- obtaining informed consent when the research offers only the prospect of a direct benefit to the fetus. A statement by the Committee on Ethics of the American College of Obstetricians and Gynecologists notes a concern that the recognition of distinct paternal rights before the birth of a child might undercut the mother's autonomy. Therefore, if the research would be of direct benefit to the woman and the fetus, only the mother's informed consent is required.

Regulations for Protecting Human Subjects of Research

Two issues that deserve focus because of the applicability of 45 CFR 46, Subpart B, are research at the threshold of viability and the ability of adolescent pregnant women to consent to research. In the 2001 revision to Subpart B, the term *neonate* was used as applied to research involving pregnant women, human fetuses, neonates of uncertain viability, or nonviable neonates. Subpart B defines a viable neonate as one that, given the benefit of medical therapy, is able to survive after delivery to the point of independently maintaining a heartbeat and respiration. The National Human Research Protections Advisory Committee of the DHHS Office for Human Research Protections expressed concern about this definition, pointing out that, in fact, many neonatal patients are of uncertain viability and are kept alive for days, weeks, and perhaps months and that depending on how this definition is applied, some infants would now be considered premature under this definition (see Box 13-2 for a further discussion.)

Institutional review boards (IRBs) are struggling with how to apply the concept discussed in Box 13-2, particularly the differences between minimal risk and no added risk.

---

[5]Note that 45 CFR 46, Subpart B, applies only to research that is funded or supported by DHHS.

In reviewing the clinical causes of prematurity, the adolescent pregnant woman is an important subpopulation of interest. There are two basic approaches to obtaining informed consent from an adolescent woman, particularly if the parent is not involved. The first are the so-called mature minor state statutes, and the second is emancipation. A mature minor is someone who is thought to be able to make decisions about clinical care, including sexually transmitted diseases and family planning, without parental involvement. An emancipated individual is one who qualifies as a legal adult, even though he or she is under the usual age for attaining legal adulthood. It is unclear whether the pertinent legal statutes and principles apply to research. State law often does not address research. Therefore, researchers must rely on the interpretation of legal counsel at a particular institution about the applicability of state law, which leads to a wide degree of variability (Campbell, 2004).

When the FDA adopted the informed consent regulations that apply to the pediatric population, the agency specifically chose not to adopt the section of the DHHS research regulations that covers waivers of informed consent. Although some IRBs have allowed adolescents to provide informed consent for research in situations in which the adolescents were thought to be mature enough to make their own decisions about treatment, drug research with this population requires parental permission.

Although there is no question that protecting human subjects is important and that oversight in this area is needed, it is also clear that there is a point at which the protection processes involved may impede the ability to do meaningful and important research if the IRB bureaucratic requirements become overwhelming. Inappropriate delays can deprive patients of beneficial research advances and increase the costs to the institution, NIH, and the individual researchers. This problem is especially relevant to research on preterm births and infants born preterm.

To address these issues, some institutions have formed a specific IRB subcommittee related to pregnancy and neonatology that comprises experts in pregnancy and neonatology who review research protocols only in those areas of study. This recent innovation has streamlined the process, but it is not known how common this practice is at universities that perform obstetric and neonatal research with many participants. However, concerns remain that the regulatory demands that have been imposed on clinical researchers over the last 5 to 10 years are making it extremely difficult to conduct large-scale, multi-institutional clinical care-related research on the problems of preterm birth and those encountered by infants born preterm.

450

BOX 13-2
Research Involving Pregnant Women and Neonates

Pregnant women or fetuses may be involved in research if all of the conditions that are listed in the federal regulations at 45 CFR 46.204 are met. There should be sufficient preclinical and clinical data to assess potential risks to pregnant women and fetuses. Absent the prospect of direct benefit for either the pregnant woman or the fetus, the risk to the fetus must be minimal and the knowledge to be obtained must be important and unobtainable by any other means. The definition of minimal risk is defined in 45 CFR 46 as follows: "Minimal risk means that the probability and magnitude of harm or discomfort anticipated in the research are not greater in and of themselves than those ordinarily encountered in daily life or during the performance of routine physical or psychological examinations or tests." If the research holds out the prospect of direct benefit solely to the fetus, then the consent of the pregnant woman and the consent of the father are obtained in accord with the informed consent provisions of 45 CFR 46, Subpart A, except that the father's consent need not be obtained if he is unable to consent because of "unavailability, incompetence, or temporary incapacity or the pregnancy resulted from rape or incest." Otherwise, the consent of the pregnant woman is sufficient. For children who are pregnant, assent and permission must be obtained in accord with the provisions of Subpart D of 45 CFR 46.

In addition, there must be an independent assessment of the viability of the neonate. Neonates of uncertain viability and nonviable neo-

---

Liability Issues

Obstetricians and gynecologists are charged significantly higher premiums for liability insurance than physicians in other specialties (MacLennan et al., 2005). When clinical departments must pay $150,000 or $165,000 a year for a faculty member's malpractice insurance, as they are in Pennsylvania and Alabama, respectively, it absorbs resources that might otherwise be available to support research. The AAMC *Report on Medical School Faculty Salaries, 2003–2004* (AAMC, 2005b) shows that the mean compensation for an assistant professor of maternal-fetal medicine breaks down by region as follows: $205,000 for the Northeast, $220,000 for the South, $234,000 for the Midwest, and $196,000 for the West. The addition of the annual compensation and the annual liability insurance premium in New Jersey and Florida, for example, gives total costs of $308,235 and $411,700, respectively, illustrating just how expensive it is to provide protected time

nates may be involved in research if the following conditions are met: neonates of uncertain viability may not be involved in research unless the research holds out the prospect of enhancing the probability of survival of the neonate to the point of viability and any risk is the least possible for achieving that objective, or the purpose of the research is the development of important biomedical knowledge that cannot be obtained by other means and there will be no added risk to the neonate resulting from the research. If neither parent is able to consent because of unavailability, incompetence, or temporary incapacity, the legally effective informed consent of either parent's legally authorized representative can be obtained.

After delivery a nonviable neonate may not be involved in research unless all of the following additional conditions are met: (1) the vital functions of the neonate will not be artificially maintained; (2) the research will not terminate the heartbeat or respiration of the neonate; (3) there will be no added risk to the neonate resulting from the research; (4) the purpose of the research is the development of important biomedical knowledge that cannot be obtained by other means; and (5) the legally effective informed consent of both parents of the neonate is obtained (unless either parent is unable to consent because of unavailability, incompetence, or temporary incapacity, or the consent of the father need not be obtained if the pregnancy resulted from rape or incest). The consent of a legally authorized representative of either or both of the parents of a nonviable neonate will not suffice.

SOURCE: G. R. Baer and R. M. Nelson, A Review of Ethical Issues Involved in Premature Birth (Appendix C of this report).

for research (Gibbons, 2005). Decreased reimbursement from government and third part payers also contributes to the decreased ability of clinical departments to support investigators.

NIH research grants pay a relatively small percentage of the expense of the research enterprise. The remainder primarily comes from funds generated from patient care, and if those funds are being used for liability insurance, little is left to support the academic department's research infrastructure. The individual obstetrician and gynecologist trying to conduct research must earn enough income to pay for malpractice insurance. This requires 4 or 5 days of patient care services each week, which leaves virtually no time for clinical research (Chauchan et al., 2005).

Support mechanisms by which insurance issues can be minimized should be considered. Aside from federal or state action to limit medical liability awards, other solutions could come in the form of increased grant support or through changes in insurance company liability policies. For example, grant supports could share part of the liability insurance costs for the time investigators spend in clinical research. Two changes in insurance company liability policies that would be helpful are known as "split positions" and "split assignments." A split position involves two doctors each working half time and each paying half of a premium instead of a full one. A split assignment occurs when one doctor spends 50 percent of her or his time in clinical research and the other 50 percent of her or his time taking care of patients. In such a case it would be helpful if that doctor could pay half the full-time premium or if the premium could be significantly reduced.

All of these obstacles to research in this area contribute to the mood of the faculty and the culture of the institution, which are much more negative than they have been in the past. It is not surprising that students and residents who listen to clinical researchers in obstetrics and gynecology talk about liability issues, the difficulties involved in working with IRBs, and increased regulations become unenthusiastic about doing clinical research in obstetrics and gynecology.

LEADERSHIP CHALLENGES AND NEEDS

Preterm delivery is a complex problem, with genetic, immunologic, infectious disease, environmental, social, and psychological dimensions. It produces a syndrome that is hidden until its manifestation as preterm labor; however, the events responsible for preterm labor might have occurred at any time before its initiation, even as far back as the development of the mother as a fetus. Because of its complexity, few inroads into the prevention and treatment of preterm birth have been made. However, there have been successes in gaining a better understanding of some of the mechanisms implicated in preterm birth. These could lead the way to more treatment trials. Such trials, however, must be more specific and focused on smaller and more well-defined cohorts.

Despite the efforts of the research community to develop new strategies to prevent and treat preterm labor, they have been insufficient. At the federal level, the Advisory Committee on Infant Mortality, established to advise the DHHS secretary on the department's programs to reduce infant mortality and improve the health of pregnant women and infants, called attention to the problem of preterm delivery and recommended the establishment of an interagency working group on low birth weight and preterm birth to stimulate multidisciplinary research, scientific exchange, and collaboration among DHHS agencies (ACIM, 2001).

NIH-sponsored individual research grants are an important component in progress, but more concerted and concentrated efforts must be made to build multidisciplinary investigative teams and develop new investigators mentored and led by more experienced investigators in specialized centers that focus on the problems related to preterm birth. This will require a higher level of funding than is currently available and funding sustained over a period of time that allows a research infrastructure to be created and sustained so that new knowledge can be developed. Medical schools and academic medical centers should facilitate and encourage research programs in their obstetrics departments. In addition, obtaining R01 grants are seen as critical for judging junior faculty for appointments and promotions. Given the importance of multidisciplinary approaches in research and availability of other funding sources such as U grants, K grants, and other contracts, these should also be viewed as important in the promotion process.

A few universities have built active research programs by reallocating research dollars obtained from clinical revenues. This approach allows the creation of an infrastructure that can focus on obtaining future funds through grants. This is essential to identifying and recruiting basic scientists and physician scientists with expertise in statistics, epidemiology, nutrition, immunology, muscle physiology, molecular biology, microbiology, and other relevant disciplines. Building such a program requires a sustained commitment on the part of the department chair. Once the program is established, clinical data sets must be created and maintained. These data sets can then be used for the preparation of grant applications. The collection of baseline data provides resources for analysis by young investigators, which facilitates the development of new ideas. This may involve relationships with large clinical care providers to provide access to more data. A few programs have advanced from a retrospective database or chart review approach to include analysis of existing biological samples, prospective cohort studies, randomized trials, and multidisciplinary, multicenter studies. Trainees are more likely to be drawn to such centers because of the strength and vitality of the clinical research program.

Challenges in Building a Sustainable Research Enterprise

Research progress on preterm birth and infants born preterm will require scientists from many disciplines working in concert. Physician scientists from obstetrics and gynecology are an important component of such teams. What is needed is a paradigm shift in the field of obstetrics and gynecology to provide clinical investigators who can translate the research findings that come from basic science laboratories or pharmaceutical companies into new clinical diagnostic and treatment knowledge. The research training of such individuals is a high priority. It is estimated that only 50 physicians in departments of obstetrics and gynecology received NIH training or career development support between 1980 and 1990. During that same time period, 112 obstetricians and gynecologists were funded with

R01 grants, an average of 12 a year. The track record has been worse for training grants. However, there has been some progress. In 2004, 31 departments of obstetrics and gynecology had more than five NIH awards.

There needs to be increased recognition of the importance of research in obstetrics, whether it is done in a basic science department or a clinical department in the context of an academic medical center. In addition to neonatology, pediatrics, and obstetrics and gynecology departments, other departments need to include investigations of preterm birth in their research programs. Importantly, deans of medical schools should expect their obstetric and gynecology departments to develop research programs that address preterm birth and should support them in those efforts.

Medical schools and research institutions need to create opportunities for physician scientists to conduct research on preterm birth by providing protected time, funds, and appropriate ethical guidance and oversight. Obstetrics research is difficult for obstetricians and gynecologists because they must spend large amounts of time in practice. Therefore, an infrastructure like those that exist in research-intensive departments is also needed to assist with manuscript preparation, grant applications, and administrative activities that support clinical practice and research.

Appropriate leadership, administrative structures, and organizations will facilitate the changes that are needed to make more progress on reducing the rates of preterm birth. This may require the creation of a center of excellence that is outside of departments of obstetrics and gynecology but that is associated with them and that has an administrative structure different from that of departments of clinical medicine. Although NIH has helped to build faculties in obstetrics and gynecology in schools of medicine, NIH cannot provide complete support for faculty members. Serious research programs must be prepared to share the costs for the faculty time and the resources needed to attract and train talented investigators who are committed to careers in biomedical research on preterm birth and its consequences.

Finding 13-1: There is need for a major focus on the problem of preterm birth. This will require the efforts of individuals from a broad spectrum of clinical, basic, and social science disciplines; the recruitment of more investigators; and increased funding. There are special barriers to the recruitment and participation of physician scientists who are trained in obstetrics and gynecology, such as a paucity of departments of intensive research in obstetrics and gynecology, the length of time required for combined clinical and research training, and the cost of liability insurance that is not proportional to clinical activity.

14

Public Policies Affected by Preterm Birth

ABSTRACT

Because many public entitlement and benefit programs target minority individuals and individuals of low socioeconomic condition, who are at increased risk of delivering infants preterm, the burden of illness associated with preterm birth falls disproportionately on the public sector. The consequences of preterm birth have implications not only for medical costs but also for a broader range of services and social programs, such as early intervention programs, special education, income support (including the Supplemental Security Income program and Temporary Assistance to Needy Families), Title V Maternal and Child Health Programs, foster care programs, and the juvenile justice system. Little is known about the magnitude of the public burden, aside from the costs associated with medical expenditures for preterm birth paid for by Medicaid. It is not possible to assign dollar costs associated with prematurity to other services and programs because of a lack of data. There may be potential for public policy to reduce the rate of preterm birth and improve the outcomes for children and families through the financing of health care, the organization of health care, improvements in the quality of care, and other social policies. However, effective public policies will require a better understanding of the determinants of preterm birth.

This chapter discusses two aspects of preterm birth and the public sector. The first aspect is the burden of illness associated with preterm birth and its effects on public entitlement and benefit programs. Because preterm birth occurs disproportionately among populations of low socioeconomic condition, the costs associated with prematurity generate a considerable burden on public programs, many of which target low-income and other vulnerable populations. This chapter thus reviews some of the major public programs that incur costs because of preterm birth. In addition, because the consequences of premature birth may last a lifetime, public programs are potentially affected for many decades. Thus, the burden of illness in association with preterm birth to the public sector is long term, highlighting the importance of prevention of premature birth.

The second aspect is the potential for public policy to be used to reduce the rate of preterm birth and improve the health outcomes for infants born preterm. For instance, a recommendation from the 1985 Institute of Medicine report *Preventing Low Birthweight* (IOM, 1985) was that generous eligibility standards should be set to maximize the possibility that poor women may qualify for Medicaid coverage and thus be able to obtain prenatal care. The chapter thus discusses the evidence from policy initiatives, such as the expansions of Medicaid, and discusses future policy options that can be used to reduce the rate of preterm birth.

PUBLIC PROGRAM EXPENDITURES ASSOCIATED WITH PRETERM BIRTH

Preterm birth occurs disproportionately in populations of low socioeconomic condition. Because many public programs target these populations, the costs of preterm birth to the public are substantial. For example, 40 percent of the medical costs associated with preterm births are paid for by Medicaid (Russell et al., 2005). The costs of preterm birth, however, extend far beyond the medical costs associated with birth. As has been documented in previous chapters, preterm birth has significant lifetime consequences for many infants born preterm. These costs and the associated public burden can extend far into the future—an average of 77 years on the basis of today's life expectancies (NCHS, 2004a).

The consequences of preterm birth span a broad range of services and social supports, along with their associated costs, including medical costs, educational costs, income supports, and costs for other public programs, such as the foster care system. Little is known about the magnitude of the public burden for infants born preterm, aside from the costs associated with the medical expenditures paid for by Medicaid. On the basis of the estimates in Chapter 12 of the medical costs for the first 7 years of life (in present discounted value) for infants born preterm, Medicaid costs for the cohort born in 2005 are estimated to be at least $6.4 billion.[1] It should be noted that this is a lower bound on Medicaid expenditures, as it represents only the health care costs in the first 7 years of life. Quantification of the public burden of preterm birth would thus be useful in determining the potential reductions in public expenditures that could be achieved by reducing the rate of preterm birth. However, on the basis of the very high medical costs associated with preterm birth, the burden on public programs is clearly very high. If effective interventions can be found to reduce the rate of preterm birth, the potential for large savings to the public sector exist. Therefore, investments in the research necessary to find effective interventions for preterm birth—whether they are clinical or are related to the quality, financing, and organization of medical care or to changes in social policy—will generate large returns to the public sector.

The public programs most affected by preterm birth are listed in Table 14-1. These span a broad range of medical, educational, income support, and other public programs. Total program expenditures in 2004 are listed in the last column of the table. It is not possible, however, to assign the dollar amounts associated with preterm birth to each of these programs because of a lack of available data. For many programs, no information on the number of beneficiaries who were born with low birth weights is available.

The programs listed in Table 14-1 have different eligibility and benefits arrangements; and most allow substantial state variations in program structure, benefits, eligibility, and enrollment. Of the programs discussed here, only educational and maternal and child health programs have no means testing. Federal standards for eligibility and benefits are in effect for only one program, Supplemental Security Income (SSI).

Health Insurance

Medicaid pays for a large share (40 percent) of the medical costs associated with preterm birth (Russell et al., 2005). Because low-income pregnant women are eligible for Medicaid, Medicaid pays for about a third of all deliveries in the United States (Rosenbaum, 2002).

Most children in the United States receive health insurance through a parent's employment. The next most common sources of health insurance for children are the Medicaid program and the State Children's Health Insurance Program (SCHIP), two public programs that combine federal and state revenues.

---

[1]Data are based on the medical costs reported in Chapter 12 and assume that 40 percent of infants born preterm are covered by Medicaid over the first 7 years of life.

TABLE 14-1 Selected Public Programs Affected by Preterm Birth

Program	Income Eligibility	State Options for Eligibility	Total Budgetary Expenses, Fiscal Year 2004
Health insurance Medicaid	✓	✓	$471 billion
State Children's Health Insurance Program	✓	✓	$11.2 billion
Supplemental Security Income	✓		$36.4 million
Education (early intervention and special education services)		✓	$11.1 million
Temporary Assistance to Needy Families	✓	✓	$19.6 million
Title V Maternal and Child Health Programs		✓	$730 million
Other Foster care Juvenile justice			$6.8 million $336 thousand

SOURCES: ACF (2005), 45 CFR § 1355.57 (2005), CMS (2005a,c), DOE (2005, 2006), DOJ (2005), HRSA (2000, 2004), OJJDP (2005), and SSA (2005a,b,c,d).

Recent changes in Medicaid eligibility (and eligibility for a number of other public programs) have made it more difficult for individuals who are not U.S. citizens to receive Medicaid coverage. Until reforms were enacted in the late 1990s, most legal immigrants had access to Medicaid coverage, although undocumented immigrants did not. With the reforms, even legal immigrants face substantial barriers to access. As of 2004, half of all states covered pregnant immigrants using state funds (http://kff.org/uninsured/upload/Health-Coverage-for-Immigrants-Fact-Sheet.pdf), partly through recognition of the fact that the infants will be citizens of the state, and so states seek to help improve the outcomes of all pregnancies (Kaiser Family Foundation, 2004).

The original purpose of private health insurance programs was to share the risk associated with unpredictable serious health events and their treatment, and private health insurance benefits have broadened greatly over the decades to include a good deal of preventive care. Nonetheless, private health insurance typically limits substantially the benefits that it provides for children with long-term health conditions. Coverage for rehabilitation services, for example, is usually limited to 3 months after an acute event that usually requires hospitalization. Thus, the notion of ongoing treatment to maintain or limit the loss of functioning has little place in private health insurance models. In addition, various cost-sharing mechanisms in private health insurance programs can severely strain the resources of families raising children with chronic health conditions, who must frequently make substantial copayments for health care.

In contrast, public health insurance, especially Medicaid, has relatively generous long-term health care benefits, partly reflecting the high degree of dependence of many older citizens on Medicaid for nursing home care. Thus, Medicaid includes a relatively generous package of benefits for long-term care, including coverage for specialized therapies and durable medical equipment (although states have much flexibility in the scope and the amount of services that they will cover and in the payments that they provide for services).

Another public program, the Medicaid Early and Periodic Screening, Diagnosis, and Treatment (EPSDT) program, requires states to provide the full range of federally approved services (even if the state's Medicaid plan does not routinely cover these services) for conditions identified in a visit paid for through the EPSDT program.

SCHIP covers children in households with incomes that are not necessarily below the poverty level. In the development of SCHIP, the U.S. Congress considered whether it should include the same benefits package available through Medicaid but ultimately decided to require a less generous package for status, choosing to develop a new program, SCHIP, rather than simply expanding the state Medicaid programs. Thus, although SCHIP covers increasing numbers of children in households with incomes above the Medicaid eligibility levels, SCHIP may not offer many long-term-care services.

Children with chronic health conditions access Medicaid through several mechanisms. Children who receive public assistance through the Temporary Assistance to Needy Families (TANF) program are automatically eligible for Medicaid. Over the past 2 to 3 decades, Medicaid eligibility has been increasingly separated from eligibility for public assistance, mainly through increases in the maximum incomes for eligibility. Nonetheless, substantial numbers of children who became eligible under the more generous income criteria never enrolled in the program. Other routes to Medicaid eligibility include the SSI disability program and spend-down mechanisms (by which a person becomes eligible for Medicaid if health care expenses bring the household income down to Medicaid income eligibility levels).

Importantly, the long-term benefits provided through Medicaid can pay for the highly needed specialized treatments over time for children with chronic conditions following preterm birth.

Education

Through the Individuals with Disabilities Education Act (IDEA; which was renewed in 2004) (DOE, 2005), children with long-term health conditions receive a variety of services. The original legislation underlying these programs called for assuring "the free appropriate public education in the least restrictive environment." The two main IDEA programs include early intervention services and special education. Early intervention services cover children from birth to 3 years of age, at which point eligible children enter the special education system. Early intervention services typically provide in-home services for very young children. These services are mainly directed toward strengthening parents' skills to provide treatments or stimulation for their children. These services also include group programs for older children (1- and 2-year-olds). States vary in their eligibility requirements for early intervention services; for example, some states include children at risk of a developmental disability, whereas others require documentation of developmental delay before they provide services.

Special education services are directed toward ameliorating health and developmental conditions that may interfere with the child's ability to learn. Some services are directly educational; that is, children are placed in a specialized classroom part time or full time to maximize their educational development. Other services may be directed to the treatment of problems that may interfere with the child's ability to participate in regular or specialized classrooms; for example, speech and language services and physical and occupational therapy are provided. Other services that are provided may include social work or psychological counseling.

Early intervention and special education services may therefore greatly aid children and youth with chronic conditions, but they also account for substantial public expenditures.

Supplemental Security Income

The SSI program provides cash assistance to low-income people with substantial disabilities. SSI recipients in almost all states gain access to Medicaid coverage, even when their incomes may be above the usual state requirements for eligibility for the program. Nonetheless, SSI also has financial eligibility requirements, although household incomes can range up to as much as twice the federal poverty level. The maximum income support is currently about $6,000 per year; this money can be used for any need that a child may have. SSI sets a fairly severe standard of disability for eligibility: estimates are that only about 1 to 2 percent of U.S. children would meet the disability standards, well below estimates of the numbers of children with health-related limitations of activity (the current estimate is that 7 to 8 percent of U.S. children have health-related limitations of activity) (NCCD, 1995). Current presumptive eligibility criteria include a birth weight of less than 1,200 grams for a child claimant less than 1 year of age, with a planned reevaluation at 12 months of age to determine ongoing clinical severity. In 2004, 16,349 children were approved for the receipt of SSI under the presumptive eligibility criterion of a birth weight of less than 1,200 grams. An additional 2,452 children with birth weights between 1,200 and 2,000 grams were also enrolled in the program (SSA, 2005a; Title XVI Only Disabled Child claims applications filed 1995–2004; Title XVI Disability Research File, obtained from the SSA Office of Disability Programs).

The eligibility determination process can be complex, with the person (or family) applying to the Social Security Administration, which then refers the case to the state's Disability Determination Service, which operates under rules established by the federal government. The state staff, who are usually lay personnel, review the child's medical records and supporting evidence to determine whether the child meets SSA's listed criteria for eligibility. The determination of eligibility can be difficult, especially for very young children.

SSI expenditures for children grew rapidly in the early 1990s, after major expansions in clinical eligibility for SSI (with new allowable diagnoses) as well as other efforts to improve the access of children with disabilities to the program were implemented. SSI (and related Medicaid) expenditures thus represent another high-cost item for children with disabilities and range from $12 billion to $15 billion per year (Mashaw et al., 1996).

For children who are severely disabled, SSI eligibility can continue into adulthood. Under the SSI program, a redetermination of eligibility status for SSI is undertaken by use of the eligibility criteria for adults when the child reaches age 18. In contrast to the criteria for children (that the impairment results in severe functional limitations), the criteria for adults require proof that the individual cannot sustain gainful employment. If an improvement is possible but cannot be predicted, the case will be reviewed about once every 3 years and is then reviewed every 7 years if improvement is not expected.

Although it is not known how many individuals enrolled in the SSI programs for adults and children were born preterm, preterm birth and its possible adverse long-term health outcomes generate public costs through the SSI program. These public costs can extend far into the future for any child born preterm, potentially for the entire life course. The latter may span many decades, as the average life expectancy is 77 years for children born in 2005.

Temporary Assistance to Needy Families

Income supports for low-income families are also provided through the TANF program, which replaced the Aid to Families with Dependent Children (AFDC) program in 1997. In 1996, the U.S. Congress passed the Personal Responsibility Work Opportunity and Reconciliation Act (PRWORA), known as "welfare reform," (PRWORA, 1996) which ended the long-standing federal entitlement to cash assistance for the poor (AFDC). Federal mandates imposed a 5-year lifetime cap on benefits for individuals, required recipients to work for their benefits ("workfare") within 2 years of receiving assistance, and prohibited eligibility among certain groups (drug felons and noncitizens). Half of all states, however, have exemptions to the 5-year time limit for the care of a disabled child.

PRWORA separated the administration of the TANF program from that of Medicaid, with the intention of maintaining Medicaid enrollment for this population. However, the delinkage of Medicaid from the TANF program did not work as intended, and researchers have documented decreases in Medicaid enrollment among TANF program (AFDC) enrollees (Gold, 1999; Klein and Fish-Parcham, 1999; Mann and Schott, 1999; Wellstone et al., 1999) and among women of reproductive age (Boonstra and Gold, 2002; Mann, 2003) in the general population.

Title V Maternal and Child Health Programs

The Title V Maternal and Child Health programs provide a variety of services for children with chronic health conditions. Approximately 85 percent of the federal funds from Title V Maternal and Child Health programs go directly to the states, which are given wide flexibility in their use for maternal and child health programs. About one-third of the state allocations go to programs for children with special health care needs; about 50 percent of the funds are used for preventive programs in maternal and child health (Lesser, 1985). The remaining 15 percent of the federal funds support a variety of special programs of regional and national significance in maternal and child health. These vary from the provision of support for professional training programs, a small research program, and targeted programs in areas such as improving health insurance coverage for children with special health care needs and grants to support the development of regional systems of care for various health conditions. Recent renewals of the Title V enabling legislation have charged the federal Maternal and Child Health Bureau with the responsibility of supporting the development of systems of care for children with special health care needs. The federal response to the U.S. Supreme Court *Olmstead* decision furthered this responsibility by again defining the bureau as the lead agency for community service systems, helping to ensure the integration of children with special health care needs into communities (New Freedom Initiative). These community service programs are meant to help organize the complex variety of services that children with chronic conditions may need.

Foster Care and Juvenile Justice Programs

Children in foster care have particularly high rates of chronic health problems, both primary mental health conditions and a variety of chronic physical conditions (Chernoff et al., 1994; Halfon et al., 1992, 1995). Many of these children were born preterm, although the contribution of preterm birth to the numbers of children in foster care is not clear. Many children also experienced disorganized homes in which their parents' own conditions limited their ability to nurture them, with child abuse and neglect common among children who are subsequently placed in foster care (Chipungu and Bent-Goodley, 2003).

Children in the juvenile justice system have demographics and clinical characteristics similar to those of children in foster care (although their median age is higher). They also have high levels of chronic health conditions, especially mental health conditions (particularly attention deficit-hyperactivity disorder) (Chernoff et al., 1994).

A recent report from the Urban Institute highlights the interactions among disability, dependence on public income support, and other programs by noting that almost half of adolescents with SSI support transitioning to young adulthood have dropped out of school, and a third have been arrested or have been reported to have some troubles that resulted in their participation in the court system (Loprest and Wittenburg, 2005). Although the increased risk of chronic health conditions and behavioral problems would appear to place children and adolescents born preterm at greater risk for foster care placement and delinquent behavior, the limited literature does not appear to support this concern (Hack et al., 2002; Leventhal, 1981; Leventhal et al., 1984). However, studies have not examined whether preterm birth incurs added costs in foster care and juvenile justice systems.

Finding 14-1: The distribution of the costs of preterm birth between the public and the private sectors and among constituencies within these sectors has not been determined. Children born preterm may require a wide array of publicly supported services.

ROLE OF PUBLIC POLICY AND PROGRAMS IN REDUCING PRETERM BIRTH AND ENSURING HEALTHY OUTCOMES

Public policy and programs have the potential to reduce the rate of preterm birth and ensure healthy outcomes for infants who were born preterm through the provision of guidance on how to formulate effective public policies to reduce the rate of preterm birth. The provision of guidance can be difficult, however, because, as documented throughout this report, a great deal of uncertainty regarding the mechanisms through which preterm birth occurs still exists and relatively little evidence regarding effective interventions is available. The provision of guidance on how to improve the outcomes for children who were born preterm is somewhat less problematic, however, as the evidence on the positive effects of social and other policies on the health of children is stronger. Effective policy recommendations, however, will require more research to identify effective clinical interventions; to determine the role of the quality, financing, and organization of the health care delivery system on outcomes; and to identify the role of social policies on the health of mothers and children.

The lack of data that can be used to inform policies has been reported elsewhere. In 2001, the Advisory Committee on Infant Mortality published a report that reviewed the current literature and concluded that the findings from the literature justified "considerable investment in research programs, and policies focused on the goal of decreasing the incidence of preterm delivery, and thus of low birth weight and infant mortality" (ACIM, 2001, p. 15). The Committee on Infant Mortality called for research efforts in areas of disparities, smoking prevention and cessation, promotion of health education and healthy behaviors, and understanding the causes of preterm labor and premature rupture of membranes. It also recommended investigation of the health care delivery system and its effects on birth outcomes.

The remainder of this section discusses selected policy options for the financing of health care, the organization and quality of care, and other social policies and their possible roles in reducing the rate of preterm birth and ensuring healthy outcomes for infants.

Financing of Health Care

Policy makers have focused on the expansion of access to prenatal care since the 1980s in an effort to improve birth outcomes in general, including a reduction in the rate of preterm birth. These efforts have primarily been achieved through an expansion of Medicaid eligibility for pregnant women at the state level. States have the option of extending eligibility to those with incomes greater than 133 percent of the federal poverty level, and the majority of states do so. A direct link between increased insurance coverage and the receipt of early prenatal care was demonstrated in a study by the RAND Corporation of Medicaid eligibility expansion in Florida (Long and Marquis, 1998). When Medicaid eligibility expanded to include those with incomes at 185 percent of the federal poverty level, the numbers of women who sought prenatal care in the first trimester rose, with more than 80 percent of pregnant women receiving care early in their pregnancies (Schlesinger and Kornesbusch, 1990).[2]

Alternatively, states can increase access to prenatal care outside of the confines of Medicaid by expanding programs that target uninsured pregnant women to provide them with access to prenatal care through Maternal and Child Health program block grants (Schlesinger and Kronebusch, 1990). Coverage of prenatal services has also been extended through expansion of SCHIP [Title XXI of the Social Security Act, Pub I, No. 74-271 (49 Stat 620) (1935)].

Evaluations of the results of the Medicaid expansions have not found reduced rate of preterm birth or improvements in maternal outcomes in association with these increases in insurance coverage for pregnant women, however (Piper et al., 1990), despite increases in the levels of enrollments in Medicaid and the use of prenatal care. Some evidence suggests, however, that the expansions may have been associated with decreases in the rate of infant mortality (Currie and Gruber, 1996).

One reason that the expansions may not have been effective in reducing the rate of preterm birth may be that current prenatal care is focused on risks other than preterm birth (see Chapter 9). This is in part due to the uncertainty regarding the mechanisms through which preterm birth occurs and the existence of relatively little evidence on effective interventions for the prevention of preterm birth (see Chapters 6 and 9). In fact, an increasing number of studies challenge the role of prenatal care in the prevention of preterm birth (Alexander and Kotelchuck, 2001; Lu and Halfon, 2003). Even when prenatal care is initiated early in the first trimester, prenatal care has not been demonstrated to decrease the rate of preterm birth (Fiscella, 1995). Intensive prenatal care programs[3] targeted at women identified to be at high risk for preterm delivery have also not been demonstrated to be effective when they have been evaluated in randomized control trials (Fiscella, 1995), nor does access to early prenatal care eliminate the disparities in the rate of preterm birth by race and ethnicity (CDC, 2005i). Studies

---

[2]Other authors disagree, noting an overall increase in the number of prenatal visits (by an average of one additional visit per mother) associated with Medicaid eligibility expansions without a coincident shift in earlier care.

[3]Preterm birth prevention programs have a variety of features, including early and frequent visits, weekly or biweekly cervical ultrasounds, case management, and education regarding the warning signs of preterm labor.

of Medicaid programs with enhanced prenatal benefits such as outreach or care coordination have demonstrated that these programs have only modest effects on birth outcomes (Joyce, 1998). Nonetheless, prenatal care provides the mechanism through which maternal risks can be identified and referrals to appropriate hospitals for care can be made. It further provides the framework through which other interventions can be implemented and thus plays an important role in the potential to reduce the rate of preterm birth. Prenatal care is necessary, but not sufficient to reduce rates of preterm birth.

The Medicaid eligibility of pregnant women generally ends at 60 days postpartum. It is unknown whether the provision of health insurance for all women of child-bearing age or those at high risk of preterm birth would have an effect on reducing the rate of preterm birth or improving maternal outcomes. However, women who had a preterm birth are at risk for a recurrence in a subsequent pregnancy (Adams et al., 2000; Iams et al., 1998; Krymko et al., 2004), possibly because many of the biobehavioral risk factors for preterm birth are carried from one pregnancy to the next.

The interpregnancy period offers an important window of opportunity for addressing these risk factors and optimizing women's health before their next pregnancy. At present, access to health care in the interpregnancy period is limited for many women, particularly low-income women, whose pregnancy-related Medicaid coverage generally terminates at 60 days postpartum (Gold, 1997). Expansion of Medicaid coverage to low-income women who had a preterm birth (e.g., through a Medicaid waiver) is one policy option for improving health care access for these women in the interpregnancy period. Several demonstration programs on interconception care have been completed or are ongoing (Dunlop and Brann, 2005; IHPIT, 2003); however, their effectiveness in preventing a recurrence of preterm birth has not been conclusively established. More research will be required to define the contents and demonstrate the effectiveness and cost-effectiveness of interconception care before policy recommendations can be made.

Organization and Quality of Perinatal and Neonatal Care

Beyond the content of prenatal care, little is known about the quality of care throughout the reproductive spectrum. There are also few indicators of the quality of care that infants born preterm receive in neonatal intensive care units (NICUs). As discussed below, however, the potential to reduce the rate of infant mortality in association with preterm birth is high if such measures could be developed.

Knowledge of the quality of care received during pregnancy and delivery also has the potential to reduce the rate of preterm birth. However, few quality measures related to the perinatal period have been developed. Reporting systems such as the National Center on Quality Assurance's Health Plan Employer Data and Information Set measures (www.ncqa.org/Programs/HEDIS) contain only a few basic indicators related to the timing and content of prenatal care and the birth outcome. Better measures of the quality of health care therefore need to be developed to enable the implementation of quality improvement efforts and to guide public policy.

The organization of the health care delivery system has long been viewed as a key determinant of birth outcomes. In the 1970s, the March of Dimes developed practice guidelines advocating for the regionalization of perinatal care in the United States (Committee on Perinatal Health, 1976). These recommendations were the result of research during the previous decade linking the regionalization of neonatal care with improved neonatal survival and improved overall outcomes. As the program was initially envisioned, regionalized perinatal care involved the designation of three levels of care based on the clinical conditions of the patients, both the mother and the infant. Level I centers were able to provide basic or routine obstetric and newborn care. Level II centers had the capability to care for patients of moderate risk, and Level III centers were reserved for high-risk cases requiring the most specialized care. In addition to the designation of levels of care, regionalized perinatal care was to include the coordination of care among the region's hospitals through maternal risk evaluation, consultative services, maternal transport, neonatal transport, long-term follow-up, and when appropriate, transport back to centers that provide lower levels of care.

In the early 1980s the Robert Wood Johnson Foundation sponsored a multicenter program to evaluate the benefits of regionalized perinatal-neonatal care (McCormick et al., 1985). That project documented the increase in the regionalization of care with a concomitant marked improvement in neonatal survival. By the latter half of the decade, however, the emphasis on the regionalization of perinatal care was being replaced by interhospital competition driven by the reimbursement policies of an increasingly managed care environment. To compete for managed care contracts and to maintain and attract obstetric patients, smaller community hospitals were hiring neonatalogists and building new NICUs, even in the absence of increased obstetric patient volumes or the ability to provide comprehensive neonatal care services.

In 1988, in a follow-up to the initial Robert Wood Johnson Foundation demonstration project, the foundation sponsored a review of the regionalization of perinatal care (Cooke et al., 1988). Contrary to the first report, that review highlighted a reversal in regionalization, increased competition between hospitals, and blurred distinctions between levels of care. The negative impact of such deregionalization was documented in a more recent review of the experience in Missouri (Yeast et al., 1998). The effect of deregionalization during the time period between 1982 and 1986 was compared with that during the time period between 1990 and 1994. An increase in the number of self-designated Level II facilities occurred over this time period, with a concomitant decrease in the number of Level I institutions. However, the relative risk of neonatal mortality for infants born with very low birth weights was twofold higher in Level II centers than in Level III centers.

More recently, the private sector has begun a trend toward moving patients to high-quality hospitals through evidence-based selective referral. Evidence-based hospital referral in its broadest sense means that health care providers make sure that patients with high-risk conditions are treated in hospitals that provide care at levels that result in the best outcomes. This approach has been adopted by the Leapfrog Group, an organization founded by the largest employers in the United States to improve value-based purchasing of health care (www.leapfroggroup.org). Evidence-based hospital referral standards for infants born with very low birth weights required that infants who had an expected birth weight of less than 1,500 grams, a gestational age of less than 32 weeks, or correctable major birth defects be delivered at a regional NICU with an average daily census of 15 or more.

Several studies have focused on the role of volume in the outcomes of care in a NICU (Phibbs et al., 1996; Rogowski et al., 2004a). One of those studies (Rogowski et al., 2004a) addressed the appropriateness of the use of the volume and the level of care for the selective referral of patients. That study demonstrated that the NICU volume and the level of care provided in the NICU explain very little of the variation among hospitals in the rates of mortality among infants born with very low birth weights, although volume and the level of care provided in the NICU were statistically significant determinants of outcomes. The NICU volume, the level of care provided in the NICU, and other readily available data on hospital characteristics explained at most 16 percent of the variation in the rates of mortality among a large sample of hospitals in the Vermont Oxford Network (which operates 400 NICUs in the United States).

In general, large variations in outcomes exist among NICUs that cannot be explained by patient mix or other readily observable hospital characteristics, such as volume and level of care. Recent research has suggested a role for the organizational and management structures of NICUs in ensuring good patient outcomes (Pollack et al., 1998). There is evidence that adult ICUs that these factors are associated with higher quality of care (Shortell et al., 1994). Given the high level of nursing intensity required in NICUs, it will be important to determine the role of nursing in providing high-quality care, which has been demonstrated to be important in studies of adult populations (Tourangeau et al., 2006). There is also evidence that other NICU staff, such as nutritionists, contribute to high-quality care

(Olsen et al., 2002). In summary, more research on the determinants of high-quality care will be needed so that patients can be sent to the best hospitals.

Although previous strategies for the regionalization of neonatal health care provision were primarily based on the level of NICU care required, recent approaches to moving patients to appropriate hospitals have focused more broadly on high-quality hospitals. However, the identification of high-quality hospitals is difficult, and methods that can be use to identify high-quality hospitals will require further research. Nonetheless, the rate of mortality among infants born preterm could decline dramatically by focusing policies on improving the quality of hospital care. A recent study demonstrated that for the Vermont Oxford Network, if all hospitals achieved risk-adjusted mortality rates of the highest performing quintile, the overall mortality rate for very low birth weight infants would decrease by 24 percent (Rogowski et al., 2004b).

Finding 14-2: The literature on the environment for the perinatal and neonatal management of infants born preterm is evolving from a strict reliance on a limited characterization of levels of care to more clinically relevant responses to patient needs. However, the optimal deployment of resources for specific types of preterm delivery is not yet established.

Early Intervention and Coordination of Programs for High-Risk Children

Early intervention programs have been demonstrated to be effective, at least in the short term, in improving the cognitive outcomes for at least some children born preterm (see Chapter 11). They also have the potential to lead to important improvements in family functioning (Berlin et al., 1998; Majnemer, 1998; McCormick et al., 1998; Ramey and Ramey, 1999; Ramey et al., 1992). Evidence on the long term-effects, however, is inconclusive. The early intervention programs studied varied in the severity of the conditions affecting children with disabilities, as did the intensity and the extent of the services provided. The establishment of quality standards for these programs holds promise for improving the outcomes for children born preterm.

The coordination of care and other social programs for children born preterm may also improve outcomes, as children with special needs encounter many gaps in coverage for services in both the private and the public sectors. As noted earlier in this chapter, however, the public programs aimed at caring for these children are a patchwork, with little coordination between programs. A unified approach to providing the medical, educational, and other needs of these children may ensure healthy outcomes. Such a coordinated approach may also benefit all children with special needs, whether they were born preterm or not. A unified approach would require both the elimination of the patchwork nature of the programs and the provision of comprehensive health care, educational, and other benefits to these children.

Other Social Programs

Because preterm birth is a complex cluster of problems and considerable uncertainty on the mechanisms of occurrence of preterm birth exists, it is difficult to provide guidance on how public policy can be used to reduce the rate of preterm birth, beyond those already discussed.

A number of countries have addressed preterm births by instituting policies. For example, as discussed in Chapter 5, Belgium and Sweden instituted policies regarding coverage of services for IVF to encourage single embryo transfers. As a result the percentage of multiple births, which carry a significant risk for preterm birth, has significantly decreased. In the 1970s, France instituted a perinatal health policy to prevent preterm birth (for review see Papiernik and Goffinet, 2004). A reduction in the proportion of preterm deliveries (before 37 weeks for singleton pregnancies) has been reported over the past 30 years. The proportion decreased from 8.3 percent in 1972 to 6.8 percent in 1976, to 5.6 percent in 1982, to 4.9 percent in 1988. This decrease was more notable for preterm births less than 34 weeks. In addition, spontaneous preterm births decreased, while indicated preterm births increased. It has been difficult to replicate these results in other countires. As discussed in Chapter 1, it is difficult to draw comparisons of preterm birth rates among various countries because of differences in measurement of gestational age, reporting of fetal deaths and live births which affect preterm birth rates, and variations in maternal characteristics and behaviors, social environment, and health services.

A growing body of evidence suggests potential directions for policy on the basis of the individual, interpersonal, neighborhood, and environmental factors that have been shown to be associated with preterm birth. More research on the determinants of preterm birth will be required, however, before any recommendations can be made.

Among individual characteristics, poverty is one of the strongest predictors of preterm birth (see Chapter 4). Poverty is a complex problem that can be influenced directly by income support programs for low-income people, such as the TANF program, or indirectly through mechanisms such as minimum wage policies; housing policies; the Food Program for Women, Infants, and Children; and educational policies. Little evidence that directly links specific policies to a reduced rate of premature birth is currently available, however. Poor women are also at risk of more stressful life events and more chronic stress (Lu et al., 2005; Peacock, 1993).

On the employment side, it is worth noting that the literature provides some evidence that work that is physically demanding, work that requires prolonged standing, shift or night work, or work that creates high cumulative levels of fatigue is associated with an increased risk for preterm birth (Mozuekewich et al., 2000). The work requirements of the TANF program might need to be examined more closely if stronger evidence emerges linking certain types of jobs and preterm labor.

Pregnancy in unmarried women has been associated with a higher risk of preterm birth. Public policies can influence family formation. For example, the "marriage penalty" under current Earned Income Tax Credits (EITC) or TANF programs and state child support policies may discourage family formation among unmarried couples (McLanahan et al., 2001). Public policies can be used to encourage family formation and partner involvement, such as allowing deductions on the second earner's income for EITC, eliminating the distinction between single-parent and two-parent families in determining eligibility for the TANF program, and experimentation with child support amnesty programs. Whether such policies will lead to greater family formation and lower preterm birth rates among unmarried couples remains to be determined.

In addition to operating at the individual level, socioeconomic condition operates at the group and the community levels in potentially important ways, also suggesting a potential role for public policy (see Chapter 4). In particular, policies affecting neighborhood context hold the potential for reducing the disparities in birth outcomes between whites and African Americans because of the clear patterns of residential segregation that result in unequal exposures to adverse neighborhood conditions among different racial and ethnic groups. Concentrated poverty and associated neighborhood disadvantages, including a lack of goods and services, decreased access to primary care physicians and obstetricians (Fossett et al., 1992), a lack of recreational opportunities, poor housing quality, and high crime rates, are more common features of African-American than white neighborhoods (Massey and Denton, 1993; Wilson, 1987). However, further research is needed to understand the roles of these factors in preterm birth.

Beyond segregation, there is some evidence that racism and discrimination have also been associated with poorer pregnancy outcomes. Public policies affecting housing, segregation, discrimination, and the built environment may hold promise for reducing the rate of preterm birth and reducing the disparities in the rates of preterm birth by race and ethnicity.

It has also been discussed in this report that abstention from drugs, particularly cocaine, may play a role in reducing preterm birth. Public health programs such as educational interventions could potentially be used to address these issues. Further, some evidence suggests that healthy diets and exercise may be important. Educational interventions may also be useful in promoting healthy behaviors. As noted above, changes in the built environment of disadvantaged neighborhoods, such as the presence of safe parks and grocery stores, could also potentially reduce the rate of preterm birth by promoting healthy behaviors.

Finally, environmental exposures may play a role in preterm birth, as discussed in Chapter 8. Reducing such exposures could be addressed by targeted environmental policies. However, further evidence needs to be developed before specific recommendations related to environmental exposures can be made.

Finding 14-3: Effective public policies that will reduce the rates of preterm birth and improve the outcomes for infants born preterm will require a better understanding of the determinants of preterm birth and the determinants of healthy outcomes for infants born preterm and better information on effective interventions. Preterm birth is associated with large expenditures across a wide range of public programs, including those for health care, education, and income support. Public investment in reducing the rate of preterm birth has the potential to result in large cost savings not only to society as a whole but also to the public sector.

Section V

Research and Policy

RECOMMENDATIONS

Recommendation V-1: *The National Institutes of Health and private foundations should establish integrated multidisciplinary research centers. The objective of these centers will be to focus on understanding the causes of preterm birth and the health outcomes for women and their infants who were born preterm.*

Consistent with the Roadmap initiative of the National Institutes of Health, these activities should include the following:

• Basic, translational, and clinical research involving the clinical, basic, and behavioral and social science disciplines is needed. This research should include but not be limited to investigations covered by recommendations pertaining to the etiologies of preterm birth; the psychosocial, behavioral, sociodemographic, and environmental toxicant exposure-related risk factors associated with preterm birth; the disparities in the rates of preterm birth by race and ethnicity; the identification and treatment of women at risk of preterm labor; quality of health care provided to infants born preterm; and health services research.
• Sustained intellectual leadership of these research activities is essential to make progress in understanding and improving the outcomes for women and their infants who have been born preterm.

• Mentored research training programs should be integral parts of these centers. Fostering the development of basic and clinical researchers, including facilitating opportunities for funding and promotion, is critical.

• Funding agencies should provide ample and sustained funds to allow these centers to investigate the complex syndrome of preterm birth, analogous to programs developed to study cancer and cardiovascular disease.

Recommendation V-2: *Establish a quality agenda. Investigators, professional societies, state agencies, payors, and funding agencies should establish a quality agenda with the intent of maximizing outcomes with current technology for infants born preterm.*

This agenda should

• define quality across the full spectrum of providers who treat women delivering preterm and infants born preterm;

• identify efficacious interventions for preterm infants and identify the quality improvement efforts that are needed to incorporate these interventions into practice; and

• analyze variations in outcomes for preterm infants among institutions.

Recommendation V-3: *Conduct research to understand the impact of the health care delivery system on preterm birth. The National Institutes of Health, the Agency for Healthcare Quality and Research, and private foundations should conduct and support research to understand the consequences of the organization and financing of the health care delivery system on access, quality, cost, and the outcomes of care as they relate to preterm birth throughout the full reproductive and childhood spectrum.*

Recommendation V-4: *Study the effects of public programs and policies on preterm birth. The National Institutes of Health, the Centers for Medicare and Medicaid Services, and private foundations should conduct and/or support research on the role of social programs and policies on the occurrence of preterm birth and the health of children born preterm.*

Recommendation V-5: *Conduct research that will inform public policy. In order to formulate effective public policies to reduce preterm birth and assure healthy outcomes for infants, public and private funding agencies and organizations, state agencies, payors, professional societies, and researchers will need to work to imple-*

ment all of the previous recommendations. Research in the areas of better defining the problem of preterm birth, clinical investigations, and etiologic and epidemiologic investigations is critical to conduct before policy makers can create policies that will successfully address this problem.

15

A Research Agenda to
Investigate Preterm Birth

The purpose of this report has been to assess the state of the science on the causes of preterm birth; address the health, social-emotional, and economic consequences of preterm birth for children born preterm and their families; and establish a framework for action in addressing the range of priority issues, including a research and policy agenda for the future. The preceding chapters have provided an overview of the current knowledge on the measurement of maturity in infants; the range of causes of preterm birth; the diagnosis and treatment of preterm labor; the health and neurodevelopmental consequences for infants born preterm; and the impact of preterm birth on family, societal costs, and public programs.

The committee evaluated this evidence to identify gaps in knowledge and recommend areas for future research. In its review of the evidence, the committee finds that understanding of the conditions and the mechanisms that lead to preterm labor is limited and that despite the availability of several interventions that are designed to inhibit preterm labor, preterm birth remains a significant barrier to the health of newborns. It is clear that a variety of disciplines working in concert will be needed to address this problem.

Resolution of many of the complex questions about preterm birth will require large-scale, prospective studies. The National Children's Study, a large-scale prospective study that has been proposed, has the potential to provide such data. The study will examine the effects of environmental influences on the health and development of more than 100,000 U.S. children and will monitor these children longitudinally from before birth to age 21. The environmental factors that will be assessed include natural and artificial environmental factors, geographic locations, physical surroundings, social factors, cultural and family influences and differences, behavioral influences and outcomes, biological and chemical factors, and genetics. The study will analyze the interactions of these factors and how they might affect children's health. Many of these factors have been discussed in this report as potential causes of preterm birth. Such a cohort study will be of great value in helping to provide an understanding of the causes and consequences of preterm birth. Therefore, if the study is conducted, data should be collected in a manner consistent with the committee's recommendations.

This final chapter organizes the recommendations and findings presented in previous sections into a research agenda. The agenda is presented to help focus and direct research efforts. The recommendations are grouped and prioritized and therefore presented in a different sequence than they appear in the full report; however, their numeric designation remains the same.

Priority areas are grouped as follows:

I.   **Establish Multidisciplinary Research Centers**

II.   **Priority Areas for Research**

- *Better define the problem of preterm birth with improved data*
  Recommendations included in this category pertain to the need for improved collection of surveillance and descriptive data in order to better define the nature and scope of the problem of preterm birth.
  1. Improve national data
  2. Study the economic outcomes for infants born preterm

- *Conduct clinical and health services research investigations*
  Recommendations in this category pertain to the need to examine and improve the clinical treatment of women who deliver preterm and infants born preterm and the health care systems that care for them.
  1. Improve the methods of identifying and treating women at risk for preterm labor
  2. Study the acute and the long-term outcomes for infants born preterm
  3. Study infertility treatments and institute guidelines to reduce the number of multiple gestations
  4. Improve the quality of care for women at risk for preterm labor and infants born preterm
  5. Investigate the impact of the health care delivery system on

preterm birth

- *Conduct etiologic and epidemiologic investigations*
  Recommendations in this category pertain to the need to examine
  the potential causes of preterm birth and its distribution in the population.
  1. Investigate the etiologies of preterm birth
  2. Study the multiple psychosocial, behavioral, and environmental risk factors associated with preterm birth simultaneously
  3. Investigate racial-ethnic and socioeconomic disparities in the
  rates of preterm birth

III. **Study and Inform Public Policy**
      Recommendations in this final group pertain to the need to under-
      stand the impact of preterm birth on various public programs poli-
      cies and how policies can be used to reduce rates of preterm birth.

Categories under group II are not prioritized because the committee
believes that they are actions that should occur simultaneously. However,
recommendations within the categories are prioritized. The policy recommendations are listed last, as information resulting from previous recommendations will be needed in order to analyze and improve policies pertaining to preterm birth.

The findings and recommendations presented in this report are intended
to assist policy makers, academic researchers, funding agencies and organizations, insurers, and health care professionals with prioritizing research
and to inform the public about the problem of preterm birth. The ultimate
goal of the committee's efforts is to work toward improved outcomes for
the children who have been born preterm and their families.

I. ESTABLISH MULTIDISCIPLINARY RESEARCH CENTERS

The committee finds that there is need for a major focus on the problem
of preterm birth. This will require the efforts of individuals from a broad
spectrum of clinical, basic, and social science disciplines; the recruitment of
more investigators; and increased funding. There are special barriers to the
recruitment and participation of physician scientists who are trained in obstetrics and gynecology, such as a paucity of departments of intensive research in obstetrics and gynecology, the length of time required for combined clinical and research training, and the cost of liability insurance that
is not proportional to clinical activity (Finding 13-1).

Therefore, the committee recommends the establishment of multidisciplinary research centers to study preterm pregnancy and preterm infants.

Recommendation V-1: *The National Institutes of Health and private foundations should establish integrated multidisciplinary research centers. The objective of these centers will be to focus on understanding the causes of preterm birth and the health outcomes for women and their infants who were born preterm.*

Consistent with the Roadmap initiative of the National Institutes of Health, these activities should include the following:

• Basic, translational, and clinical research involving the clinical, basic, and behavioral and social science disciplines is needed. This research should include but not be limited to investigations covered by recommendations pertaining to the etiologies of preterm birth; the psychosocial, behavioral, sociodemographic, and environmental toxicant exposure-related risk factors associated with preterm birth; the disparities in the rates of preterm birth by race and ethnicity; the identification and treatment of women at risk of preterm labor; quality of health care provided to infants born preterm; and health services research.

• Sustained intellectual leadership of these research activities is essential to make progress in understanding and improving the outcomes for women and their infants who have been born preterm.

• Mentored research training programs should be integral parts of these centers. Fostering the development of basic and clinical researchers, including facilitating opportunities for funding and promotion, is critical.

• Funding agencies should provide ample and sustained funds to allow these centers to investigate the complex syndrome of preterm birth, analogous to programs developed to study cancer and cardiovascular disease.

II. PRIORITY AREAS FOR RESEARCH

Better Define the Problem of Preterm Birth with Improved Data

The committee finds that there is a need to define more clearly the problem of preterm birth to better understand and study its causes and consequences. Two areas for research that can accomplish this are improved national data on preterm birth and studies of the economic outcomes for infants born preterm.

1. Improve National Data

Birth weight is an incomplete surrogate for gestational age for determination of the risk of perinatal morbidity and mortality (Finding 2-1).

The establishment of reliable gestational age estimates by ultrasound early in pregnancy facilitates both research and practice on the identification of multiple gestations; the diagnosis of preterm labor; the need for tocolysis, the administration of steroids, the elective induction of labor; determination of the mode of delivery, the hospital where the birth will take place, whether resuscitation will be needed in the delivery room; and the adequacy of fetal growth (Finding 2-2).

Neither gestational age nor birth weight is a sufficient or complete indicator of the level of immaturity of a newborn (Finding 2-3).

Recommendation I-1: *Promote the collection of improved perinatal data. The National Center for Health Statistics of the Centers for Disease Control and Prevention should promote and use a national mechanism to collect, record, and report perinatal data.*

The following key elements should be included:

• The quality of gestational age measurements in vital records should be evaluated. Vital records should indicate the accuracy of the gestational age determined by ultrasound early in pregnancy (less than 20 weeks of gestation).
• Birth weight for gestational age should be considered one measure of the adequacy of fetal growth.
• Perinatal mortality and morbidity should be reported by gestational age, birth weight, and birth weight for gestational age.
• A categorization or coding scheme that reflects the heterogeneous etiologies of preterm birth should be developed and implemented.
• Vital records should also state whether fertility treatments (including in vitro fertilization and ovulation promotion) were used. The committee recognizes that the nature of these data is private and sensitive.

Recommendation I-2: *Encourage the use of ultrasound early in pregnancy to establish gestational age. Because it is recognized that more precise measures of gestational age are needed to move the field forward, professional societies should encourage the use of ultrasound early in pregnancy (less than 20 weeks of gestation) to establish gestational age and should establish standards of practice and recommendations for the training of personnel to improve the reliability and the quality of ultrasound data.*

Recommendation I-3: *Develop indicators of maturational age. Funding agencies should support and investigators should develop reliable and precise perinatal (prenatal and postnatal) standards as indicators of maturational age.*

2. Study Economic Outcomes for Infants Born Preterm

The medical costs of preterm birth during infancy, particularly during the neonatal period, are high and the medical needs are relatively well understood. The long-term medical, educational, productivity, and productivity costs borne by the individual, as well as by the family and society, are not well understood (Finding 12-1).

The distribution of the costs of preterm birth between the public and the private sectors and among constituencies within these sectors has not been determined. Children born preterm may require a wide array of publicly supported services (Finding 14-1).

The variance in the costs associated with preterm birth is large, even within gestational age groups. Sufficient knowledge about the factors that explain this variance is not available (Finding 12-2).

Recommendation IV-2: *Investigate the economic consequences of preterm birth. Researchers should investigate the gaps in understanding of the economic consequences of preterm birth to establish the foundation for accurate economic evaluation of the relative value of policies directed at prevention and guidelines for treatment.*

This research should

- assess the long-term educational, social, productivity, and medical costs associated with preterm birth, as well as the distributions of such costs;
- undertake multivariate modeling to refine the understanding of what drives the large variance of the economic burden, even by gestational age at birth;
- be ongoing to provide the basis for ongoing assessments; and
- establish the basis for refined economic assessment of policies and interventions that would reduce the economic burden.

Conduct Clinical and Health Services Research Investigations

The committee finds that in addition to improvements in data collection to obtain a better understanding of the scope and the nature of the problem of preterm birth, five clinical and health services areas warrant investigation: the identification and treatment of women at risk for preterm labor, study of acute and long-term outcomes for infants born preterm, study of and guidelines for infertility treatments, improvements in the quality of care for women at risk for preterm labor and infants born preterm, and investigation of the impact of the health care delivery system.

1. Improve the Methods of Identification and Treatment of Women at Risk for Preterm Labor

Preterm parturition has heterogeneous origins that result in common biological pathways and that lead to relatively few clinical presentations (e.g., preterm labor, preterm rupture of membranes, and cervical insufficiency) (Finding 6-1).

Current methods for the identification of women at risk for preterm birth by the use of demographic, behavioral, and biological risk factors have low sensitivities. Although the sensitivities increase as pathways and clinical syndromes are identified, the efficacies of interventions decline as the parturitional process progresses (Finding 9-2).

Current methods for the diagnosis and treatment of women at risk of an imminent preterm birth are not sufficiently evidence based (Finding 9-4).

The goal of prevention of preterm birth is subordinate to the goal of improved perinatal morbidity and mortality outcomes. This goal is important, because the continuation of pregnancy in women with preterm parturition in some instances may increase the health risk for the mother or the fetus, or both (Finding 9-5).

Recommendation III-1: *Improve methods for the identification and treatment of women at increased risk of preterm labor. Researchers should investigate ways to improve methods to identify and treat women with an increased risk of preterm labor.*

Specifically:

• The content and structure of prenatal care should include an assessment of the risk of preterm labor.

• Improved methods for the identification of women at increased risk of preterm labor both before pregnancy and in the first and second trimesters are needed.

• Combinations of known markers of preterm labor (e.g., a prior preterm birth, ethnicity, a short cervix, and biochemical and biophysical markers) and potential new markers (e.g., genetic markers) should be studied to allow the creation of an individualized composite assessment of risk.

• More accurate methods are needed to

 o diagnose preterm labor,

 o assess fetal health to identify women and fetuses that are and that are not candidates for the arrest of labor, and

 o arrest labor.

• The success of perinatal care during preterm birth should be based primarily on perinatal morbidity and mortality rates as well as the rate of preterm birth, the numbers of infants born with low birth weights, or neonatal morbidity and mortality.

2. Study Acute and Long-Term Outcomes for Infants Born Preterm

The knowledge and beliefs of health care providers influence their attitudes toward and their management of mothers with threatened preterm delivery and their infants (Finding 9-6).

Studies of intervention strategies for the prevention of preterm birth have had preterm birth as their only outcome variable. The study samples have not been large enough for sufficient investigations of morbidity, mortality, and neurological morbidity (Finding 9-3).

Most studies of the outcomes of preterm birth use birth weight criteria for the selection of study participants. Few studies report on the outcomes for preterm infants by gestational age. In addition to infants born preterm, studies with samples of infants with birth weights less than 2,500 grams include full-term infants who are small for gestational age (Finding 11-1).

There is tremendous variation in the outcomes reported for individuals born preterm. Much of this variation is due to a lack of uniformity in study sample selection criteria, the study methodologies used, the age of evaluation, and the measurement tools and cutoffs used (Finding 11-2).

Few long-term studies of adolescents and adults born preterm have been conducted. Good indicators of the functional development of the central nervous system of preterm infants in neonatal intensive care units are lacking, and predictors of long-term neurodevelopmental and health outcomes are inadequate (Finding 11-3).

Few postnatal intervention strategies that can be used to improve outcomes for children born preterm have been evaluated, and such intervention strategies are needed, especially for more immature preterm infants (Finding 10-1).

Recommendation IV-1: *Develop guidelines for the reporting of infant outcomes. The National Institutes of Health, the U.S. Department of Education, other funding agencies, and investigators should develop guidelines for determining and reporting outcomes for infants born preterm that better reflect their health, neurodevelopmental, educational, social, and emotional outcomes across the life span and conduct research to determine methods that can be used to optimize these outcomes.*

Specifically,

• Outcomes should be reported by gestational age categories, in addition to birth weight categories; and better methods of measuring fetal and infant maturity should be devised.

• Obstetrics-perinatology departments and pediatrics-neonatology departments should work together to establish guidelines to achieve a more uniform approach to evaluating and reporting outcomes, including ages of evaluation, measurement tools, and the minimum duration of follow-up. The measurement tools should cover a broad range of outcomes and should include quality of life and the elicitation of outcome preferences from adolescents and adults born preterm and their families.

• Long-term outcome studies should be conducted into adolescence and adulthood to determine the extent of recovery, if any, and to monitor individuals who were born preterm for the onset of disease during adulthood as a result of being born preterm.

• Research should identify better neonatal predictors of neurodevelopmental disabilities, functional outcomes, and other long-term outcomes. These will allow improved counseling of the parents, enhance the safety of trials of interventions for mothers and their infants by providing more immediate feedback on infant development, and facilitate planning for the use of comprehensive follow-up and early intervention services.

• Follow-up and outcome evaluations for infants involved in maternal trials of prenatal means of prevention or treatment of threatened preterm delivery and infant trials of means of prevention and treatment of organ injury not only should report the infant's gestational age at delivery and any neonatal morbidity but also should include neurological and cognitive outcomes. Specific outcomes should be tailored to answer the study questions.

• Research should identify and evaluate the efficacies of postnatal interventions that improve outcomes.

3. Study Infertility Treatments and Institute Guidelines to Reduce the Number of Multiple Gestations

Fertility treatments are a significant contributor to preterm birth among both multiple and singleton pregnancies (Finding 5-2).

The mechanisms by which conditions of infertility, subfertility, and fertility treatments increase the risk of preterm birth, particularly among singleton pregnancies, are unknown. The mechanisms may be markedly different from the mechanisms suggested when racial and socioeconomic causes of preterm birth are considered (Finding 5-3).

The prevalence of the use of superovulation with or without artificial insemination is unknown, and no systematic mechanisms are in place to collect these data (Finding 5-1).

Recommendation II-4: *Investigate the causes of and consequences for preterm births that occur because of fertility treatments. The National Institutes of Health and other agencies, such as the Centers for Disease Control and Prevention and the Agency for Healthcare Research and Quality, should provide support for researchers to conduct investigations to obtain an understanding of the mechanisms by which fertility treatments, such as assisted reproductive technologies and ovulation promotion, may increase the risk for preterm birth. Studies should also be conducted to investigate the outcomes for mothers who have received fertility treatments and who deliver preterm and the outcomes for their infants.*

Specifically, those conducting work in this area should attempt to achieve the following:

• Develop comprehensive registries for clinical research, with particular emphasis on obtaining data on gestational age and birth weight, whether the preterm birth was indicated or spontaneous, the outcomes for the newborns, and perinatal mortality and morbidity. These registries must distinguish multiple gestations from singleton gestations and link multiple infants from a single pregnancy.

• Conduct basic biological research to identify the mechanisms of preterm birth relevant to fertility treatments and the underlying causes of infertility or subfertility that may contribute to preterm delivery.

• Investigate the outcomes for preterm infants as well as all infants whose mothers received fertility treatments.

• Understand the impact of changing demographics on the use and outcomes of fertility treatments.

• Assess the short- and long-term economic costs of various fertility treatments.

• Investigate ways to improve the outcomes of fertility treatments, including ways to identify high-quality gametes and embryos to optimize success through the use of single embryos and improve ovarian stimulation protocols that lead to monofollicular development.

Recommendation II-5: *Institute guidelines to reduce the number of multiple gestations. The American College of Obstetricians and Gynecologists, the American Society for Reproductive Medicine, and state and federal public health agencies should institute guidelines that will reduce the number of multiple gestations. Particular* *attention should be paid to the transfer of a single embryo and the restricted use of superovulation drugs and other nonassisted reproductive technologies for infertility treatments. In addition to mandatory reporting to the Centers for Disease Control and Prevention by centers and individual physicians who use assisted reproductive technologies, the use of superovulation therapies should be similarly reported.*

4. Improve the Quality of Care for Women at Risk for Preterm Labor and Infants Born Preterm

Prenatal care was designed to address one complication of pregnancy; namely, preeclampsia. The proper timing of visits and the appropriate content of prenatal care for the detection or management of preterm delivery are not known (Finding 9-1).

The literature on the environment for the perinatal and neonatal management of infants born preterm is evolving from a strict reliance on a limited characterization of levels of care to more clinically relevant responses to patient needs. However, the optimal deployment of resources for specific types of preterm delivery is not yet established (Finding 14-2).

Substantial interinstitutional variations in the complication rates for infants born preterm have been documented, and some outcomes, like physical growth, remain suboptimal (Finding 10-2).

Early childhood educational and other therapeutic research interventions have been demonstrated to improve outcomes for some infants born preterm; however, it is critical to determine the appropriate intensity, type of service, personnel, and curricula to achieve improvement in interventions (Finding 11-4).

Recommendation V-2: *Establish a quality agenda. Investigators, professional societies, state agencies, payors, and funding agencies should establish a quality agenda with the intent of maximizing outcomes with current technology for infants born preterm.*

This agenda should

• define quality across the full spectrum of providers who treat women delivering preterm and infants born preterm;
• identify efficacious interventions for preterm infants and identify the quality improvement efforts that are needed to incorporate these interventions into practice; and
• analyze variations in outcomes for preterm infants among institutions.

5. Investigate the Role of the Health Care Delivery System

Recommendation V-3: *Conduct research to understand the impact of the health care delivery system on preterm birth.* The National Institutes of Health, the Agency for Healthcare Quality and Research, and private foundations should conduct and support research to understand the consequences of the organization and financing of the health care delivery system on access, quality, cost, and the outcomes of care as they relate to preterm birth throughout the full reproductive and childhood spectrum.

Conduct Etiologic and Epidemiologic Investigations

The committee highlights three specific research areas pertaining to the etiology and epidemiology of preterm birth: investigations that will provide an understanding of the etiology of preterm birth, studies of multiple risk factors, and studies that will provide a better understanding of the racial-ethnic and socioeconomic disparities in the rates of preterm birth.

1. Investigate the Etiologies of Preterm Birth

The committee finds that the lack of success of public health and clinical interventions to date is due, in large measure, to the limited understanding of the heterogeneous etiologies of preterm birth.

Recommendation II-1: *Support research on the etiologies of preterm birth.* Funding agencies should be committed to sustained and vigorous support for research on the etiologies of preterm birth to fill critical knowledge gaps.

Areas to be supported should include the following:

• The physiological and pathologic mechanisms of parturition across the entire gestational period as well as the pregestational period should be studied.
• The role of inflammation and its regulation during implantation and parturition should be studied. Specifically, perturbations to the immunologic and inflammatory pathways caused by bacterial and viral infections, along with the specific host responses to these pathogens, should be addressed.
• Preterm birth should be defined as a syndrome of multiple pathophysiological pathways, with refinement of the phenotypes of preterm birth

that recognizes and accurately reflects the heterogeneity of the underlying etiology.

• Animal models, in vitro systems, and computer models of human implantation, placentation, parturition, and preterm birth should be studied.

• Simple genetic and more complex epigenetic causes of preterm birth should be studied.

• Gene-environment interactions and environmental factors should be considered broadly to include the physical and social environments.

• Biological targets and the mechanisms and biological markers of exposure to environmental pollutants should be studied.

2. Study the Multiple Psychosocial, Behavioral, Sociodemographic, and Environmental Risk Factors Associated with Preterm Birth Simultaneously

The committee finds that psychosocial, behavioral, and sociodemographic risk factors for preterm birth tend to cooccur; and the potentially powerful and complex interactions among these factors have been understudied. When they are studied independently, each of these risk factors tends to have a weak and inconsistent association with the risk of preterm birth. The committee acknowledges that with each additional potential interaction sought, the sample size required to retain an adequate statistical power to reveal meaningful differences increases.

Limited data suggest that some environmental pollutants, such as lead and tobacco smoke, and air pollution may contribute to the risk of preterm birth; but most environmental pollutants have not been investigated. In addition, the interactions between environmental toxicant exposures with other behavioral, psychosocial, and sociodemographic attributes have been understudied (Finding 8-1).

Independent of the individual-level attributes that are risk factors for preterm birth, adverse neighborhood conditions such as poverty and crime are risk factors for preterm birth. These data suggest that intervention strategies may need to expand from focusing exclusively on the individual to including the contributions of social structural factors to the risk of preterm birth (Finding 4-2).

Recommendation II-2: *Study multiple risk factors to facilitate the modeling of the complex interactions associated with preterm birth. Public and private funding agencies should promote and researchers should conduct investigations of multiple risk factors for preterm birth simultaneously rather than investigations of the individual risk factors in isolation. These studies will facilitate the mod-*

eling of these complex interactions and aid with the development and evaluation of more refined interventions tailored to specific risk profiles.

Specifically, these studies should achieve the following:

• Develop strong theoretical models of the pathways from psychosocial factors, including stress, social support, and other resilience factors, to preterm delivery as a basis for ongoing observational research. These frameworks should include plausible biological mechanisms. Comprehensive studies should include psychosocial, behavioral, medical, and biological data.

• Incorporate understudied exposures, such as the characteristics of employment and work contexts, including work-related stress; the effects of domestic or personal violence during pregnancy; racism; and personal resources, such as optimism, mastery and control, and pregnancy intendedness. These studies should also investigate the potential interactions of these exposures with exposure to environmental toxicants.

• Emphasize culturally valid measures in studies of stress and preterm delivery to consider the unique forms of stress that individuals in different racial and ethnic groups experience. Measurement of stress should also include specific constructs such as anxiety.

• Expand the study of neighborhood-level effects on the risk of preterm birth by including novel data in multilevel models. Data that address this information should be made more available to researchers for such activities. Interagency agreements for the sharing of data should be reached to support the development of cartographic modeling of neighborhoods.

• Work toward the development of primary strategies for the prevention of preterm birth. When there is evidence of modest effects of multiple causes, interventions that address all of these factors should be considered.

• Have designs that are common enough to allow for pooling of data and samples, and consider studying high-risk populations to increase the power of the study.

3. Investigate Racial-Ethnic and Socioeconomic Disparities in the Rates of Preterm Birth

A particular focus of sociodemographic studies of preterm birth should be on disparities by race-ethnicity and socioeconomic condition, as significant differences in the rates of preterm birth by race-ethnicity and socioeconomic condition continue to exist in the United States. The causes of these persisting disparities remain largely unexplained (Finding 4-1).

Recommendation II-3: *Expand research into the causes and methods for the prevention of the racial-ethnic and socioeconomic disparities in the rates of preterm birth. The National Institutes of Health and other funding agencies should expand current efforts in and expand support for research into the causes and methods for the prevention of the racial-ethnic and socioeconomic disparities in the rates of preterm birth. This research agenda should continue to prioritize efforts to understand factors contributing to the high rates of preterm birth among African American infants and should also encourage investigation into the disparities among other racial-ethnic subgroups.*

This research should be guided by an integrative approach that takes into account the cooccurrence and interactions among the multiple determinants of disparities in preterm birth, including racism, which operates at multiple levels and across the life course.

III. STUDY AND INFORM PUBLIC POLICY

Finally, the committee finds that effective public policies that will reduce the rates of preterm birth and improve the outcomes for infants born preterm will require a better understanding of the determinants of preterm birth and the determinants of healthy outcomes for infants born preterm and better information on effective interventions. Preterm birth is associated with large expenditures across a wide range of public programs, including those for health care, education, and income support. Public investment in reducing the rate of preterm birth has the potential to result in large cost savings not only to society as a whole but also to the public sector (Finding 14-3).

Recommendation V-4: *Study the effects of public programs and policies on preterm birth. The National Institutes of Health, the Centers for Medicare and Medicaid Services, and private foundations should conduct and/or support research on the role of social programs and policies on the occurrence of preterm birth and the health of children born preterm.*

Recommendation V-5: *Conduct research that will inform public policy. In order to formulate effective public policies to reduce preterm birth and assure healthy outcomes for infants, public and private funding agencies and organizations, state agencies, payors, professional societies, and researchers will need to work to imple-*

ment all of the previous recommendations. Research in the areas of better defining the problem of preterm birth, clinical investigations, and etiologic and epidemiologic investigations is critical to conduct before policy makers can create policies that will successfully address this problem.

References

AAMC (Association of American Medical Colleges). 2005a. *Faculty Roster.* Presented by Diane Magrane, MD, at IOM Committee on Understanding Premature Birth and Assuring Heatlhy Outcomes Workshop, August 10, 2005. Washington, DC: IOM.

AAMC. 2005b. *Report on Medical School Faculty Salaries, 2003-2004.* Presented by Diane Magrane, MD, at IOM Committee on Understanding Premature Birth and Assuring Healthy Outcomes Workshop, August 10, 2005. Washington, DC: IOM.

AAMR (American Association of Mental Retardation). 2005. *Definition of Mental Retardation.* [Online]. Available: http://www.aamr.org/Policies/faq_mental_retardation.shtml [accessed February 13, 2006].

AAP (American Academy of Pediatrics). 1993. Committee on Substance Abuse and Committee on Children with Disabilities: Fetal alcohol syndrome and fetal alcohol effects. *Pediatrics* 9:1004-1006.

AAP. 2006. *AAP Red Book.* [Online]. Available: http://aapredbook.aappublications.org [accessed March 8, 2006].

Abbasi S, Hirsch D, Davis J, Tolosa J, Stouffer N, Debbs R, Gerdes JS. 2000. Effect of single versus multiple courses of antenatal corticosteroids on maternal and neonatal outcome. *American Journal of Obstetrics and Gynecology* 182:1243.

Abdolmaleky HM, Thiagalingam S, Wilcox M. 2005. Genetics and epigenetics in major psychiatric disorders: Dilemmas, achievements, applications, and future scope. *American Journal of PharmacoGenomics* 5:149-160.

ACF (Administration for Children and Families). 2005. [Online]. Available: http://www.acf.hhs.gov [accessed January 30, 2006].

ACIM (Advisory Committee on Infant Mortality). 2001. *Low Birth Weight: Report and Recommendations.* Final report to the Secretary of Health and Human Services.

ACOG (American College of Obstetricians and Gynecologists). 2001. Assessment of risk factors for preterm birth. ACOG Practice Bulletin No. 31. *Obstetrics and Gynecology* 98:709-716.

ACOG. 2003. Management of preterm labor. *ACOG Practice Bulletin No. 431.* 101:1039-1047.

ACOG. 2004. Ultrasonography in pregnancy. *ACOG Practice Bulletin No. 58.* 104:1449-1458.

Adams MM, Delaney KM, Stupp PW, McCarthy BJ, Rawlings JS. 1997. The relationship of interpregnancy interval to infant birthweight and length of gestation among low-risk women, Georgia. *Paediatric and Perinatal Epidemiology* 1:48-62.

Adams MM, Elam-Evans LD, Wilson HG, Gilbertz DA. 2000. Rates of and factors associated with recurrence of preterm delivery. *JAMA* 283:1591-1596.

Adashi EY, Ekins MN, LaCoursiere Y. 2004. On the discharge of Hippocratic obligations: Challenges and opportunities. *American Journal of Obstetrics and Gynecology* 190(4): 885-893.

Aggazzotti G, Righi E, Fantuzzi G, Biasotti B, Ravera G, Kanitz S, Barbone F, Sansebastiano G, Battaglia MA, Leoni V, Fabiani L, Triassi M, Sciacca S. 2004. Chlorination by-products (CBPs) in drinking water and adverse pregnancy outcomes in Italy. *Journal of Water and Health* 2:233-247.

Aghajafari F, Murphy K, Matthews S, Ohlsson A, Amankwah K, Hannah M. 2002. Repeated doses of antenatal corticosteroids in animals: A systematic review. *American Journal of Obstetrics and Gynecology* 186(4):843-849.

Ahlborg G Jr., Bodin L. 1991. Tobacco smoke exposure and pregnancy outcome among working women. A prospective study at prenatal care centers in Orebro County, Sweden. *American Journal of Epidemiology* 133:338-347.

Ahlborg G Jr., Bodin L, Hogstedt C. 1990. Heavy lifting during pregnancy—A hazard to the fetus? A prospective study. *International Journal of Epidemiology* 19(1):90-97.

Ahluwalia IB, Grummer-Strawn L, and Scanlon KS. 1997. Exposure to environmental tobacco smoke and birth outcome: Increased effects on pregnant women aged 30 years or older. *American Journal of Epidemiology* 146:42-47.

Ahmad SA, Sayed MH, Barua S, Khan MH, Faruquee MH, Jalil A, Hadi SA, Talukder HK. 2001. Arsenic in drinking water and pregnancy outcomes. *Environmental Health Perspectives* 109:629-631.

AHRQ (Agency for Health Care Research and Quality). 2002. *Criteria for Determining Disability in Infants and Children: Low Birth Weight.* [Online]. Available: http://www.ahrq. gov/clinic/epcsums/lbwdissum.htm [accessed March 9, 2006].

Al-Aweel I, Pursley DM, Rubin LP, Shah B, Weisberger S, Richardson DK. 2001. Variation in prevalence of hypotension, hypertension and vasopressor use in NICUs. *Journal of Perinatology* 21:272-278.

Albertine KH, Jones GP, Starcher BC, Bohnsack JF, Davis PL, Cho S, Carlton DP, Bland RD. 1999. Chronic lung injury in preterm lambs. *American Journal of Respiratory and Critical Care Medicine* 159:945-958.

Albertsen K, Hannerz H, Borg V, Burr H. 2003. The effect of work environment and heavy smoking on the social inequalities in smoking cessation. *Public Health* 117(6):383-388.

Albertsen K, Andersen A-M N, Olsen J, Grønbaek M. 2004. Alcohol consumption during pregnancy and the risk of preterm delivery. *American Journal of Epidemiology* 159: 155-161.

Alexander GR, Allen MC. 1996. Conceptualization, measurement, and use of gestational age. I. Clinical and public health practice. *Journal of Perinatology: Official Journal of the California Perinatal Association* 16(1):53-59.

Alexander GR, Kotelchuck M. 2001. Assessing the role and effectiveness of prenatal care: History, challenges, and directions for future research. *Public Health Reports* 116(4): 306-316.

Alexander GR, Slay M. 2002. Prematurity at birth: Trends, racial disparities, and epidemiology. *Mental Retardation & Developmental Disabilities Research Reviews* 8(4):215-220.

Alexander GR, De Caunes F, Hulsey TC, Tompkins ME, Allen M. 1992. Validity of postnatal assessments of gestational age: A comparison of the method of Ballard et al. and early ultrasonography. *American Journal of Obstetrics and Gynecology* 166(3):891-895.

Alexander GR, Tompkins ME, Petersen DJ, Hulsey TC, Mor J. 1995. Discordance between LMP-based and clinically estimated gestational age: Implications for research, programs, and policy. *Public Health Reports* 110(4):395-402.

Alexander GR, Himes JH, Kaufman RB, Mor J, Kogan M. 1996. A United States national reference for fetal growth. *Obstetrics and Gynecology* 87(2 I):163-168.

Alexander GR, Kogan M, Martin J, Papiernik E . 1998. What are the fetal growth patterns of singletons, twins, and triplets in the United States? *Clinical Obstetrics and Gynecology* 41(1):115-125.

Alexander GR, Kogan MD, Himes JH. 1999. 1994-1996 U.S. singleton birth weight percentiles for gestational age by race, Hispanic origin, and gender. *Maternal and Child Health Journal* 3(4):225-231.

Alexander GR, Kogan M, Bader D, Carlo W, Allen M, Mor J. 2003. U.S. birth weight/ gestational age-specific neonatal mortality: 1995-1997 rates for whites, hispanics, and blacks. *Pediatrics* 111(1):e61-e66.

Alexander S, Buekens P, Blondel B, Kaminski M. 1990. Is routine antenatal booking vaginal examination necessary for reasons other than cervical cytology if ultrasound examination is planned? *British Journal of Obstetrics and Gynaecology* 97(4):365-366.

Al-Jasmi F, Al-Mansoor F, Alsheiba A, Carter AO, Carter TP, Hossain MM. 2002. Effect of interpregnancy interval on risk of spontaneous preterm birth in Emirati women, United Arab Emirates. *Bulletin of the World Health Organization* 80:871-875.

Allen MC. 2002. Overview: Prematurity. *Mental Retardation & Developmental Disabilities Research Reviews* 8(4):213-214.

Allen MC. 2005a. Assessment of gestational age and neuromaturation. *Mental Retardation and Developmental Disabilities Research Reviews* 11(1):21-33.

Allen MC. 2005b. Risk assessment and neurodevelopmental outcomes. In: Taeusch HW, Ballard RA, Gleason CA eds. *Avery's Diseases of the Newborn*, 8th edition. Philadelphia, PA: Elsevier Saunders. Pp. 1026-1042.

Allen MC, Capute AJ. 1986. Assessment of early auditory and visual abilities of extremely premature infants. *Developmental Medicine and Child Neurology* 28(4):458-466.

Allen MC, Capute AJ. 1989. Neonatal neurodevelopmental examination as a predictor of neuromotor outcome in premature infants. *Pediatrics* 83(4):498-506.

Allen MC, Donohue PK, Dusman AE. 1993. The limit of viability—Neonatal outcome of infants born at 22 to 25 weeks' gestation. *New England Journal of Medicine* 329(22): 1597-1601.

Allen MC, Alexander GR, Tompkins ME, Hulsey TC. 2000. Racial differences in temporal changes in newborn viability and survival by gestational age. *Paediatric and Perinatal Epidemiology* 14(2):152-158.

Als H. 1998. Developmental care in the newborn intensive care unit. *Current Opinion in Pediatrics* 10(2):138-142.

Als H, Duffy FH, McAnulty GB, Rivkin MJ, Vajapeyam S, Mulkern RV, Warfield SK, Huppi PS, Butler SC, Conneman N, Fischer C, Eichenwald EC. 2004. Early experience alters brain function and structure. *Pediatrics* 113(4 I):846-857.

Althuisius SM, Dekker GA, Hummel P, Bekedam DJ, Van Geijn HP. 2001. Final results of the cervical incompetence prevention randomized cerclage trial (CIPRACT): Therapeutic cerclage with bed rest versus bed rest alone. *American Journal of Obstetrics and Gynecology* 185(5):1106-1112.

Altman DG, Chitty LS. 1994. Charts of fetal size: I. Methodology. *British Journal of Obstetrics and Gynaecology* 101(1):29-34.

Altman D, Powers WJ, Perlman JM, Herscovitch P, Volpe SL, Volpe JJ. 1988. Cerebral blood flow requirement for brain viability in newborn infants is lower than adults. *Annals of Neurology* 24:218-226.

Amaro H, Fried LE, Cabral H, Zuckerman B. 1990. Violence during pregnancy and substance use. *American Journal of Public Health* 80(5):575-579.

Amiel-Tison C. 1968. Neurological evaluation of the maturity of newborn infants. *Archives of Disease in Childhood* 43(227):89-93.

Amiel-Tison C. 1980. Possible acceleration of neurological maturation following high-risk pregnancy. *American Journal of Obstetrics and Gynecology* 138(3):303-306.

Amiel-Tison C, Gosselin J. 2001. *Neurologic Development from Birth to 6 Years*. Baltimore, MD: Johns Hopkins University Press.

Amiel-Tison C, Grenier A. 1986. *Neurologic Assessment During the First Year of Life*. New York: Oxford.

Amiel-Tison C, Pettigrew AG. 1991. Adaptive changes in the developing brain during intrauterine stress. *Brain and Development* 13(2):67-76.

Amiel-Tison C, Allen MC, Lebrun F, Rogowski J. 2002. Macropremies: Underprivileged newborns. *Mental Retardation & Developmental Disabilities Research Reviews* 8(4): 281-292.

Amiel-Tison C, Cabrol D, Denver R, Jarreau P-H, Papiernik E, Piazza PV. 2004a. Fetal adaptation to stress. I. Acceleration of fetal maturation and earlier birth triggered by placental insufficiency in humans. *Early Human Development* 78(1):15-27.

Amiel-Tison C, Cabrol D, Denver R, Jarreau P-H, Papiernik E, Piazza PV. 2004b. Fetal adaptation to stress: II. Evolutionary aspects; Stress-induced hippocampal damage; long-term effects on behavior; consequences on adult health. *Early Human Development* 78(2): 81-94.

Amini SB, Catalano PM, Dierker LJ, Mann LI. 1996. Births to teenagers: Trends and obstetric outcomes. *Obstetrics and Gynecology* 87(5 I):668-674.

Anand KJS. 1998. Clinical importance of pain and stress in preterm neonates. *Biology of the Neonate* 73(1):1-9.

Anand KJS, Abu-Saad HH, Aynsley-Green A, Bancalari E, Benini F, Champion GD, Craig KD, Dangel TS, Fournier-Charrière E, Franck LS, Grunau RE, Hertel SA, Jacqz-Aigrain E, Jorch G, Kopelman BI, Koren G, Larsson B, Marlow N, McIntosh N, Ohlsson A, Olsson G, Porter F, Richter R, Stevens B, Taddio A. 2001. Consensus statement for the prevention and management of pain in the newborn. *Archives of Pediatrics and Adolescent Medicine* 155(2):173-180.

Ananth CV, Joseph KS, Oyelese Y, Demissie K, Vintzileos AM. 2005. Trends in preterm birth and perinatal mortality among singletons: United States, 1989 through 2000. *Obstetrics and Gynecology* 105(5 I):1084-1091.

Anderson AN, Gianaroli L, Felberbaum R, de Mouzon J. 2005. Assisted reproductive technology in Europe, 2001. Results generated from European register by ESHRE. *Human Reproduction* 20(5):1158-1176.

Anderson P, Doyle LW. 2003. Neurobehavioral outcomes of school-age children born extremely low birth weight or very preterm in the 1990s. *JAMA* 289(24):3264-3272.

Anderson RT, Sorlie P, Backlund E, Johnson N, Kaplan GA. 1996. Mortality effects of community socioeconomic status. *Epidemiology* 8(1): 42-47.

Ando M, Takashima S, Mito T. 1988. Endotoxin, cerebral blood flow, amino acids and brain damage in young rabbits. *Brain and Development* 10(6):365-370.

Andrews KW, Savitz DA, Hertz-Picciotto I. 1994. Prenatal lead exposure in relation to gestational age and birth weight: A review of epidemiologic studies. *American Journal of Industrial Medicine* 26:13-32.

Andrews WW, Goldenberg RL. 2003. What we have learned from an antibiotic trial in fetal fibronectin positive women. *Seminars in Perinatology* 27(3):231-238.

Andrews WW, Hauth JC, Goldenberg RL. 2000. Infection and preterm birth. *American Journal of Perinatology* 17:357-365.

Andrews WW, Sibai BM, Thom EA, Dudley D, Ernest JM, McNellis D, Leveno KJ, Wapner R, Moawad A, O'Sullivan MJ, Caritis SN, Iams JD, Langer O, Miodovnik M, Dombrowski M. 2003. Randomized clinical trial of metronidazole plus erythromycin to prevent spontaneous preterm delivery in fetal fibronectin-positive women. *Obstetrics and Gynecology* 101(5):847-855.

Andrews WW, Goldenberg RL, Hauth JC, Cliver SP, Copper R, Conner M. 2006. Interconceptional antibiotics to prevent spontaneous preterm birth: A randomized clinical trial. *American Journal of Obstetrics and Gynecology* 194(3):617-623.

Annells M, Hart P, Mullighan C, Heatley S, Robinson J, Bardy P, McDonald H. 2004. Interleukins-1, -4, -6, -10, tumor necrosis factor, transforming growth factor-beta, FAS, and mannose-binding protein C gene polymorphisms in Australian women: Risk of preterm birth. *American Journal of Obstetrics and Gynecology* 191(6):2056-2067.

Anotayanonth S, Subhedar NV, Garner P, Neilson JP, Harigopal S. 2004. Betamimetics for inhibiting preterm labour. *Cochrane Database of Systematic Reviews* (4).

Arechavaleta-Velasco F, Koi H, Strauss JF 3rd, Parry S. 2002. Viral infection of the trophoblast: Time to take a serious look at its role in abnormal implantation and placentation? *Journal of Reproductive Immunology* 55:113-121

Arias F, Rodriquez L, Rayne SC, Kraus FT. 1993. Maternal placental vasculopathy and infection: Two distinct subgroups among patients with preterm labor and preterm ruptured membranes. *American Journal of Obstetrics and Gynecology* 168:585-591.

Ashbaugh JB, Leick-Rude MK, Kilbride HW. 1999. Developmental care teams in the neonatal intensive care unit: Survey on current status. *Journal of Perinatology* 19(1):48-52.

Asrat T. 2001. Intra-amniotic infection patients with preterm prelabor rupture of membranes. Pathophysiology, detection and management. *Clinicial Perinatology* 28:735-751.

Asrat T, Lewis DF, Garitie TJ, Major CA, Nageotte MP, Towers CV, Montgomery DM, Dorchester WA. 1991. Rate of recurrence of preterm premature rupture of membranes in consecutive pregnancies. *American Journal of Obstetrics and Gynecology* 165(a Pt1): 1111-1115.

Astolfi P, Zonta LA. 2002. Delayed maternity and risk at delivery. *Paediatric and Perinatal Epidemiology* 16(1):67-72.

Aucott S, Donohue PK, Atkins E, Allen MC. 2002. Neurodevelopmental care in the NICU. *Mental Retardation and Developmental Disabilities Research Reviews* 8(4):298-308.

Avchen RN, Scott KG, Mason CA. 2001. Birth weight and school-age disabilities: A population-based study. *American Journal of Epidemiology* 154(10):895-901.

Avery GB, Fletcher AB, Kaplan M, Brudno DS. 1985. Controlled trial of dexamethasone in respirator-dependent infants with bronchopulmonary dysplasia. *Pediatrics* 75(1): 106-111.

Avery ME, Tooley WH, Keller JB, Hurd SS, Bryan MH, Cotton RB, et al. 1987. Is chronic lung disease in low birth weight infants preventable? A survey of eight centers. *Pediatrics* 79:26-30.

Aylward GP. 2002a. Cognitive and neuropsychological outcomes: More than IQ scores. *Mental Retardation and Developmental Disabilities Research Reviews* 8(4):234-240.

Aylward GP. 2002b. Methodological issues in outcome studies of at-risk infants. *Journal of Pediatric Psychology* 27(1):37-45.

Aylward GP. 2005. Neurodevelopmental outcomes of infants born prematurely. *Journal of Developmental and Behavioral Pediatrics* 26(6):427.

Aylward GP, Pfeiffer SI, Wright A, Verhulst SJ. 1989. Outcome studies of low birth weight infants published in the last decade: A metaanalysis. *Journal of Pediatrics* 115(4): 515-520.

Aziz K, McMillan DD, Andews W, Pendray M, Qiu Z, Karuri S, et al. 2005. Variations in rates of nosocomial infection among Canadian neonatal intensive care units may be practice related. *BMC Pediatrics* 5:22.

Bachmann LM, Coomarasamy A, Honest H, Khan KS. 2003. Elective cervical cerclage for prevention of preterm birth: A systematic review. *Acta Obstetricia et Gynecologica Scandinavica* 82(5):398-404.

Back SA. 2005. Congenital malformations of the central nervous system. In: Taeusch HW, Ballard RA, Gleason CA eds. *Avery's Diseases of the Newborn*, 8th edition. Philadelphia, PA: Elsevier Saunders. Pp. 1471-1483.

Back SA, Rivkees SA. 2004. Emerging concepts in periventricular white matter injury. *Seminars in Perinatology* 28:405-414.

Back SA, Gan X, Li Y, Rosenberg PR, Volpe JJ. 1998. Maturation-dependent vulnerability of oligodendrocytes to oxidative stress-induced death caused by glutathione depletion. *Journal of Neuroscience* 18:6241-6253.

Back SA, Luo NL, Borenstein NS, Levine JM, Volpe JJ, Kinney HC. 2001. Late oligodendrocyte progenitors coincide with the developmental window of vulnerability for human perinatal white matter injury. *Journal of Neuroscience* 21:1302-1312.

Back SA, Han BH, Luo NL, Chricton CA, Xanthoudakis S, Tam J, Arvin KL, Holtzman DL. 2002. Selective vulnerability of late oligodendrocyte progenitors to hypoxia-ischemia. *Journal of Neuroscience* 22:455-463.

Bae J, Peters-Golden M, Loch-Caruso R. 1999a. Stimulation of pregnant rat uterine contraction by the polychlorinated biphenyl (PCB) mixture aroclor 1242 may be mediated by arachidonic acid release through activation of phospholipase A2 enzymes. *Journal of Pharmacology and Experimental Therapeutics* 289(2):1112-1120.

Bae J, Stuenkel EL, Loch-Caruso R. 1999b. Stimulation of oscillatory uterine contraction by the PCB mixture Aroclor 1242 may involve increased [Ca2+]i through voltage-operated calcium channels. *Toxicology and Applied Pharmacology* 155(3):261-272.

Bagenholm R, Nilsson A, Kjellmer I. 1997. Formation of free radicals in hypoxic ischemic brain damage in the neonatal rat, assessed by an endogenous spin trap and lipid peroxidation. *Brain Research* 773:132-138.

Bagenholm R, Nilsson A, Gotborg CW, Kjellmer I. 1998. Free radicals are formed in the brain of fetal sheep during reperfusion after cerebral ischemia. *Pediatrics Research* 43:271-275.

Baird TM. 2004. Clinical correlates, natural history and outcome of neonatal apnoea. *Seminars in Neonatology* 9(3):205-211.

Baker JP. 2000. The incubator and the medical discovery of the premature infant. *Journal of Perinatology* 20(5):321-328.

Bakketeig LS, Hoffman HJ. 1981. Epidemiology of preterm birth: Results from a longitudinal study of births in Norway. In: Elder MG, Hendricks CH eds. *Preterm Labor*. London, UK, and Boston, MA: Butterworth. Pp. 17-46.

Bakketeig LS, Hoffman HJ, Harley EE. 1979. The tendency to repeat gestational age and birth weight in successive births. *American Journal of Obstetrics and Gynecology* 135(8):1086-1103.

Ballard JL, Novak KK, Driver M. 1979. A simplified score for assessment of fetal maturation of newly born infants. *Journal of Pediatrics* 95(5 I):769-774.

Ballard JL, Khoury JC, Wedig K, Wang L, Eilers-Walsman BL, Lipp R. 1991. New Ballard Score, expanded to include extremely premature infants. *Journal of Pediatrics* 119(3): 417-423.

Bamshad M. 2005. Genetic influences on health: Does race matter. *JAMA* 294:937-946.

Bancalari E. 2002. Neonatal chronic lung disease. In: Fanaroff AA, Martin RJ eds. *Neonatal Perinatal Medicine*, 7th edition. St. Loius, MO: Mosby-Year Book. P. 1057.

Barbaras, AP. 1966. Ehlers-Danlos syndrome: Associated with prematurity and premature rupture of foetal membranes; possible increase in incidence. *British Medical Journal* 5515: 682-684.

Barbieri RL. 2005. Too many embryos for one woman: What counts as success or failure in ART? *OBG Management* 17(7):8-9.

Barker DJ, Winter PD, Osmond C, Margetts B, Simmonds SJ. 1989a. Weight in infancy and death from ischaemic heart disease. *Lancet* 2(8663):577-580.

Barker DJ, Osmond C, Golding J, Kuh D, Wadsworth ME. 1989b. Growth in utero, blood pressure in childhood and adult life, and mortality from cardiovascular disease. *British Medical Journal* 298(6673):564-567.

Barker DJ, Hales CN, Fall CH, Osmond C, Phipps K, Clark PM. 1993a. Type 2 (non-insulin-dependent) diabetes mellitus, hypertension and hyperlipidaemia (syndrome X): Relation to reduced fetal growth. *Diabetologia* 36(1):62-67.

Barker DJ, Osmond C, Simmonds SJ, Wield GA. 1993b. The relation of small head circumference and thinness at birth to death from cardiovascular disease in adult life. *British Medical Journal* 306(6875):422-426.

Barker DJP. 1998. In utero programming of chronic disease. *Clinical Science* 95(2):115-128.

Barnard KE, Bee HL. 1983. The impact of temporally patterned stimulation on the development of preterm infants. *Child Development* 54(5):1156-1167.

Barnett WS. 1995. Long-term effects of early childhood programs on cognitive and school outcomes. *Future of Children* 5(3):25-50.

Barrington KJ. 2001a. The adverse neuro-developmental effects of postnatal steroids in the preterm infant: A systematic review of RCTs. *BMC Pediatrics* 1.

Barrington KJ. 2001b. Postnatal steroids and neurodevelopmental outcomes: A problem in the making. *Pediatrics* 107(6):1425-1426.

Basso O, Baird DD. 2003. Infertility and preterm delivery, birthweight, and caesarean section: A study within the Danish National Birth Cohort. *Human Reproduction* 18(11):2478-2484.

Basso O, Olsen J, Knudsen LB, Christensen K. 1998. Low birth weight and preterm birth after short interpregnancy intervals. *American Journal of Obstetrics and Gynecology* 178: 259-263.

Battaglia FC, Lubchenco LO. 1967. A practical classification of newborn infants by weight and gestational age. *Journal of Pediatrics* 71(2):159-163.

Baud O, Foix-L'Helias L, Kaminski M, Audibert F, Jarreau P-H, Papiernik E, Huon C, Lepercq J, Dehan M, Lacaze-Masmonteil T. 1999. Antenatal glucocorticoid treatment and cystic periventricular leukomalacia in very premature infants. *New England Journal of Medicine* 341(16):1190-1196.

Bavdekar A, Yajnik CS, Fall CH, Bapat S, Pandit AN, Deshpande D, Bhave S, Kellingray SD, Joglekar C. 1999. Insulin resistance syndrome in 8-year-old Indian children: Small at birth, big at 8 years, or both? *Diabetes* 48(12):2422-2429.

Beck LF, Morrow B, Lipscomb LE, Johnson CH, Gaffield ME, Rogers M, Gilbert BC. 2002. Prevalence of selected maternal behaviors and experiences, Pregnancy Risk Assessment Monitoring System (PRAMS), 1999. *Morbidity and Mortality Weekly Report: Surveillance Summaries* 51(2):1-27.

Becker G, Castrillo M, Jackson R, Nachtigall RD. 2006. Infertility among low-income latinos. *Fertility and Sterility* 85(4):882-887.

Beckerman KP. 2005. Identification, evaluation, and care of the human immunodeficiency virus-exposed neonate. In: Taeusch HW, Ballard RA, Gleason CA eds. *Avery's Diseases of the Newborn*, 8th edition. Philadelphia, PA: Elsevier Saunders.

Beckman PJ, Pokorni JL. 1988. A longitudinal study of families of preterm infants: Changes in stress and support over the first two years. *Journal of Special Education* 22(1):55-65.

Beddhu S. 2004. The body mass index paradox and an obesity, inflammation, and atherosclerosis syndrome in chronic kidney disease. *Seminars in Dialysis* 17:229-232.

Bejar R, Curbelo V, Davis C, Gluck L. 1981. Premature labor. II. Bacterial sources of phospholipase. *Obstetrics and Gynecology* 57(4):479-482.

Bejar R, Wozniak P, Allard M, Benirschke K, Vaucher Y, Coen R. 1988. Antenatal origin of neurologic damage in newborn infants. I. Preterm infants. *American Journal of Obstetrics and Gynecology* 159:357-363.

Belej-Rak T, Okun N, Windrim R, Ross S, Hannah ME. 2003. Effectiveness of cervical cerclage for a sonographically shortened cervix: A systematic review and meta-analysis. *American Journal of Obstetrics and Gynecology* 189(6):1679-1687.

Belfield CR, Nores M, Barnett S, Schweinhart L. 2006. The High/Scope Perry Preschool Program: Cost-benefit analysis using data from the age-40 followup. *Journal of Human Resources* 41(1):162-190.

Bellinger D. 2004. Assessing environmental neurotoxicant exposures and child neurobehavior Confounded by confounding? *Epidemiology* 15:383-384.

Bellu R, de Waal KA, Zanini R. 2005. Opioids for neonates receiving mechanical ventilation. *Cochrane Database of Systematic Reviews: Early Human Development* 81(3):293-302.

Berghella V, Tolosa JE, Kuhlman K, Weiner S, Bolognese RJ, Wapner RJ. 1997. Cervical ultrasonography compared with manual examination as a predictor of preterm delivery. *American Journal of Obstetrics and Gynecology* 177(4):723-730.

Berghella V, Odibo AO, Tolosa JE. 2004. Cerclage for prevention of preterm birth in women with short cervix found on transvaginal ultrasound examination: A randomized trial. *American Journal of Obstetrics and Gynecology* 191:1311-1317.

Berghella V, Odibo AO, To MS, Rust DA, Althuisius SM. 2005. Cerclage for short cervix on ultrasonography. Meta-analysis of trials using individual patient-level data. *Obstetrics and Gynecology* 106:181-189.

Berkman ND, Thorp JM, Lohr KN, et al. 2003. Tocolytic treatment for the management of preterm labor: A review of the evidence. *American Journal of Obstetrics and Gynecology* 188:1648-1659.

Berkowitz GS, Kasl SV. 1983. The role of psychosocial factors in spontaneous preterm delivery. *Journal of Psychosomatic Research* 27(4):283-290.

Berkowitz GS, Papiernik E. 1993. Epidemiology of preterm birth. *Epidemiologic Reviews* 15(2):414-443.

Berkowitz GS, Lapinski RH, Wolff MS. 1996. The role of DDE and polychlorinated biphenyl levels in preterm birth. *Archives of Environmental Contamination and Toxicology* 30:139-141.

Berkowitz GS, Blackmore-Prince C, Lapinski RH, Savitz DA. 1998. Risk factors for preterm birth subtypes. *Epidemiology* 9:279-285.

Berkowitz R, Davis J. 2006. Introduction: Health disparities in infertility. *Fertility and Sterility* 85(4):842-843.

Berlin LJ, Brooks-Gunn J, McCarton C, McCormick MC. 1998. The effectiveness of early intervention: Examining risk factors and pathways to enhanced development. *Preventive Medicine* 27(2):238-245.

Bernstein IM. 2003. The assessment of newborn size. *Pediatrics* 111(6 I):1430-1431.

Bernstein IM, Meyer MC, Capeless EL. 1994. "Fetal growth charts": Comparison of crosssectional ultrasound examinations with birth weight. *Journal of Maternal-Fetal Medicine* 3(4):182-186.

Berseth CL. 2005. Developmental anatomy and physiology of the gastrointestinal tract. In: Taeusch HW, Ballard RA, Gleason CA eds. *Avery's Diseases of the Newborn*, 8th edition. Philadelphia, PA: Elsevier Saunders. Pp. 12-34.

Bhargava SK, Sachdev HS, Fall CH, Osmond C, Lakshmy R, Barker DJ, Biswas SK, Ramji S, Prabhakaran D, Reddy KS. 2004. Relation of serial changes in childhood body-mass index to impaired glucose tolerance in young adulthood. *New England Journal of Medicine* 350(9):865-875.

Bhutta AT, Cleves MA, Casey PH, Cradock MM, Anand KJS. 2002. Cognitive and behavioral outcomes of school aged children who were born preterm: A meta analysis. *JAMA* 288(6):128-737.

Bhutta T, Henderson-Smart DJ. 2002. Rescue high frequency oscillatory ventilation versus conventional ventilation for pulmonary dysfunction in preterm infants. *Cochrane Reviews.* Issue 3.

Bhutta T, Ohlsson A. 1998. Systematic review and meta-analysis of early postnatal dexamethasone for prevention of chronic lung disease. *Archives of Disease in Childhood: Fetal and Neonatal Edition* 79:F26-F33.

Bian J, Sun Y. 1997. Transcriptional activation by p53 of thehuman type IV collagenase (gelatinase A or the matrix metalloproteinase2) promoter. *Molecular and Cellular Biology* 17:6330-6318.

Binkin NJ, Yip R, Fleshood L, Trowbridge FL. 1988. Birth weight and childhood growth. *Pediatrics* 82:828-834.

Bin-Nun A, Bromiker R, Wilschanski M, Kaplan M, Rudensky B, Caplan M, Hammerman C. 2005. Oral probiotics prevent necrotizing enterocolitis in very low birth weight neonates. *Journal of Pediatrics* 147(2):192-196.

Birnholz JC, Benacerraf BR. 1983. The development of human fetal hearing. *Science* 222(4623):516-518.

Bishop EH. 1964. Pelvic scoring for elective induction. *Obstetrics and Gynecology* 24: 266-268.

Bitler M, Schmidt L. 2006. Health disparities and infertility: Impacts of state-level insurance mandates. *Fertility and Sterility* 85(4):858-865.

Bitto A, Gray RH, Simpson JL, Queenan JT, Kambic RT, Perez A, Mena P, Barbato M, Li C, Jennings V. 1997. Adverse outcomes of planned and unplanned pregnancies among users of natural family planning: A prospective study. *American Journal of Public Health* 87(3):338-343.

Bjerager M, Steensberg J, Greisen G. 1995. Quality of life among young adults born with very low birthweights. *Acta Paediatrica, International Journal of Paediatrics* 84(12):1339-1343.

Bjorklund LJ, Ingimarsson J, Curstedt T, John J, Robertson B, Werner O, Vilstrup CT. 1997. Manual ventilation with a few large breaths at birth compromises the therapeutic effect of subsequent surfactant replacement in immature lambs. *Pediatrics Research* 42: 348-355.

Blackmore-Prince C, Harlow SD, Gargiullo P, Lee MA, Savitz DA. 1999. Chemical hair treatments and adverse pregnancy outcome among Black women in central North Carolina. *American Journal of Epidemiology* 149:712-716.

Blackmore-Prince C, Iyasu S, Kendrick JS, Strauss LT, Kugaraj KA, Gargiullo PM, Atrash HK. 2000. Are interpregnancy intervals between consecutive live births among black women associated with infant birth weight? *Ethnicity and Disease* 10(1):106-112.

Blackwell MT, Eichenwald EC, McAlmon K, Petit K, Linton PT, McCormick MC, Richardson DK. 2005. Interneonatal intensive care unit variation in growth rates and feeding practices in healthy moderately premature infants. *Journal of Perinatology* 25:478-485.

Blauw-Hospers CH, Hadders-Algra M. 2005. A systematic review of the effects of early intervention on motor development. *Developmental Medicine and Child Neurology* 47(6): 421-432.

Blondel B. 1998. Social and medical support during pregnancy: An overview of the randomized controlled trials. *Prenatal and Neonatal Medicine* 3:141-144.

Blondel B, Zuber M-C. 1988. Marital status and cohabitation during pregnancy: Relationship with social conditions, antenatal care and pregnancy outcome in France. *Paediatric and Perinatal Epidemiology* 2(2):125-137.

Bloom SL, Spong CY, Weiner SJ, Landon MB, Rouse DJ, Varner MW, Moawad AH, Caritis SN, Harper M, Wapner RJ, Sorokin Y, Miodovnik M, O'Sullivan MJ, Sibai B, Langer O, Gabbe SG. 2005. Complications of anesthesia for cesarean delivery. *Obstetrics and Gynecology* 106(2):281-287.

Bloomfield FH, Oliver MH, Hawkins P, Campbell M, Phillips DJ, Gluckman PD, Challis JR. 2003. A periconceptional nutritional origin for noninfectious preterm birth. *Science* 300:606.

Blumenthal I. 2004. Periventricular leucomalacia: A review. *European Journal of Pediatrics* 163:435-442.

Bobak, M. 2000. Outdoor air pollution, low birth weight, and prematurity. *Environmental Health Perspectives* 108:173-176.

Boggess KA, Lieff S, Murtha AP, Moss K, Beck J, Offenbacher S. 2003. Maternal periodontal disease is associated with an increased risk for preeclampsia. *Obstetrics and Gynecology* 101:227-231.

Boggess KA, Madianos PN, Preisser JS, Moise KJ, Offenbacher S. 2005a. Chronic maternal and fetal Porphyromonas gingivalis exposure during pregnancy in rabbits. *American Journal of Obstetrics and Gynecology* 192:554-557.

Boggess KA, Moss K, Madianos P, Murtha AP, Beck J, Offenbacher SD. 2005b. Fetal immune response to oral pathogens and risk of preterm birth. *American Journal of Obstetrics and Gynecology* 193(3):1121-1126.

Bohm SK, McConalogue K, Kong W, Bunnett NW. 1998. Proteinase-activated receptors: New functions for old enzymes. *News in Physiological Sciences* 13:231-240.

Bol KA, Collins JS, Kirby RS. 2006. Survival of infants with neural tube defects in the presence of folic acid fortification. *Pediatrics* 117(3):803-813.

Boonstra H, Gold RB. 2002. Overhauling welfare: Implications for reproductive health policy in the United States. *Journal of the American Medical Women's Association* 57(1):41-46.

Botting N, Powls A, Cooke RWI, Marlow N. 1998. Cognitive and educational outcome of very-low-birthweight children in early adolescence. *Developmental Medicine and Child Neurology* 40(10):652-660.

Botto LD, Khoury MJ. 2001. Commentary: Facing the challenge of gene-environment interaction: The two-by-two table and beyond. *American Journal of Epidemiology* 153:1016-1020.

Bottoms SF, Paul RH, Iams JD, Mercer BM, Thom EA, Roberts JM, Caritis SN, Moawad AH, Van Dorsten JP, Hauth JC, Thurnau GR, Miodovnik M, Meis PM, McNellis D, MacPherson C, Norman GS, Jones P, Mueller-Heubach E, Swain M, Goldenberg RL, Copper RL, Bain R, Rowland E, Lindheimer M, Menard MK, Collins BA, Stramm S, Siddiqi TA, Elder N, Carey JC, Meuer A, Fisher M, Yaffe SJ, Catz C, Klebanoff M, Harger JH, Landon MB, Johnson F, Kovacs BW, Rabello Y, Sibai BM, Ramsey R, Dombrowski MP, Lacey D. 1997. Obstetric determinants of neonatal survival: Influence of willingness to perform cesarean delivery on survival of extremely low-birth-weight infants. *American Journal of Obstetrics and Gynecology* 176(5):960-966.

Bove F, Shim Y, Zeitz P. 2002. Drinking water contaminants and adverse pregnancy outcomes: A review. *Environmental Health Perspectives* 110(Suppl 1):61-74.

Boyce WT, Schaefer C, Uitti C. 1985. Permanence and change: Psychosocial factors in the outcome of adolescent pregnancy. *Social Science and Medicine* 21(11):1279-1287.

Boyce WT, Schaefer C, Harrison HR, Haffner WH, Lewis M, Wright AL. 1986. Social and cultural factors in pregnancy complications among Navajo women. *American Journal of Epidemiology* 124(2):242-253.

Bracci R. 1997. Free oxygen radicals and surfactant. *Biology of the Neonate* 71(Suppl 1): 23-27.

Bracewell M, Marlow N. 2002. Patterns of motor disability in very preterm children. *Mental Retardation and Developmental Disabilities Research Reviews* 8(4):241-248.

Brandon DH, Holditch-Davis D, Belyea M. 2002. Preterm infants born at less than 31 weeks' gestation have improved growth in cycled light compared with continuous near darkness. *Journal of Pediatrics* 140(2):192-199.

Brandt LP, Nielsen CV. 1992. Job stress and adverse outcome of pregnancy: A causal link or recall bias? *American Journal of Epidemiology* 135(3):302-311.

Brant K, Caruso RL. 2005. Late-gestation rat myometrial cells express multiple isoforms of phospholipase A2 that mediate PCB 50-induced release of arachidonic acid with coincident prostaglandin production. *Toxicological Sciences* 88(1):222-230.

Brant K, Guan W, Tithof P, Loch Caruso R. 2006a. Gestation age-related increase in 50 kDa rat uterine calcium-independent phospholipase A2 expression influences uterine sensitivity to polychlorinated biphenyl stimulation. *Biology of Reproduction* (in press).

Brant KA, Thiex NW, Caruso RL. 2006b. Polybrominated diphenyl ethers stimulate the release of pro-inflammatory cytokines from term human gestational membranes. *Toxicologist* 90:Abstract 1553.

Branum AM, Schoendorf KC. 2005. The influence of maternal age on very preterm birth of twins: Differential effects by parity. *Paediatric and Perinatal Epidemiology* 19(5): 399-404.

Bremer DL, Palmer EA, Fellows RR, Baker JD, Hardy RJ, Tung B, Rogers GL. 1998. Strabismus in premature infants in the first year of life. *Archives of Ophthalmology* 116(3): 329-333.

Breslau N. 1995. Psychiatric sequelae of low birth weight. *Epidemiologic Reviews* 17(1): 96-106.

Breslau N, Klein N, Allen L. 1988. Very low birthweight: Behavioral sequelae at nine years of age. *Journal of the American Academy of Child and Adolescent Psychiatry* 27(5): 605-612.

Breslau N, DelDotto JE, Brown GG, Kumar S, Ezhuthachan S, Hufnagle KG, Peterson EL. 1994. A gradient relationship between low birth weight and IQ at age 6 years. *Archives of Pediatrics and Adolescent Medicine* 148(4):377-383.

Brett KM, Strogatz DS, Savitz DA. 1997. Employment, job strain, and preterm delivery among women in North Carolina. *American Journal of Public Health* 87(2):199-204.

Bricker L, Neilson JP. 2000. Routine doppler ultrasound in pregnancy. *Cochrane Database of Systematic Reviews* 2.

Brion LP, Bell EF, Raghuveer TS. 2003. Vitamin E supplementation for prevention of morbidity and mortality in preterm infants. *Cochrane Database of Systematic Reviews (Online: Update Software)* 3.

Brocklehurst P, Hannah M, McDonald H. 2000. Interventions for treating bacterial vaginosis in pregnancy. *Cochrane Database of Systematic Reviews* 2.

Brody DJ, Bracken MB. 1987. Short interpregnancy interval: A risk factor for low birthweight. *American Journal of Perinatology* 4:50-54.

Brookes AJ. 1999. The essence of SNPs. *Gene* 234:177-186.

Brooks-Gunn J. 1991. Stress and support during pregnancy: What do they tell us about low birthweight? In: *Advances in the Prevention of Low Birth Weight: An International Symposium.* Berendes HW, Kessel S, Yaffee S eds. Washington, DC: National Center for Education in Maternal and Child Health. Pp. 39-57.

Brooks-Gunn J, Duncan GJ. 1997. The effects of poverty on children. *Future of Children* 7(2):55-87.

Brooks-Gunn J, Gross RT, Kraemer HC, Spiker D, Shapiro S. 1992a. Enhancing the cognitive outcomes of low birth weight, premature infants: For whom is the intervention most effective? *Pediatrics* 89(6 Suppl):1209-1215.

Brooks-Gunn J, Liaw F-R, Kato Klebanov P. 1992b. Effects of early intervention on cognitive function of low birth weight preterm infants. *Journal of Pediatrics* 120(3):350-359.

Brooks-Gunn J, McCarton CM, Casey PH, McCormick MC. 1994. Early intervention in low-birth-weight premature infants: Results through age 5 years from the Infant Health and Development Program. *JAMA* 272(16):1257-1262.

Brown HL, Britton KA, Brizendine EJ, Hiett AK, Ingram D, Turnquest MA, Golichowski AM, Abernathy MP. 1999. A randomized comparison of home uterine activity monitoring in the outpatient management of women treated for preterm labor. *American Journal of Obstetrics and Gynecology* 180(4):798-805.

Brown P. 1995. Race, class, and environmental health: A review and systematization of the literature. *Environmental Research* 69:15-30.

Bruce FC, Fiscella K, Kendrick JS. 2000. Vaginal douching and preterm birth: An intriguing hypothesis. *Medical Hypotheses* 54(3):448-452.

Bruce FC, Kendrick JS, Kieke BA Jr., Jagielski S, Joshi R, Tolsma DD. 2002. Is vaginal douching associated with preterm delivery? *Epidemiology* 13(3):328-333.

Buck GM, Msall ME, Schisterman EF, Lyon NR, Rogers BT. 2000. Extreme prematurity and school outcomes. *Paediatric and Perinatal Epidemiology* 14(4):324-331.

Buekens P, Delvoye P, Wollast E, Robyn C. 1984. Epidemiology of pregnancies with unknown last menstrual period. *Journal of Epidemiology and Community Health* 38(1):79-80.

Buhimschi IA, Christner R, Buhimschi CS. 2005. Proteomic biomarker analysis of amniotic fluid for identification of intra-amniotic inflammation. *British Journal of Obstetrics and Gynaecology* 112(2):173-181.

Buka SL, Brennan RT, Rich-Edwards JW, Raudenbush SW, Earls F. 2003. Neighborhood support and the birth weight of urban infants. *American Journal of Epidemiology* 157(1):1-8.

Bukowski J, Somers G, Bryanton J. 2001a. Agricultural contamination of groundwater as a possible risk factor for growth restriction or prematurity. *Journal of Occupational and Environmental Medicine* 43:377-383.

Bukowski R, Gahn D, Denning J, Saade G. 2001b. Impairment of growth in fetuses destined to deliver preterm. *American Journal of Obstetrics and Gynecology* 185:463-467

Burdjalov VF, Baumgart S, Spitzer AR. 2003. Cerebral function monitoring: A new scoring system for the evaluation of brain maturation in neonates. *Pediatrics* 112(4):855-861.

Cameo P, Srisuparp S, Strakova Z, Fazleabas AT. 2004. Chorionic gonadotropin and uterine dialogue in the primate. *Reproductive Biology and Endocrinology* 2.

Campbell AT. 2004. State regulation of medical research with children and adolescents: An overview and analysis. In: *Ethical Conduct of Clinical Research Involving Children*. Field MJ, Behrman RE eds. Washington, DC: The National Academies Press.

Campbell FA, Pungello EP, Miller-Johnson S. 2002. The development of perceived scholastic competence and global self-worth in African American adolescents from low-income families: The roles of family factors, early educational intervention, and academic experience. *Journal of Adolescent Research* 17(3):277-302.

Campbell S, Warsof SL, Little D, Cooper DJ. 1985. Routine ultrasound screening for the prediction of gestational age. *Obstetrics and Gynecology* 65(5):613-620.

Canick JA, Saller DN Jr., Lambert-Messerlian GM. 2003. Prenatal screening for Down syndrome: current and future methods. *Clinics in Laboratory Medicine* 23:395-411.

Capone AJ, Accardo PJ. 1996. *Developmental Disabilities in Infancy and Childhood*, 2nd edition. Baltimore, MD: Paul H. Brookes. Pp. 23-37.

Caravale B, Tozzi C, Albino G, Vicari S. 2005. Cognitive development in low risk preterm infants at 3-4 years of life. *Archives of Disease in Childhood: Fetal and Neonatal* 90(6):F474-F479.

Cardoso WV, Williams MC. 2000. Basic mechanisms of lung development: Eighth Woods Hole Conference on Lung Cell Biology. *American Journal of Respiratory Cell and Molecular Biology* 25:137.

Carey JC, Klebanoff MA. 2003. National Institute of Child Health and Human Development Maternal-Fetal Medicine Units Network: What have we learned about vaginal infections and preterm birth? *Seminars in Perinatology* 27:212-216.

Carey JC, Klebanoff MA, Hauth JC, Hillier SL, Thom EA, Ernest JM, Heine RP, Nugent RP, Fischer ML, Leveno KJ, Wapner R, Varner M, Trout W, Moawad A, Sibai BM, Miodovnik M, Dombrowski M, O'Sullivan MJ, VanDorsten JP, Langer O, Roberts J. 2000. Metronidazole to prevent preterm delivery in pregnant women with asymptomatic bacterial vaginosis. *New England Journal of Medicine* 342(8):534-540.

Caritis SN, Edelstone DI, Mueller-Heubach E. 1979. Pharmacologic inhibition of preterm labor. *American Journal of Obstetrics and Gynecology* 133:557-578.

Caritis SN, Chiao JP, Moore JJ, Ward SM. 1987. Myometrial desensitization after ritodrine infusion. *American Journal of Physiology* 253.

Caritis SN, Chiao JP, Kridgen P. 1991. Comparison of pulsatile and continuous ritodrine administration: Effects on uterine contractility and beta-adrenergic receptor cascade. *American Journal of Obstetrics and Gynecology* 164:1005-1011.

Carlton DP, Albertine KH, Cho SC, Lont M, Bland RD. 1997. Role of neutrophils in lung vascular injury and edema after premature birth in lambs. *Journal of Applied Physiology* 83:1307-1317.

Carmichael S, Abrams B. 1997. A critical review of the relationship between gestational weight gain and preterm delivery. *Obstetrics and Gynecology* 89(5):865-873.

Carmichael SL, Iyasu S. 1998. Changes in the black-white infant mortality gap from 1983 to 1991 in the United States. *American Journal of Preventive Medicine* 15(3):220-227.

Carr-Hill RA, Hall MH. 1985. The repetition of spontaneous preterm labour. *British Journal of Obstetrics and Gynaecology* 92(9):921-928.

Casey ML, MacDonald PC. 1988. Biomolecular processes in the initiation of parturition: Decidual activation. *Clinical Obstetrics and Gynecology* 31:533-552.

Casey PH, Kraemer HC, Bernbaum J, Yogman MW, Sells JC. 1991. Growth status and growth rates of a varied sample of low birth weight, preterm infants: A longitudinal cohort from birth to three years of age. *Journal of Pediatrics* 119:599-605.

Casper RF, Lye SJ. 1986. Myometrial desensitization to continuous but not to intermittent β-adrenergic agonist infusion in the sheep. *American Journal of Obstetrics and Gynecology* 154(2):301-305.

Cassel J. 1976. The contribution of the social environment to host resistance: The Fourth Wade Hampton Frost Lecture. *American Journal of Epidemiology* 104:107-123.

Castillo-Durán C, Weisstaub G. 2003. Zinc supplementation and growth of the fetus and low birth weight infant. *Journal of Nutrition* 133(5 Suppl 2):1494S-1568S.

Cats BP, Tan KEWP. 1989. Prematures with and without regressed retinopathy of prematurity: Comparison of long-term (6-10 years) ophthalmological morbidity. *Journal of Pediatric Ophthalmology and Strabismus* 26(6):271-275.

Caulfield LE, Zavaleta N, Shankar AH, Merialdi M. 1998. Potential contribution of maternal zinc supplementation during pregnancy to maternal and child survival. *American Journal of Clinical Nutrition* 68(2 Suppl):499S-508S.

Cavalier S, Escobar GJ, Fernbach SA, Queensberry CP, Chellino M. 1996. Postdischarge utilization of medical services by high-risk infants. Experience in a large managed care organization. *Pediatrics* 97:693-699.

CDC (Centers for Disease Control and Prevention). 1999a. Impact of multiple births on low birthweight—Massachusetts. *Morbidity and Mortality Weekly Report* 48 (14):289-292.

CDC. 1999b. *Trends in Twin and Triplet Births, 1980-1997*. [Online]. Available: http://www.cdc.gov/nchs/data/nvsr47/nvs47_24.pdf [accessed March 22, 2006].

CDC. 2000. *Nonmarital Childbearing in the United States, 1940-1999*. [Online]. Available: http://www.cdc.gov/nchs/data/nvsr/nvsr48/nvs48_16.pdf [accessed March 22, 2006].

CDC. 2001. *Births: Final Data for 1999*. [Online]. Available: http://www.cdc.gov/nchs/data/nvsr/nvsr49/nvsr49_01.pdf [accessed August 30, 2005].

CDC. 2002a. *Births: Final Data for 2000*. [Online]. Available: http://www.cdc.gov/nchs/data/nvsr/nvsr50/nvsr50_05.pdf [accessed August 30, 2005].

CDC. 2002b. *National Survey on Family Growth*. [Online]. Available: http://www.cdc.gov/nchs/nsfg.htm [accessed March 1, 2006].

CDC. 2002c. *Births: Final Data for 2002*. [Online]. Available: http://www.cdc.gov/nchs/data/nvsr/nvsr50/nvsr50_05.pdf [accessed October 17, 2005].

CDC. 2003a. *Supplemental Analyses of Recent Trends in Infant Mortality*. National Center for Health Statistics. [Online]. Available: http://www.cdc.gov/nchs/products/pubs/pubd/hestats/infantmort/infantmort.htm [accessed February 5, 2006].

CDC. 2003b. *2001 Assisted Reproductive Technology Success Rates*. National Summary and Fertility Clinic Reports. [Online]. Available: http://www.cdc.gov/reproductivehealth/ART01/PDF/ART2001.pdf [accessed February 4, 2004].

CDC. 2003c. Births: Final data for 2002. *National Vital Statistics Reports: From the Centers for Disease Control and Prevention, National Center for Health Statistics, National Vital Statistics System* 52(10):1-113.

CDC. 2003d. *Births: Final Data for 2002*. [Online]. Available: http://www.cdc.gov/nchs/data/nvsr/nvsr52/nvsr52_10.pdf [accessed January 10, 2006].

CDC. 2004a. *Births: Preliminary Data for 2003*. [Online]. Available: http://www.cdc.gov/nchs/data/nvsr/nvsr53/nvsr53_09.pdf [accessed August 30, 2005].

CDC. 2004b. *Birth Edit Specifications for the 2003 Proposed Revision of the U.S. Standard Certificate of Birth*. [Online]. Available: http://permanent.access.gpo.gov/websites/www.cdc.gov/nchs/data/dvs/MasterSpec9-10-02-acc.pdf [accessed February 13, 2006].

CDC. 2004c. Economic costs associated with mental retardation, cerebral palsy, hearing loss, and vision impairment—United States, 2003. *Morbidity and Mortality Weekly Report* 53(3):57-59.

CDC. 2004d. *Births: Final Data for 2003*. [Online]. Available: http://www.cdc.gov/nchs/data/nvsr/nvsr53_09.pdf [accessed May 22, 2006].

CDC. 2004e. *NCHS Definitions: Fetal Death*. [Online]. Available: http://www.cdc.gov/nchs/datawh/nchsdefs/fetaldeath.htm [accessed May 26, 2006].

CDC. 2004f. *Births, Marriages, Divorces, and Deaths: Provisional Data for January 2004*. [Online]. Available: http://www.cdc.gov/nchs/data/nvsr/nvsr53/nvsr53_01.pdf [accessed June 2, 2006].

CDC. 2005a. *Preliminary Births for 2004*. [Online]. Available: http://www.cdc.gov/nchs/products/pubs/pubd/hestats/prelimbirths04/prelimbirths/04health.htm [accessed November 17, 2005].

CDC. 2005b. Birth rates by age of mother 1993-2003. In: *Births: Final Data for 2003*. [Online]. Available: http://www.cdc.gov/nchs/data/nvsr54/nvsr54_02.pdf [accessed October 3, 2005].

CDC. 2005c. Explaining the 2001-02 infant mortality increase: Data from the linked birth/infant death data set. *National Vital Statistics Reports* 53(12).

CDC. 2005d. *Linked Birth and Infant Death Data.* [Online]. Available: http://www.cdc.gov/nchs/linked.htm [accessed February 27, 2006].

CDC. 2005e. *Supplemental Analyses of Recent Trends in Infant Mortality.* [Online]. Available: http://www.cdc.gov/nchs/products/pubs/pubd/hestats/infantmort/infantmort.htm [accessed January 31, 2006].

CDC. 2005f. *Assisted Reproductive Technology Success Rates 2003: National Summary and Fertility Clinic Reports.* [Online]. Available: http://www.cdc.govART/aRT2003/DF/ART2003.pdf [accessed March 10, 2006].

CDC. 2005g. Assisted reproductive technology surveillance—United States, 2002 and malaria surveillance—United States. *Morbidity and Mortality Weekly Report* 54, No.SS-2.

CDC. 2005h. Annual summary of vital statistics-2003. *Pediatrics* 115(3):619-635.

CDC. 2005i. *Births: Final Data for 2003.* National Vital Statistics Reports 54(2). Hyattsville, MD: National Center for Health Statistics.

CFN (Committee on Fetus and Newborn). 2004. Age terminology during the perinatal period. *Pediatrics* 114(5):1362-1364.

Chaikand S, Corman H. 1991. The impact of low birthweight on special education costs. *Journal of Health Economics* 10(3):291-311.

Chakravarti A, Little P. 2003. Nature, nurture and human disease. *Nature* 421(6921): 412-414.

Challis JR, Sloboda DM, Alfaidy YN, Lye SJ, Gibb W, Patel FA. 2002. Prostaglandins and mechanisms of preterm birth. *Reproduction* 124:1-17.

Challis JRG. 1994. Characteristics of parturation. In: Creas, RK, Resnik, R (eds. *Maternal Fetal Medicine: Principles and Practice.* Philadelphia, PA: W.B. Saunders Company. Pp. 482-493.

Challis JRG. 2000. Mechanism of parturition and preterm labor. *Obstetrics and Gynecology Survey* 55:650-660.

Challis JRG, Matthews SG, Gibb W, Lye SJ. 2000. Endocrine and paracrine regulation of birth at term and preterm. *Endocrine Reviews* 21:514-550.

Chambers JG, Shkolnik J, Perez M. 2003. *Total Expenditure for Students with Disabilities, 1999-2000: Spending Variation by Disability.* Special Education Expenditure Project, Report 5. Washington, DC: American Institutes for Research.

Chang Y-J, Lin C-H, Lin L-H. 2001. Noise and related events in a neonatal intensive care unit. *Acta Paediatrica Taiwanica* 42(4):212-217.

Charpak N, Ruiz-Peláez JG, De Calume ZF. 1996. Current knowledge of kangaroo mother intervention. *Current Opinion in Pediatrics* 8(2):108-112.

Chauchan SP, et al. 2005. Professional liability claims and Central Association of Obstetricians and Gynecologist members: Myth versus reality. *American Journal of Obstetrics and Gynecology* 192:1820-1828.

Chernoff R, Combs-Orme T, Risley-Curtiss C, Heisler A. 1994. Assessing the health status of children entering foster care. *Pediatrics* 93(4):594-601.

Chervenak FA, Skupski DW, Romero R, Myers MK, Smith-Levitin M, Rosenwaks Z, Thaler HT, Hobbins JC, Spinnato JA. 1998. How accurate is fetal biometry in the assessment of fetal age? *American Journal of Obstetrics and Gynecology* 178(4):678-687.

Cheschier N. 2003. Bulletins-Obstetrics ACoP. ACOG practice bulletin. Neural tube defects. Number 44, July 2003. (Replaces committee opinion number 252, March 2001). *International Journal of Gynaecology and Obstetrics* 83:123-133.

Chien PF, Khan KS, Ogston S, Owen P. 1997. The diagnostic accuracy of cervico-vaginal fetal fibronectin in predicting preterm delivery: An overview. *British Journal of Obstetrics and Gynaecology* 104:436-444.

Chipungu SS, Bent-Goodley TB. 2003. Meeting the challenges of contemporary foster care. *Future of Children* 14:75-93.

Chiumello D, Pristine G, Slutsky AS. 1999. Mechanical ventilation affects local and systemic cytokines in an animal model of acute respiratory syndrome. *American Journal of Respiratory Critical Care Medicine* 160:109-116.

Chow LC, Wright KW, Sola A, CSMC Oxygen Administration Study Group. 2003. Can changes in clinical practice decrease the incidence of severe retinopathy of prematurity in very low birth weight infants? *Pediatrics* 111:339-345.

CHUMS (Collaborative Home Uterine Monitoring Study Group). 1995a. A multicenter randomized trial of home uterine activity monitoring. *American Journal of Obstetrics and Gynecology* 172:253.

CHUMS. 1995b. A multicenter randomized controlled trial of home uterine monitoring: Active versus sham device. *American Journal of Obstetrics and Gynecology* 173:1120-1127.

Cifuentes J, Bronstein J, Phibbs CS, Phibbs RH, Schmitt SK, Carlo WA. 2002. Mortality in low birth weight infants according to level of neonatal care at hospital of birth. *Pediatrics* 109(5):745-751.

Clark R, Powers R, White R, Bloom B, Sanchez P, Benjamin Jr. DK. 2004. Prevention and treatment of nosocomial sepsis in the NICU. *Journal of Perinatology* 24(7):446-453.

Clark RH, Gerstmann DR, Jobe AH, Moffitt ST, Slutsky AS, Yoder BA. 2001. Lung injury in neonates: Causes, strategies for prevention, and long-term consequences. *Journal of Pediatrics* 139:478-486.

Clausson B, Lichtenstein P, Cnattingius S. 2000. Genetic influence on birthweight and gestational length determined by studies in offspring of twins. *British Journal of Obstetrics and Gynaecology* 107(3):375-381.

Clements KM, Barfield WD, Ayadi MF, Wilber N. 2007. Preterm birth-associated cost of early intervention services: An analysis by gestational age. *Pediatrics* 119(4):(in press).

CMS (Centers for Medicare and Medicaid Services). 2005a. *Medicaid Program—General Information.* [Online]. Available: http://www.cms.hhs.gov/MedicaidGenInfo/ [accessed January 30, 2006].

CMS. 2005b. *Net Reported Medicaid and SCHIP Expenditures.* [Online]. Available: http://www.cms.hhs.gov/MedicaidBudgetExpendSystem/Downloads/2004to1997.pdf [accessed May 10, 2006].

Cnattingius S. 2004. The epidemiology of smoking during pregnancy: Smoking prevalence, maternal characteristics, and pregnancy outcomes. *Nicotine and Tobacco Research* 6(Suppl 2):S125-S140.

Cnattingius S, Forman MR, Berendes HW, Isotalo L. 1992. Delayed childbearing and risk of adverse perinatal outcome: A population-based study. *JAMA* 268(7):886-890.

Cnattingius S, Forman MR, Berendes HW, Graubard BI, Isotalo L. 1993. Effect of age, parity, and smoking on pregnancy outcome: A population-based study. *American Journal of Obstetrics and Gynecology* 168(1 I):16-21.

Cnattingius S, Granath F, Petersson G, Harlow BL. 1999. The influence of gestational age and smoking habits on the risk of subsequent preterm deliveries. *New England Journal of Medicine* 341(13):943-948.

Coalson JJ, Winter VT, Siler-Khodr T, Yoder BA. 1999. Neonatal chronic lung disease in extremely immature baboons. *American Journal of Respiratory Critical Care Medicine* 160:1333-1346.

Coates PM, Brown SA, Sonawane BR, Koldovsky O. 1983. Effect of early nutrition on serum cholesterol levels in adult rats challenged with high fat diet. *Journal of Nutrition* 113(5):1046-1050.

Coats DK, Paysse EA, Steinkuller PG. 2000. Threshold retinopathy of prematurity in neonates less than 25 weeks' estimated gestational age. *Journal of American Association for Pediatric Opthalmology and Strabismus* 4(3):183-185.

Cohen S. 1988. Psychosocial models of the role of social support in the etiology of physical disease. *Health Psychology* 7(3):269-297.

Cohen S. 1995. *Measuring Stress: A Guide for Health and Social Scientists.* New York: Oxford University Press.

Cohen S. 2000. *Social Support Measurement and Intervention.* Oxford, UK: Oxford University Press.

Cohen BA, Siegfried EC. 2005. Newborn skin: Development and basic concepts. In: Taeusch HW, Ballard RA, Gleason CA eds. *Avery's Diseases of the Newborn,* 8th edition. Philadelphia, PA: Elsevier Saunders. Pp. 1471-1483.

Cohen S, Syme SL. 1985. Issues in the study and application of social support. In: Cohen S, Syme SL eds. *Social Support and Health.* Orlando, FL: Academic Press. Pp. 3-22.

Cohen S, Kessler R, Gordon LU. 1995. *Measuring Stress: A Guide for Health and Social Scientists.* New York: Oxford University Press.

Coker AL, Sanderson M, Dong B. 2004. Partner violence during pregnancy and risk of adverse pregnancy outcomes. *Paediatric and Perinatal Epidemiology* 18(4):260-269.

Collaborative Group on Preterm Birth Prevention. 1993. Multicenter randomized controlled trial of a preterm birth prevention program. *American Journal of Obstetrics and Gynecology* 169(2 Pt 1):352-366.

Collins FS. 2004a. What we do and don't know about "race," "ethnicity," genetics and health at the down of the genome era. *Nature Genetics* 36(Suppl):S13-S15.

Collins FS. 2004b. The case for a U.S. prospective cohort study of genes and environment. *Nature* 429(6990):475-477.

Collins JW Jr., David RJ. 1990. The differential effect of traditional risk factors on infant birthweight among Blacks and Whites in Chicago. *American Journal of Public Health* 80(6):679-681.

Collins JW Jr., David RJ. 1997. Urban violence and African-American pregnancy outcome: An ecologic study. *Ethnicity and Disease* 7(3):184-190.

Collins JW Jr., Hawkes EK. 1997. Racial differences in post-neonatal mortality in Chicago: What risk factors explain the black infant's disadvantage? *Ethnicity and Health* 2(1-2):117-125.

Collins JW Jr., David RJ, Symons R, Handler A, Wall S, Andes S. 1998. African-American mothers' perception of their residential environment, stressful life events, and very low birthweight. *Epidemiology* 9(3):286-289.

Collins JW Jr., David RJ, Symons R, Handler A, Wall SN, Dwyer L. 2000. Low-income African-American mothers' perception of exposure to racial discrimination and infant birth weight. *Epidemiology* 11(3):337-339.

Collins JW Jr., David RJ, Handler A, Wall S, Andes S. 2004. Very low birthweight in African American infants: The role of maternal exposure to interpersonal racial discrimination. *American Journal of Public Health* 94(12):2132-2138.

Collins MP, Lorenz JM, Jetton JR, Paneth N. 2001. Hypocapnia and other ventilation-related risk factors for cerebral palsy in low birth weight infants. *Pediatric Research* 50(6):712-719.

Collins NL, Dunkel-Schetter C, Lobel M, Scrimshaw SC. 1993. Social support in pregnancy: Psychosocial correlates of birth outcomes and postpartum depression. *Journal of Personality and Social Psychology* 65(6):1243-1258.

Colver AF, Gibson M, Hey EN, Jarvis SN, Mackie PC, Richmond S. 2000. Increasing rates of cerebral palsy across the severity spectrum in north-east England 1964-1993. *Archives of Disease in Childhood: Fetal and Neonatal Edition* 83(1):F7-F12.

Committee on Perinatal Health. 1976. Toward improving the outcome of pregnancy: Recommendations for the regional development of maternal and perinatal health services. *Toward Improving the Outcome of Pregnancy No. 1.* White Plains, NY: March of Dimes National Foundation.

Conde-Agudelo A, Diaz-Rossello JL, Belizan JM. 2003. Kangaroo mother care to reduce morbidity and mortality in low birthweight infants. *Cochrane Database of Systematic Reviews* 2:CD002771.

Conde-Agudelo A, Belizan JM, Norton MH, Rosas-Bermudez A. 2005. Effect of the interpregnancy interval on perinatal outcomes in Latin America. *Obstetrics and Gynecology* 106:359-366.

Cone T. 1985. Myth and appalling morality. In: *History of the Care and Feeding of the Premature Infant*. Boston, MA: Little, Brown, & Company. Pp. 1-12.

Conner JM, Soll RF, Edwards WH. 2003. Topical ointment for preventing infection in preterm infants. *Cochrane Reviews* 4.

Cook TD, Campbell DT. 1979. *Quasi-Experimentation: Design and Analysis Issues for Field Settings*. Chicago, IL: Rand McNally.

Cooke L, Steer P, Woodgate P. 2003. Indomethacin for asymptomatic patent ductus arteriosus in preterm infants. *Cochrane Database of Systematic Reviews (Online: Update Software)* (2).

Cooke RWI. 1999. Trends in incidence of cranial ultrasound lesions and cerebral palsy in very low birthweight infants 1982-93. *Archives of Disease in Childhood: Fetal and Neonatal Edition* 80(2): F115-F117.

Cooke RWI. 2004. Health, lifestyle, and quality of life for young adults born very preterm. *Archives of Disease in Childhood* 89(3):201-206.

Cooke RWI, Foulder-Hughes L, Newsham D, Clarke D. 2004. Ophthalmic impairment at 7 years of age in children born very preterm. *Archives of Disease in Childhood: Fetal and Neonatal Edition* 89(3):F249-F253.

Cooke SA, Schwartz RM, Gagnon DE. 1988. *The Perinatal Partnership: An Approach to Organizing Care in the 1990s*. Project #12129. Providence, RI: The National Perinatal Information Center.

Cools F, Offringa M. 2005. Neuromuscular paralysis for newborn infants receiving mechanical ventilation. *Cochrane Reviews* 2.

Cooper RS, Kaufman JS, Ward R. 2003. Race and genomics. *New England Journal of Medicine* 348:1166-1170.

Copper RL, Goldenberg, RL, Davis RO, Cutter GR, Dubard MB, Corliss DK, Andrews JB. 1990. Warning symptoms, uterine contractions, and cervical examination: Findings in women at risk of preterm delivery. *American Journal of Obstetrics and Gynecology* 162(3):748-754.

Copper RL, Goldenberg RL, Das A, Elder N, Swain M, Norman G, Ramsey R, Cotroneo P, Collins BA, Johnson F, Jones P, Meier AM. 1996. The preterm prediction study: Maternal stress is associated with spontaneous preterm birth at less than thirty-five weeks' gestation. National Institute of Child Health and Human Development Maternal-Fetal Medicine Units Network. *American Journal of Obstetrics and Gynecology* 175(5):1286-1292.

Costeloe K, Hennessy E, Gibson AT, Marlow N, Wilkinson AR, for the EPICure Study Group. 2000. The EPICure Study: Outcomes to discharge from hospital for infants born at the threshold of viability. *Pediatrics* 106(4):659-671.

Cotterrell M, Balázs R, Johnson AL. 1972. Effects of corticosteroids on the biochemical maturation of rat brain: Postnatal cell formation. *Journal of Neurochemistry* 19(9):2151-2167.

Courtney SE, Long W, McMillan D, Walter D, Thompson T, Sauve R, Conway B, Bard H. 1995. Double-blind 1-year follow-up of 1540 infants with respiratory distress syndrome randomized to rescue treatment with two doses of synthetic surfactant or air in four clinical trials. *Journal of Pediatrics* 126(5 II):S43-S52.

Coussons-Read ME, Okun ML, Schmitt MP, Giese S. 2005. Prenatal stress alters cytokine levels in a manner that may endanger human pregnancy. *Psychosomatic Medicine* 67(4):625-631.

Cox ED, Hoffmann SC, Dimercurio BS, Wesley RA, Harlan DM, Kirk AD, Blair PJ. 2001. Cytokine polymorphic analyses indicate ethnic differences in the allelic distribution of interleukin-2 and interleukin-6. *Transplantation* 72(4):720-726.

Cox SM, Sherman ML, Leveno KJ. 1990. Randomized investigation of magnesium sulfate for prevention of preterm birth. *American Journal of Obstetrics and Gynecology* 163(3): 767-772.

Cramer JC. 1995. Racial and ethnic differences in birthweight: The role of income and financial assistance. *Demography* 32(2):231-247.

Criniti A, Thyer A, Chow G, Lin P, Klein N, Soules M. 2005. Elective single blastocyst transfer reduces twin rates without compromising pregnancy rates. *Fertility and Sterility* 84(6): 1613-1619.

Cronin CM, Shapiro CR, Casiro OG, Cheang MS. 1995. The impact of very low-birth-weight infants on the family is long lasting: A matched control study. *Archives of Pediatrics and Adolescent Medicine* 149(2):151-158.

Crowley PA. 1999. Prophylactic corticosteroids for preterm birth. *Cochrane Reviews* 2.

Crowther CA, Henderson-Smart DJ. 2003. Phenobarbital prior to preterm birth for preventing neonatal periventricular haemorrhage. *Cochrane Reviews* 3.

Crowther CA, Hiller JE, Doyle LW. 2002. Magnesium sulphate for preventing preterm birth in threatened preterm labour. *Cochrane Database of Systematic Reviews (Online: Update Software)* 4.

Crowther CA, Hiller JE, Doyle LW, Haslam RR. 2003. Effect of magnesium sulfate given for neuroprotection before preterm birth: A randomized controlled trial. *JAMA* 290(20): 2669-2676.

Crowther CA, Alfirevic Z, Haslam RR. 2004. Thyrotropin-releasing hormone added to corticosteroids for women at risk of preterm birth for preventing neonatal respiratory disease. *Cochrane Database of Systematic Reviews* 2.

CRPCG (Cryotherapy for Retinopathy of Prematurity Cooperative Group). 1988. Multicenter trial of cryotherapy for retinopathy of prematurity: Preliminary results. *Archives of Ophthalmology* 106(4):471-479.

CRPCG. 1994. The natural ocular outcome of premature birth and retinopathy. Status at 1 year. Cryotherapy for Retinopathy of Prematurity Cooperative Group. *Archives of Ophthalmology* 112(7):903-912.

Cubbin C, LeClere FB, Smith GS. 2000. Socioeconomic status and injury mortality: Individual and neighborhood determinants. *Journal of Epidemiology and Community Health* 54: 517-524.

Culhane JF, Rauh V, McCollum KF, Hogan VK, Agnew K, Wadhwa PD. 2001. Maternal stress is associated with bacterial vaginosis in human pregnancy. *Maternal and Child Health Journal* 5(2):127-134.

Cummins SK, Nelson KB, Grether JK, Velie EM. 1993. Cerebral palsy in four northern California counties, births 1983 through 1985. *Journal of Pediatrics* 123(2):230-237.

Cunningham FG, Leveno KJ, Bloom SL, Hauth JC, Gilstrap L, Wenstrom KD. 2005. *Williams Obstetrics*, 22nd edition. New York: McGraw-Hill. Pp. 5, 232.

Cunze T, Rath W, Osmers R, Martin M, Warneke G, Kuhn W. 1995. Magnesium and calcium concentration in the pregnant and non-pregnant myometrium. *International Journal of Gynaecology and Obstetrics* 48:9-13.

Currie J, Gruber J. 1996. Saving babies: The efficacy and cost of recent changes in Medicaid eligibility of pregnant women. *Journal of Political Economy* 104(6):1263-1296.

Cutler DM, Meara E. 2000. The technology of birth: Is it worth it? In: Alan Garber ed. *Frontiers in Health Policy Research*, Volume 3. Cambridge, MA: MIT Press. Pp. 33-67.

Czeizel AE, Dudas I, Metneki J. 1994. Pregnancy outcomes in a randomised controlled trial of periconceptional multivitamin supplementation. Final report. *Archives of Gynecology and Obstetrics* 255(3):131-139.

Da Fonseca EB, Bittar RE, Carvalho MH, et al. 2003. Prophylactic administration of progesterone by vaginal suppository to reduce the incidence of spontaneous preterm birth in
women at increased risk: A randomized placebo-controlled double-blind study. *American Journal of Obstetrics and Gynecology* 188:419-424.

Dafopoulos KC, Galazios GC, Tsikouras PN, Koutlaki NG, Liberis VA, Anastasiadis PG.
2002. Interpregnancy interval and the risk of preterm birth in Thrace, Greece. *European
Journal of Obstetrics, Gynecology, and Reproductive Biology* 103:14-17.

Daikoku T, Tranguch S, Friedman DB, Das SK, Smith DF, Dey SK. 2005. Proteomic analysis
identifies immunophilin FK506 binding protein 4 (FKBP52) as a downstream target of
Hoxa10 in the periimplantation mouse uterus. *Molecular Endocrinology* 19(3):683-697.

Dammann O, Leviton A. 1998. Infection remote from the brain, neonatal white matter damage, and cerebral palsy in the preterm infant. *Seminars in Pediatric Neurology* 5(3):
190-201.

Dammann O, Kuban KCK, Leviton A. 2002. Perinatal infection, fetal inflammatory response,
white matter damage, and cognitive limitations in children born preterm. *Mental Retardation and Developmental Disabilities Research Reviews* 8(1):46-50.

Dammann O, Leviton A, Gappa M, Dammann CE. 2005. Lung and brain damage in preterm
newborns, and their association with gestational age, prematurity subgroup, infection/
inflammation and long term outcome. *British Journal of Obstetrics and Gynaecology*
112(Suppl 1):4-9.

Dar E, Kanarek MS, Anderson HA, Sonzogni WC. 1992. Fish consumption and reproductive
outcomes in Green Bay, Wisconsin. *Environmental Research* 59:189-201.

Darlow BA, Graham PJ. 2002. Vitamin A supplementation for preventing morbidity and mortality in very low birthweight infants. *Cochrane Database of Systematic Reviews (Online:
Update Software)* 4.

Darlow BA, Hutchinson JL, Simpson JM, Henderson-Smart DJ, Donoghue DA, Evans NJ.
2005. Variation in rats of severe retinopathy of prematurity among neonatal intensive
care units in the Australian and New Zealand Neonatal Network. *British Journal of
Ophthalmology* 89:1592-1596.

Darrah J, Piper M, Byrne P, Watt MJ. 1994. The use of waterbeds for very low-birthweight
infants: Effects on neuromotor development. *Developmental Medicine and Child Neurology* 36(11):989-999.

David RJ. 1980. The quality and completeness of birthweight and gestational age data in
computerized birth files. *American Journal of Public Health* 70(9):964-973.

Davis L, Edwards H, Mohay H, Wollin J. 2003. The impact of very premature birth on the
psychological health of mothers. *Early Human Development* 73(1-2):61-70.

Dayan J, Creveuil C, Herlicoviez M, Herbel C, Baranger E, Savoye C, Thouin A. 2002. Role of
anxiety and depression in the onset of spontaneous preterm labor. *American Journal of
Epidemiology* 155(4):293-301.

De Groot L, Hopkins B, Touwen B. 1995. Muscle power, sitting unsupported and trunk
rotation in pre-term infants. *Early Human Development* 43(1):37-46.

Dejmek J, Selevan SG, Sram RJ. 1996. [The environment, life style and pregnancy outcome].
Cas Lek Cesk 135:510-515.

Demissie K, Rhoads G, Ananth C, Alexander G, Kramer M, Kogan M, Joseph K. 2001. Trends
in preterm birth and neonatal mortality among Blacks and Whites in the United States
from 1989-1997. *American Journal of Epidemiology* 154(4):307-315.

Deng W, Wang H, Rosenberg PA, Volpe JJ, Jensen FE. 2004. Role of metabotropic glutamate
receptors in oligodendrocytes excitotoxicity and oxidative stress. *Proceedings of the National Academy of Sciences USA* 101:7751-7756.

De Roos AJ, Smith MT, Chanock S, Rothman N. 2004. Toxicological considerations in the application and interpretation of susceptibility biomarkers in epidemiological studies. *IARC Scientific Publications* 157:105-125.

Devaney BL, Ellwood MR, Love JM. 1997. Programs that mitigate the effects of poverty on children. *Future of Children* 7(2):88-112.

De Vries LS, Groenendaal F. 2002. Neuroimaging in the preterm infant. *Mental Retardation and Developmental Disabilities Research Reviews* 8(4):273-280.

De Vries LS, Liem KD, Van Dijk K, Smit BJ, Sie L, Rademaker KJ, Gavilanes AWD. 2002. Early versus late treatment of posthaemorrhagic ventricular dilatation: Results of a retrospective study from five neonatal intensive care units in The Netherlands. *Acta Paediatrica, International Journal of Paediatrics* 91(2):212-217.

De Weerth C, Buitelaar JK. 2005. Physiological stress reactivity in human pregnancy—a review. *Neuroscience and Biobehavioral Reviews* 29(2):295-312.

Dey SK, Lim H, Das SK, Reese J, Paria BC, Daikoku T, Wang H. 2004. Molecular cues to implantation. *Endocrine Review* 25:345-373.

Deykin EY, MacMahon B. 1980. Pregnancy, delivery, and neonatal complications among autistic children. *American Journal of Diseases of Children* 134(9):860-864.

DHHS (U.S. Department of Health and Human Services). 2004 (unpublished). *Inventory of Research and Databases Pertaining to Low Birth Weight, Preterm Birth, and Sudden Infant Death Syndrome*. Washington, DC: HHS Interagency Coordinating Council on Low Birth Weight and Preterm Birth.

DHHS. 2005. *Budget in Brief FY 2005*. [Online]. Available: http://www.hhs.gov/budget/05budget/fy2005bibfinal.pdf.

Diez-Roux A. 1999. Bringing context back into epidemiology: Variables and fallacies in multilevel analysis. *American Journal of Public Health* 88:216-222.

Diez-Roux A, Nieto FJ, Muntaner C, Tyroler HA, Comstock GW, Shahar E, Cooper LS, Watson RL, Szklo M. 1997. Neighborhood environments and coronary heart disease: A multilevel analysis. *American Journal of Epidemiology* 146(1):48-63.

Diez-Roux AV, Merkin SS, Hannan P, Jacobs DR, Kiefe CI. 2003. Area characteristics, individual-level socioeconomic indicators, and smoking in young adults: the coronary artery disease risk development in young adults study. *American Journal of Epidemiology* 157(4):315-326.

Dinesen SJ, Greisen G. 2001. Quality of life in young adults with very low birth weight. *Archives of Disease in Childhood: Fetal and Neonatal Edition* 85(3):F165-F169.

DiPietro JA. 2005. Neurobehavioral assessment before birth. *Mental Retardation and Developmental Disabilities Research Reviews* 11(1):4-13.

DiPietro JA, Hilton SC, Hawkins M, Costigan KA, Pressman EK. 2002. Maternal stress and affect influence fetal neurobehavioral development. *Developmental Psychology* 38(5):659-668.

Dizon-Townson DS, Major H, Varner M, Ward K. 1997. A promoter mutation that increases transcription of the tumor necrosis factor-alpha gene is not associated with preterm delivery. *American Journal of Obstetrics and Gynecology* 177(4):810-813.

Dodd JM, Crowther CA, Cincotta R, et al. 2005. Progesterone supplementation for preventing preterm birth: A systemic review and meta-analysis. *Acta Obstetricia et Gynecologica Scandinavica* 84:526-533.

DOE (U.S. Department of Education). 2005. *Special Education and Rehabilitative Services— IDEA 2004 Resources*. [Online]. Available: http://www.ed.gov/policy/speced/guid/idea/idea2004.html [accessed January 30, 2006].

DOE. 2006. *Summary of Discretionary Funds Fiscal Years 2001-2007*. [Online]. Available: http://www.ed.gov/about/overview/budget/budget07/summary/appendix1.pdf [accessed May 10, 2006].

DOJ (U.S. Department of Justice). 2005. *Office of Justice Programs—Juvenile Justice Programs.* [Online]. Available: http://www.usdoj.gov/jmd/2005summary/pdf/p167-169.pdf [accessed May 10, 2006].

DOL (U.S. Department of Labor). 2004. *Women in the Labor Force: A Databook.* [Online]. Available: http://www.bls.gov/cps/wlf-databook.htm [accessed September 29, 2005].

DOL. 2005. *Employment Characteristics of Families.* [Online]. Available: http://www.bls.gov/news.release/famee.toc.htm [accessed February 27, 2006].

Dole N, Savitz DA, Hertz-Picciotto I, Siega-Riz AM, McMahon MJ, Buekens P. 2003. Maternal stress and preterm birth. *American Journal of Epidemiology* 157(1):14-24.

Dolk H, Pattenden S, Johnson A. 2001. Cerebral palsy, low birthweight and socio-economic deprivation: Inequalities in a major cause of childhood disability. *Paediatric and Perinatal Epidemiology* 15(4):359-363.

Donohue, P. 2002. Health-related quality of life of preterm children and their caregivers. *Mental Retardation and Developmental Disabilities* 8:293-297.

Downey G, Coyne JC. 1990. Children of depressed parents: An integrative review. *Psychology Bulletin* 1:50-76.

Doyle LW. 2001. Outcome at 5 years of age of children 23 to 27 weeks' gestation: Refining the prognosis. *Pediatrics* 108(1):134-141.

Doyle LW, Anderson PJ. 2005. Improved neurosensory outcome at 8 years of age of extremely low birthweight children born in Victoria over three distinct eras. *Archives of Disease in Childhood: Fetal and Neonatal Edition* 90(6):F484-F488.

Doyle LW, Casalaz D. 2001. Outcome at 14 years of extremely low birthweight infants: A regional study. *Archives of Disease in Childhood: Fetal and Neonatal Edition* 85(3):F159.

Doyle LW, Callanan C, Carse E, Charlton MP, Drew J, Ford G, Fraser S, Hayes M, Kelly E, Knoches A, McDougall P, Rickards A, Watkins A, Woods H, Yu V. 1995. Neurosensory outcome at 5 years and extremely low birthweight. *Archives of Disease in Childhood* 73(5 Suppl):F143-F146.

Doyle LW, Faber R, Callanan C, Morley R. 2003a. Blood pressure in late adolescence and very low birth weight. *Pediatrics* 111:252-257.

Doyle LW, Ford G, Davis N. 2003b. Health and hospitalisations after discharge in extremely low birth weight infants. *Seminars in Neonatology* 8(2):137-145.

Doyle LW, Bowman E, Callanan C, Davis NM, Ford GW, Kelly E, Rickards AL, Stewart M, Casalaz D, Fraser S, Watkins A, Woods H, Carse EA, Charlton MP, Hayes M, Yu V, Halliday J. 2004a. Changing availability of neonatal intensive care for extremely low birthweight infants in Victoria over two decades. *Medical Journal of Australia* 181(3):136-139.

Doyle LW, Faber B, Callanan C, Ford GW, Davis NM. 2004b. Extremely low birth weight and body size in early adulthood. *Archives of Disease in Childhood* 89(4):347-350.

Doyle LW, Halliday HL, Ehrenkranz RA, Davis PG, Sinclair JC. 2005. Impact of postnatal systemic corticosteroids on mortality and cerebral palsy in preterm infants: Effect modification by risk for chronic lung disease. *Pediatrics* 115(3):655-661.

Drakeley AJ, Roberts D, Alfirevic Z. 2003. Cervical stitch (cerclage) for preventing pregnancy loss in women. *Cochrane Database Systematic Reviews* 1.

Drey EA, Kang M-S, McFarland W, Darney PD. 2005. Improving the accuracy of fetal foot length to confirm gestational duration. *Obstetrics and Gynecology* 105(4):773-778.

Drillien CM, Thomson AJM, Burgoyne K. 1980. Low-birthweight children at early school-age: A longitudinal study. *Developmental Medicine and Child Neurology* 22(1):26-47.

Drummond MF, O'Brien B, Stoddart GL, Torrance GW. 2003. *Methods for the Economic Evaluation of Health Care Programmes,* 2nd edition. New York: Oxford University Press.

Dubowitz LM. 1979. A study of visual function in the premature infant. *Child: Care, Health and Development* 5(6):399-404.

Dubowitz LM, Dubowitz V, Goldberg C. 1970. Clinical assessment of gestational age in the newborn infant. *Journal of Pediatrics* 77(1):1-10.

Dubowitz LMS, Goldberg C. 1981. Assessment of gestation by ultrasound in various stages of pregnancy in infants differing in size and ethnic origin. *British Journal of Obstetrics and Gynaecology* 88(3):255-259.

Dubowitz LMS, Dubowitz V, Morante A, Verghote M. 1980. Visual function in the preterm and fullterm newborn infant. *Developmental Medicine and Child Neurology* 22(4): 465-475.

Dubowitz V, Dubowitz LM. 1985. (in reply to letter) Inadequacy of Dubowitz Gestational Age in low birthweight infants. *Obstetrics and Gynecology* 65:601-602.

Dudley DJ, Branch DW, Edwin SS, Mitchell MD. 1996. Induction of preterm birth in mice by RU486. *Biology of Reproduction* 55(5):992-995.

Dunkel-Schetter C. 1998. Maternal stress and preterm delivery. *Prenatal and Neonatal Medicine* 3:39-42.

Dunlop A, Brann A. 2005, June 21. African American women at Grady Memorial Hospital (GMH). Presented at the National Summit on Preconception Care. Atlanta, GA.

Dunn MS, Shennan AT, Hoskins EM, Lennox K, Enhorning G. 1988. Two-year follow-up of infants enrolled in a randomized trial of surfactant replacement therapy for prevention of neonatal respiratory distress syndrome. *Pediatrics* 82(4):543-547.

Dye TD, Oldenettel D. 1996. Physical activity and the risk of preterm labor: An epidemiological review and synthesis of recent literature. *Seminars in Perinatology* 20(4):334-339.

Dyson DC, Danbe KH, Bamber JA, et al. 1998. Monitoring women at risk for preterm birth. *New England Journal of Medicine* 338:15-19.

Eaton WW, Mortensen PB, Thomsen PH, Frydenberg M. 2001. Obstetric complications and risk for severe psychopathology in childhood. *Journal of Autism and Developmental Disorders* 31(3):279-285.

Ecker JL, Chen KT, Cohen AP, Riley LE, Lieberman ES. 2001. Increased risk of cesarean delivery with advancing maternal age: Indications and associated factors in nulliparous women. *American Journal of Obstetrics and Gynecology* 185(4):883-887.

Edwards CH, Cole OJ, Oyemade UJ, Knight EM, Johnson AA, Westney OE, Laryea H, West W, Jones S, Westney LS. 1994. Maternal stress and pregnancy outcomes in a prenatal clinic population. *Journal of Nutrition* 124(6 Suppl):1006S-1021S.

Egarter C, Leitich H, Husslein P, Kaider A, Schemper M. 1996. Adjunctive antibiotic treatment in preterm labor and neonatal morbidity: A meta-analysis. *Obstetrics and Gynecology* 88(2):303-309.

Eichenwald EC, Blackwell M, Lloyd JS, Tran T, Wilder RE, Richardson DK. 2001. Interneonatal intensive care unit variation in discharge timing: Influence of apnea and feeding management. *Pediatrics* 108:928-933.

Einspieler C, Prechtl HFR. 2005. Prechtl's assessment of general movements: A diagnostic tool for the functional assessment of the young nervous system. *Mental Retardation and Developmental Disabilities Research Reviews* 11(1):61-67.

Eisengart S, Singer LT, Fulton S, Baley JE. 2003. Coping and psychological distress in mothers of very low birth weight young children. *Parenting: Science and Practice* 3(1):49-72.

Eiser C, Morse R. 2001. Can parents rate their child's health-related quality of life? Results of a systematic review. *Quality of Life Research* 10:347-357.

Ekwo EE, Moawad A. 1998. The relationship of interpregnancy interval to the risk of preterm births to black and white women. *International Journal of Epidemiology* 7:68-73.

Ekwo EE, Gosselink CA, Moawad A. 1992. Unfavorable outcome in penultimate pregnancy and premature rupture of membranes in successive pregnancy. *Obstetrics and Gynecology* 80:166.

Elbourne D, Oakley A. 1991. An overview of trials of social support during pregnancy. In: Berends HW, Kessel S, Yaffee S eds. *Advances in the Prevention of Low Birth Weight: An International Symposium*. Washington, DC: National Center for Education in Maternal and Child Health. Pp. 203-223.

Elbourne D, Oakley A, Chalmers I. 1989. Social and psychological support during pregnancy. In: Chalmers I, Enkin M, Keirse M eds. *Effective Care in Pregnancy and Childbirth*. Oxford, UK: Oxford University Press. Pp. 16-32.

Elbourne D, Ayers S, Dellagrammaticas H, Johnson A, Leloup M, Lenoir-Piat S. 2001. Randomised controlled trial of prophylactic etamsylate: Follow up at 2 years of age. *Archives of Disease in Childhood: Fetal and Neonatal Edition* 84(3):F183-F187.

Elder HA, Santamarina BA, Smith S, Kass EH. 1971. The natural history of asymptomatic bacteriuria during pregnancy: The effect of tetracycline on the clinical course and the outcome of pregnancy. *American Journal of Obstetrics and Gynecology* 111(3):441-462.

Elo IT, Rodgriguez G, Lee H. 2001. Racial and neighborhood disparities in birth weight in Philadelphia. Annual Meeting of the Populations Association of America, Washington DC. Paper presented, under revision for publication.

Elovitz MA, Mrinalini C. 2004. Animal models of preterm birth. *Trends in Endocrinology and Metabolism* 15:479-487.

Elovitz MA, Mrinalini C. 2005. Can medroxyprogesterone acetate alter Toll-like receptor expression in a mouse model of intrauterine inflammation? *American Journal of Obstetrics and Gynecology* 193(3 Suppl):1149-1155.

Elovitz MA, Ascher-Landsberg J, Saunders T, Phillippe M. 2000. The mechanisms underlying the stimulatory effects of thrombin on myometrial smooth muscle. *American Journal of Obstetrics and Gynecology* 183:674-681.

Elovitz MA, Baron J, Phillipe M. 2001. The role of thrombin in preterm parturition. *American Journal of Obstetrics and Gynecology* 185:1059-1063.

El-Sayed YY, Riley ET, Holbrook RH Jr., Cohen SE, Chitkara U, Druzin ML. 1999. Randomized comparison of intravenous nitroglycerin and magnesium sulfate for treatment of preterm labor. *Obstetrics and Gynecology* 93:79-83.

Emsley HCA, Wardle SP, Sims DG, Chiswick ML, D'Souza SW. 1998. Increased survival and deteriorating developmental outcome in 23 to 25 week old gestation infants, 1990-1994 compared with 1984-1989. *Archives of Disease in Childhood: Fetal and Neonatal Edition* 78(2):F99-F104.

Engel S, Olshan A, Savitz D, Thorp J, Erichsen H, Chanock S. 2005b. Risk of small-for-gestational age is associated with common anti-inflammatory cytokine polymorphisms. *Epidemiology* 16(4):478-486.

Engel SAM, Erichsen HC, Savitz DA, Thorp J, Chanock SJ, Olshan AF. 2005a. Risk of spontaneous preterm birth is associated with common proinflammatory cytokine polymorphisms. *Epidemiology* 16(4):469-477.

England LJ, Levine RJ, Qian C, Morris CD, Sibai BM, Catalano PM, Curet LB, Klebanoff MA. 2002. Smoking before pregnancy and risk of gestational hypertension and preeclampsia. *American Journal of Obstetrics and Gynecology* 186(5):1035-1040.

EOP (Executive Office of the President of the United States). 1995. *Standards for the Classification of Federal Data on Race and Ethnicity*. [Online]. Available: http://www.whitehouse.gov/OMB/fedreg/race-ethnicity.html [accessed February 27, 2006].

Erickson JD, Bjerkedal T. 1978. Interpregnancy interval. Association with birth weight, stillbirth, and neonatal death. *Journal of Epidemiology and Community Health* 32:124-130.

Ericson A, Kallen B. 1998. Very low birthweight boys at the age of 19. *Archives of Disease in Childhood: Fetal and Neonatal Edition* 78(3):F171-F174.

Ericksson JG, Forsen T, Tumilehto J, Winter PD, Osmond C, Barker DJ. 1999. Catch-up growth in childhood and death from coronary heart disease: Longitudinal study. *British Medical Journal* 318 (7181):427-431.

Eriksson JG, Forsen T, Tuomilehto J, Osmond C, Barker DJ. 2001. Early growth and coronary heart disease in later life: Longitudinal study. *British Medical Journal* 322 (7292):949-953.

Eschenbach DA, Nugent RP, Rao AV, Cotch MF, Gibbs RS, Lipscomb KA, Martin DH, Pastorek JG, Rettig PJ, Carey JC, Regan JA, Geromanos KL, Lee MLF, Poole WK, Edelman R, Yaffe SJ, Catz Rhoads CSGG, McNellis D. 1991. A randomized placebo-controlled trial of erythromycin for the treatment of Ureaplasma urealyticum to prevent premature delivery. *American Journal of Obstetrics and Gynecology* 164(3):734-742.

Escobar GJ, Littenberg B, Petitti DB. 1991. Outcome among surviving very low birthweight infants: A meta-analysis. *Archives of Disease in Childhood* 66(2):204-211.

Escobar GJ, Joffe S, Gardner MN, Armstrong MA, Folck BF, Carpenter DM. 1999. Rehospitalization in the first two weeks after discharge from the neonatal intensive care unit. *Pediatrics* 104(1):e2. [Online]. Available: http://www.pediatrics.org/cgi/content/full/104/1/e2.

Escobar GJ, Greene JD, Hulac P, Kincannon E, Bischoff K, Gardneer MN, Armstrong MA, France EK. 2005. Rehospitalisation after birth hospitalization: Patterns among all gestations. *Archives of Disease in Childhood* 90:111-112.

Escobar GJ, McCormick MC, Zupancic JAF, Coleman-Phox K, Armstrong MA, Greene DJ, Eichenwald EC, Richardson DK. In press. Unstudied infants: Outcomes of moderately premature infants in the NICU. *Archives of Disease in Childhood*.

Eskenazi B, Mocarelli P, Warner M, Chee WY, Gerthoux PM, Samuels S, Needham LL, Patterson DG, Jr. 2003. Maternal serum dioxin levels and birth outcomes in women of Seveso, Italy. *Environmental Health Perspectives* 111:947-953.

Eskenazi B, Harley K, Bradman A, Weltzien E, Jewell NP, Barr DB, Furlong CE, Holland NT. 2004. Association of in utero organophosphate pesticide exposure and fetal growth and length of gestation in an agricultural population. *Environmental Health Perspectives* 112:1116-1124.

Evans DJ, Levene MI. 2001. Evidence of selection bias in preterm survival studies: A systematic review. *Archives of Disease in Childhood: Fetal and Neonatal Edition* 84(2): F79-F84.

Evans RG, Stoddart GL. 1990. Producing health, consuming health care. *Social Science and Medicine* 31(12):1347-1363.

Evenson KR, Siega-Riz AM, Savitz DA, Leiferman JA, Thorp JM Jr. 2002. Vigorous leisure activity and pregnancy outcome: The Pregnancy, Infection, and Nutrition Study. *Epidemiology* 13:653-659.

Fagher U, Laudanski T, Schutz A, Sipowicz M, Akerlund M. 1993. The relationship between cadmium and lead burdens and preterm labor. *International Journal of Gynaecology and Obstetrics* 40:109-114.

Falcon M, Vinas P, Luna A. 2003. Placental lead and outcome of pregnancy. *Toxicology* 185(12):59-66.

Farhang L, Weintraub JM, Petreas M, Eskenazi B, Bhatia R. 2005. Association of DDT and DDE with birth weight and length of gestation in the child health and development studies, 1959-1967. *American Journal of Epidemiology* 162(8):717-725.

Farr V, Kerridge DF, Mitchell RG. 1966. The value of some external characteristics in the assessment of gestational age at birth. *Developmental Medicine and Child Neurology* 8(6):657-660.

Fazleabas AT, Kim JJ, Strakova Z. 2004. Implantation: Embryonic signals and the modulation of the uterine environment: A review. *Placenta* 18:S26-S31.

Feeny D, Furlong W, Barr RD, Torrance GW, Rosenbaum P, Weitzman S. 1992. A comprehensive multiattribute system for classifying the health status of survivors of childhood cancer. *Journal of Clinical Oncology* 10(6):923-928.

Feeny D, Furlong W, Saigal S, Sun J. 2004. Comparing directly measured standard gamble scores to HUI2 and HUI3 utility scores: Group- and individual-level comparisons. *Social Science and Medicine* 58:799-809.

Fein GG, Jacobson JL, Jacobson SW, Schwartz PM, Dowler JK. 1984. Prenatal exposure to polychlorinated biphenyls: Effects on birth size and gestational age. *Journal of Pediatrics* 105:315-320.

Feinberg EC, Larsen FW, Catherino WH, Zhang J, Armstrong AY. 2006. Comparison of assisted reproductive technology utilization and outcomes between Caucasian and African American patients in an equal-access-to-care setting. *Fertility and Sterility* 85(4):888-894.

Feingold E, Sheir-Neiss G, Melnychuk J, Bachrach S, Paul D. 2002. HRQL and severity of brain ultrasound findings in a cohort of adolescents who were born preterm. *Journal of Adolescent Health* 31(3):234-239.

Fekkes M, Theunissen NCM, Brugman E, Veen S, Verrips E. 2000. Development and psychometric evaluation of the TAPQOL: A health-related quality of life instrument for 1-5-year-old children. *Quality of Life Research* 9:961-972.

Feldman PJ, Dunkel-Schetter C, Sandman CA, Wadhwa PD. 2000. Maternal social support predicts birth weight and fetal growth in human pregnancy. *Psychosomatic Medicine* 62(5):715-725.

Fernell E, Hagberg G, Hagberg B. 1994. Infantile hydrocephalus epidemiology: An indicator of enhanced survival. *Archives of Disease in Childhood* 70(2 Suppl):F123-F128.

Ferrand PE, Parry S, Sammel M, Macones GA, Kuivaniemi H, Romero R, Strauss JF 3rd. 2002. A polymorphism in the matrix metalloproteinase-9 promoter is associated with increased risk of preterm premature rupture of membranes in African Americans. *Molecular Human Reproduction* 8(5):494-501.

Ferraz EM, Gray RH, Fleming PL, Maia TM. 1988. Interpregnancy interval and low birth weight: Findings from a case-control study. *American Journal of Epidemiology* 28:1111-1116.

Fewtrell MS, Doherty C, Cole TJ, Stafford M, Hales CN, Lucas A. 2000. Effects of size at birth, gestational age and early growth in preterm infants on glucose and insulin concentrations at 9-12 years. *Diabetologia* 43(6):714-717.

Fewtrell MS, Lucas A, Cole TJ, Wells JC. 2004. Prematurity and reduced body fatness at 8-12 y of age. *American Journal of Clinical Nutrition* 80(2):436-440.

Filicori M, Cognigni GE, Gamberini E, Troilo E, Parmegiani L, Bernardi S. 2005. Impact of medically assisted fertility on preterm birth. *BJOG: An International Journal of Obstetrics and Gynaecology* 112(Suppl 1):113-117.

Finegan JA, Quarrington B. 1979. Pre-, peri-, and neonatal factors and infantile autism. *Journal of Child Psychology and Psychiatry and Allied Disciplines* 20(2):119-128.

Finer NN, Higgins R, Kattwinkel J, Martin RJ. 2006. Summary proceedings from the apnea of prematurity group. *Pediatrics* 117:47-51.

Finnstrom O. 1972. Studies on maturity in newborn infants. VI. Comparison between different methods for maturity estimation. *Acta Paediatrica Scandinavica* 61(1):33-41.

Finnstrom O, Otterblad Olausson P, Sedin G, Serenius F, Svenningsen N, Thiringer K, Tunell R, Wesstrom G. 1998. Neurosensory outcome and growth at three years in extremely low birthweight infants: Follow-up results from the Swedish national prospective study. *Acta Paediatrica, International Journal of Paediatrics* 87(10):1055-1060.

Fiscella K. 1995. Does prenatal care improve birth outcomes? A critical review. *Obstetrics and Gynecology* 85(30):468-480.

Fiscella K. 2005. Race, genes, and preterm delivery. *Journal of the National Medical Association* 97(11):1516-1526.

Fiscella KMM, Franks PM, Kendrick JSM, Meldrum SM, Kieke BA Jr. 2002. Risk of preterm birth that is associated with vaginal douching. *American Journal of Obstetrics and Gynecology* 186(6):1345-1350.

Fitzgerald JF, Levin SC, Naulty JS, Collins JG. 1999. Evaluation of intrathecal phenol injection using a rat model: Scientific abstracts. *Regional Anesthesia and Pain Medicine* 24(3 Suppl 1):40.

Fledelius HC, Greisen G. 1993. Very pre-term birth and visual impairment: A retrospective investigation of 411 infants of gestational age 30 weeks or less, 1983-89 Rigshospitalet, Copenhagen. *Acta Ophthalmologica Supplement* 210:63-65.

Flegal KM, Harlan WR, Landis JR. 1988. Secular trends in body mass index and skinfold thickness with socioeconomic factors in young adult women. *American Journal of Clinical Nutrition* 48(3):535-543.

Fletcher JM, Francis DJ, Thompson NM, Brookshire BL, Bohan TP, Landry SH, Davidson KC, Miner ME. 1992. Verbal and nonverbal skill discrepancies in hydrocephalic children. *Journal of Clinical and Experimental Neuropsychology* 14(4):593-609.

Floyd RC, McLauglin BN, Perry KG Jr., Martin RW, Sullivan CA, Morrison JC. 1995. Magnesium sulfate or nifedipine hydrochloride for acute tocolysis of preterm labor: Efficacy and side effects. *Journal of Maternal-Fetal Investigation* 5(1):25-29.

Flynn JR. 1999. Searching for justice: The discovery of IQ gains over time. *American Psychologist* 54(1):5-20.

Follett PL, Koh S, Fu JM, Volpe JJ, Jensen FE. 2000. Protective effects of topiramate in a rodent model of periventricular leukomalacia. *Annals of Neurology* 48:34A.

Ford GW, Doyle LW, Davis NM, Callanan C. 2000. Very low birth weight and growth into adolescence. *Archives of Pediatrics and Adolescent Medicine* 154(8):778-784.

Fortier I, Marcoux S, Brisson J. 1995. Maternal work during pregnancy and the risks of delivering a small-for-gestational-age or preterm infant. *Scandinavian Journal of Work, Environment, and Health* 21(6):412-418.

Fortunato SJ, Menon R, Lombardi SJ. 1999. MMP/TIMP imbalance in the amniotic fluid during PROM: An indirect support for endogenous pathway to membrane rupture. *Journal of Perinatal Medicine* 27:362-368.

Fortunato SJ, Menon R, Bryant C, Lombardi SJ. 2000a. Programmed cell death (apoptosis) as a possible pathway to metalloproteinase activation and fetal membrane degradation in premature rupture of membranes. *American Journal of Obstetrics and Gynecology* 182:1468-1476.

Fortunato, SJ, Menon, R, Lombardi, SJ. 2000b. Amniochorion gelatinase-gelatinase inhibitor imbalance in virto: A possible infectious pathway to rupture. *Obstetrics and Gynecology* 95:240-244.

Fossett JW, Perloff JD, Kletke PR, Peterson JA. 1992. Medicaid and access to child health care in Chicago. *Journal of Health Politics, Policy, and Law* 17(2):273-298.

Fowlie PW. 2005. Managing the baby with a patent ductus arteriosus. More questions than answers? *Archives of Disease in Childhood: Fetal and Neonatal Edition* 90(3):F190.

Fowlie PW, Davis PG. 2002. Prophylactic intravenous indomethacin for preventing mortality and morbidity in preterm infants. *Cochrane Database of Systematic Reviews (Online: Update Software)* 3.

Fox MD, Allbert JR, McCaul JF, Martin RW, McLaughlin BN, Morrison JC. 1993. Neonatal morbidity between 34 and 37 weeks' gestation. *Journal of Perinatology: Official Journal of the California Perinatal Association* 13(5):349-353.

Franck LS, Boyce WT, Gregory GA, Jemerin J, Levine J, Miaskowski C. 2000. Plasma norepinephrine levels, vagal tone index, and flexor reflex threshold in premature neonates receiving intravenous morphine during the postoperative period: A pilot study. *Clinical Journal of Pain* 16(2):95-104.

Fraser AM, Brockert JE, Ward RH. 1995. Association of young maternal age with adverse reproductive outcomes. *New England Journal of Medicine* 332(17):1113-1117.

French JI, McGregor JA, Draper D, Parker R, McFee J. 1999. Gestational bleeding, bacterial vaginosis, and common reproductive tract infections: Risk for preterm birth and benefit of treatment. *Obstetrics and Gynecology* 93(5):715-724.

Fuentes-Afflick E, Hessol NA. 2000. Interpregnancy interval and the risk of premature infants. *Obstetrics and Gynecology* 95:383-390.

Fujimoto T, Parry S, Urbanek M, Sammel M, Macones G, Kuivaniemi H, Romero R, Strauss III JF. 2002. A single nucleotide polymorphism in the matrix metalloproteinase-1 (MMP-1) promoter influences amnion cell MMP-1 expression and risk for preterm premature rupture of the fetal membranes. *Journal of Biological Chemistry* 277(8):6296-6302.

Gabbard SA, Schryer J. 2003. Early amplification options. *Mental Retardation and Developmental Disabilities Research Reviews* 9(4):236-242.

Gaebler CP, Hanzlik JR. 1996. The effects of a prefeeding stimulation program on preterm infants. *American Journal of Occupational Therapy* 50(3):184-192.

Gagliardi L, Cavazza A, Brunelli A, Battaglioli M, Merazzi D, Tandoi F, Cella D, Perotti GF, Pelti M, Stucchi I, Frisone F, Avanzini A, Bell R. 2004. Assessing mortality risk in very low birthweight infants: A comparison of CRIB, CRIB-II, and SNAPPE-II. *Archives of Disease in Childhood: Fetal and Neonatal Edition* 89(5):F419-F422.

Gamsu HR, Mullinger BM, Donnai P, Dash CH. 1989. Antenatal administration of betamethasone to prevent respiratory distress syndrome in preterm infants: Report of a UK multicentre trial. *British Journal of Obstetrics and Gynaecology* 96(4):401-410.

Gan XD, Back SD, Rosenberg PA, Volpe JJ. 1997. Stage-specific vulnerability of rat oligodendrocytes in culture to non-NMDA receptor-mediated toxicity. *Social Neuroscience* 2(Abstr):17420.

Gappa M, Berner MM, Hohenschild S, Dammann CEL, Bartmann P. 1999. Pulmonary function at school-age in surfactant-treated preterm infants. *Pediatric Pulmonology* 27(3):191-198.

Gardosi JO. 2005. Prematurity and fetal growth restriction. *Early Human Development* 81(1):43-49.

Gardosi J, Kady SM, McGeown P, Francis A, Tonks A, Ben-Tovim D, Phillips PA, Crotty M. 2005. Classification of stillbirth by relevant condition at death (ReCoDe): Population based cohort study. *British Medical Journal* 331(7525):1113-1117.

Garfield RE. 1988. Structural and functional studies of the control of myometrial contractility and labour. In: McNellis D, Challis JRG, MacDonald PC, Nathanielsz PW, Roberts JM eds. *The Onset of Labour: Cellular and Integrative Mechanisms.* Ithaca, NY: Perinatology Press. Pp. 55-80.

Garfield RE, Gasc JM, Baulieu EE. 1987. Effects of the antiprogesterone RU 486 on preterm birth in the rat. *American Journal of Obstetrics and Gynecology* 157(5):1281-1285.

Garite TJ, Clark R, Thorp JA. 2004. Intrauterine growth restriction increases morbidity and mortality among premature neonates. *American Journal of Obstetrics and Gynecology* 191(2):481-487.

Gariti DL, Zollinger TW, Look KY. 2005. Factors detracting students from applying for an obstetrics and gynecology residency. *American Journal of Obstetrics and Gynecology* 193:289-293.

Gatts JD, Wallace DH, Glasscock GF, McKee E, Cohen RS. 1994. A modified newborn intensive care unit environment may shorten hospital stay. *Journal of Perinatology: Official Journal of the California Perinatal Association* 14(5):422-427.

Genc MR, Gerber S, Nesin M, Witkin SS. 2002. Polymorphism in the interleukin-1 gene complex and spontaneous preterm delivery. *American Journal of Obstetrics and Gynecology* 187(1):157-163.

Genc MR, Onderdonk AB, Vardhana S, Delaney ML, Norwitz ER, Tuomala RE, Paraskevas L-R, Witkin SS. 2004. Polymorphism in intron 2 of the interleukin-1 receptor antagonist gene, local midtrimester cytokine response to vaginal flora, and subsequent preterm birth. *American Journal of Obstetrics and Gynecology* 191(4):1324-1330.

Georgieff MK, Bernbaum JC. 1986. Abnormal shoulder girdle muscle tone in premature infants during their first 18 months of life. *Pediatrics* 77(5):664-669.

Geronimus AT. 1992. The weathering hypothesis and the health of African-American women and infants: Evidence and speculations. *Ethnicity and Disease* 2(3):207-221.

Geronimus AT. 1996. Black/white differences in the relationship of maternal age to birthweight: A population-based test of the weathering hypothesis. *Social Science and Medicine* 42:589-597.

Gibbons JM. 2005. *Academic Costs*. Presentation to IOM Committee on Understanding Premature Birth and Assuring Healthy Outcomes Workshop, August 10, 2005. Data from Medical Liability Monitor, October 2004, 29(10). Washington, DC: IOM.

Gibbs RS, Romero R, Hillier SL, Eschenbach DA, Sweet RL. 1992. A review of premature birth and subclinical infection. *American Journal of Obstetrics and Gynecology* 166(5): 1515-1528.

Gibson D, Sheps S, Uh S, Schechter M, McCormick A. 1990. Retinopathy of prematurity-induced blindness: Birth weight-specific survival and the new epidemic. *Pediatrics* 86(3):405-412.

Gichangi PB, Ndinya-Achola JO, Ombete J, Nagelkerke NJ, Temmerman M. 1997. Antimicrobial prophylaxis in pregnancy: A randomized, placebo-controlled trial with cefetamet-pivoxil in pregnant women with a poor obstetric history. *American Journal of Obstetrics and Gynecology* 177(3):680-684.

Gilbert WM, Nesbitt TS, Danielsen B. 2003. The cost of prematurity: Quantification by gestational age and birth weight. *Obstetrics and Gynecology* 102(3):488-492.

Gilbert WS, Quinn GE, Dobson V, Reynolds J, Hardy RJ, Palmer EA. 1996. Partial retinal detachment at 3 months after threshold retinopathy of prematurity. Long-term structural and functional outcome. Multicenter Trial of Cryotherapy for Retinopathy of Prematurity Cooperative Group. *Archives of Ophthalmology* 114(9):1085-1091.

Gilkerson L, Gorski PA, Panitz P, Meisels SJ, Shonkoff JP. 1990. *Hospital-Based Intervention for Preterm Infants and Their Families*. New York: Cambridge.

Gill TM, Feinstein AR. 1994. A critical appraisal of the quality of quality-of-life measurements. *JAMA* 272(8):619-626.

Gilles FH, Leviton A, Kerr CS. 1976. Endotoxin leucoencephalopathy in the telencephalon of the newborn kitten. *Journal of Neurological Sciences* 27(2):183-191.

Gilles FH, Leviton A, Dooling EC. 1983. *The Developing Human Brain: Growth and Epidemiologic Neuropathology*. Boston, MA: John Wright, Inc. Pp. 244-315.

Giscombe CL, Lobel M. 2005. Explaining disproportionately high rates of adverse birth outcomes among African Americans: The impact of stress, racism, and related factors in pregnancy. *Psychology Bulletin* 131(5):662-683.

Gleason CA, Back SA. 2005. Developmental physiology of the central nervous system. In: Taeusch HW, Ballard RA, Gleason CA eds. *Avery's Diseases of the Newborn*, 8th edition. Philadelphia, PA: Elsevier Saunders. Pp. 903-907.

Gluck L. 1971. Biochemical development of the lung: Clinical aspects of surfactant development, RDS and the intrauterine assessment of lung maturity. *Clinical Obstetrics and Gynecology* 14(3):710-721.

Gluck L, Kulovich MV. 1973a. Fetal lung development. Current concepts. *Pediatric Clinics of North America* 20(2):367-379.

Gluck L, Kulovich MV. 1973b. Lecithin-sphingomyelin ratios in amniotic fluid in normal and abnormal pregnancy. *American Journal of Obstetrics and Gynecology* 115(4):539-546.

Gluck L, Chez RA, Kulovich MV. 1974. Comparison of phospholipid indicators of fetal lung maturity in the amniotic fluid of the monkey (Macaca mulatta) and baboon (Papio papio). *American Journal of Obstetrics and Gynecology* 120(4):524-530.

Glynn LM, Wadhwa PD, Dunkel-Schetter C, Chicz-Demet A, Sandman CA. 2001. When stress happens matters: Effects of earthquake timing on stress responsivity in pregnancy. *American Journal of Obstetrics and Gynecology* 184(4):637-642.

Glynn LM, Schetter CD, Wadhwa PD, Sandman CA. 2004. Pregnancy affects appraisal of negative life events. *Journal of Psychosomatic Research* 56(1):47-52.

Goepfert AR, Goldenberg RL, Andrews WW, Hauth JC, Mercer B, Iams J, Meis P, Moawad A, Thom E, VanDorsten JP, Caritis SN, Thurnau G, Miodovnik M, Dombrowski M, Roberts J, McNellis D, National Institute of Child Health and Human Development Maternal-Fetal Medicine Units Network. 2001. The Preterm Prediction Study: Association between cervical interleukin 6 concentration and spontaneous preterm birth. National Institute of Child Health and Human Development Maternal-Fetal Medicine Units Network. *American Journal of Obstetrics and Gynecology* 184(3):483-488.

Goepfert AR, Jeffcoat MK, Andrews WW, Faye-Petersen O, Cliver SP, Goldenberg RL, Hauth JC. 2004. Periodontal disease and upper genital tract inflammation in early spontaneous preterm birth. *Obstetrics and Gynecology* 104(4):777-783.

Gold MR, Siegel JE, Russell LB, Weinstein MC. 1996. *Cost-Effectiveness in Health and Medicine*. New York: Oxford University Press.

Gold RB. 1997. Latest Medicaid waivers break new ground for family planning. *State Reproductive Health Monitor* 8:8-9.

Gold RB. 1999. Implications for family planning of post-welfare reform insurance trends. *Guttmacher Report on Public Policy* 2:1-7.

Goldenberg R, Cliver S, Bronstein J, Cutter G, Andrews W, Mennemeyer S. 1994. Bed rest in pregnancy. *Obstetrics and Gynecology* 84(1):131-136.

Goldenberg RL, Andrews WW. 1996. Intrauterine infection and why preterm prevention programs have failed. *American Journal of Public Health* 86:781-783.

Goldenberg RL, Rouse DJ. 1999. Interventions to prevent prematurity. In: McCormick MC, Siegel J eds. *Prenatal Care: Effectiveness and Implementation*. Cambridge, UK: Cambridge University Press. Pp. 105-138.

Goldenberg RL, Davis RO, Cutter GR, Hoffman HJ, Brumfield CG, Foster JM. 1989. Prematurity, postdates, and growth retardation: The influence of use of ultrasonography on reported gestational age. *American Journal of Obstetrics and Gynecology* 160(2): 462-470.

Goldenberg RL, Patterson ET, Freese MP. 1992. Maternal demographic, situational and psychosocial factors and their relationship to enrollment in prenatal care: A review of the literature. *Women and Health* 19(2-3):133-151.

Goldenberg RL, Tamura T, Neggers Y, Copper RL, Johnston KE, DuBard MB, Hauth JC. 1995. The effect of zinc supplementation on pregnancy outcome. *JAMA* 274(6):463-468.

Goldenberg RL, Cliver SP, Mulvihill FX, Hickey CA, Hoffman HJ, Klerman LV, Johnson MJ. 1996a. Medical, psychosocial, and behavioral risk factors do not explain the increased risk for low birth weight among black women. *American Journal of Obstetrics and Gynecology* 175(5):1317-1324.

Goldenberg RL, Mercer BM, Meis PJ, Copper RL, Das A, McNellis D. 1996b. The preterm prediction study: Fetal fibronectin testing and spontaneous preterm birth. *Obstetrics and Gynecology* 87(5 I):643-648.

Goldenberg RL, Thom E, Moawad AH, Johnson F, Roberts J, Caritis SN. 1996c. The preterm prediction study: Fetal fibronectin, bacterial vaginosis, and peripartum infection. *Obstetrics and Gynecology* 87(5 I):656-660.

Goldenberg RL, Mercer BM, Iams JD, Moawad AH, Meis PJ, Das A, McNellis D, Miodovnik M, Menard MK, Caritis SN, Thurnau GR, Bottoms SF, Klebanoff M, Yaffe S, Catz C, Fischer M, Thom E, Hauth JC, Copper R, Northen A, Mueller-Heubach E, Swain M, Frye A, Lindheimer M, Jones P, Elder N, Siddiqi TA, Harger JH, Cotroneo M, Landon MB, Johnson F, Carey JC, Meier A, Van Dorsten JP, Collins BA, LeBoeuf F, Newman RB, Sibai B, Ramsey R, Fricke J, Norman GS. 1997. The preterm prediction study: Patterns of cervicovaginal fetal fibronectin as predictors of spontaneous preterm delivery. *American Journal of Obstetrics and Gynecology* 177(1):8-12.

Goldenberg RL, Iams JD, Mercer BM, Meis PJ, Moawad AH, Copper RL, Das A, Thom E, Johnson F, McNellis D, Miodovnik M, Van Dorsten JP, Caritis SN, Thurnau GR, Bottoms SF. 1998. The preterm prediction study: The value of new vs standard risk factors in predicting early and all spontaneous preterm births. *American Journal of Public Health* 88(2):233-238.

Goldenberg RL, Hauth JC, Andrews WW. 2000. Intrauterine infection and preterm delivery. *New England Journal of Medicine* 342:1500-1507.

Goldenberg RL, Iams JD, Mercer BM, Meis PJ, Moawad A, Das A, Miodovnik M, VanDorsten PJ, Caritis SN, Thurnau G, Dombrowski MP. 2001. The Preterm Prediction Study: Toward a multiple-marker test for spontaneous preterm birth. *American Journal of Obstetrics and Gynecology* 185(3):643-651.

Goldenberg RL, Culhane JF, Johnson DC. 2005. Maternal infection and adverse fetal and neonatal outcomes. *Clinics in Perinatology* 32(3):523-559.

Golding J, Rowland A, Greenwood R, Lunt P. 1991. Aluminium sulphate in water in north Cornwall and outcome of pregnancy. *British Medical Journal* 302:1175-1177.

Goldstein I, Lockwood C, Belanger K, Hobbins J. 1988. Ultrasonographic assessment of gestational age with the distal femoral and proximal tibial ossification centers in the third trimester. *American Journal of Obstetrics and Gynecology* 158(1):127-130.

Gomez R, Romero R, Medina L, et al. 2005. Cervicovaginal fibronectin improves the prediction of preterm delivery based on sonographic cervical length in patients with preterm uterine contractions and intact membranes. *American Journal of Obstetrics and Gynecology* 192:350-359.

Goodman M, Rothberg AD, Houston-McMillan JE. 1985. Effect of early neurodevelopmental therapy in normal and at-risk survivors of neonatal intensive care. *Lancet* 2(8468):1327-1330.

Goodwin MM, Gazmararian JA, Johnson CH, Gilbert BC, Saltzman LE. 2000. Pregnancy intendedness and physical abuse around the time of pregnancy: Findings from the pregnancy risk assessment monitoring system, 1996-1997. PRAMS Working Group. Pregnancy Risk Assessment Monitoring System. *Maternal and Child Health Journal* 4(2):85-92.

Goodwin TM, Valenzuela G, Silver H, Hayashi R, Creasy GW, Lane R. 1996. Treatment of preterm labor with the oxytocin antagonist atosiban. *American Journal of Perinatology* 13:143-146.

Gordts S, Campo R, Puttemans P, Brosens I, Valkenburg M, Norre J, Renier M, Coeman D. 2005. Belgian legislation and the effect of elective single embryo transfer on IVF outcome. *Reproductive BioMedicine Online* 10(4):436-441.

Gorsuch RL, Key MK. 1974. Abnormalities of pregnancy as a function of anxiety and life stress. *Psychosomatic Medicine* 36(4):352-362.

Gosselin J, Gahagan S, Amiel-Tison C. 2005. The Amiel-Tison Neurological Assessment at Term: Conceptual and methodological continuity in the course of follow-up. *Mental Retardation and Developmental Disabilities Research Reviews* 11(1):34-51.

Gould JB, Gluck L, Kulovich MV. 1977. The relationship between accelerated pulmonary maturity and accelerated neurological maturity in certain chronically stressed pregnancies. *American Journal of Obstetrics and Gynecology* 127(2):181-186.

Goyen T-A, Lui K, Woods R. 1998. Visual-motor, visual-perceptual, and fine motor outcomes in very-low-birthweight children at 5 years. *Developmental Medicine and Child Neurology* 40(2):76-81.

Graham YP, Heim C, Goodman SH, Miller AH, Nemeroff CB. 1999. The effects of neonatal stress on brain development: Implications for psychopathology. *Developmental Psychopathology* 11(3):545-565.

Grand RJ, Turnell AS, Grabham PW. 1996. Cellular consequences of thrombin-receptor activation. *Biochemical Journal* 313:353-368.

Grandjean P, Bjerve KS, Weihe P, Steuerwald U. 2001. Birthweight in a fishing community: Significance of essential fatty acids and marine food contaminants. *International Journal of Epidemiology* 30:1272-1278.

Grant A, Glazener CM. 2001. Elective caesarean section versus expectant management for delivery of the small baby. *Cochrane Reviews* 2.

Gravel JS, O'Gara J. 2003. Communication options for children with hearing loss. *Mental Retardation and Developmental Disabilities Research Reviews* 9(4):243-251.

Graves CG, Matanoski GM, and Tardiff RG. 2001. Weight of evidence for an association between adverse reproductive and developmental effects and exposure to disinfection by-products: A critical review. *Regulatory Toxicology and Pharmacology* 34:103-124.

Gravett MG, Novy MJ. 1997. Endocrine-immune interactions in pregnant non-human primates with intrauterine infection. *Infectious Diseases in Obstetrics and Gynecology* 5:142-153.

Gravett MG, Witkin SS, Haluska GJ, Edwards JL, Cook MJ, Novy MJ. 1994. An experimental model for intraamniotic infection and preterm labor in rhesus monkeys. *American Journal of Obstetrics and Gynecology* 171(6):1660-1667.

Gravett MG, Haluska GJ, Cook MJ, Novy MJ. 1996. Fetal and maternal endocrine responses to experimental intrauterine infection in rhesus monkeys. *American Journal of Obstetrics and Gynecology* 174:1725-1733.

Gravett MG, Hitti J, Hess DL, Eschenbach DA. 2000. Intrauterine infection and preterm delivery: Evidence for activation of the fetal hypothalamic-pituitary-adrenal axis. *American Journal of Obstetrics and Gynecology* 182:1404-1413.

Gravett MG, Sadowsky D, Witkin S, Novy M. 2003. Immunomodulators plus antibiotics to prevent preterm delivery in experimental intra-amniotic infection (IAI). *American Journal of Obstetrics and Gynecology* 189 (Suppl):S56.

Gravett MG, Novy MJ, Rosenfeld RG, Reddy AP, Jacob T, Turner M, McCormack A, Lapidus JA, Hitti J, Eschenbach DA, Roberts CT Jr., Nagalla SR. 2004. Diagnosis of intra-amniotic infection by proteomic profiling and identification of novel biomarkers. *JAMA* 292(4):462-469.

Gray DJ, Robinson HB, Malone J, Thomson RB Jr. 1992. Adverse outcome in pregnancy following amniotic fluid isolation of Ureaplasma urealyticum. *Prenatal Diagnosis* 12(2):111-117.

Gray RF, Indurkhya A, McCormick MC. 2004. Prevalence, stability and predictors of clinically significant behavior problems in low birth weight children at 3,5, and 8 years of age. *Pediatrics* 114:736-743.

Greber S, Vial Y, Hohlfeld P, Witkin SS. 2003. Detection of Ureaplasma urealyticum in second-trimester amniotic fluid by polymerase chain reaction correlates with subsequent preterm labor and delivery. *Journal of Infectious Diseases* 187:518-521.

Green NS, Damus K, Simpson JL, Iams J, Reece EA, Hobel CJ, Merkatz IR, Greene MF, Schwarz RH, the March of Dimes Scientific Advisory Committee on Prematurity. 2005. Research agenda for preterm birth: Recommendations from the March of Dimes. *American Journal of Obstetrics and Gynecology* 193(3):626-635.

Greisen G. 1986. Cerebral blood flow in preterm infants during the first week of life. *Acta Paediatrica Scandinavica* 75:43-51.

Grether JK, Nelson KB. 1997. Maternal infection and cerebral palsy in infants of normal birth weight. *JAMA* 278:207-211.

Grether J, Hirtz D, McNellis D, Nelson K, Rouse DJ. 1998. Tocolytic magnesium sulphate and paediatric mortality. *Lancet* 351(9098):292.

Grether JK, Hoogstrate J, Walsh-Greene E, Nelson KB. 2000. Magnesium sulfate for tocolysis and risk of spastic cerebral palsy in premature children born to women without preeclampsia. *American Journal of Obstetrics and Gynecology* 183(3):717-725.

Grigsby PL, Poore KR, Hirst JJ, Jenkin G. 2000. Inhibition of premature labor in sheep by a combined treatment of nimesulide, a prostaglandin synthase type 2 inhibitor, and atosiban, an oxytocin receptor antagonist. *American Journal of Obstetrics and Gynecology* 183(3):649-657.

Gross SJ, Mettelman BB, Dye TD, Slagle TA. 2001. Impact of family structure and stability on academic outcome in preterm children at 10 years of age. *Journal of Pediatrics* 138(2): 169-175.

Grosse SD. 2003. Productivity loss tables (Appendix). In: Haddix AC, Teutsch SM, Corso PA eds. *Prevention Effectiveness: A Guide to Decision Analysis and Economic Evaluation*, 2nd edition. London, UK: Oxford University Press.

Grunau RE, Whitfield MF, Petrie J. 1998. Children's judgements about pain at age 8-10 years: Do extremely low birthweight (< 1000 g) children differ from full birthweight peers. *Journal of Child Psychology and Psychiatry and Allied Disciplines* 39(4):587-594.

Grunau RE, Oberlander TF, Whitfield MF, Fitzgerald C, Lee SK. 2001. Demographic and therapeutic determinants of pain reactivity in very low birth weight neonates at 32 weeks' postconceptional age. *Pediatrics* 107(1):105-112.

Grunau RE, Whitfield MF, Davis C. 2002. Pattern of learning disabilities in children with extremely low birth weight and broadly average intelligence. *Archives of Pediatrics and Adolescent Medicine* 156(6):615-620.

Grunau RE, Whitfield MF, Fay TB. 2004. Psychosocial and academic characteristics of extremely low birth weight (800 g) adolescents who are free of major impairment compared with term-born control subjects. *Pediatrics* 114(6):e725-e732.

Grunau RE, Holsti L, Haley DW, Oberlander T, Weinberg J, Solimano A, Whitfield MF, Fitzgerald C, Yu W. 2005. Neonatal procedural pain exposure predicts lower cortisol and behavioral reactivity in preterm infants in the NICU. *Pain* 113(3):293-300.

Guendelman S, English PB. 1995. Effect of United States residence on birth outcomes among Mexican immigrants: An exploratory study. *American Journal of Epidemiology* 142(9 Suppl):S30-S38.

Guinn DA, Goepfert AR, Owen J, Brumfield C, Hauth JC. 1997. Management options in women with preterm uterine contractions: A randomized clinical trial. *American Journal of Obstetrics and Gynecology* 177(4):814-818.

Guinn DA, Goepfert AR, Owen J, Wenstrom KD, Hauth JC. 1998. Terbutaline pump maintenance therapy for prevention of preterm delivery: A double-blind trial. *American Journal of Obstetrics and Gynecology* 179(4):874-878.

Guinn DA, Atkinson MW, Sullivan L, Lee M, MacGregor S, Parilla BV, Davies J, Hanlon-Lundberg K, Simpson L, Stone J, Wing D, Ogasawara K, Muraskas J. 2001. Single vs. weekly courses of antenatal corticosteroids for women at risk of preterm delivery: A randomized controlled trial. *JAMA* 286(13):1581-1587.

Guise J-M, Mahon SM, Aickin M, Helfand M, Peipert JF, Westhoff C. 2001. Screening for bacterial vaginosis in pregnancy. *American Journal of Preventive Medicine* 20(3 Suppl):62-72.

Guyatt GH, Cook DJ. 1994. Health status, quality of life, and the individual: Commentary. *JAMA* 272:630-631.

Guzzetta F, Shackelford GD, Volpe S. 1986. Periventricular intraparenchymal echodensities in the premature newborn: Critical determinant of neurologic outcome. *Pediatrics* 78(6): 995-1006.

Gyetvai K, Hannah ME, Hodnett ED, Ohlsson A. 1999. Tocolytics for preterm labor: A systematic review. *Obstetrics and Gynecology* 94:869-877.

Haas JS, Udvarhelyi S, et al. 1993. The effect of health coverage for uninsured pregnant women on maternal health and the use of cesarean section. *JAMA* 270(1):61-64.

Hack M. 1999. Consideration of the use of health status, functional outcome, and quality-of-life to monitor neonatal intensive care practice. *Pediatrics* 103:319-328.

Hack M, Fanaroff AA. 1999. Outcomes of children of extremely low birthweight and gestational age in the 1990's. *Early Human Development* 53(3):193-218.

Hack M, Taylor HG. 2000. Perinatal brain injury in preterm infants and later neurobehavioral function. *JAMA* 284:1973-1974.

Hack M, Mostow A, Miranda SB. 1976. Development of attention in preterm infants. *Pediatrics* 58(5):669-674.

Hack M, Muszynski SY, Miranda SB. 1981. State of awakeness during visual fixation in preterm infants. *Pediatrics* 68(1):87-92.

Hack M, Merkatz IR, McGrath SK. 1984. Catch-up growth in very-low-birth-weight infants. Clinical correlates. *American Journal of Diseases of Children* 138(4):370-375.

Hack M, Weissman B, Breslau N, Klein N, Borawski-Clark E, Fanaroff A. 1993. Health of very low birth weight children during their first eight years. *Journal of Pediatrics* 122:887-892.

Hack M, Taylor HG, Klein N, Eiben R, Schatschneider C, Mercuri-Minich N. 1994. School-age outcomes in children with birth weights under 750 g. *New England Journal of Medicine* 331(12):753-759.

Hack M, Weissman B, Borawski-Clark E. 1996. Catch-up growth during childhood among very-low-birth-weight children. *Archives of Pediatrics and Adolescent Medicine* 150(11): 1122-1129.

Hack M, Wilson-Costello D, Friedman H, Taylor GH, Schluchter M, Fanaroff AA. 2000. Neurodevelopment and predictors of outcomes of children with birth weights of less than 1000 g 1992-1995. *Archives of Pediatrics and Adolescent Medicine* 154(7):725-731.

Hack M, Flannery DJ, Schluchter M, Cartar L, Borawski E, Klein N. 2002. Outcomes in young adulthood for very-low-birth-weight infants. *New England Journal of Medicine* 346(3):149-157.

Hack M, Schluchter M, Cartar L, Rahman M, Cuttler L, Borawski E. 2003. Growth of very low birth weight infants to age 20 years. *Pediatrics* 112(1 Pt 1):e30-e38.

Hack M, Youngstrom EA, Cartar L, Schluchter M, Gerry Taylor H, Flannery D, Klein N, Borawski E. 2004. Behavioral outcomes and evidence of psychopathology among very low birth weight infants at age 20 years. *Pediatrics* 114(4):932-940.

Hack M, Schluchter M, Cartar L, Rahman M. 2005a. Blood pressure among very low birth weight (<1.5 kg) young adults. *Pediatrics Research* 58(4):677-684.

Hack M, Taylor HG, Drotar D, Schluchter M, Cartar L, Wilson-Costello D, Klein N, Friedman H, Mercuri-Minich N, Morrow M. 2005b. Poor predictive validity of the Bayley Scales of Infant Development for cognitive function of extremely low birth weight children at school age. *Pediatrics* 116(2):333-341.

Hadders-Algra M. 2002. Two distinct forms of minor neurological dysfunction: Perspectives emerging from a review of data of the Groningen Perinatal Project. *Developmental Medicine and Child Neurology* 44(8):561-571.

Hadlock FP, Harrist RB, Carpenter RJ. 1984. Sonographic estimation of fetal weight. The value of femur length in addition to head and abdomen measurements. *Radiology* 150(2):535-540.

Hadlock FP, Harrist RB, Shah YP. 1987. Estimating fetal age using multiple parameters: A prospective evaluation in a racially mixed population. *American Journal of Obstetrics and Gynecology* 156(4):955-957.

Hadlock FP, Shah YP, Kanon DJ, Lindsey JV. 1992. Fetal crown-rump length: Reevaluation of relation to menstrual age (5-18 weeks) with high-resolution real-time use. *Radiology* 182(2):501-505.

Hagberg B, Hagberg G, Olow I, V Wendt L. 1996. The changing panorama of cerebral palsy in Sweden. VII. Prevalence and origin in the birth year period 1887-90. *Acta Paediatrica, International Journal of Paediatrics* 85(8):954-960.

Hagberg H, Peebles D, Mallard C. 2002. Models of white matter injury: Comparison of infectious, hypoxic-ischemic, and excitotoxic insults. *Mental Retardation and Developmental Disabilities Research Reviews* 8:30-38.

Hagberg H, Mallard C, Jacobsson B. 2005. Role of cytokines in preterm labour and brain injury. *BJOG: An International Journal of Obstetrics and Gynaecology* 112(Suppl 1):16-18.

Hager RME, Daltveit AK, Hofoss D, Nilsen ST, Kolaas T, Oian P, Henriksen T. 2004. Complications of cesarean deliveries: Rates and risk factors. *American Journal of Obstetrics and Gynecology* 190(2):428-434.

Haig D. 2004. The (dual) origin of epigenetics. *Cold Spring Harbor Symposia on Quantitative Biology* 69:67-70.

Hakansson S, Farooqi A, Holmgren PA, Serenius F, Hogberg U. 2004. Proactive management promotes outcome in extremely preterm infants: A population-based comparison of two perinatal management strategies. *Pediatrics* 114(1):58-64.

Halfon N, Berkowitz G, Klee L. 1992. Mental health service utilization by children in foster care in California. *Pediatrics* 89(6 Suppl):1238-1244.

Halfon N, Mendonca A, Berkowitz G. 1995. Health status of children in foster care: The experience of the Center for the Vulnerable Child. *Archives of Pediatrics and Adolescent Medicine* 149(4):386-392.

Hall A, McLeod A, Counsell C, Thomson L, Mutch L. 1995. School attainment, cognitive ability, and motor function in a total Scottish very-low-birthweight population at eight years: A controlled study. *Developmental Medicine and Child Neurology* 37(12):1037-1050.

Halliday HL. 1999. Clinical trials of postnatal corticosteroids: Inhaled and systemic. *Biology of the Neonate* 76(Suppl 1):29-40.

Halliday HL. 2004. Postnatal steroids and chronic lung disease in the newborn. *Paediatric Respiratory Reviews* 5(Suppl A):S245-S248.

Halliday HL, Ehrenkranz RA. 2001a. Delayed (>3 weeks) postnatal corticosteroids for chronic lung disease in preterm infants. *Cochrane Database of Systematic Reviews (Online: Update Software)* 2.

Halliday HL, Ehrenkranz RA. 2001b. Early postnatal (<96 hours) corticosteroids for preventing chronic lung disease in preterm infants. *Cochrane Database of Systematic Reviews (Online: Update Software)* 1.

Halliday HL, Ehrenkranz RA. 2001c. Moderately early (7-14 days) postnatal corticosteroids for preventing chronic lung disease in preterm infants. *Cochrane Database of Systematic Reviews (Online: Update Software)* 1.

Halsey CL, Collin MF, Anderson CL. 1993. Extremely low birth weight children and their peers: A comparison of preschool performance. *Pediatrics* 91(4):807-811.

Halsey CL, Collin MF, Anderson CL. 1996. Extremely low-birth-weight children and their peers: A comparison of school-age outcomes. *Archives of Pediatrics and Adolescent Medicine* 150(8):790-794.

Haluska GJ, Kaler CA, Cook MJ, Novy MJ. 1994. Prostaglandin production during spontaneous labor and after treatment with RU486 in pregnant rhesus macaques. *Biology of Reproduction* 51(4):760-765.

Hampton T. 2004. Panel reviews health effects data for assisted reproductive technologies. *JAMA* 292(24):2961-2962.

Hamvas A, Wise PH, Yang RK, Wampler NS, Noguchi A, Maurer MM, Walentik CA, Schramm WF, Cole FS. 1996. The influence of the wider use of surfactant therapy on neonatal mortality among blacks and whites. *New England Journal of Medicine* 334(25): 1635-1640.

Hanke W, Kalinka J, Florek E, Sobala W. 1999. Passive smoking and pregnancy outcome in central Poland. *Human and Experimental Toxicology* 18:265-271.

Hansen BM, Greisen G. 2004. Is improved survival of very-low-birthweight infants in the 1980s and 1990s associated with increasing intellectual deficit in surviving children? *Developmental Medicine and Child Neurology* 46(12):812-815.

Hansen D, Lou HC, Olsen J. 2000. Serious life events and congenital malformations: A national study with complete follow-up. *Lancet* 356(9233):875-880.

Hao K, Wang X, Niu T, Xu X, Li A, Chang W, Wang L, Li G, Laird N, Xu X. 2004. A candidate gene study of preterm delivery: Application of high-throughput genotyping technology and advanced statistical methods. *Human Molecular Genetics* 13:683-691.

Hard A-L, Niklasson A, Svensson E, Hellstrom A. 2000. Visual function in school-aged children born before 29 weeks of gestation: A population-based study. *Developmental Medicine and Child Neurology* 42(2):100-105.

Harding JE, Pang J-M, Knight DB, Liggins GC. 2001. Do antenatal corticosteroids help in the setting of preterm rupture of membranes? *American Journal of Obstetrics and Gynecology* 184(2):131-139.

Hardy RJ, Palmer EA, Schaffer DB, Phelps DL, Davis BR, Cooper CJ. 1997. Outcome-based management of retinopathy of prematurity. *Journal of the American Association for Pediatric Opthalmology and Strabismus* 1(1):46-54.

Harger JH. 2002. Cerclage and cervical insufficiency: An evidence-based analysis. *Obstetrics and Gynecology* 100(6):1313-1327.

Harger JH, Hsing AW, Tuomala RE, Gibbs RS, Mead PB, Eschenbach DA, Knox GE, Polk BF. 1990. Risk factors for preterm premature rupture of fetal membranes: A multicenter case-control study. *American Journal of Obstetrics and Gynecology* 163(1 I):130-137.

Harrison H. 2001. Making lemonade: A parent's view of "quality of life" studies. *Journal of Clinical Ethics* 12(3):239-250.

Hasegawa K, Yoshioka H, Sawada T, Nishikawa H. 1993. Direct measurement for free radicals in the neonatal mouse brain subjected to hypoxia: An electron spin resonance spectroscopic study. *Brain Research* 607:161-166.

Hassan MI, Aschner Y, Manning CH, Xu J, Aschner JL. 2003. Racial differences in selected cytokine Allelic and genotypic frequencies among healthy, pregnant women in North Carolina. *Cytokine* 21:10-16.

Haumont D. 2005. Management of the neonate at the limits of viability. *BJOG: An International Journal of Obstetrics and Gynaecology* 112(Suppl 1): 64-66.

Hauth JC, Goldenberg RL, Andrews WW, DuBard MB, Copper RL. 1995. Reduced incidence of preterm delivery with metronidazole and erythromycin in women with bacterial vaginosis. *New England Journal of Medicine* 333:1732-1736.

Hauth JC, Andrews WW, Goldenberg RL. 1998. Infection-related risk factors predictive of spontaneous preterm birth. *Prenatal and Neonatal Medicine* 3:86-90.

Hay PE, Lamont RF, Taylor-Robinson D, et al. 1994. Abnormal bacterial colonisation of the genital tract and subsequent preterm delivery and late miscarriage. *British Medical Journal* 308:295-298.

Hayes D. 2003. Screening methods: Current status. *Mental Retardation and Developmental Disabilities Research Reviews* 9(2):65-72.

Hedegaard M, Henriksen TB, Sabroe S, Secher NJ. 1993. Psychological distress in pregnancy and preterm delivery. *British Medical Journal* 307(6898):234-239.

Hedegaard M, Henriksen TB, Secher NJ, Hatch MC, Sabroe S. 1996. Do stressful life events affect duration of gestation and risk of preterm delivery? *Epidemiology* 7(4):339-345.

Hediger ML, Scholl TO, Schall JL, Krueger PM. 1997. Young maternal age and preterm labor. *Annals of Epidemiology* 7(6):400-406.

Hediger ML, Overpeck MD, Ruan WJ, Troendle JF. 2002. Birthweight and gestational age effects on motor and social development. *Paediatric and Perinatal Epidemiology* 16(1): 33-46.

Heinrichs SC, Koob GF. 2004. Corticotropin-releasing factor in brain: A role in activation, arousal, and affect regulation. *Journal of Pharmacology and Experimental Therapeutics* 311(2):427-440.

Heins HC Jr., Nance NW, McCarthy BJ, Efird CM. 1990. A randomized trial of nurse-midwifery prenatal care to reduce low birth weight. *Obstetrics and Gynecology* 75(3 Pt 1):341-345.

Helders PJM, Cats BP, Debast S. 1989. Effects of a tactile stimulation/range-finding programme on the development of VLBW-neonates during the first year of life. *Child: Care, Health and Development* 15(6):369-379.

Helgeson VS, Cohen S. 1996. Social support and adjustment to cancer: Reconciling descriptive, correlational, and intervention research. *Health Psychology* 15(2):135-148.

Hellerstedt WL, Himes JH, Story M, Edwards LE. 1997. The effects of cigarette smoking and gestational weight change on birth outcomes in obese and normal-weight women. *American Journal of Public Health* 87:591-596.

Henderson-Smart DJ, Osborn DA. 2002. Kinesthetic stimulation for preventing apnea in preterm infants. *Cochrane Reviews* 1.

Henderson-Smart D, Steer P. 2004. Doxapram treatment for apnea in preterm infants. *Cochrane Database of Systematic Reviews (Online: Update Software)* 4.

Henderson-Smart DJ, Pettigrew AG, Edwards DA. 1985. Prenatal influences on the brainstem development of preterm infants. In: Jones CT, Nathanielz PW eds. *Physiological Development of the Fetus and Newborn.* Oxford, UK: Academic Press. Pp. 627-631.

Hendler I, Goldenberg RL, Mercer BM, Iams JD, Meis PJ, Moawad AH, MacPherson CA, Caritis SN, Miodovnik M, Menard KM, Thurnau GR, Sorokin Y. 2005. The Preterm Prediction Study: Association between maternal body mass index and spontaneous and indicated preterm birth. *American Journal of Obstetrics and Gynecology* 192(3): 882-886.

Henikoff S, McKittrick E, Ahmad K. 2004. Epigenetics, histone H3 variants, and the inheritance of chromatin states. *Cold Spring Harbor Symposia on Quantitative Biology* 69: 235-243.

Henriksen TB, Hedegaard M, Secher NJ. 1994. The relation between psychosocial job strain, and preterm delivery and low birthweight for gestational age. *International Journal of Epidemiology* 23(4):764-774.

Henriksen TB, Baird DD, Olsen J, Hedegaard M, Secher NJ, Wilcox AJ. 1997. Time to pregnancy and preterm delivery. *Obstetrics and Gynecology* 89(4):594-599.

Herron MA, Katz M, Creasy RK. 1982. Evaluation of a preterm birth prevention program: Preliminary report. *Obstetrics and Gynecology* 59(4):452-456.

Hille ETM, Den Ouden AL, Bauer L, Van den Oudenrijn C, Brand R, Verloove-Vanhorick SP. 1994. School performance at nine years of age in very premature and very low birth weight infants. Perinatal risk factors and predictors at five years of age. *Journal of Pediatrics* 125(3):426-434.

Hillier SL, Martius J, Krohn MA, Kiviat NB, Holmes KK, Eschenbach DA. 1988. A case-control study of chorioamnionitis in prematurity. *New England Journal of Medicine* 319:972-978.

Hillier SL, Nugent RP, Eschenbach DA, Krohn MA, Gibbs RS, Martin DH, Cotch MF, Edelman R, Pastorek JG 2nd, Rao AV, McNellis D, Regan J, Carey JC, Klebanoff MA. 1995. Association between bacterial vaginosis and preterm delivery of a low-birth-weight infant. The Vaginal Infections and Prematurity Study Group. *New England Journal of Medicine* 333:1737-1742.

Hintz SR, Kendrick DE, Vohr BR, Poole WK, Higgins RD, for the National Institute of Child Health and Human Development Neonatal Research Network. 2005. Changes in neuro-developmental outcomes at 18 to 22 months' corrected age among infants of less than 25 weeks' gestational age born in 1993-1999. *Pediatrics* 115(6):1645-1651.

Hirsch E, Wang H. 2005. The molecular pathophysiology of bacterially induced preterm labor: Insights from the murine model. *Journal of the Society for Gynecologic Investigation* 12:145-155.

Hittner HM, Hirsch NJ, Rudolph AJ. 1977. Assessment of gestational age by examination of the anterior vascular capsule of the lens. *Journal of Pediatrics* 91(3):455-458.

Hittner HM, Gorman WA, Rudolph AJ. 1981. Examination of the anterior vascular capsule of the lens: II. Assessment of gestational age in infants small for gestational ages. *Journal of Pediatric Ophthalmology and Strabismus* 18(2):52-54.

Ho S, Saigal S. 2005. Current survival and early outcomes of infants of borderline viability. *NeoReviews* 6(3):e123-e132.

Hobel CJ, Dunkel-Schetter C, Roesch S. 1998. Maternal stress as a signal to the fetus. *Prenatal and Neonatal Medicine* 3:116-120.

Hobel CJ, Dunkel-Schetter C, Roesch SC, Castro LC, Arora CP. 1999. Maternal plasma corticotropin-releasing hormone associated with stress at 20 weeks' gestation in pregnancies ending in preterm delivery. *American Journal of Obstetrics and Gynecology* 180(1 Pt 3):S257-S263.

Hodnett ED, Fredericks S. 2003. Support during pregnancy for women at increased risk of low birthweight babies. *Cochrane Database of Systematic Reviews* 3:CD000198.

Hoffman S, Hatch MC. 1996. Stress, social support and pregnancy outcome: A reassessment based on recent research. *Paediatric and Perinatal Epidemiology* 10(4):380-405.

Hoffman S, Hatch MC. 2000. Depressive symptomatology during pregnancy: Evidence for an association with decreased fetal growth in pregnancies of lower social class women. *Health Psychology* 19(6):535-543.

Hoffmann SC, Stanley EM, Cox ED, DiMercurio BS, Koziol DE, Harlan DM, Kirk AD, Blair PJ. 2002. Ethnicity greatly influences cytokine gene polymorphism distribution. *American Journal of Transplantation* 2(6):560-567.

Hofman PL, Regan F, Harris M, Robinson E, Jackson W, Cutfield WS. 2004a. The metabolic consequences of prematurity. *Growth Hormone and IGF Research* 14(Suppl A): S136-S139.

Hofman PL, Regan F, Jackson WE, Jefferies C, Knight DB, Robinson EM, Cutfield WS. 2004b. Premature birth and later insulin resistance. *New England Journal of Medicine* 351(21): 2179-2186.

Hofstetter MK. 2005. Fungal infections in the neonatal intensive care unit. In: Taeusch HW, Ballard RA, Gleason CA eds. *Avery's Diseases of the Newborn*, 8th edition. Philadelphia, PA: Elsevier Saunders. Pp. 595-600.

Hogue CJ, Bremner JD. 2005. Stress model for research into preterm delivery among black women. *American Journal of Obstetrics and Gynecology* 192(5 Suppl):S47-S55.

Hogue CJ, Vasquez C. 2002. Toward a strategic approach for reducing disparities in infant mortality. *American Journal of Public Health* 92(4):552-556.

Hollander D. 2005. Women in their 30s are the most likely to experience adverse birth outcomes if jailed during pregnancy. *Perspectives on Sexual and Reproductive Health* 37(1):48-49.

Holling EE, Leviton A. 1999. Characteristics of cranial ultrasound white-matter echolucencies that predict disability: A review. *Developmental Medicine and Child Neurology* 41(2): 136-139.

Holsti L, Grunau RE, Oberlander TF, Whitfield MF. 2005. Prior pain induces heightened motor responses during clustered care in preterm infants in the NICU. *Pediatrics* 114(1):65-72.

Holt VL, Danoff NL, Mueller BA, Swanson MW. 1997. The association of change in maternal marital status between births and adverse pregnancy outcomes in the second birth. *Paediatric and Perinatal Epidemiology* 11(Suppl 1):31-40.

Holzman C, Paneth N. 1994. Maternal cocaine use during pregnancy and perinatal outcomes. *Epidemiologic Reviews* 16(2):315-334.

Holzman C, Paneth N, Fisher R, the MSU Prematurity Group. 1998. Rethinking the concept of risk factors for preterm delivery: Antecedents, markers and mediators. *Prenatal and Neonatal Medicine* 3(1):47-52.

Holzman C, Bullen B, Fisher R, Paneth N, Reuss L. 2001. Pregnancy outcomes and community health: The POUCH study of preterm delivery. *Paediatric and Perinatal Epidemiology* 15(Suppl 2):136-158.

Homer CJ, Beresford SA, James SA, Siegel E, Wilcox S. 1990. Work-related physical exertion and risk of preterm, low birthweight delivery. *Paediatric and Perinatal Epidemiology* 4(2):161-174.

Honest H, Bachman LM, Coomarasamy A, et al. 2003. Accuracy of cervical transvaginal sonography in predicting preterm birth: A systematic review. *Ultrasound Obstetrics and Gynecology* 22:305-322.

Honest H, Bachmann LM, Knox EM, Gupta JK, Kleijnen J, Khan KS. 2004. The accuracy of various tests for bacterial vaginosis in predicting preterm birth: A systematic review. *BJOG: An International Journal of Obstetrics and Gynaecology* 111(5):409-422.

Honest H, Bachmann LM, Ngai C, Gupta JK, Kleijnen J, Khan KS. 2005. The accuracy of maternal anthropometry measurements as predictor for spontaneous preterm birth—a systematic review. *European Journal of Obstetrics and Gynecology and Reproductive Biology* 119(1):11-20.

Honeycutt AA, Grosse SD, Dunlap LJ, et al. 2003. Economic costs of mental retardation, cerebral palsy, hearing loss, and vision impairment. In: Altman BM, Barnartt SN, Hendershot G, Larson S eds. *Using Survey Data to Study Disability: Results from the National Health Interview Survey on Disability*. London, UK: Elsevier Science Ltd. Pp. 207-228.

Hong EJ, West AE, Greenberg ME. 2005. Transcriptional control of cognitive development. *Current Opinion in Neurobiology* 15:21-28.

Honnor MJ, Zubrick SR, Stanley FJ. 1994. The role of life events in different categories of preterm birth in a group of women with previous poor pregnancy outcome. *European Journal of Epidemiology* 10(2):181-188.

Hooker D. 1952. *The Prenatal Origin of Behavior*. New York: Hafner Publishing Co. P. 143.

Hooker D, Hare C. 1954. Early human fetal behavior, with a preliminary note on double simultaneous fetal stimulation. *Research Publications—Association for Research in Nervous and Mental Disease* 33:98-113.

Horbar JD, Plsek PE, Leahy K. 2003. NIC/Q 2000: Establishing habits for improvement in neonatal intensive care units. *Pediatrics* 111(4 Pt2):e397-e410.

Hourani L, Hilton S. 2000. Occupational and environmental exposure correlates of adverse live-birth outcomes among 1032 U.S. Navy women. *Journal of Occupational and Environmental Medicine* 42:1156-1165.

House JS. 1981. *Work Stress and Social Support* Reading, MA: Addison-Wesley.

House JS, Landis KR, Umberson D. 1988. Social relationships and health. *Science* 241(4865): 540-555.

Hovi P, Andersson S, Eriksson JG, Kajantie E. 2005, May. Elevated fasting serum insulin in young adults born with very low birth weight. Abstract #5535. PAS Annual Meeting, Washington, DC.

HRSA (Health Resources and Services Administration). 2000. *Understanding Title V of the Social Security Act.* [Online]. Available: ftp://ftp.hrsa.gov/mchb/titlevtoday/UnderstandingTitleV.pdf [accessed January 30, 2006].

HRSA. 2004. *HRSA FY 2004 Budget.* [Online]. Available: http://newsroom.hrsa.gov/NewsBriefs/2004/FY04-HRSA-Budget.htm [accessed May 10, 2006]. P. 88.

Hsieh TT, Chen SF, Shau WY, Hsieh CC, Hsu JJ, Hung TH. 2005. The impact of interpregnancy interval and previous preterm birth on the subsequent risk of preterm birth. *Journal of the Society for Gynecologic Investigation* 12:202-207.

Huang WL, Beazley LD, Quinlivan JA, Evans SF, Newnham JP, Dunlop SA. 1999. Effect of corticosteroids on brain growth in fetal sheep. *Obstetrics and Gynecology* 94:213.

Huddy CLJ, Johnson A, Hope PL. 2001. Educational and behavioural problems in babies of 32-35 weeks gestation. *Archives of Disease in Childhood* 85(1):F23-F28.

Hueston WJ. 1998. Preterm contractions in community settings: II. Predicting preterm birth in women with preterm contractions. *Obstetrics and Gynecology* 92:43-46.

Hueston WJ, Knox MA, Eilers G, Pauwels J, Lonsdorf D. 1995. The effectiveness of preterm-birth prevention educational programs for high-risk women: A meta-analysis. *Obstetrics and Gynecology* 86(4 II Suppl):705-712.

Huizink AC, de Medina PG, Mulder EJ, Visser GH, Buitelaar JK. 2002. Psychological measures of prenatal stress as predictors of infant temperament. *Journal of the American Academy of Child and Adolescent Psychiatry* 41(9):1078-1085.

Huizink AC, Robles de Medina PG, Mulder EJ, Visser GH, Buitelaar JK. 2003. Stress during pregnancy is associated with developmental outcome in infancy. *Journal of Child Psychology and Psychiatry* 44(6):810-818.

Huizink AC, Mulder EJ, Buitelaar JK. 2004. Prenatal stress and risk for psychopathology: Specific effects or induction of general susceptibility? *Psychology Bulletin* 130(1): 115-142.

Hulsey TC, Alexander GR, Robillard PY, Annibale DJ, Keenan A. 1993. Hyaline membrane disease. The role of ethnicity and maternal risk characteristics. *American Journal of Obstetrics and Gynecology* 168(2):572-576.

Hultman CM, Sparen P, Cnattingius S. 2002. Perinatal risk factors for infantile autism. *Epidemiology* 13(4):417-423.

Humphrey T. 1964. Some correlations between the appearance of human fetal reflexes and the development of the nervous system. *Progress in Brain Research* 4:93-135.

Huxley R, Neil A, Collins R. 2002. Unravelling the fetal origins hypothesis: Is there really an inverse association between birthweight and subsequent blood pressure? *Lancet* 360(9334):659-665.

Iams JD. 2003. Prediction and early detection of preterm labor. *Obstetrics and Gynecology* 101:402-412.

Iams JD, Johnson FF, O'Shaughnessy RW. 1990. Ambulatory uterine activity monitoring in the posthospital care of patients with preterm labor. *American Journal of Perinatology* 7:170-173.

Iams JD, Johnson FF, Parker M. 1994. A prospective evaluation of the signs and symptoms of preterm labor. *Obstetrics and Gynecology* 84:227.

Iams JD, Johnson FF, Sonek J, Sachs L, Gebauer C, Samuels P. 1995. Cervical competence as a continuum: A study of ultrasonographic cervical length and obstetric performance. *American Journal of Obstetrics and Gynecology* 172(4 I):1097-1106.

Iams JD, Goldenberg RL, Meis PJ, Mercer BM, Moawad A, Das A, Thom E, McNellis D, Copper RL, Johnson F, Roberts JM, Hauth JC, Northern A, Neely C, Mueller-Heubach E, Swain M, Frye A, Lindheimer M, Jones P. 1996. The length of the cervix and the risk of spontaneous premature delivery. *New England Journal of Medicine* 334(9):567-572.

Iams JD, Goldenberg RL, Mercer BM, Moawad A, Thom E, Meis PJ, McNellis D, Caritis SN, Miodovnik M, Menard MK, Thurnau GR, Bottoms SE, Roberts JM. 1998. The Preterm Prediction Study: Recurrence risk of spontaneous preterm birth. National Institute of Child Health and Human Development Maternal-Fetal Medicine Units Network. *American Journal of Obstetrics and Gynecology* 178(5):1035-1040.

Iams JD, Newman RB, Thom EA, Goldenberg RL, Mueller-Heubach E, Moawad A, Sibai BM, Caritis SN, Miodovnik M, Paul RH, Dombrowski MP, McNellis D. 2002. Frequency of uterine contractions and the risk of spontaneous preterm delivery. *New England Journal of Medicine* 346(4):250-255.

IHPIT (The Interconception Health Promotion Initiative Team). 2003. *Interconception Health Promotion Initiative Final Report.* Denver: Colorado Trust. [Online]. Available: http://www.coloradotrust.org/repository/publications/pdfs/IHPIFinalReport04.pdf [accessed January 9, 2006].

Ikegami M, Polk D, Jobe A. 1996. Minimum interval from fetal betamethasone treatment to postnatal lung responses in preterm lambs. *American Journal of Obstetrics and Gynecology* 174:1408-1413.

Ikegami M, Jobe AH, Newnham J, Polk DH, Willet KE, Sly P. 1997. Repetitive prenatal-glucocorticoids improve lung function and decrease growth in preterm lambs. *American Journal of Respiratory and Critical Care Medicine* 156:178-184.

Inder T. 2005. Abnormal cerebral structure is present at term in premature infants. *Pediatrics* 115(2):286-295.

Inder T, Neil J, Yoder B, Rees S. 2004. Non-human primate models of neonatal brain injury. *Seminars in Perinatology* 28:396-404.

Indredavik MS, Vik T, Heyerdahl S, Kulseng S, Fayers P, Brubakk A-M. 2004. Psychiatric symptoms and disorders in adolescents with low birth weight. *Archives of Disease in Childhood: Fetal and Neonatal Edition* 89(5):F445-F450.

Inhorn MC, Fakih MH. 2006. Arab Americans, African Americans, and infertility: Barriers to reproduction and medical care. *Fertility and Sterility* 85(4):844-852.

The International HapMap Consortium. 2003. The International HapMap Project. *Nature* 426:789-796.

Ioannidis JP, Ntzani EE, Trikalinos TA. 2004. "Racial" differences in genetic effects for complex diseases. *Nature Genetics* 36(12):1243-1244.

IOM (Institute of Medicine). 1985. *Preventing Low Birthweight.* Washington, DC: National Academy Press.

IOM. 1988. *Prenatal Care: Reaching Mothers, Reaching Infants.* Washington, DC: National Academy Press.

IOM. 1989. *Medical Professional Liability and the Delivery of Obstetrical Care: Volume I.* Washington, DC: National Academy Press.

IOM. 1992. *Strengthening Research in Academic OB/GYN Departments.* Washington, DC: National Academy Press.

IOM. 1994. *Careers in Clinical Research: Obstacles and Opportunities.* Washington, DC: National Academy Press.

IOM. 1995. *The Best Intentions: Unintended Pregnancy and the Well-Being of Children and Families*. Washington, DC: National Academy Press.

IOM. 2000. *Promoting Health: Intervention Strategies from Social and Behavioral Research*. Washington, DC: National Academy Press.

IOM. 2003. *The Role of Environmental Hazards in Premature Birth*: A Workshop Summary. Washington, DC: The National Academies Press.

IOM. 2006. *Valuing Health for Regulatory Cost-Effectiveness Analysis*. Washington, DC: The National Academies Press.

Irgens A, Kruger K, Skorve AH, Irgens LM. 1998. Reproductive outcome in offspring of parents occupationally exposed to lead in Norway. *American Journal of Independent Medicine* 34:431-437.

Irving RJ, Belton NR, Elton RA, Walker BR. 2000. Adult cardiovascular risk factors in premature babies. *Lancet* 355(9221):2135-2136.

Irwin M. 1999. Immune correlates of depression. *Advances in Experimental Medicine and Biology* 461:1-24.

Istvan J. 1986. Stress, anxiety, and birth outcomes: A critical review of the evidence. *Psychology Bulletin* 100(3):331-348.

Jaakkola JJ, Jaakkola N, Zahlsen K. 2001. Fetal growth and length of gestation in relation to prenatal exposure to environmental tobacco smoke assessed by hair nicotine concentration. *Environmental Health Perspectives* 109:557-561.

Jackson R. 2004. Perinatal outcomes in singletons following in vitro fertilization: A meta-analysis. *Obstetrics and Gynecology*. 103(3):551-563.

Jackson GM, Ludmir J, Bader TJ. 1992. The accuracy of digital examination and ultrasound in the evaluation of cervical length. *Obstetrics and Gynecology* 79:214.

Jackson K, Schollin J, Bodin L, Ternestedt BM. 2001. Utilization of healthcare by very-low-birthweight infants during their first year of life. *Acta Paediatrica* 90:213-217.

Jackson RA, Gibson KA, Wu YW, Croughan MS. 2004. Perinatal outcomes in singletons following in vitro fertilization: A meta-analysis. *Obstetrics and Gynecology* 103(3): 551-563.

Jacob S, Moley KH. 2005. Gametes and embryo epigenetic reprogramming affect developmental outcome: Implication for assisted reproductive technologies. *Pediatric Research* 58(3):437-446.

Jacob SV, Coates AL, Lands LC, MacNeish CF, Riley SP, Hornby L, Outerbridge EW, Davis GM, Williams RL. 1998. Long-term pulmonary sequelae of severe bronchopulmonary dysplasia. *Journal of Pediatrics* 133(2):193-200.

Jacobs SE, O'Brien K, Inwood S, Kelly EN, Whyte HE. 2000. Outcome of infants 23-26 weeks' gestation pre and post surfactant. *Acta Paediatrica, International Journal of Paediatrics* 89(8):959-965.

Jain T. 2006. Socioeconomic and racial disparities among infertility patients seeking care. *Fertility and Sterility* 85(4):876-881.

James AT, Bracken MB, Cohen AP, Saftlas A, Lieberman E. 1999. Interpregnancy interval and disparity in term small for gestational age births between black and white women. *Obstetrics and Gynecology* 93:109-112.

James SA. 1993. Racial and ethnic differences in infant mortality and low birth weight: A psychosocial critique. *Annals of Epidemiology* 3:130-136.

Jamie WE, Edwards RK, Ferguson RJ, Duff P. 2005. The interleukin-6 -174 single nucleotide polymorphism: Cervical protein production and the risk of preterm delivery. *American Journal of Obstetrics and Gynecology* 192(4):1023-1027.

Jannet D, Abankwa A, Guyard B, Carbonne B, Marpeau L, Milliez J. 1997. Nicardipine versus salbutamol in the treatment of premature labor. A prospective randomized study. *European Journal of Obstetrics Gynecology and Reproductive Biology* 73(1):11-16.

Jeffcoat MK, Geurs NC, Reddy MS, Cliver SP, Goldenberg RL. Hauth JC. 2001a. Periodontal infection and preterm birth: Results of a prospective study. *Journal of the American Dental Association* 132:875-880.

Jeffcoat MK, Geurs NC, Reddy MS, Goldenberg RL, Hauth JC. 2001b. Current evidence regarding periodontal disease as a risk factor in preterm birth. *Annals of Periodontology/ The American Academy of Periodontology* 6(1):183-188.

Jeffcoat MK, Hauth JC, Geurs NC, Reddy MS, Cliver SP, Hodgkins PM, Goldenberg RL. 2003. Periodontal disease and preterm birth: Results of a pilot intervention study. *Journal of Periodontology* 74:1214-1218.

Jenney M, Campbell S. 1997. Measuring quality of life. *Archives of Disease in Childhood* 77:347-354.

Jesse DE, Seaver W, Wallace DC. 2003. Maternal psychosocial risks predict preterm birth in a group of women from Appalachia. *Midwifery* 19(3):191-202.

Jiang YH, Bressler J, Beaudet AL. 2004. Epigenetics and human disease. *Annual Review of Genomics and Human Genetics* 5:479-510.

Jobe AH. 1993. Pulmonary surfactant therapy. *New England Journal of Medicine* 328:861.

Jobe AH. 1999. The new BPD: An arrest of lung development. *Pediatrics Research* 46: 641-643.

Jobe AH, Bancalari E. 2001. NICHD/NHLBI/ORD Workshop Summary. Bronchopulmonary dysplasia. *American Journal of Respiratory and Critical Care Medicine* 163:1723-1729.

Jobe AH, Ikegami M. 2001. Biology of surfactant. *Clinical Perinatology* 28:655.

Jobe AH, Wada N, Berry LM, Ikegami M, Ervin MG. 1998. Single and repetitive maternal glucocorticoid exposures reduce fetal growth in sheep. *American Journal of Obstetrics and Gynecology* 178(5):880-885.

Joesoef MR, Hillier SL, Wiknjosastro G, Sumampouw H, Linnan M, Norojono W, Idajadi A, Utomo B. 1995. Intravaginal clindamycin treatment for bacterial vaginosis: Effects on preterm delivery and low birth weight. *American Journal of Obstetrics and Gynecology* 173(5):1527-1531.

Joffe M, Li Z. 1994. Association of time to pregnancy and the outcome of pregnancy. *Fertility and Sterility* 62(1):71-75.

Joffe S, Escobar GJ, Black SB, Armstrong MA, Lieu TA. 1999. Rehospitalization for respiratory syncytial virus among premature infants. *Pediatrics* 104:894-899.

Johansson B, Wedenberg E, Westin B. 1992. Fetal heart rate response to acoustic stimulation in relation to fetal development and hearing impairment. *Acta Obstetricia et Gynecologica Scandinavica* 71(8):610-615.

Johnsen SL, Rasmussen S, Sollien R, Kiserud T. 2005. Fetal age assessment based on femur length at 10-25 weeks of gestation, and reference ranges for femur length to head circumference ratios. *Acta Obstetricia et Gynecologica Scandinavica* 84(8):725-733.

Johnson AA, Knight EM, Edwards CH, Oyemade UJ, Cole OJ, Westney OE, Westney LS, Laryea H, Jones S. 1994. Selected lifestyle practices in urban African American women— Relationships to pregnancy outcome, dietary intakes and anthropometric measurements. *Journal of Nutrition* 124(6 Suppl):963S-972S.

Johnson JWC, Mitzner W, London WT, Palmer AE, Scott R, Kearney K. 1978. Glucocorticoids and the rhesus fetal lung. *American Journal of Obstetrics and Gynecology* 130: 905-916.

Johnson JWC, Mitzner W, Beck JC, London WT, Sly DL, Lee PA, Khouzami VA, Cavalieri RL. 1981. Long-term effects of betamethasone on fetal development. *American Journal of Obstetrics and Gynecology* 141:1053-1061.

Johnson S, Ring W, Anderson P, Marlow N. 2005. Randomised trial of parental support for families with very preterm children: Outcome at 5 years. *Archives of Disease in Childhood* 90(9):909-915.

Jones RAK, on behalf of the Collaborative Dexamethasone Trial Follow-up Group. 2005. Randomized, controlled trial of Dexamethasone in Neonatal Chronic Lung Disease: 13- to 17-year follow-up study: II. Respiratory status, growth, and blood pressure. *Pediatrics* 116(2):379-384.

Joseph KS, Kramer MS. 1996. Review of the evidence on fetal and early childhood antecedents of adult chronic disease. *Epidemiologic Reviews* 18(2):158-174.

Joseph KS, Kramer MS, Marcoux S, Ohlsson A, Wen SW, Allen A, Platt R. 1998. Determinants of preterm birth rates in Canada from 1981 through 1983 and from 1992 through 1994. *New England Journal of Medicine* 339(20):1434-1439.

Joyce T. 1998. Impact of augmented prenatal care on birth outcomes of Medicaid recipients in New York City. *Journal of Health Economics* 18:31-67.

Juberg DR, Loch-Caruso R. 1992. Investigation of the role of estrogenic action and prostaglandin E2 in DDT-stimulated rat uterine contractions ex vivo. *Toxicology* 74(2-3): 161-172.

Juberg DR, Stuenkel EL, Loch-Caruso R. 1995. DDE chlorinated insecticide 1,1-dichloro-2,2-bis(4-chlorophenyl)ethane (p,p'-DDD) increases intracellular calcium in rat myometrial smooth muscle cells. *Toxicology and Applied Pharmacology* 135(1):147-155.

Juul SE. 2005. Developmental biology of the hematologic system. In: Taeusch HW, Ballard RA, Gleason CA eds. *Avery's Diseases of the Newborn*. 8th edition. Philadelphia, PA: Elsevier Saunders. Pp. 112-132.

Juurlink BHJ. 1997. Response of glial cells to ischemia: Roles of reactive oxygen species and glutathione. *Neuroscience and Biobehavioral Reviews* 21:151-166.

Kahn DJ, Richardson DK, Billett HH. 2003. Inter-NICU variation in the rates and management of thrombocytopenia among very low birth-weight infants. *Journal of Perinatology* 23:312-316.

Kaiser Family Foundation. 2004. *Health Coverage for Immigrants*. [Online]. Available: http://kff.org/uninsured/upload/Health-Coverage-for-Immigrants-Fact-Sheet.pdf [accessed June 2, 2006].

Kaiser J, Gauss CH, Williams DK. 2005. The effects of hypercapnia on cerebral autoregulation in ventilated very low birth weight infants. *Pediatric Research* 58(5):931-935.

Kaiser RS, Trese MT, Williams GA, Cox MS Jr. 2001. Adult retinopathy of prematurity: Outcomes of rhegmatogenous retinal detachments and retinal tears. *Ophthalmology* 108(9):1647-1653.

Kalantar-Zadeh K, Block G, Horwich T, Fonarow GC. 2004. Reverse epidemiology of conventional cardiovascular risk factors in patients with chronic heart failure. *Journal of the American College of Cardiology* 43:1439-1444.

Kalish RB, Thaler HT, Chasen ST, Gupta M, Berman SJ, Rosenwaks Z, Chervenak FA. 2004. First- and second-trimester ultrasound assessment of gestational age. *American Journal of Obstetrics and Gynecology* 191(3):975-978.

Källén B, Finnstrom O, Nygren KG, Olausson PO. 2005. Temporal trends in multiple births after in vitro fertilisation in Sweden, 1982-2001: A register study. *British Medical Journal* 331(7513):382-383.

Kallan JE. 1992. Effects of interpregnancy intervals on preterm birth, intrauterine growth retardation, and fetal loss. *Social Biology* 39:231-245.

Kallan JE. 1997. Reexamination of interpregnancy intervals and subsequent birth outcomes: Evidence from U.S. linked birth/infant death records. *Social Biology* 44:205-212.

Kamlin CO, Davis PG. 2004. Long versus short inspiratory times in neonates receiving mechanical ventilation. *Cochrane Database of Systematic Reviews (Online: Update Software)* 4.

Kato I, Toniolo P, Koenig KL, Shore RE, Zeleniuch-Jacquotte A, Akhmedkhanov A, Riboli E. 1999. Epidemiologic correlates with menstrual cycle length in middle aged women. *European Journal of Epidemiology* 15(9):809-814.

Kaufman D, Boyle R, Hazen KC, Patrie JT, Robinson M, Donowitz LG. 2001. Fluconazole prophylaxis against fungal colonization and infection in preterm infants. *New England Journal of Medicine* 345(23):1660-1666.

Kaufman JS, Cooper RF, McGee DL. 1997. Socioeconomic status and health in blacks and whites: The problem of residual confounding and the resiliency of race. *Epidemiology* 8(6):621-628.

Kavanaugh K, Meier P, Zimmermann B, Mead L. 1997. The rewards outweigh the efforts: Breastfeeding outcomes for mothers of preterm infants. *Journal of Human Lactation* 13(1):15-21.

Kawachi I. 2000. Income inequality and health. In: Berkman LF, Kawachi I eds. *Social Epidemiology*. New York: Oxford University Press. Pp. 76-94.

Kayisli UA, Guzeloglu-Kayisli O, Arici A. 2004. Endocrine-immune interactions in human endometrium. *Annals of the New York Academy of Sciences* 1034:50-63.

Keene DJ, Wimmer JE Jr., Mathew OP. 2000. Does supine positioning increase apnea, bradycardia, and desaturation in preterm infants? *Journal of Perinatology* 20(1):17-20.

Keirse MJ. 1990. Progestogen administration in pregnancy may prevent preterm delivery. *British Journal of Obstetrics and Gynaecology* 97(2):149-154.

Kekki M, Kurki T, Pelkonen J, Kurkinen-Raty M, Cacciatore B, Paavonen J. 2001. Vaginal clindamycin in preventing preterm birth and peripartal infections in asymptomatic women with bacterial vaginosis: A randomized, controlled trial. *Obstetrics and Gynecology* 97(5 Pt 1):643-648.

Kelada SN, Eaton DL, Wang SS, Rothman NR, Khoury MJ. 2003. The role of genetic polymorphisms in environmental health. *Environmental Health Sciences* 111:1055-1164.

Kelly RW. 1994. Pregnancy maintainance and parturition: The role of prostaglandin in manipulating the immune and inflammatory response. *Endocrine Reviews* 15:684-706.

Kelly RW, King AE, Critchley HOD. 2001. Cytokine control in human endometrium. *Reproduction* 121:3-19.

Kenyon SL, Taylor DJ, Tarnow-Mordi W. 2001a. Broad-spectrum antibiotics for spontaneous preterm labour: The ORACLE II randomised trial. *Lancet* 357(9261):989-994.

Kenyon SL, Taylor DJ, Tarnow-Mordi W, ORACLE Collaborative Group. 2001b. Broad-spectrum antibiotics for preterm, prelabour rupture of fetal membranes: The ORACLE I randomised trial. ORACLE Collaborative Group. *Lancet* 357(9261):979-988.

Kenyon S, Boulvain M, Neilson J. 2004. Antibiotics for preterm rupture of the membranes: A systematic review. *Obstetrics and Gynecology* 104(5 I):1051-1057.

Kesmodel U, Olsen SF, Secher NJ. 2000. Does alcohol increase the risk of preterm delivery? *Epidemiology* 11(5):512-518.

Kesson AM, Henderson-Smart DJ, Pettigrew AG, Edwards DA. 1985. Peripheral nerve conduction velocity and brainstem auditory evoked responses in small for gestational age preterm infants. *Early Human Development* 11(3-4):213-219.

Khader YS, Ta'ani Q. 2005. Periodontal diseases and the risk of preterm birth and low birth weight: A meta-analysis. *Journal of Periodontology* 76:161-165.

Khadilkar V, Tudehope D, Burns Y, O'Callaghan M, Mohay H. 1993. The long-term neurodevelopmental outcome for very low birthweight (VLBW) infants with "dystonic" signs at 4 months of age. *Journal of Paediatrics and Child Health* 29(6):415-417.

Kharrazi M, DeLorenze GN, Kaufman FL, Eskenazi B, Bernert JT Jr., Graham S, Pearl M, Pirkle J. 2004. Environmental tobacco smoke and pregnancy outcome. *Epidemiology* 15:660-670.

Khoury MJ, Cohen BH. 1987. Genetic heterogeneity of prematurity and intrauterine growth retardation: clues from the Old Order Amish. *American Journal of Obstetrics and Gynecology* 157(2):400-410.

Kimberlin DF, Andrews WW. 1998. Bacterial vaginosis: association with advers pregnancy outcome. *Seminars in Perinatology* 22:242-249.

King JF, Grant A, Keirse MJNC. 1988. Beta-mimetics in preterm labour: An overview of the randomized controlled trials. *British Journal of Obstetrics and Gynaecology* 95:211.

King TE Jr. 2002. Racial disparities in clinical trials. *New England Journal of Medicine* 346(18):1400-1402.

Kiss H, Pichler E, Petricevic L, Husslein P. 2004. Cost effectiveness of a screen-and-treat program for asymptomatic vaginal infections in pregnancy: Towards a significant reduction in the costs of prematurity. *European Journal of Obstetrics and Gynecology and Reproductive Biology.*

Klassen AF, Lee SK, Parminder R, Chan HWP, Matthew D, Brabyn D. 2004. Health status and health-related quality of life in a population-based sample of neonatal intensive care unit graduates. *Pediatrics* 113:594-600.

Klebanoff MA. 1988. Short interpregnancy interval and the risk of low birthweight. American *Journal of Public Health* 78:667-670.

Klebanoff MA, Nugent RP, Rhoads GG. 1984. Coitus during pregnancy: Is it safe? *Lancet* 2(8408):914-917.

Klebanoff MA, Shiono PH, Berendes HW, Rhoads GG. 1989. Facts and artifacts about anemia and preterm delivery. *JAMA* 262(4):511-515.

Klebanoff MA, Regan JA, Rao V, Nugent RP, Blackwelder WC, Eschenbach DA, Pastorek II JG, Williams S, Gibbs RS, Carey JC, Yaffe SJ, Catz CS, Rhoads GG, McNellis D, Berendes HW, Reed G, Edelman R, Kaslow RA, Cotch MF. 1995. Outcome of the vaginal infections and prematurity study: Results of a clinical trial of erythromycin among pregnant women colonized with group B streptococci. *American Journal of Obstetrics and Gynecology* 172(5):1540-1545.

Klebanoff MA, Carey JC, Hauth JC, Hillier SL, Nugent RP, Thom EA, Ernest JM, Heine RP, Wapner RJ, Trout W, Moawad A, Leveno KJ, Copper RL, Northen A, Andrews WW, Jones P, Lindheimer MD, Elder N, Siddiqi TA, MacPherson C, Leindecker S, Fischer ML, Caritis SN, Cotroneo M, Camon T, Beydoun S, Alfonso C, Doyle F, Catz C, Yaffe SJ, Iams JD, Johnson F, Landon MB, Thurnau G, Meier A, Collins BA, LeBeouf F, Newman RB, Mercer BM, Ramsey R, Berkus M, Nicholson S, Sherman ML, Bloom S, DiVito M, Tolosa J, Dudley D, Reynolds L, Meis P, Mueller-Heubach E, Swain M, Bottoms SF, Norman GS. 2001. Failure of metronidazole to prevent preterm delivery among pregnant women with asymptomatic Trichomonas vaginalis infection. *New England Journal of Medicine* 345(7):487-493.

Klebanoff MA, Hillier SL, Nugent RP, MacPherson CA, Hauth JC, Carey JC, for the National Institute of Child Health and Human Development Maternal-Fetal Medicine Units Network. 2005. Is bacterial vaginosis a stronger risk factor for preterm birth when it is diagnosed earlier in gestation? *American Journal of Obstetrics and Gynecology* 192: 470-477.

Klebanov PK, Brooks-Gunn J, McCormick MC. 1994. School achievement and failure in very low birth weight children. *Journal of Developmental and Behavioral Pediatrics* 15(4): 248-256.

Klebanov PK, Brooks-Gunn J, McCormick MC. 2001. Maternal coping strategies and emotional distress: Results of an early intervention program for low birth weight young children. *Developmental Psychology* 37(5).

Klein R, Fish-Parcham C. 1999. *Losing Health Insurance: Unintended Consequences of Welfare Reform.* Washington, DC: Families USA.

Klein TE, Chang JT, Cho MK, Easton KL, Fergerson R, Hewett M, Lin Z, Liu Y, Liu S Oliver DE, Rubin DL, Shafa F, Stuart JM, Altman RB. 2001. Intergrating genotype and phenotype information: An overview of the PharmGKB project. *The Pharmacogenomics Journal* 1:167-170.

Kleinman JC, Kessel SS. 1987. Racial differences in low birth weight. Trends and risk factors. *New England Journal of Medicine* 317(12):749-753.

Klerman LV, Cliver SP, Goldenberg RL. 1998. The impact of short interpregnancy intervals on pregnancy outcomes in a low-income population. *American Journal of Public Health* 88:1182-1185.

Klerman LV, Ramey SL, Goldenberg RL, Marbury S, Hou J, Cliver SP. 2001. A randomized trial of augmented prenatal care for multiple-risk, Medicaid-eligible African American women. *American Journal of Public Health* 91(1):105-111.

Klimach VJ, Cooke RWI. 1988. Maturation of the neonatal somatosensory evoked response in preterm infants. *Developmental Medicine and Child Neurology* 30(2):208-214.

Kline J, Ng SKC, Schittini M, Levin B, Susser M. 1997. Cocaine use during pregnancy: Sensitive detection by hair assay. *American Journal of Public Health* 87(3):352-358.

Klip H, Van Leeuwen F, Burger C. 2000. Risk of ovarian cancer after use of fertility drugs [Risico op ovariumcarcinoom na gebruik van fertiliteitsbevorderende geneesmiddelen]. *Tijdschrift voor Fertiliteitsonderzoek* 14(1):16-21.

Kneyber MCJ, Plotz FB, Kimpen JLL. 2005. Bench to bedside review: Paediatric viral lower respiratory tract disease necessitating mechanical ventilation-should we use exogenous surfactant? *Critical Care* 9:550-555.

Kok JH, Briet JM, Van Wassenaer AG. 2001. Postnatal thyroid hormone replacement in very preterm infants. *Seminars in Perinatology* 25(6):417-425.

Kollee LAA, Verloove-Vanhorick PP, Verwey RA, Brand R, Ruys JH. 1988. Maternal and neonatal transport: Results of a national collaborative survey of preterm and very low birth weight infants in the Netherlands. *Obstetrics and Gynecology* 72(5):729-732.

Koller H, Lawson K, Rose SA, Wallace I, McCarton C. 1997. Patterns of cognitive development in very low birth weight children during the first six years of life. *Pediatrics* 99(3):383-389.

Konishi Y, Mikawa H, Suzuki J. 1986. Asymmetrical head-turning of preterm infants: Some effects on later postural and functional lateralities. *Developmental Medicine and Child Neurology* 28(4):450-457.

Konishi Y, Kuriyama M, Mikawa H, Suzuki J. 1987. Effect of body position on later postural and functional lateralities of preterm infants. *Developmental Medicine and Child Neurology* 29(6):751-757.

Konishi Y, Takaya R, Kimura K, Takeuchi K, Saito M, Konishi K. 1997. Laterality of finger movements in preterm infants. *Developmental Medicine and Child Neurology* 39(4): 248-252.

Konte JM, Creasy RK, Laros RK Jr. 1988. California North Coast Preterm Birth Prevention Project. *Obstetrics and Gynecology* 71(5):727-730.

Koroukian SM. 2004. Relative risk of postpartum complications in the Ohio medicaid population: Vaginal versus cesarean delivery. *Medical Care Research and Review* 61(2): 203-224.

Kost K, Landry DJ, Darroch JE. 1998. Predicting maternal behaviors during pregnancy: Does intention status matter? *Family Planning Perspectives* 30(2):79-88.

Koupilova I, Vagero D, Leon DA, Pikhart H, Prikazsky V, Holcik J, Bobak M. 1998. Social variation in size at birth and preterm delivery in the Czech Republic and Sweden, 1989-1991. *Paediatric and Perinatal Epidemiology* 12(1):7-24.

Koy C, Heitner JC, Woisch R, Kreutzer M, Serrano-Fernandez P, Gohlke R, Reimer T, Glocker MO. 2005. Cryodetector mass spectrometry profiling of plasma samples for HELLP diagnosis: An exploratory study. *Proteomics* 5(12):3079-3087.

Kramer M. 1987. Determinants of low birth weight: Methodological assessment and metaanalysis. *Bulletin of the World Health Organization.* 65:663-737.

Kramer MS, McLean FH, Boyd ME, Usher RH. 1988. The validity of gestational age estimation by menstrual dating in term, preterm, and postterm gestations. *JAMA* 260(22):3306-3308.

Kramer MS, Coates AL, Michoud M-C, Dagenais S, Hamilton EF, Papageorgiou A. 1995. Maternal anthropometry and idiopathic preterm labor. *Obstetrics and Gynecology* 86(5):744-748.

Kramer MS, Seguin L, Lydon J, Goulet L. 2000. Socio-economic disparities in pregnancy outcome: Why do the poor fare so poorly? *Paediatric and Perinatal Epidemiology* 14(3):194-210.

Kramer MS, Goulet L, Lydon J, Seguin L, McNamara H, Dassa C, Platt RW, Chen MF, Gauthier H, Genest J, Kahn S, Libman M, Rozen R, Masse A, Miner L, Asselin G, Benjamin A, Klein J, Koren G. 2001a. Socio-economic disparities in preterm birth: Causal pathways and mechanisms. *Paediatric and Perinatal Epidemiology* 15(Suppl 2):104-123.

Kramer MS, Platt RW, Wen SW, Joseph KS, Allen A, Abrahamowicz M, Blondel B, Breart G. 2001b. A new and improved population-based Canadian reference for birth weight for gestational age. *Pediatrics* 108(2):E35.

Krieger JN. 2002. Urinary tract infections: What's new? *Journal of Urology* 168(6):2351-2358.

Krieger N. 1990. Racial and gender discrimination: Risk factors for high blood pressure? *Social Science and Medicine* 30(12):1273-1281.

Krieger N. 2000. Discrimination and health. In: Berkman L, Kawachi I eds. *Social Epidemiology*. Oxford, UK: Oxford University Press. Pp. 36-75.

Krieger N, Sidney S. 1996. Racial discrimination and blood pressure: The CARDIA Study of young black and white adults. *American Journal of Public Health* 86(10):1370-1378.

Krieger N, Rowley DL, Herman AA, Avery B, Phillips MT. 1993. Racism, sexism, and social class: Implications for studies of health, disease and well-being. *American Journal of Preventive Medicine* 9:82-122.

Krieger N, Chen JT, Waterman PD, Rehkopf DH, Subramanian SV. 2003. Race/ethnicity, gender, and monitoring socioeconomic gradients in health: Comparison of area-based socioeconomic measures—The Public Health Disparities Geocoding Project. *American Journal of Public Health* 93(10):1655-1671.

Kristensen P, Irgens LM, Daltveit AK, Andersen A. 1993. Perinatal outcome among children of men exposed to lead and organic solvents in the printing industry. *American Journal of Epidemiology* 137:134-144.

Kristensen P, Irgens LM, Andersen A, Bye AS, Sundheim L. 1997. Gestational age, birth weight, and perinatal death among births to Norwegian farmers, 1967-1991. *American Journal of Epidemiology* 146:329-338.

Krymko H, Bashiri A, Smolin A, Sheiner E, Bar-David J, Shoham-Vardi I, Vardi H, Mazor M. 2004. Risk factors for recurrent preterm delivery. *European Journal of Obstetrics, Gynecology, and Reproductive Biology* 113:160-163.

Kumarasamy V, Mitchell MD, Bloomfield FH, Oliver MH, Campbell ME, Challis JR, Harding JE. 2005. Effects of periconceptional undernutrition on the initiation of parturition in sheep. *American Journal of Physiology. Regulatory, Integrative, and Comparative Physiology* 288(1):R67-R72.

Kurki T, Hiilesmaa V, Raitasalo R, Mattila H, Ylikorkala O. 2000. Depression and anxiety in early pregnancy and risk for preeclampsia. *Obstetrics and Gynecology* 95(4):487-490.

Kurkinen-Raty M, Ruokonen A, Vuopala S, Koskela M, Rutanen EM, Karkkainen T, Jouppila P. 2001. Combination of cervical interleukin-6 and -8, phosphorylated insulin-like growth factor-binding protein-1 and transvaginal cervical ultrasonography in assessment of the risk of preterm birth. *British Journal of Obstetrics and Gynaecology* 108(8):875-881.

Kuvacic I, Skrablin S, Hodzic D, Milkovic G. 1996. Possible influence of expatriation on perinatal outcome. *Acta Obstetricia et Gynecologica Scandinavica* 75(4):367-371.

Lachman ME, Weaver SL. 1998. The sense of control as a moderator of social class differences in health and well-being. *Journal of Personality and Social Psychology* 74(3):763-773.

Laird PW. 2005. Cancer epigenetics. *Human Molecular Genetics* 15(Suppl 1):R65-R76.

Lam F, Bergauer NK, Jacques D, Coleman SK, Stanziano GJ. 2001. Clinical and cost-effectiveness of continuous subcutaneous terbutaline versus oral tocolytics for treatment of recurrent preterm labor in twin gestations. *Journal of Perinatology* 21(7):444-450.

Lamont RF, Duncan SL, Mandal D, Bassett P. 2003. Intravaginal clindamycin to reduce preterm birth in women with abnormal genital tract flora. *Obstetrics and Gynecology* 101(3):516-522.

Lander E S, Linton LM, Birren B, Nusbaum C, Zody MC, Baldwin J. 2001. Initial sequencing and analysis of the human genome. *Nature* 409:860-921.

Landgraf JM, Abetz L, Ware JE. 1999. *The CHQ User's Manual*. Boston, MA: Health Act.

Landgren, O. 1996. Environmental pollution and delivery outcome in southern Sweden: A study with central registries. *Acta Paediatrica* 85:1361-1364.

Landsbergis PA, Hatch MC. 1996. Psychosocial work stress and pregnancy-induced hypertension. *Epidemiology* 7(4):346-351.

Lang JM, Lieberman E, Ryan KJ, Monson RR. 1990. Interpregnancy interval and risk of preterm labor. *American Journal of Epidemiology* 132:304-309.

Lang JM, Lieberman E, Cohen A. 1996. A comparison of risk factors for preterm labor and term small-for-gestational-age birth. *Epidemiology* 7(4):369-376.

Laplante DP, Barr RG, Brunet A, Galbaud du Fort G, Meaney ML, Saucier JF, Zelazo PR, King S. 2004. Stress during pregnancy affects general intellectual and language functioning in human toddlers. *Pediatrics Research* 56(3):400-410.

Laptook A, Jackson GL. 2006. Cold stress and hypoglycemia in the late preterm ("near-term") infant: Impact on nursery of admission. *Seminars in Perinatology* 30(1):24-27.

Larroque B. 1992. Alcohol and the fetus. *International Journal of Epidemiology* 21(90001): 8S-16S.

Larsson HJ, Eaton WW, Madsen KM, Vestergaard M, Olesen AV, Agerbo E, Schendel D, Thorsen P, Mortensen PB. 2005. Risk factors for autism: Perinatal factors, parental psychiatric history, and socioeconomic status. *American Journal of Epidemiology* 161(10): 916-925.

Latini G, De Felice C, Presta G, Del Vecchio A, Paris I, Ruggieri F, Mazzeo P. 2003. In utero exposure to di-(2-ethylhexyl)phthalate and duration of human pregnancy. *Environmental Health Perspectives* 111(14):1783-1785.

Latini G, Massaro M, De Felice C. 2005. Prenatal exposure to phthalates and intrauterine inflammation: A unifying hypothesis. *Toxicological Sciences* 85(1):743.

Lawson CC, Schnorr TM, Whelan EA, Deddens JA, Dankovic DA, Piacitelli LA, Sweeney MH, Connally LB. 2004. Paternal occupational exposure to 2,3,7,8-tetrachlorodibenzo-p-dioxin and birth outcomes of offspring: Birth weight, preterm delivery, and birth defects. *Environmental Health Perspectives* 112:1403-1408.

Lazarus RS, Folkman S. 1984. *Stress, Appraisal, and Coping*. New York: Springer.

Le TN, Johansson A. 2001. Impact of chemical warfare with agent orange on women's reproductive lives in Vietnam: A pilot study. *Reproductive Health Matters* 9:156-164.

Leaf AA, Green CR, Esack A, Costeloe KL, Prior PF. 1995. Maturation of electroretinograms and visual evoked potentials in preterm infants. *Developmental Medicine and Child Neurology* 37(9):814-826.

Lederman RP. 1986. Maternal anxiety in pregnancy: Relationship to fetal and newborn health status. *Annual Review of Nursing Research* 4:3-19.

Lederman SA, Rauh V, Weiss L, Stein JL, Hoepner LA, Becker M, Perera FP. 2004. The effects of the World Trade Center event on birth outcomes among term deliveries at three lower Manhattan hospitals. *Environmental Health Perspectives* 112(17):1772-1778.

Lee SK, Penner PL, Cox M. 1991. Impact of very low birth weight infants on the family and its relationship to parental attitudes. *Pediatrics* 88(1):105-109.

Lee SK, McMillan DD, Ohlsson A, Pendray M, Synnes A, Whyte R, Chien L-Y, Sale J. 2000. Variations in practice and outcomes in the Canadian NICU network: 1996-1997. *Pediatrics* 106(5 I):1070-1079.

Lees CC, Lojacono A, Thompson C. 1999. Glyceryl trinitrate and ritodrine in tocolysis: An international multicenter randomized study. GTN Preterm Labour Investigation Group. *Obstetrics and Gynecology* 94:403-408.

Leeson CP, Kattenhorn M, Morley R, Lucas A, Deanfield JE. 2001. Impact of low birth weight and cardiovascular risk factors on endothelial function in early adult life. *Circulation* 103(9):1264-1268.

Lefebvre F, Glorieux J, St-Laurent-Gagaon T. 1996. Neonatal survival and disability rate at age 18 months for infants born between 23 and 28 weeks of gestation. *American Journal of Obstetrics and Gynecology* 174(3):833-838.

Lefebvre F, Mazurier E, Tessier R. 2005. Cognitive and educational outcomes in early adulthood for infants weighing 1000 grams or less at birth. *Acta Paediatrica, International Journal of Paediatrics* 94(6):733-740.

Leitich H, Brunbauer M, Kaider A, Egarter C, Husslein P. 1999a. Cervical length and dilatation of the internal cervical os detected by vaginal ultrasonography as markers for preterm delivery: A systematic review. *American Journal of Obstetrics and Gynecology* 181(6): 1465-1472.

Leitich H, Egarter C, Kaider A, Hoblagschwandtner M, Berghammer P, Husslein P. 1999b. Cervicovaginal fetal fibronectin as a marker for preterm delivery: A meta-analysis. *American Journal of Obstetrics and Gynecology* 180(5):1169-1176.

Lemancewicz A, Laudanska H, Laudanski T, Karpiuk A, Batra S. 2000. Permeability of fetal membranes to calcium and magnesium: Possible role in preterm labour. *Human Reproduction* 15:2018-2022.

Lemons JA, Bauer CR, Oh W, Korones SB, Papile LA, Stoll BJ, Verter J, Temprosa M, Wright LL, Ehrenkranz RA, Fanaroff AA, Stark A, Carlo W, Tyson JE, Donovan EF, Shankaran S, Stevenson DK. 2001. Very low birth weight outcomes of the National Institute of Child Health and Human Development Neonatal Research Network, January 1995 through December 1996. *Pediatrics* 107:E1.

Leppert PC, Takamoto N, Yu SY. 1996. Apoptosis in fetal membranes may predispose them to rupture. *Journal of the Society for Gynecologic Investigation* 3:128a.

Lesser AJ. 1985. The origin and development of maternal and child health programs in the United States. *American Journal of Public Health* 75:590-598.

Leung TN, Chung TK, Madsen G, McLean M, Chang AM, Smith R. 1999. Elevated midtrimester maternal corticotrophin-releasing hormone levels in pregnancies that delivered before 34 weeks. *British Journal of Obstetrics and Gynaecology* 106:1041-1046.

Levi R, Lundberg U, Hanson U, Frankenhaeuser M. 1989. Anxiety during pregnancy after Tschernobyl accident is related to obstetric outcome. *Journal of Psychosomatic Obstetrics and Gynecology* 10:221-230.

Leviton A. 1993. Preterm birth and cerebral palsy: Is tumor necrosis factor the missing link? *Developmental Medicine and Child Neurology* 35:553-558.

Levitt NS, Lambert EV, Woods D, Seckl JR, Hales CN. 2005. Adult BMI and fat distribution but not height amplify the effect of low birthweight on insulin resistance and increased blood pressure in 20-year-old South Africans. *Diabetologia* 48(6):1118-1125.

Levy DL, Noelke K, Goldsmith JP. 1981. Maternal and infant transport program in Louisiana. *Obstetrics and Gynecology* 57(4):500-504.

Levy F. 1994. Attention deficit disorder. *Australian and New Zealand Journal of Psychiatry* 28(4):693.

Lewis DF, Brody K, Edwards MS, Brouillette RM, Burlison S. 1996. London SNPreterm premature ruptured membranes: A randomized trial of steroids after treatment with antibiotics. *Obstetrics and Gynecology* 88:801.

Ley D, Wide-Swensson D, Lindroth M, Svenningsen N, Marsal K. 1997. Respiratory distress syndrome in infants with impaired intrauterine growth. *Acta Paediatrica, International Journal of Paediatrics* 86(10):1090-1096.

Lichtenberger EO. 2005. General measures of cognition for the preschool child. *Mental Retardation and Developmental Disabilities Research Reviews* 11(3):197-208.

Liggins GC, Thorburn GD. 1994. Initiation of parturition. In: Lamming GE ed. *Marshall's Physiology of Reproduction*. London, UK: Chapman and Hall. Pp. 863-1002.

Lin MC, Chiu HF, Yu HS, Tsai SS, Cheng BH, Wu TN, Sung FC, Yang CY. 2001. Increased risk of preterm delivery in areas with air pollution from a petroleum refinery plant in Taiwan. *Journal of Toxicology and Environmental Health* A(64):637-644.

Link BG, Phelan JC. 1995. Social conditions as fundamental causes of disease. *Journal of Health and Social Behavior*. Extra Issue:80-94.

Lithell HO, McKeigue PM, Berglund L, Mohsen R, Lithell UB, Leon DA. 1996. Relation of size at birth to non-insulin dependent diabetes and insulin concentrations in men aged 50-60 years. *British Medical Journal* 312(7028):406-410.

Little J, Bradley L, Bray MS, Clyne M, Dorman J, Ellsworth DL, Hanson J, Khoury M, Lau J, O'Brien TR, Rothman N, Stroup D, Taioli E, Thomas D, Vainio H, Wacholder S, Weinberg C. 2002. Reporting, appraising, and integrating data on genotype prevalence and gene-disease associations. *American Journal of Epidemiology* 156(4):300-310.

Liu H, Giasson B, Mushynski W, Almazan G. 2002. AMPA receptor-mediated toxicity in oligodendrocyte progenitors involves free radical generation and activation of JNK, calpain and caspase 3. *Journal of Neurochemistry* 82:398-409.

Liu S, Krewski D, Shi Y, Chen Y, Burnett RT. 2003. Association between gaseous ambient air pollutants and adverse pregnancy outcomes in Vancouver, Canada. *Environmental Health Perspectives* 111:1773-1778.

Liu S, Heaman M, Joseph KS, Liston RM, Huang L, Sauve R, Kramer MS. 2005. Risk of maternal postpartum readmission associated with mode of delivery. *Obstetrics and Gynecology* 105(4):836-842.

Liu Y, Gold EB, Lasley BL, Johnson WO. 2004. Factors affecting menstrual cycle characteristics. *American Journal of Epidemiology* 160(2):131-140.

Liu YL, Nwosu UC, Rice PJ. 1998. Relaxation of isolated human myometrial muscle by beta2-adrenergic receptors but not beta1-adrenergic receptors. *American Journal of Obstetrics and Gynecology* 179:895-898.

Livingston JC, Maxwell BD, Sibai BM. 2003. Chronic hypertension in pregnancy. *Minerva Ginecologica* 55(1):1-13.

Lobel M. 1994. Conceptualizations, measurement, and effects of prenatal maternal stress on birth outcomes. *Journal of Behavioral Medicine* 17(3):225-272.

Lobel M, Dunkel-Schetter C, Scrimshaw SC. 1992. Prenatal maternal stress and prematurity: A prospective study of socioeconomically disadvantaged women. *Health Psychology* 11(1):32-40.

Lobel M, DeVincent CJ, Kaminer A, Meyer BA. 2000. The impact of prenatal maternal stress and optimistic disposition on birth outcomes in medically high-risk women. *Health Psychology* 19(6):544-553.

Lockwood CJ. 1999. Stress-associated preterm delivery: The role of corticotropin-releasing hormone. *American Journal of Obstetrics and Gynecology* 180(1 Pt 3):S264-S266.

Lockwood CJ, Kuczynski E. 2001. Risk stratification and pathological mechanisms in preterm delivery. *Paediatric and Perinatal Epidemiology* Jul(15 Suppl 2):78-89.

Lockwood CJ, Senyei AE, Dische MR, Casal D, Shah KD, Thung SN, Jones L, Deligdisch L, Garite TJ. 1991. Fetal fibronectin in cervical and vaginal secretions as a predictor of preterm delivery. *New England Journal of Medicine* 325(10):669-674.

Lockwood CJ, Toti P, Arcuri F, Paidas M, Buchwalder L, Krikun G, Schatz F. 2005. Mechanisms of abruption-induced premature rupture of the fetal membranes: Thrombin-enhanced interleukin-8 expression in term decidua. *American Journal of Pathology* 167(5): 1443-1449.

Long SH, Marquis MS. 1998. The effects of Florida's Medicaid eligibility expansion for pregnant women. *American Journal of Public Health* 88(3):371-376.

Longnecker MP, Klebanoff MA, Zhou H, Brock JW. 2001. Association between maternal serum concentration of the DDT metabolite DDE and preterm and small-for-gestational-age babies at birth. *Lancet* 358:110-114.

Longnecker MP, Klebanoff MA, Brock JW, Guo X. 2005. Maternal levels of polychlorinated biphenyls in relation to preterm and small-for-gestational-age birth. *Epidemiology* 16:641-647.

Loprest PJ, Wittenburg D. 2005. *Choices, Challenges, and Options: Child SSI Recipients Preparing for the Transition to Adult Life.* [Online]. Available: http://www.urban.org/url.cfm?ID=411168 [accessed May 23, 2005].

Lorenz E, Hallman M, Marttila R, Haataja R, Schwartz DA. 2002. Association between the Asp299Gly Polymophosms in the Toll-like receptor 4 and premature births in the Finnish population. *Pediatric Research* 52(3):373-376.

Lorenz JM, Paneth N. 2000. Treatment decisions for the extremely premature infant. *Journal of Pediatrics* 137(5):593-595.

Lorenz JM, Paneth N, Jetton JR, Den Ouden L, Tyson JE. 2001. Comparison of management strategies for extreme prematurity in New Jersey and the Netherlands: Outcomes and resource expenditure. *Pediatrics* 108(6):1269-1274.

Lou HC, Hansen D, Nordentoft M, Pryds O, Jensen F, Nim J, Hemmingsen R. 1994. Prenatal stressors of human life affect fetal brain development. *Developmental Medicine and Child Neurology* 36(9):826-832.

Loudon JA, Sooranna SR, Bennett PR, Johnson MR. 2004. Mechanical stretch of human uterine smooth muscle cells increases IL-8 mRNA expression and peptide synthesis. *Molecular Human Reproduction* 10:895-899.

Lowe J, Woodward B, Papile L-A. 2005. Emotional regulation and its impact on development in extremely low birth weight infants. *Journal of Developmental and Behavioral Pediatrics* 26(3):209-213.

Lu MC, Chen B. 2004. Racial and ethnic disparities in preterm birth: The role of stressful life events. *American Journal of Obstetrics and Gynecology* 191(3):691-699.

Lu MC, Halfon N. 2003. Racial and ethnic disparities in birth outcomes: A life-course perspective. *Maternal and Child Health Journal* 7(1):13-30.

Lu Q, Lu MC, Dunkel Schetter C. 2005. Learning from success and failure in psychosocial intervention: An evaluation of low birth weight prevention trials. *Journal of Health Psychology* 10(2):185-195.

Lubchenco L, Hansman C, Dressler M, Boyd E. 1963. Intrauterine growth as estimated from liveborn birth-weight data at 24 to 42 weeks of gestation. *Pediatrics* 32(5):793-800.

Lubchenco LO, Butterfield LJ. 1983. Graduates of neonatal intensive care units—long-term prognosis in varying degrees of maturity. *Medical Section Proceedings of the Annual Meeting of the Medical Section of the American Council of Life Insurance* 47-58.

Lubs M-LE. 1973. Racial differences in maternal smoking effects on the newborn infant. *American Journal of Obstetrics and Gynecology* 115:66-76.

Lucey JF, Rowan CA, Shiono P, Wilkinson AR, Kilpatrick S, Payne NR, Horbar J, Carpenter J, Rogowski J, Soll RF. 2004. Fetal infants: The fate of 4172 infants with birth weights of 401 to 500 grams—The Vermont Oxford Network experience (1996-2000). *Pediatrics* 113(6 I):1559-1566.

Lukassen HGM, Braat DD, Wetzels AMM, Zielhuis GA, Adang EMM, Scheenjes E, Kremer JAM. 2005. Two cycles with single embryo transfer versus one cycle with double embryo transfer: A randomized controlled trial. *Human Reproduction* 20(3):702-708.

Luke B. 1996. Reducing fetal deaths in multiple births: Optimal birthweights and gestational ages for infants of twin and triplet births. *Acta Geneticae Medicae et Gemellologiae* 45(3):333-348.

Lumley JM. 2003. Unexplained antepartum stillbirth in pregnancies after a caesarean delivery. *Lancet* 362(9398):1774-1775.

Lundsberg LS, Bracken MB, Saftlas AF. 1997. Low-to-moderate gestational alcohol use and intrauterine growth retardation, low birthweight, and preterm delivery. *Annals of Epidemiology* 7(7):498-508.

Luo ZC, Wilkins R, Platt RW, Kramer MS. 2004. Risks of adverse pregnancy outcomes among Inuit and North American Indian women in Quebec, 1985-1997. *Paediatric and Perinatal Epidemiology* 18(1):40-50.

Lyall F, Lye SJ, Teoh TG, Cousin F, Milligan G, Robson SC. 2002. Expression of Gsα, Connexin-43, Connexin-26, and EP1, 3, and 4 receptors in myometrium of prelabor singleton versus multiple gestations and the effects of mechanical stretch and steroids on Gsÿ. *Journal of the Society for Gynecologic Investigation* 9:299-307.

Lye SJ, Ou CW, Teoh TG, Erb G, Stevens Y, Casper R, Patel F and Challis JRG. 1998. The molecular basis of labour and tocolysis. *Fetal and Maternal Medicine Review* 121-136.

Lynch CM, Kearney R, Turner MJ. 2003. Maternal morbidity after elective repeat caesarean section after two or more previous procedures. *European Journal of Obstetrics Gynecology and Reproductive Biology* 106(1):10-13.

MacDonald LD, Peacock JL, Anderson HR. 1992. Marital status: Association with social and economic circumstances, psychological state and outcomes of pregnancy. *Journal of Public Health Medicine* 14(1):26-34.

MacDorman MF, Martin JA, Matthews TA. 2005. Explaining the 2001-02 infant mortality increase: Data from the linked birth/infant death data set. *National Vital Statistics Reports* 53(12). Hyattsville, MD: National Center for Health Statistics.

Macey TJ, Harmon RJ, Easterbrooks MA. 1987. Impact of premature birth on the development of the infant in the family. *Journal of Consulting and Clinical Psychology* 55(6): 846-852.

MacGillivray I, Campbell DM. 1995. The changing pattern of cerebral palsy in Avon. *Paediatric and Perinatal Epidemiology* 9(2):146-155.

MacGregor JA, French JI, Lawellin D, Franco-Buff A, Smith C, Todd JK. 1987. Bacterial protease-induced reduction of chorioamniotic membrane strength and elasticity. *Obstetrics and Gynecology* 69:167-174.

Machemer R. 1993. Late traction detachment in retinopathy of prematurity or ROP-like cases. *Graefe's Archive for Clinical and Experimental Ophthalmology* 231(7):389-394.

Macintyre S, Ellaway A, Cummins S. 2002. Place effects on health: How can we conceptualize, operationally and measure them? *Social Science and Medicine* 55:125-139.

Mackenzie AP, Schatz F, Krikun G, Funai EF, Kadner S, Lockwood CJ. 2004. Mechanisms of abruption-induced premature rupture of the fetal membranes: Thrombin enhanced decidual matrix metalloproteinase-3 (stromelysin-1) expression. *American Journal of Obstetrics and Gynecology* 191:1996-2001.

MacLennan A, et al. 2005. Who will delivery our grandchildren? Implications of Cerebral Palsy litigation. *JAMA* 294(13):1688-1690.

MacNaughton MC, Chalmers IG, Dubowitz V, Dunn PM, Grant AM, Mcpherson K, et al. 1993. Final report of the Medical Research Council/Royal College of Obstetrics and Gynaecology multicentre randomised trial of cervical cerclage. *British Journal of Obstetrics and Gynaecology* 100:516.

Macones GA, Segel SY, Stamilio DM, Morgan MA. 1999a. Predicting delivery within 48 hours in women treated with parenteral tocolysis. *Obstetrics and Gynecology* 93(3): 432-436.

Macones GA, Segel SY, Stamilio DM, Morgan MA. 1999b. Prediction of delivery among women with early preterm labor by means of clinical characteristics alone. *American Journal of Obstetrics and Gynecology* 181(6):1414-1418.

Macones GA, Parry S, Elkousy M, Clothier B, Ural SH, Strauss III JF. 2004. A polymorphism in the promoter region of TNF and bacterial vaginosis: Preliminary evidence of gene-environment interaction in the etiology of spontaneous preterm birth. *American Journal of Obstetrics and Gynecology* 190(6):1504-1508.

Madan A, Good WV. 2005. Disorders of the eye. In: Taeusch HW, Ballard RA, Gleason CA eds. *Avery's Diseases of the Newborn*, 8th edition. Philadelphia, PA: Elsevier Saunders. Pp. 1471-1483, 1539-1555.

Madan A, Jan JE, Good WV. 2005. Visual development in preterm infants. *Developmental Medicine and Child Neurology* 47(4):276-280.

Maichuk GT, Zahorodny W, Marshall R. 1999. Use of positioning to reduce the severity of neonatal narcotic withdrawal syndrome. *Journal of Perinatology* 19(7):510-513.

Main DM, Gabbe SG. 1987. Risk scoring for preterm labor: Where do we go from here? *American Journal of Obstetrics and Gynecology* 157(4 Pt 1):789-793.

Main DM, Gabbe SG, Richardson D, Strong S. 1985. Can preterm deliveries be prevented? *American Journal of Obstetrics and Gynecology* 151(7):892-898.

Main DM, Richardson D, Gabbe SG. 1987. Prospective evaluation of a risk scoring system for predicting preterm delivery in black inner city women. *Obstetrics and Gynecology* 69(1):61-66.

Main, Meis, Mueller H. 1993. Collaborative group on preterm birth prevention: Multicenter randomized controlled trial of a preterm birth prevention program. *American Journal of Obstetrics and Gynecology* 169:352-357.

Maisonet M, Correa A, Misra D, and Jaakkola JJ. 2004. A review of the literature on the effects of ambient air pollution on fetal growth. *Environmental Research* 95:106-115.

Majnemer A. 1998. Benefits of early intervention for children with developmental disabilities. *Seminars in Pediatric Neurology* 5(1):62-69.

Majnemer A, Snider L. 2005. A comparison of developmental assessments of the newborn and young infant. *Mental Retardation and Developmental Disabilities Research Reviews* 11(1):68-73.

Major CA, de Veciana M, Lewis DF. 1995. Preterm premature rupture of membranes and abruption placentae: Is there an association between these pregnancy complications? *American Journal of Obstetrics and Gynecology* 172:672.

Malak T, Bell SC. 1994. Structural characteristics of term human fetal membranes: A novel zone of extreme morphological alteration within the rupture site. *British Journal of Obstetrics and Gynaecology* 101(5):375-386.

Malusky SK. 2005. A concept analysis of family-centered care in the nicu. *Neonatal Network* 24(6):25-32.

Malviya M, Ohlsson A, Shah S. 2006. Surgical versus medical treatment with cyclooxygenase inhibitors for symptomatic patent ductus arteriosus in preterm infants. *Cochrane Reviews* 1.

Mamelle N, Laumon B, Lazar P. 1984. Prematurity and occupational activity during pregnancy. *American Journal of Epidemiology* 119(3):309-322.

Mammel MC, Johnson DE, Green TP, Thompson TR. 1983. Controlled trial of dexamethasone therapy in infants with bronchopulmonary dysplasia. *Lancet* 1(8338):1356-1358.

Mancuso RA, Dunkel Schetter C, Rini CM, Roesch SC, Hobel CJ. 2004. Maternal prenatal anxiety and corticotropin-releasing hormone associated with timing of delivery. *Psychosomatic Medicine* 66(5):762-769.

Manderbacka K, Merilainen J, Hemminki E, Rahkonen O, Teperi J. 1992. Marital status as a predictor of perinatal outcome in Finland. *Journal of Marriage and the Family* 54(3): 508-515.

Mann C. 2003. The flexibility factor: Finding the right balance. *Health Affairs* 22:62-76.

Mann C, Schott L. 1999. Ensuring that eligible families receive Medicaid when cash assistance is denied or terminated. *Policy and Practice of Public Human Services* 57:6-10.

Manning FA. 1995. Fetal assessment in low-risk pregnancy. *Current Opinion in Obstetrics and Gynecology* 7(6):461-464.

Manton WI, Cook JD. 1984. High accuracy (stable isotope dilution) measurements of lead in serum and cerebrospinal fluid. *British Journal of Independent Medicine* 41:313-319.

Maradny EE, Kanayama N, Halim A, Maehara K, Terao T. 1996. Stretching of fetal membranes increases the concentration of interleukin-8 and collagenase activity. *American Journal of Obstetrics and Gynecology* 174:843-849.

Marivate M, de Villiers KQ, Fairbrother P. 1977. Effect of prophylactic outpatient administration of fenoterol on the time of onset of spontaneous labor and fetal growth rate in twin pregnancy. *American Journal of Obstetrics and Gynecology* 128(7):707-708.

Markowitz J. 2004. Part C updates: Sixth in a series of updates on selected aspects of the early intervention program for infants and toddlers with disabilities. In: Danaher J ed. *Synthesis Brief: The National Early Intervention Longitudinal Study (NEILS): Child and Family Outcomes at 36 Months*. Washington, DC: Department of Education.

Marlow N, Wolke D, Bracewell MA, Samara M, the EPICure Study Group. 2005. Neurologic and developmental disability at six years of age after extremely preterm birth. *New England Journal of Medicine* 352(1):9-19.

Maroziene L, Grazuleviciene R. 2002. Maternal exposure to low-level air pollution and pregnancy outcomes: A population-based study. *Environmental Health* 1:6.

Martens PJ, Derksen S, Gupta S. 2004. Predictors of hospital readmission of Manitoba newborns within six weeks postbirth discharge: A population-based study. *Pediatrics* 114: 708-713.

Martin J, Hamilton BE, Sutton PD, Ventura SJ, Menacker F, Munson ML. 2003. *Births: Final Data for 2002*. Hyattsville, MD: Centers for Disease Control and Prevention. Pp. 1-116.

Martin JA, Hoyert DL. 2002. The national fetal death file. *Seminars in Perinatology* 26(1): 3-11.

Martius J, Eschenbach DA. 1990. The role of bacterial vaginosis as a cause of amniotic fluid infection, chorioamnionitis and prematurity—a review. *Archives of Gynecology and Obstetrics* 247:1-13.

Martyn CN, Gale CR, Jespersen S, Sherriff SB. 1998. Impaired fetal growth and atherosclerosis of carotid and peripheral arteries. *Lancet* 352(9123):173-178.

Marzi M, Vigano A, Trabattoni D, Villa ML, Salvaggio A, Clerici E, Clerici M. 1996. Characterization of type 1 and type 2 cytokine production profile in physiologic and pathologic human pregnancy. *Clinical and Experimental Immunology* 106:127-133.

Maschoff KL, Baldwin HS. 2005. Embryology and development of the cardiovascular system. In: Taeusch HW, Ballard RA, Gleason CA eds. *Avery's Diseases of the Newborn*, 8th edition. Philadelphia, PA: Elsevier Saunders. Pp. 156-167.

Mashaw JL, Perrin JM, Reno VP eds. 1996. *Restructuring the SSI Disability Program for Children and Adolescents.* [Online]. Available: http://www.nasi.org/usr_doc/Restructuring_SSI.pdf [accessed January 30, 2006].

Mason GC, Maresh MJA. 1990. Alterations in bladder volume and the ultrasound appearance of the cervix. *British Journal of Obstetrics and Gynecology* 97:457-458.

Mason-Brothers A, Ritvo ER, Pingree C, Petersen PB, Jenson WR, McMahon WM, Freeman BJ, Jorde LB, Spencer MJ, Mo A, Ritvo A. 1990. The UCLA-University of Utah epidemiologic survey of autism: Prenatal, perinatal, and postnatal factors. *Pediatrics* 86(4): 514-519.

Massaro DJ, Massaro GD. 2000. The regulation of the formation of pulmonary alveoli. In: Bland RD, Coalson JJ eds. *Chronic Lung Disease in Early Infancy.* New York: Marcel Dekker. Pp. 479-492.

Massett HA, Greenup M, Ryan CE, Staples DA, Green NS, Maibach EW. 2003. Public perceptions about prematurity: A national survey. *American Journal of Preventitive Medicine* 24:120-127.

Massey DS, Denton NA. 1993. *American Apartheid: Segregation and the Making of the Underclass.* Boston, MA: Harvard University Press.

Mathews TJ, Menacker F, MacDoman MF. 2002. *Infant Mortality Statistics from the 2000 Period Linked Birth/Infant Death Data Sets.* National Vital Statistics Reports 50(12). Hyattsville, MD: National Center for Health Statistics.

Matsuda T, Okuyama K, Cho K, Hoshi N, Matsumoto Y, Kobayashi Y, Fujimoto S. 1999. Induction of antenatal periventricular leukomalacia by hemorrhagic hypotension in the chronically instrumented fetal sheep. *American Journal of Obstetrics and Gynecology* 181(3):725-730.

Matthews KA, Rodin J. 1992. Pregnancy alters blood pressure responses to psychological and physical challenge. *Psychophysiology* 29(2):232-240.

Mattison DR, Damus K, Fiore E, Petrini J, Alter C. 2001. Preterm delivery: A public health perspective. *Paediatric and Perinatal Epidemiology* 15(Suppl 2):7-16.

McCain GC. 1990. Family functioning 2 to 4 years after preterm birth. *Journal of Pediatric Nursing* 5(2):97-104.

McCarton CM, Brooks-Gunn J, Wallace IF, Bauer CR, Bennett FC, Bernbaum JC, Broyles RS, Casey PH, McCormick MC, Scott DT, Tyson J, Tonascia J, Meinert CL. 1997. Results at age 8 years of early intervention for low-birth-weight premature infants: The infant health and development program. *JAMA* 277(2):126-132.

McCool WF, Dorn LD, Susman EJ. 1994. The relation of cortisol reactivity and anxiety to perinatal outcome in primiparous adolescents. *Research in Nursing and Health* 17(6): 411-420.

McCormick MC. 1997. The outcomes of very low birth weight infants: Are we asking the right questions? *Pediatrics* 99:869-876.

McCormick MC, Richardson DK. 1995. Access to neonatal intensive care. *The Future of Children/Center for the Future of Children, the David and Lucile Packard Foundation* 5(1):162-175.

McCormick MC, Shapiro S, Starfield B. 1980. Rehospitalization in the first year of life for high-risk survivors. *Pediatrics* 66:991-999.

McCormick MC, Shapiro S, Starfield CH. 1985. The regionalization of perinatal services: Summary of the evaluation of a demonstration program. *JAMA* 253:799-804.

McCormick MC, Stemmler MM, Bernbaum JC, Farran AC. 1986. The very low birth weight transport goes home: Impact on the family. *Journal of Developmental and Behavioral Pediatrics* 7(4):217-223.

McCormick MC, Bernbaum JC, Eisenberg JM, Kustra SL, Finnegan E. 1991. Costs incurred by parents of very low birth weight infants after the initial neonatal hospitalization. *Pediatric* 88:533-541.

McCormick MC, Brooks-Gunn J, Workman-Daniels K. 1992. The health and developmental status of very-low-birth-weight children at school age. *JAMA* 267:2204-2208.

McCormick MC, Workman-Daniels K, Brooks-Gunn J, Peckham GJ. 1993. Hospitalization of very low birth weight children at school age. *Journal of Pediatrics* 122:360-365.

McCormick MC, Workman-Daniels K, Brooks-Gunn J. 1996. The behavioral and emotional well-being of school-age children with different birth weights. *Pediatrics* 97(1):18-25.

McCormick MC, McCarton C, Brooks-Gunn J, Belt P, Gross RT. 1998. The Infant Health and Development Program: Interim summary. *Journal of Developmental and Behavioral Pediatrics* 19(5):359-370.

McCormick MC, Escobar GJ, Zheng Z, Richardson DK. 2006. Place of birth and variations in management of late preterm ("near-term") infants. *Seminars in Perinatology* 30(1): 44-47.

McCubbin JA, Lawson EJ, Cox S, Sherman JJ, Norton JA, Read JA. 1996. Prenatal maternal blood pressure response to stress predicts birth weight and gestational age: A preliminary study. *American Journal of Obstetrics and Gynecology* 175(3 Pt 1):706-712.

McDonald AD, Armstrong BG, Sloan M. 1992. Cigarette, alcohol, and coffee consumption and prematurity. *American Journal of Public Health* 82:87-90.

McDonald H, Brocklehurst P, Parsons J. 2005. Antibiotics for treating bacterial vaginosis in pregnancy. *Cochrane Database of Systematic Reviews* 1.

McDonald HM, O'Loughlin JA, Vigneswaran R, Jolley PT, McDonald PJ. 1994. Bacterial vaginosis in pregnancy and efficacy of short-course oral metronidazole treatment: a randomized controlled trial. *Obstetrics and Gynecology* 84(3):343-348.

McDonald HM, O'Loughlin JA, Vigneswaran R, Jolly PT, Harvery JA, Bof A, McDonald PJ. 1997. Impact of metronidazole therapy on preterm birth in women with bacterial vaginosis flora (Gardnerella vaginalis): A randomized, placebo controlled trial. *British Journal of Obstetrics and Gynaecology* 104(12):1391-1397.

McDonald WH, Yates JR III. 2002. Shotgun proteomics and biomarker discovery. *Disease Markers* 18:99-105.

McEwen BS, Biron CA, Brunson KW, Bulloch K, Chambers WH, Dhabhar FS, Goldfarb RH, Kitson RP, Miller AH, Spencer RL, Weiss JM. 1997. The role of adrenocorticoids as modulators of immune function in health and disease: Neural, endocrine and immune interactions. *Brain Research Reviews* 23:79-133.

McGauhey PJ, Starfield B, Alexander C, Ensminger ME. 1991. Social environment and vulnerability of low birth weight children: A social-epidemiological perspective. *Pediatrics* 88:943-953.

McGovern PG, Llorens AJ, Skurnick JH, Weiss G, Goldsmith LT. 2004. Increased risk of preterm birth in singleton pregnancies resulting from in vitro fertilization-embryo transfer or gamete intrafallopian transfer: A meta-analysis. *Fertility and Sterility* 82(6):1514-1520.

McGrady GA, Sung JFC, Rowley DL, Hogue CJR. 1992. Preterm delivery and low birth weight among first-born infants of black and white college graduates. *American Journal of Epidemiology* 136(3):266-276.

McGuire W, Fowlie PW. 2002. Treating extremely low birthweight infants with prophylactic indomethacin. *British Medical Journal* 324(7329):60-61.

McLanahan S, Garfinkel I, Mincy RB. 2001. *Fragile Families, Welfare Reform, and Marriage.* Policy Brief No. 10. Washington, DC: The Brookings Institution.

McLaughlin F, Rusen ID, Liu SL. 1999. *Canadian Surveillance System: Preterm Birth Fact Sheet.* [Online]. Available: http://www.phac-aspc.gc.ca/rhs-ssg/factshts/pterm_e.html [accessed March 2, 2006].

McLean M, Smith R. 1999. Corticotropin-releasing hormone in human pregnancy and parturition. *Trends in Endocrinology and Metabolism* 10:174-178.

McLean M, Bisits A, Davies J, Walters W, Hackshaw A, De Voss K, Smith R. 1999. Predicting risk of preterm delivery by second-trimester measurement of maternal plasma corticotropin-releasing hormone and alpha-fetoprotein concentrations. *American Journal of Obstetrics and Gynecology* 181:207-215.

Medstat. 2004. *Report: The Costs of Prematurity to U.S. Employers.* March of Dimes. Available: http://www.marchofdimes.cm/prntableArticles/15341_15349.asp [accessed January 3, 2007].

Meier PP. 2001. Breastfeeding in the special care nursery: Prematures and infants with medical problems. *Pediatric Clinics of North America* 48(2):425-442.

Meis PJ. 2005. 17 Hydroxyprogesterone for the prevention of preterm delivery. *Obstetrics and Gynecology* 105(5):1128-1135.

Meis PJ, Ernest JM, Moore ML. 1987. Causes of low birth weight births in public and private patients. *American Journal of Obstetrics and Gynecology* 156(5):1165-1168.

Meis PJ, Goldenberg RL, Mercer BM. 1995. The preterm prediction study: Significance of vaginal infections. *American Journal of Obstetrics and Gynecology* 173:1231.

Meis PJ, Goldenberg RL, Mercer BM, Iams JD, Moawad AH, Miodovnik M, Menard MK, Caritis SN, Thurnau GR, Bottoms SF, Das A, Roberts JM, McNellis D. 1998. The preterm prediction study: Risk factors for indicated preterm births. *American Journal of Obstetrics and Gynecology* 178(3):562-567.

Meis PJ, Goldenberg RL, Mercer BM, Iams JD, Moawad AH, Miodovnik M, Menard MK, Caritis SN, Thurnau GR, Dombrowski MP, Das A, Roberts JM, McNellis D. 2000. Preterm prediction study: Is socioeconomic status a risk factor for bacterial vaginosis in black or in white women? *American Journal of Perinatology* 17(1):41-45.

Meis PJ, Klebanoff M, Thom E, Dombrowski MP, Sibai B, Moawad AH, Spong CY, Hauth JC, Miodovnik M, Varner MW, Leveno KJ, Caritis SN, Iams JD, Wapner RJ, Conway D, O'Sullivan MJ, Carpenter M, Mercer B, Ramin SM, Thorp JM, Peaceman AM. 2003. Prevention of recurrent preterm delivery by 17 alpha-hydroxyprogesterone caproate. *New England Journal of Medicine* 348(24):2379-2385.

Menon R, Fortunato S. 2004. The role of matrix degrading enzymes and apoptosis in rupture of membranes. *Journal of the Society for Gynecologic Investigation* 11(7):427-437.

Ment LR, Vohr B, Allan W, Katz KH, Schneider KC, Westerveld M, Duncan CC, Makuch RW. 2003. Change in cognitive function over time in very low-birth-weight infants. *JAMA* 289(6):705-711.

Ment LR, Vohr BR, Makuch RW, Westerveld M, Katz KH, Schneider KC, Duncan CC, Ehrenkranz R, Oh W, Philip AGS, Scott DT, Allan WC. 2004. Prevention of intraventricular hemorrhage by indomethacin in male preterm infants. *Journal of Pediatrics* 145(6):832-834.

Mercer B, Egerman R, Beazley D, Sibai B, Carr T, Sepesi J. 2001a. Antenatal corticosteroids in women at risk for preterm birth: A randomized trial. *American Journal of Obstetrics and Gynecology* 184:S6 (SMFM Abstract 12).

Mercer B, Egerman R, Beazley D, Sibai B, Carr T, Sepesi J. 2001b. Steroids reduce fetal growth: Analysis of a prospective trial. *American Journal of Obstetrics and Gynecology* 184:S6 (SMFM Abstract 15).

Mercer BM. 2003. Preterm premature rupture of the membranes. *Obstetrics and Gynecology* 101:178-193.

Mercer BM, Goldenberg RL, Das A, Moawad AH, Iams JD, Meis PJ, Copper RL, Johnson F, Thom E, McNellis D, Miodovnik M, Menard MK, Caritis S, Thumau GR, Bottoms SF, Roberts J. 1996. The preterm prediction study: A clinical risk assessment system. *American Journal of Obstetrics and Gynecology* 174(6):1885-1893.

Mercer BM, Miodovnik M, Thurnau GR, Goldenberg RL, Das AF, Ramsey RD, Rabello YA, Meis PJ, Moawad AH, Iams JD, Van Dorsten JP, Paul RH, Bottoms SF, Merenstein G, Thom EA, Roberts JM, McNellis D. 1997. Antibiotic therapy for reduction of infant morbidity after preterm premature rupture of the membranes: A randomized controlled trial. *JAMA* 278(12):989-995.

Mercer BM, Goldenberg RL, Moawad AH, Meis PJ, Ianis JD, Das AF, Caritis SN, Miodovnik M, Menard MK, Thurnau GR, Dombrowski MP, Roberts JM, McNellis D. 1999. The Preterm Prediction Study: Effect of gestational age and cause of preterm birth on subsequent obstetric outcome. *American Journal of Obstetrics and Gynecology* 181(5 I):1216-1221.

Mercier C, Ferrelli K, Howard D, Soll R, the Vermont Oxford Network Follow-up Study Group. 2005. Severe disability in surviving extremely low birth weight infants: The Vermont Oxford Network Experience. *PAS Reporter* 57:1620.

Mercuri E, Ricci D, Pane M, Baranello G. 2005. The neurological examination of the newborn baby. *Early Human Development* 81(12):947-956.

Merialdi M, Carroli G, Villar J, Abalos E, Gulmezoglu AM, Kulier R, De Onis M. 2003. Nutritional interventions during pregnancy for the prevention or treatment of impaired fetal growth: An overview of randomized controlled trials. *Journal of Nutrition* 133(5 Suppl 1):1626S-1631S.

Mesquita B, Frijda NH. 1992. Cultural variations in emotions: A review. *Psychological Bulletin* 112(2):179-204.

Mestan KKL, Marks JD, Hecox K, Huo D, Schreiber MD. 2005. Neurodevelopmental outcomes of premature infants treated with inhaled nitric oxide. *New England Journal of Medicine* 353(1):23-32.

Michalek JE, Rahe AJ, Boyle CA. 1998. Paternal dioxin, preterm birth, intrauterine growth retardation, and infant death. *Epidemiology* 9:161-167.

Mikkola K, Ritari N, Tommiska V, Salokorpi T, Lehtonen L, Tammela O, Paakkonen L, Olsen P, Korkman M, Fellman V, for the Finnish ELBW Cohort Study Group. 2005. Neurodevelopmental outcome at 5 years of age of a National Cohort of extremely low birth weight infants who were born in 1996-1997. *Pediatrics* 116(6):1391-1400.

Mildred J, Beard K, Dallwitz A, Unwin J. 1995. Play position is influenced by knowledge of SIBS sleep position recommendations. *Journal of Paediatrics and Child Health* 31(6): 499-502.

Miller G, Heckmatt JZ, Dubowitz LMS, Dubowitz V. 1983. Use of nerve conduction velocity to determine gestational age in infants at risk and in very-low-birth-weight infants. *Journal of Pediatrics* 103(1):109-112 .

Miller JE. 1994. Birth order, interpregnancy interval and birth outcomes among Filipino infants. *Journal of Biosocial Science* 26:243-259.

Mills JL, Harlap S, Harley EE. 1981. Should coitus late in pregnancy be discouraged? *Lancet* 2(8238):136-138.

Min S-J, Luke B, Gillespie B, Min L, Newman RB, Mauldin JG, Witter FR, Salman FA, O'Sullivan MJ. 2000. Birth weight references for twins. *American Journal of Obstetrics and Gynecology* 182(5):250-1257.

Mishel L, Bernstein J. 2003. Wage inequality and the new economy in the U.S.: Does IT-led growth generate wage inequality. *Canadian Public Policy* 29(Suppl):S203-S222.

Misra DP, O'Campo P, Strobino D. 2001. Testing a sociomedical model for preterm delivery. *Paediatric and Perinatal Epidemiology* 15(2):110-122.

Misra DP, Guyer B, Allston A. 2003. Integrated perinatal health framework: A multiple determinants model with a life span approach. *American Journal of Preventive Medicine* 25(1):65-75.

Mitchell D. 1979. Accuracy of pre- and postnatal assessment of gestational age. *Archives of Disease in Childhood* 54(11):896-897.

Mitchell LE. 1997. Differentiating between fetal and maternal genetic effects, using the transmission test for linkage disequilibrium. *American Journal of Human Genetics* 60:1006-1007.

Mitchell LE, Bracken MB. 1990. Reproductive versus chronologic age as a predictor of low birth weight, preterm delivery, and intrauterine growth retardation in primiparous women. *Annals of Human Biology* 17(5):377-386.

Mitchell LE, Weinberg CR. 2005. Evaluation of offspring and maternal genetic effects on disease risk using a family-based approach: The "Pent" Design. *American Journal of Epidemiology* 162(7):676-685.

Mittendorf R, Covert R, Boman J, Khoshnood B, Lee K-S, Siegler M. 1997. Is tocolytic magnesium sulphate associated with increased total paediatric mortality? *Lancet* 350(9090): 1517-1518.

Mizuki J, Tasaka K, Masumoto N, Kasahara K, Miyake A, Tanizawa O. 1993. Magnesium sulfate inhibits oxytocin-induced calcium mobilization in human puerperal myometrial cells: Possible involvement of intracellular free magnesium concentration. *American Journal of Obstetrics and Gynecology* 169:134-139.

Mizuno K, Ueda A, Takeuchi T. 2002. Effects of different fluids on the relationship between swallowing and breathing during nutritive sucking in neonates. *Biology of the Neonate* 81(1):45-50.

Mohorovic, L. 2004. First two months of pregnancy—critical time for preterm delivery and low birthweight caused by adverse effects of coal combustion toxics. *Early Human Development* 80:115-123.

Moise KJ Jr., Huhta JC, Sharif DS, Ou C-N, Kirshon B, Wasserstrum N, Cano L. 1988. Indomethacin in the treatment of premature labor. Effects on the fetal ductus arteriosus. *New England Journal of Medicine* 319(6):327-331.

Molfese VJ, Thomson BK, Beadnell B, Bricker MC, Manion LG. 1987. Perinatal risk screening and infant outcome: Can predictions be improved with composite scales? *Journal of Reproductive Medicine* 32(8):569-576.

Molnar BE, Buka SL, Brennen RT, Holton JK, Earls F. 2003. A multilevel study of neighborhoods and parent-to-child physical aggression: Results from the Project on Human Development in Chicago neighborhoods. *Child Maltreatment* 8(2):84-97.

Mongelli M, Gardosi J. 1996. Gestation-adjusted projection of estimated fetal weight. *Acta Obstetricia et Gynecologica Scandinavica* 75(1):28-31.

Moore MT, Strang EW Schwartz M, Braddock M. 1988b. *Patterns in Special Education Service Delivery and Cost.* Washington, DC: Decision Resources Corporation.

Moore S, Ide M, Randhawa M, Walker JJ, Reid JG, Simpson NAB. 2004. An investigation into the association among preterm birth, cytokine gene polymorphisms and periodontal disease. *BJOG: An International Journal of Obstetrics and Gynaecology* 111(2): 125-132.

Moore TM, Iams JD, Creasy RK, et al. 1994. Diurnal and gestational patterns of uterine activity in normal human pregnancy. *Obstetrics and Gynecology* 83:517.

Morales LS, Staiger D, Horbar J, Carpenter J, Kenny M, Geppert J, Rogowski J. 2005. Mortality among very low-birthweight infants in hospitals serving minority populations. *American Journal of Public Health* 95(12):2206-2217.

Morales WJ, Schorr S, Albritton J. 1994. Effect of metronidazole in patients with preterm birth in preceding pregnancy and bacterial vaginosis: A placebo-controlled, double-blind study. *American Journal of Obstetrics and Gynecology* 171:345-347; discussion 348-349.

Morante A, Dubowitz LMS, Levene M, Dubowitz V. 1982. The development of visual function in normal and neurologically abnormal preterm and fullterm infants. *Developmental Medicine and Child Neurology* 24(6):771-784.

Morin I, Morin L, Zhang X, Platt RW, Blondel B, Bréart G, Usher R, Kramer MS. 2005. Determinants and consequences of discrepancies in menstrual and ultrasonographic gestational age estimates. *BJOG: An International Journal of Obstetrics and Gynaecology* 112(2):145-152.

Morley CJ. 1991. Surfactant treatment for premature babies—a review of clinical trials. *Archives of Disease in Childhood* 66(4 Suppl):445-450.

Morley R, Lister G, Leeson-Payne C, Lucas A. 1994. Size at birth and later blood pressure. *Archives of Disease in Childhood* 70(6):536-537.

Morse SB, Haywood JL, Goldenberg RL, Bronstein J, Nelson KG, Carlo WA. 2000. Estimation of neonatal outcome and perinatal therapy use. *Pediatrics* 105(5):1046-1050.

Mortensen EL, Michaelsen KF, Sanders SA, Reinisch JM. 2002. The association between duration of breastfeeding and adult intelligence. *JAMA* 287(18):2365-2371.

Moutquin JM. 2003. Socio-economic and psychosocial factors in the management and prevention of preterm labour. *BJOG: An International Journal of Obstetrics and Gynaecology* 20:56-60.

Moutquin JM, Cabrol D, Fisk NM, MacLennan AH, Marsál K, Rabinovici J. 2001. Effectiveness and safety of the oxytocin antagonist atosiban versus beta-adrenergic agonists in the treatment of preterm labour. *British Journal of Obstetrics and Gynaecology* 108(2): 133-142.

Moyer-Mileur L, Luetkemeier M, Boomer L, Chan GM. 1995. Effect of physical activity on bone mineralization in premature infants. *Journal of Pediatrics* 127(4):620-625.

Moyer-Mileur LJ, Brunstetter V, McNaught TP, Gill G, Chan GM. 2000. Daily physical activity program increases bone mineralization and growth in preterm very low birth weight infants. *Pediatrics* 106(5 I):1088-1092.

Mozuekewich EL, Luke B, Avni M. 2000. Working conditions and adverse pregnancy outcome: A meta analysis. *Obstetrics and Gynecology* 95:623-635.

Msall ME, Buck GM, Rogers BT, Catanzaro NL. 1992. Kindergarten readiness after extreme prematurity. *American Journal of Diseases of Children* 146(11):1371-1375.

Msall ME, Buck GM, Rogers BT, Duffy LC, Mallen SR, Catanzaro NL. 1993. Predictors of mortality, morbidity, and disability in a cohort of infants ≤ 28 weeks' gestation. *Clinical Pediatrics* 32(9):521-527.

Msall ME, Phelps DL, DiGaudio KM, Dobson V, Tung B, McClead RE, Quinn GE, Reynolds JD, Hardy RJ, Palmer EA. 2000. Severity of neonatal retinopathy of prematurity is predictive of neurodevelopmental functional outcome at age 5.5 years. *Pediatrics* 106(5 I):998-1005.

Mueller CR. 1996. Multidisciplinary research of multimodal stimulation of premature infants: An integrated review of the literature. *Maternal–Child Nursing Journal* 24(1):18-31.

Mueller-Heubach E, Guzick DS. 1989. Evaluation of risk scoring in a preterm birth prevention study of indigent patients. *American Journal of Obstetrics and Gynecology* 160(4): 829-837.

Mulder EJH, Derks JB, Visser GHA. 1997. Antenatal corticosteroid therapy and fetal behaviour: A randomised study of the effects of betamethasone and dexamethasone. *British Journal of Obstetrics and Gynaecology* 104(11):1239-1247.

Munster K, Schmidt L, Helm P. 1992. Length and variation in the menstrual cycle—a cross-sectional study from a Danish county. *British Journal of Obstetrics and Gynaecology* 99(5):422-429.

Muskiet FA. 2005. The importance of (early) folate status to primary and secondary coronary artery disease prevention. *Reproductive Toxicology* 20:403-410.

Mustafa G, David RJ. 2001. Comparative accuracy of clinical estimate versus menstrual gestational age in computerized birth certificates. *Public Health Reports* 116(1):15-21.

Mustillo S, Krieger N, Gunderson EP, Sidney S, McCreath H, Kiefe CI. 2004. Self-reported experiences of racial discrimination and Black-White differences in preterm and low-birthweight deliveries: The CARDIA Study. *American Journal of Public Health* 94(12): 2125-2131.

Mutale T. 1999. *Life in the Womb: The Origins of Health and Disease.* Ithaca, NY: Promethean Press.

Mutale T, Creed F, Maresh M, Hunt L. 1991. Life events and low birthweight—analysis by infants preterm and small for gestational age. *British Journal of Obstetrics and Gynaecology* 98(2):166-172.

Myers J, MacLeod M, Reed B, Harris N, Mires G, Baker P. 2004. Use of proteomic patterns as a novel screening tool in pre-eclampsia. *Journal of Obstetrics and Gynaecology* 24(8): 873-874.

Nadeau L, Tessier R, Lefebvre F, Robaey P. 2004. Victimization: A newly recognized outcome of prematurity. *Developmental Medicine and Child Neurology* 46(8):508-513.

Nageotte MP, Dorchester W, Porto M, Keegan KA, Freeman RK. 1988. Quantitation of uterine activity preceding preterm, term, and postterm labor. *American Journal of Obstetrics and Gynecology* 158(6 Pt 1):1254-1259.

Nagey DA, Bailey-Jones C, Herman AA. 1993. Randomized comparison of home uterine activity monitoring and routine care in patients discharged after treatment for preterm labor. *Obstetrics and Gynecology* 82:319.

Naik AS, Kallapur SG, Bachurski CJ, Jobe AH, Michna J, Kramer BW, Ikegami M. 2001. Effects of ventilation with different positive end-expiratory pressures on cytokine expression in the preterm lamb lung. *American Journal of Respiratory Critical Care Medicine* 164:494-498.

Nanda K, Cook LA, Gallo MF, Grimes DA. 2002. Terbutaline pump maintenance therapy after threatened preterm labor for preventing preterm birth. *Cochrane Database of Systematic Reviews (Online: Update Software)* 4.

Nathan DG. 2002. Careers in translational clinical research—historical perspectives, future challenges. *JAMA* 287(18):2424-2427.

Nathan DG, Wilson JD. 2003. Clinical research and the NIH—a report card. *New England Journal of Medicine* 349(19).

Nathanielz PW. 1999. *Life in the Womb: The Origins of Health and Disease.* Ithaca, NY: Promethean Press.

Navidi W, Lurmann F. 1995. Measurement error in air pollution exposure assessment. *Journal of Exposure Analysis and Environmental Epidemiology* 5:111-124.

NBHW (The National Board of Health and Welfare). *Official Statistics of Sweden.* [Online]. Available: http://www.sos.se [accessed March 1, 2006].

NCCD (National Commission on Childhood Disability). 1995. Executive summary of the National Commission on Childhood Disability. *Social Security Bulletin* 58(4):108-110.

NCCDPHP (National Center for Disease Prevention and Health Promotion). 2005. *Assisted Reproductive Technology Surveillance—United States, 2002.* [Online]. Available: http://www.cdc.gov/mmwr/preview/mmwrhtml/ss5402a1.htm [accessed October 3, 2005].

NCHS (National Center for Health Statistics). 2002. *Births: Preliminary Data for 2001.* [Online]. Available: http://www.cdc.gov/nchs/fastats/pdf/nvsr50_15tb34.pdf [accessed January 4, 2006].

NCHS. 2004a. *Health, United States 2004.* [Online]. Available: http://www.cdc.gov/nchs/data/hus/hus04trend.pdf#027 [accessed January 30, 2006].

NCHS. 2004b. *Provisional Tables On Births, Marriages, Divorces, and Deaths by State for 1998-2000.* 29(5). [Online]. Available: http://www.cdc.gov/nchs/datawh/statab/unpubd/nvstab49.htm#Briths%20and%20Deaths.

NCHS. (unpublished data). *1998 to 2000 U.S. Birth Cohorts.*

Nebert DW. 2002. Proposal for an allele nomenclature system based on the evolutionary divergence of the haplotypes. *Human Mutation* 20:463-472.

Needell B, Barth RP. 1998. Infants entering foster care compared to other infants using birth status indicators. *Child Abuse and Neglect* 22(12):1179-1187.

Neilson JP. 1998. Evidence-based intrapartum care: Evidence from the Cochrane Library. *International Journal of Gynecology and Obstetrics* 63(Suppl 1):S97-S102.

Neilson JP. 2000. Ultrasound for fetal assessment in early pregnancy. *Cochrane Database of Systematic Reviews* 2.

Nelson KB, Grether JK. 1995. Can magnesium sulfate reduce the risk of cerebral palsy in very low birthweight infants? *Pediatrics* 95(2):263-269.

Nelson KB, Dambrosia JM, Grether JK, Phillips TM. 1998. Neonatal cytokines and coagulation factors in children with cerebral palsy. *Annals of Neurology* 44(4):665-675.

Ness RB, Haggerty CL, Harger G, Ferrell R. 2004. Differential distribution of allelic variants in cytokine genes among African Americans and White Americans. *American Journal of Epidemiology* 160(11):1033-1038.

Neter J, Kutner MH, Wasserman W, Nachtsheim CJ, Neter J. 1996. *Applied Linear Statistical Models.* Chicago, IL: Irwin.

Newman MG, Lindsay MK, Graves W. 2001. Cigarette smoking and pre-eclampsia: Their association and effects on clinical outcomes. *Journal of Maternal-Fetal Medicine* 10(3):166-170.

Newman R. 1997. The preterm prediction study: Impact of twin discordancy on neonatal outcome. *American Journal of Obstetrics and Gynecology* 176(1 Pt 2).

Newman RB, Goldenberg RL, Moawad AH, Iams JD, Meis PJ, Das A, Miodovnik M, Caritis SN, Thurnau GR, Dombrowski MP, Roberts J. 2001. Occupational fatigue and preterm premature rupture of membranes. *American Journal of Obstetrics and Gynecology* 184(3):438-446.

Newsome CA, Shiell AW, Fall CH, Phillips DI, Shier R, Law CM. 2003. Is birth weight related to later glucose and insulin metabolism?—A systematic review. *Diabetic Medicine* 20(5):339-348.

Newton RW, Hunt LP. 1984. Psychosocial stress in pregnancy and its relation to low birth weight. *British Medical Journal (Clinical Research Edition)* 288(6425):1191-1194.

Newton RW, Webster PA, Binu PS, Maskrey N, Phillips AB. 1979. Psychosocial stress in pregnancy and its relation to the onset of premature labour. *British Medical Journal* 2(6187):411-413.

NIDS (National Institute of Neurological Disorders and Stroke). 2005. *Cerebral Palsy Information Page.* [Online]. Available: http://wwwninds.nih.gov/disorders/cerebral_palsy/cerebral_palsy.htm [accessed November 30, 2005].

Niebyl JR, Blake DA, White RD. 1980. The inhibition of premature labor with indomethacin. *American Journal of Obstetrics and Gynecology* 136(8):1014-1019.

Niemitz EL, Feinberg AP. 2004. Epigenetics and assisted reproductive technology: A call for investigation. *American Journal of Human Genetics* 74(4):599-609.

NIH (National Institutes of Health). 1994. Effect of corticosteroids for fetal maturation on perinatal outcomes. *American Journal of Obstetrics and Gynecology* 173(1):246-252.

NIH. 1997. *Director's Panel on Clinical Research. Report to the Advisory Committee to the NIH Director.* [Online]. Available: http://www.nih.gov/news/crp/97report [accessed October 22, 2004].

NIH (National Institutes of Health Consensus Development Panel). 2001. Antenatal corticosteroids revisited: Repeat courses—National Institutes of Health Consensus Development Conference Statement, August 17-18, 2000. *Obstetrics and Gynecology* 98:144-150.

Niparko JK, Blankenhorn R. 2003. Cochlear implants in young children. *Mental Retardation and Developmental Disabilities Research Reviews* 9(4):267-275.

Norbeck JS, Anderson NJ. 1989. Psychosocial predictors of pregnancy outcomes in low-income black, Hispanic, and white women. *Nursing Research* 38(4):204-209.

Norbeck JS, Tilden VP. 1983. Life stress, social support, and emotional disequilibrium in complications of pregnancy: A prospective, multivariate study. *Journal of Health and Social Behavior* 24(1):30-46.

Norbeck JS, DeJoseph JF, Smith RT. 1996. A randomized trial of an empirically-derived social support intervention to prevent low birthweight among African American women. *Social Science and Medicine* 43(6):947-954.

Norbiato G, Bevilacqua M, Vago T, Clerici M. 1997. Glucocorticoids and Th-1, Th-2 type cytokines in rheumatoid arthritis, osteoarthritis, asthma, atopic dermatitis, and AIDS. *Clinical and Experimental Rheumatology* 15:315-323.

Nordentoft M, Lou HC, Hansen D, Nim J, Pryds O, Rubin P, Hemmingsen R. 1996. Intrauterine growth retardation and premature delivery: The influence of maternal smoking and psychosocial factors. *American Journal of Public Health* 86(3):347-354.

Norwitz ER, Schust D, Fisher SJ. 2001. Implantation and the survival of early pregnancy. *New England Journal of Medicine* 345:1400-1408.

NRC (National Research Council). 1994. *The Funding of Young Investigators in the Biological and Biomedical Sciences.* Washington, DC: National Academy Press.

NRC. 2000. *Enhancing the Postdoctoral Experience for Scientists and Engineers.* Washington DC: National Academy Press.

NRC. 2001. *New Horizons in Health: An Integrative Approach.* Washington, DC: National Academy Press.

NRC. 2004. *Facilitating Interdisciplinary Research.* Washington, DC: The National Academies Press.

NRC. 2005. *Bridges to Independence: Fostering the Independence of New Investigators in the Life Sciences.* Washington, DC: The National Academies Press.

Nuckolls KB, Kaplan BH, Cassel J. 1972. Psychosocial assets, life crisis and the prognosis of pregnancy. *American Journal of Epidemiology* 95(5):431-441.

Nukui Ta, Day RDb, Sims CSc, Ness RBd, Romkes Ma. 2004. Maternal/newborn GSTT1 null genotype contributes to risk of preterm, low birthweight infants. *Pharmacogenetics* 14(9):569-576.

Nyberg DA, Abuhamad A, Ville Y. 2004. Ultrasound assessment of abnormal fetal growth. *Seminars in Perinatology* 28(1):3-22.

Oakes JM. 2004. The (mis)estimation of neighborhood effects: Causal inference for a practicable social epidemiology. *Social Science and Medicine* 58(10):1929-1952.

Oakley A. 1988. Is social support good for the health of mothers and babies? *Journal of Reproductive and Infant Psychology* 6:3-21.

Oakley A, Rajan L, Grant A. 1990. Social support and pregnancy outcome. *British Journal of Obstetrics and Gynaecology* 97(2):155-162.

Obel C, Hedegaard M, Henriksen TB, Secher NJ, Olsen J, Levine S. 2005. Stress and salivary cortisol during pregnancy. *Psychoneuroendocrinology* 30(7):647-656.

O'Callaghan MJ, Burns YR, Gray PH, Harvey JM, Mohay H, Rogers YM, Tudehope DI. 1996. School performance of ELBW children. A controlled study. *Developmental Medicine and Child Neurology* 38(10):917-926.

O'Campo P, Xue X, Wang M-C, O'Brien Caughey M. 1997. Neighborhood risk factors for low birthweight in Baltimore: A mutilvariate analysis. *American Journal of Public Health* 87:1113-1118.

O'Connor AR, Stephenson T, Johnson A, Tobin MJ, Moseley MJ, Ratib S, Ng Y, Fielder AR. 2002. Long-term ophthalmic outcome of low birth weight children with and without retinopathy of prematurity. *Pediatrics* 109(1):12-18.

Odibo AO, Talucci M, Berghella V. 2002. Prediction of preterm premature rupture of membranes by transvaginal ultrasound features and risk factors in a high-risk population. *Obstetrics and Gynecology* 20(3):245-251.

Odibo AO, Elkousy M, Ural SH, Macones GA. 2003. Prevention of preterm birth by cervical cerclage compared with expectant management: A systematic review. *Obstetrics and Gynecology Survey* 58:130-136.

Offenbacher S, Katz V, Fertik G, Collins J, Boyd D, Maynor G, McKaig R, Beck J. 1996. Periodontal infection as a possible risk factor for preterm low birth weight. *Journal of Periodontology* 67:1103-1113.

Offenbacher S, Lieff S, Boggess KA, Murtha AP, Madianos PN, Champagne CM, McKaig RG, Jared HL, Mauriello SM, Auten RL Jr., Herbert WN, Beck JD. 2001. Maternal periodontitis and prematurity. Part I: Obstetric outcome of prematurity and growth restriction. *Annals of Periodontology/The American Academy of Periodontology* 6(1):[d]164-174.

Ohlinger J, Brown MS, Laudert S, Swanson S, Fofah O, CARE Group. 2003. Development of potentially better practices for the neonatal intensive care unit as a culture of collaboration: Communication, accountability, respect and empowerment. *Pediatrics* 111(4 Pt 2):e461-e470.

OJJDP (Office of Juvenile Justice and Delinquency Prevention). 2005. *Authorizing Legislation.* [Online]. Available: http://ojjdp.ncjrs.org/about/legislation.html [accessed January 30, 2006].

Oka A, Belliveau MJ, Rosenberg PA, Volpe JJ. 1993. Vulnerability of oligodendroglia to glutamate: Pharmacology, mechanisms and prevention. *Journal of Neuroscience* 13:1441-1453.

O'Keefe M, Kafil-Hussain N, Flitcroft I, Lanigan B. 2001. Ocular significance of intraventricular haemorrhage in premature infants. *British Journal of Ophthalmology* 85(3):357-359.

Okey AB, Giannone JV, Smart W, Wong JM, Manchester DK, Parker NB, Feeley MM, Grant DL, Gilman A. 1997. Binding of 2,3,7,8-tetrachlorodibenzo-p-dioxin to AH receptor in placentas from normal versus abnormal pregnancy outcomes. *Chemosphere* 34:1535-1547.

Okun N, Gronau KA, Hannah ME. 2005. Antibiotics for bacterial vaginosis or Trichomonas vaginalis in pregnancy: A systematic review. *Obstetrics & Gynecology* 105(4):857-868.

Olah KS, Gee GH. 1992. The prevention of prematurity: Can we continue to ignore the cervix? *British Journal of Obstetrics and Gynaecology* 99:278.

Olausson PO, Haglund B, Weitoft GR, Cnattingius S. 2001. Teenage childbearing and long-term socioeconomic consequences: A case study in Sweden. *Perspectives on Sexual and Reproductive Health* 33(2):70-74.

Olden K, Wilson S. 2000. Environmental health and genomics: Visions and implications. *Nature Reviews Genetics* 1(2):149-153.

Olds DL, Kitzman H. 1993. Review of research on home visiting for pregnant women and parents of young children. *The Future of Children* 3(3):53-92.

Olds DL, Henderson CR Jr, Tatelbaum R, Chamberlin R. 1986. Improving the delivery of prenatal care and outcomes of pregnancy: A randomized trial of nurse home visitation. *Pediatrics* 77(1):16-28.

Olischar M, Klebermass K, Kuhle S, Hulek M, Kohlhauser C, Rncklinger E, Pollak A, Weninger M. 2004a. Reference values for amplitude-integrated electroencephalographic activity in preterm infants younger than 30 weeks' gestational age. *Pediatrics* 113(1 Pt 1):e61-e66.

Olischar M, Klebermass K, Kuhle S, Hulek M, Messerschmidt A, Weninger M. 2004b. Progressive posthemorrhagic hydrocephalus leads to changes of amplitude-integrated EEG activity in preterm infants. *Child's Nervous System* 20(1):41-45.

Oliver M, Shapiro T. 1995. *Black Wealth/White Wealth: A New Perspective on Racial Inequality.* New York: Routledge.

Olsen SF. 1993. Consumption of marine n-3 fatty acids during pregnancy as a possible determinant of birth weight. A review of current epidemiologic evidence. *Epidemiological Reviews* 15:399-413.

Olsen SF, Secher NJ. 2002. Low consumption of seafood in early pregnancy as a risk factor for preterm delivery: Prospective cohort study. *British Medical Journal* 324:1-5.

Olsen SF, Hansen HS, Sorensen TIA. 1986. Intake of marine fat, rich in (n-3)-polyunsaturated fatty acids, may increase birthweight by prolonging gestation. *Lancet* 2(8503):367-369.

Olsen SF, Olsen J, Frische G. 1990. Does fish consumption during pregnancy increase fetal growth? A study of the size of the newborn, placental weight and gestational age in relation to fish consumption during pregnancy. *International Journal of Epidemiology* 19:971-977.

Olsen SF, Sorensen JD, Secher NJ, Hedegaard M, Henriksen TB, Hansen HS, Grant A. 1992. Randomised controlled trial of effect of fish-oil supplementation on pregnancy duration. *Lancet* 339(8800):1003-1007.

Olsen SF, Hansen HS, Secher, NJ, Jensen B, Sandström B. 1995a. Gestation length and birth weight in relation to intake of marine *n*-3 fatty acids. *British Journal of Nutrition* 73: 397-404.

Olsen P, Laara E, Rantakallio P, Jarvelin M-R, Sarpola A, Hartikainen AL. 1995b. Epidemiology of preterm delivery in two birth cohorts with an interval of 20 years. *American Journal of Epidemiology* 142(11):1184-1193.

Olsen SF, Secher NJ, Tabor A, Weber T, Walker JJ, Gluud C. 2000. Randomised clinical trials of fish oil supplementation in high risk pregnancies. *British Journal of Obstetrics and Gynaecology* 107(3):382-395.

Olsen IE, Richardson DK, Schmid CH, Ausman LM, Dwyer JT. 2002. Intersite differences in weight growth velocity of extremely premature infants. *Pediatrics* 110:1125-1132.

Olson DM, Mijovic JE, Sadowsky DW. 1995. Control of human parturition. *Seminars in Perinatology* 19(1):52-63.

Ombelet W, De Sutter P, Van der Elst J, Martens G. 2005. Multiple gestation and infertility treatment: Registration, reflection and reaction—The Belgian project. *Human Reproduction Update* 11(1):3-14.

Oommen AM, Griffin JB, Sarath G, Zempleni J. 2005. Roles for nutrients in epigenetic events. *Journal of Nutritional Biochemistry* 16:74-77.

Oren A, Vos LE, Uiterwaal CS, Gorissen WH, Grobbee DE, Bots ML. 2003. Change in body mass index from adolescence to young adulthood and increased carotid intima-media thickness at 28 years of age: The Atherosclerosis Risk in Young Adults Study. *International Journal of Obesity and Related Metabolic Disorders* 27(11):1383-1390.

Ornstein M, Ohlsson A, Edmonds J, Asztalos E. 1991. Neonatal follow-up of very low birthweight/extremely low birthweight infants to school age: A critical overview. *Acta Paediatrica Scandinavica* 80(8-9):741-748.

Orr ST, Miller CA. 1995. Maternal depressive symptoms and the risk of poor pregnancy outcome. Review of the literature and preliminary findings. *Epidemiology Review* 17(1):165-171.

Orr ST, Miller CA. 1997. Unintended pregnancy and the psychosocial well-being of pregnant women. *Womens' Health Issues* 7(1):38-46.

Orr ST, Miller CA, James SA, Babones S. 2000. Unintended pregnancy and preterm birth. *Paediatric and Perinatal Epidemiology* 14(4):309-313.

Orr ST, James SA, Blackmore Prince C. 2002. Maternal prenatal depressive symptoms and spontaneous preterm births among African-American women in Baltimore, Maryland. *American Journal of Epidemiology* 156(9):797-802.

Osborn D. 2000. Thyroid hormones for preventing neurodevelopmental impairment in preterm infants. *Cochrane Reviews* 1.

Osborn D, Henderson-Smart D. 2006a. Kinesthetic stimulation for treating apnea in preterm infants. *Cochrane Reviews* 1.

Osborn D, Henderson-Smart D. 2006b. Kinesthetic stimulation versus theophylline for apnea in preterm infants. *Cochrane Reviews* 1.

Osborn D, Evans N, Kluckow M. 2002. Randomized trial of dobutamine versus dopamine in preterm infants with low systemic blood flow. *Journal of Pediatrics* 140(2):183-191.

O'Shea TM. 2002. Cerebral palsy in very preterm infants: New epidemiological insights. *Mental Retardation and Developmental Disabilities Research Reviews* 8(3):135-145.

O'Shea TM, Klinepeter KL, Goldstein DJ, Jackson BW, Dillard RG. 1997. Survival and developmental disability in infants with birth weights of 501 to 800 grams, born between 1979 and 1994. *Pediatrics* 100(6):982-986.

O'Shea TM, Kothadia JM, Klinepeter KL, Goldstein DJ, Jackson BG, Weaver RG. 1999. Randomized placebo-controlled trial of a 42-day tapering course of dexamethasone to reduce the duration of ventilator dependency in very low birth weight infants: Outcome of study participants at 1-year adjusted age. *Pediatrics* 104(1):15-21.

Osmond C, Barker DJ. 2000. Fetal, infant, and childhood growth are predictors of coronary heart disease, diabetes, and hypertension in adult men and women. *Environmental Health Perspectives* 108(Suppl 3):545-533.

Osmond C, Barker DJ, Winter PD, Fall CH, Simmonds SJ. 1993. Early growth and death from cardiovascular disease in women. *British Medical Journal* 307(6918):1519-1524.

Ou CW, Orsino A, Lye SJ. 1997. Expression of connexin-43 and connexin-26 in the rat myometrium during pregnancy and labor is differentially regulated by mechanical and hormonal signals. *Endocrinology* 138:5398-5507.

Ou CW, Qi S, Chen ZQ, Lye SJ. 1998. Increased expression of the rat myometrial oxytocin receptor messenger ribonucleic acid during labor requires both mechanical and hormonal signals. *Biology of Reproduction* 59:1055-1061.

Owen J, Iams JD, Hauth JC. 2003. Vaginal sonography and cervical incompetence. *American Journal of Obstetrics and Gynecology* 188(2):586-596.

Ozkur M, Dogulu F, Ozkur A, Gokmen B, Inaloz SS, Aynacioglu AS. 2002. Association of the Gln27Glu polymorphism of the beta-2-adrenergic receptor with preterm labor. *International Journal of Gynecology and Obstetrics* 77(3):209-215.

Paarlberg KM, Vingerhoets AJ, Passchier J, Dekker GA, Van Geijn HP. 1995. Psychosocial factors and pregnancy outcome: A review with emphasis on methodological issues. *Journal of Psychosomatic Research* 39(5):563-595.

Paarlberg KM, Vingerhoets AJ, Passchier J, Heinen AG, Dekker GA, van Geijn HP. 1996. Psychosocial factors as predictors of maternal well-being and pregnancy-related complaints. *Journal of Psychosomatic Obstetrics and Gynaecology* 17(2):93-102.

Paarlberg KM, Vingerhoets AJ, Passchier J, Dekker GA, Heinen AG, van Geijn HP. 1999. Psychosocial predictors of low birthweight: A prospective study. *British Journal of Obstetrics and Gynaecology* 106(8):834-841.

Page NM, Kemp CF, Butlin DJ, Lowry PJ. 2002. Placental peptides as markers of gestational disease. *Reproduction* 123(4):487-495.

Pagel MD, Smilkstein G, Regen H, Montano D. 1990. Psychosocial influences on new born outcomes: A controlled prospective study. *Social Science and Medicine* 30(5):597-604.

Pagnini DL, Reichman NE. 2000. Psychosocial factors and the timing of prenatal care among women in New Jersey's HealthStart program. *Family Planning Perspectives* 32(2):56-64.

Pallas Alonso CR, de La Cruz Bertolo J, Medina Lopez MC, Bustos Lozano G, de Alba Romero C, Simon De Las Heras R. 2000. [Age for sitting and walking in children born weighing less than 1,500 g and normal motor development and two years of age]. Article in Spanish. *Anales Españoles de Pediatría* 53(1):43-47.

Palmer EA, Hardy RJ, Davis BR, Stein JA, Mowery RL, Tung B, Phelps DL, Schaffer DB, Flynn JT, Phillips CL. 1991. Operational aspects of terminating randomization in the Multicenter Trial of Cryotherapy for Retinopathy of Prematurity. *Controlled Clinical Trials* 12(2):277-292.

Palta M, Sadek-Badawi M, Evans M, Weinstein MR, McGuinness G. 2000. Functional assessment of a multicenter very low-birth-weight cohort at age 5 years. *Archives of Pediatrics and Adolescent Medicine* 154(1):23-30.

Pan ES, Cole FS, Weintrub PS. 2005. Viral infections of the fetus and the newborn. In: Taeusch HW, Ballard RA, Gleason CA eds. 2005. *Avery's Diseases of the Newborn*, 8th edition. Philadelphia, PA: Elsevier Saunders. Pp. 495-529.

Paneth N. 1994. The impressionable fetus? Fetal life and adult health. *American Journal Public Health* 84(9):1372-1374.

Paneth N, Susser M. 1995. Early origin of coronary heart disease (the "Barker hypothesis"). *British Medical Journal* 310(6977):411-412.

Paneth N, Ahmed F, Stein A. 1996. Early nutritional origins of hypertension: A hypothesis still lacking support. *Journal of Hypertension* 14(Suppl 5):S121-S129.

Paneth N, Jetton J, Pinto-Martin J, Susser M. 1997. Magnesium sulfate in labor and risk of neonatal brain lesions and cerebral palsy in low birth weight infants. The Neonatal Brain Hemorrhage Study Analysis Group. *Pediatrics* 99(5).

Papanikolaou EG, Camus M, Kolibianakis EM, Van Landuyt L, Van Steirteghem A, Devroey P. 2006. In vitro fertilization with single blastocyst-stage versus single cleavage-stage embryos. *New England Journal of Medicine* 354(11):1139-1146.

Papatsonis DNM, Van Geijn HP, Adr HJ, Lange FM, Bleker OP, Dekker GA. 1997. Nifedipine and ritodrine in the management of preterm labor: A randomized multicenter trial. *Obstetrics and Gynecology* 90(2):230-234.

Papiernik E, Goffinet F. 2004. Prevention of preterm births, the French experience. *Clinical Obstetrics and Gynecology* 47(4):755-767.

Papile LA, Rudolph AM, Heymann MA. 1985. Autoregulation of cerebral blood flow in the preterm fetal lamb. *Pediatrics Research* 19:159-161.

Parazzini F, Chatenoud L, Surace M, Tozzi L, Salerio B, Bettoni G, Benzi G. 2003. Moderate alcohol drinking and risk of preterm birth. *European Journal of Clinical Nutrition* 57(10):1345-1349.

Pariante CM, Pearce BD, Pisell TL, Sanchez CI, Po C, Su C, Miller AH. 1999. The proinflammatory cytokine, interleukin-1alpha, reduces glucocorticoid receptor translocation and function. *Endocrinology* 140:4359-4366.

Parker B, McFarlane J, Soeken K. 1994a. Abuse during pregnancy: Effects on maternal complications and birth weight in adult and teenage women. *Obstetrics and Gynecology* 84(3):323-328.

Parker JD, Schoendorf KC, Kiely JL. 1994b. Associations between measures of socioeconomic status and low birth weight, small for gestational age, and premature delivery in the United States. *Annals of Epidemiology* 4:271-278.

Parker Dominguez T, Dunkel Schetter C, Mancuso R, Rini CM, Hobel C. 2005. Stress in African American pregnancies: Testing the roles of various stress concepts in prediction of birth outcomes. *Annals of Behavioral Medicine* 29(1):12-21.

Parkin JM, Hey EN, Clowes JS. 1976. Rapid assessment of gestational age at birth. *Archives of Disease in Childhood* 51(4):259-263.

Partridge JC, Martinez AM, Nishida H, Boo NY, Tan KW, Yeung CY, Lu JH, Yu VY. 2005. International comparison of care for very low birth weight infants: Parents' perceptions of counseling and decision-making. *Pediatrics* 116(2):e263-e271.

Patole SK, de Klerk N. 2005. Impact of standardised feeding regimens on incidence of neonatal necrotising enterocolitis: A systematic review and meta-analysis of observational studies. *Archives of Disease in Childhood: Fetal and Neonatal Edition* 90(2):F147-F151.

PC of SART and ASRM (The Practice Committee of the Society for Assisted Reproductive Technology and the American Society of Reproductive Medicine). 2004. Guidelines on the number of embryos transferred. *Fertility and Sterility* 82(3):773-774.

Peaceman AM, Andrews WW, Thorp JM, et al. 1997. Fetal fibronectin as a predictor of preterm birth in patients with symptoms: A multicenter trial. *American Journal of Obstetrics and Gynecology* 177:13-18.

Peacock JL, Bland JM, Anderson HR. 1995. Preterm delivery: Effects of socioeconomic factors, psychological stress, smoking, alcohol, and caffeine. *British Medical Journal* 311(7004):531-535.

Pearl M, Braveman P, Abrams B. 2001. The relationship of neighborhood socioeconomic characteristic to birth weight among 5 ethnic groups in California. *American Journal of Public Health* 91:1815-1824.

Pellicer A, Gayá F, Madero R, Quero J, Cabanas F. 2002. Noninvasive continuous monitoring of the effects of head position on brain hemodynamics in ventilated infants. *Pediatrics* 109(3):434-440.

Peralta-Carcelen M, Jackson DS, Goran MI, Royal SA, Mayo MS, Nelson KG. 2000. Growth of adolescents who were born at extremely low birth weight without major disability. *Journal of Pediatrics* 136(5):633-640.

Perkin MR, Bland JM, Peacock JL, Anderson HR. 1993. The effect of anxiety and depression during pregnancy on obstetric complications. *British Journal of Obstetrics and Gynaecology* 100(7):629-634.

Perri T, Cohen-Sacher B, Hod M, Berant M, Meizner I, Bar J. 2005. Risk factors for cardiac malformations detected by fetal echocardiography in a tertiary center. *Journal of Maternal–Fetal and Neonatal Medicine* 17(2):123-128.

Perry KG Jr., Morrison JC, Rust OA, Sullivan CA, Martin RW, Naef III RW. 1995. Incidence of adverse cardiopulmonary effects with low-dose continuous terbutaline infusion. *American Journal of Obstetrics and Gynecology* 173(4):1273-1277.

Personal Responsibility and Work Opportunity Reconciliation Act of 1996. 1996. Pub L No 104-193, 110 Stat 2105-2355.

Persson PH, Weldner BM. 1986. Reliability of ultrasound fetometry in estimating gestational age in the second trimester. *Acta Obstetricia et Gynecologica Scandinavica* 65(5): 481-483.

Peterson BS. 2003. Brain imaging studies of the anatomical and functional consequences of preterm birth for human brain development. *Annals of the New York Academy of Sciences* 1008:219-237.

Peterson BS, Vohr B, Staib LH, Cannistraci CJ, Dolberg A, Schneider KC, Katz KH, Westerveld M, Sparrow S, Anderson AW, Duncan CC, Makuch RW, Gore JC, Ment LR. 2000. Regional brain volume abnormalities and long-term cognitive outcome in preterm infants. *JAMA* 284(15):1939-1947.

Petersson K, Norbeck O, Westgren M, Broliden K. 2004. Detection of parvovirus B19, cytomegalovirus and enterovirus infections in cases of intrauterine fetal death. *Journal of Perinatal Medicine* 32(6):516-521.

Petraglia F, Florio P, Nappi C, Genazzani AR. 1996. Peptide signaling in human placenta and membranes: Autocrine, paracrine, and endocrine mechanisms. *Endocrine Reviews* 17:156-186.

Petrini J, Damus K, Russell R, Poschman K, Davidoff MJ, Mattison D. 2002. Contribution of birth defects to infant mortality in the United States. *Teratology* 66(Suppl 1):S3-S6.

Petrini JRP, Callaghan WMM, Klebanoff MM, Green NSM, Lackritz EMM, Howse JLP, Schwarz RHM, Damus KR. 2005. Estimated effect of 17 alpha-hydroxyprogesterone caproate on preterm birth in the United States. *Obstetrics and Gynecology* 105(2): 267-272.

Petrou S, Mehta Z, Hockley C, Cook-Mozaffari P, Henderson J, Goldacre M. 2003. The impact of preterm birth on hospital inpatient admissions and costs during the first 5 years of life. *Pediatrics* 112(6):1290-1297.

Petterson B, Nelson KB, Watson L, Stanley F. 1993. Twins, triplets, and cerebral palsy in births in Western Australia in the 1980s. *British Medical Journal* 307(6914):1239-1243.

Pettigrew AG, Edwards DA, Henderson-Smart DJ. 1985. The influence of intra-uterine growth retardation on brainstem development of preterm infants. *Developmental Medicine and Child Neurology* 27(4):467-472.

Phaneuf S, Asboth G, MacKenzie IZ, Melin P, Lopez Bernal A. 1994. Effect of oxytocin antagonists on the activation of human myometrium in vitro: Atosiban prevents oxytocin-induced desensitization. *American Journal of Obstetrics and Gynecology* 171:1627-1634.

Pharoah POD, Stevenson CJ, Cooke RWI, Stevenson RC. 1994. Clinical and subclinical deficits at 8 years in a geographically defined cohort of low birthweight infants. *Archives of Disease in Childhood* 70(4):264-270.

Pharoah POD, Stevenson CJ, West CR. 2003. General certificate of secondary education performance in very low birthweight infants. *Archives of Disease in Childhood* 88(4): 295-298.

Phelps DL. 2000. Supplemental therapeutic oxygen for prethreshold retinopathy of prematurity (STOP-ROP), a randomized, controlled trial. I: Primary outcomes. *Pediatrics* 105(2): 295-310.

Phelps DL, Watts JL. 2002. Early light reduction for preventing retinopathy of prematurity in very low birth weight infants. *Cochrane Reviews* 3.

Phibbs CS, Schmitt SK. 2006. Estimates of the cost of length of stay changes that can be attributed to one-week increases in gestational age for premature infants. *Early Human Development* 82:85-95.

Phibbs CS, Bronstein JM, Buxton E, Phibbs RH. 1996. The effects of patient volume and level of care at the hospital of birth on neonatal mortality. *JAMA* 276(13):1054-1059.

Philip AGS, Spellacy WN. 2004. Historical perspectives: Prenatal assessment of fetal lung maturity. *NeoReviews* 5(4):e131-e133.

Philip AGS, Amiel-Tison C, Amiel-Tison C. 2003. Historical perspectives: Neurologic maturation of the neonate. *NeoReviews* 4(8):e199-e205.

Phillippe M, Chien E. 1998. Intracellular signaling and phasic myometrial contractions. *Journal of the Society for Gynecological Investigations* 5:169-177.

Piecuch RE, Leonard CH, Cooper BA, Sehring SA. 1997a. Outcome of extremely low birth weight infants (500 to 999 grams) over a 12-year period. *Pediatrics* 100(4):633-639.

Piecuch RE, Leonard CH, Cooper BA, Kilpatrick SJ, Schlueter MA, Sola A. 1997b. Outcome of infants born at 24-26 weeks' gestation: II. Neurodevelopmental outcome. *Obstetrics and Gynecology* 90(5):809-814.

Pierrat V, Duquennoy C, Van Haastert IC, Ernst M, Guilley N, De Vries LS. 2001. Ultrasound diagnosis and neurodevelopmental outcome of localised and extensive cystic periventricular leucomalacia. *Archives of Disease in Childhood: Fetal and Neonatal Edition* 84(3):F151-F156.

Pinelli J, Symington A. 2006. Non-nutritive sucking for promoting physiologic stability and nutrition in preterm infants. *Cochrane Reviews* 1.

Pinto-Martin JA, Riolo S, Cnaan A, Holzman C, Susser MW, Paneth N. 1995. Cranial ultrasound prediction of disabling and nondisabling cerebral palsy at age two in a low birth weight population. *Pediatrics* 95(2):249-254.

Pinto-Martin J, Whitaker A, Feldman J, Cnaan A, Zhao H, Rosen-Bloch J, McCulloch, D Paneth N. 2004. Special education services and school performance in a regional cohort of low-birthweight infants at age nine. *Paediatric and Perinatal Epidemiology* 18(2): 120-129.

Piper JM, Ray WA, et al. 1990. Effects of a Medicaid eligibility expansion on prenatal care and pregnancy outcome in Tennessee. *JAMA* 264(17):2219-2223.

Piper MC, Kunos VI, Willis DM. 1986. Early physical therapy effects on the high-risk infant: A randomized controlled trial. *Pediatrics* 78(2):216-224.

Piven J, Simon J, Chase GA, Wzorek M, Landa R, Gayle J, Folstein S. 1993. The etiology of autism: Pre-, peri-, and neonatal factors. *Journal of the American Academy of Child and Adolescent Psychiatry* 32(6):1256-1263.

Platt RW. 2002. The effect of gestational age errors and their correction in interpreting population trends in fetal growth and gestational age-specific mortality. *Seminars in Perinatology* 26(4):306-311.

Pollack LD, Ratner IM, Lund GC. 1998. United States neonatology practice survey: Personnel, practice, hospital, and neonatal intensive care unit characteristics. *Pediatrics* 101(3 I): 398-405.

Ponce NA, Hoggatt KJ, Wilhelm M, Ritz B. 2005. Preterm birth: The interaction of traffic-related air pollution with economic hardship in Los Angeles neighborhoods. *American Journal of Epidemiology* 162:140-148.

Porter TF, Fraser AM, Hunter CY, Ward RH, Varner MW. 1997. The risk of preterm birth across generations. *Obstetrics and Gynecology* 90(1):63-67.

The President's Council on Bioethics. 2004. *Reproduction and Responsibility: The Regulation of New Biotechnologies*. Washington, DC: Department of Health and Human Services.

Pritchard CW, Teo PY. 1994. Preterm birth, low birthweight and the stressfulness of the household role for pregnant women. *Social Science and Medicine* 38(1):89-96.

Procianoy RS, Schvartsman S. 1981. Blood pesticide concentration in mothers and their newborn infants. Relation to prematurity. *Acta Paediatrica Scandinavica* 70: 925-928.

Profit J, Zupancic JAF, McCormick MC, Richardson DK, Escobar GJ, Tucker J, Tarnow-Mordi W, Parry G. 2006. Moderately premature infants in the Kaiser Permanente Medical Care Program in California are discharged home earlier than their peers in Massachusetts and the United Kingdom. *Archives of Disease in Childhood: Fetal Neonatal Edition* 91(4):F245-F250.

PRWORA (Personal Responsibility Work Opportunity and Reconciliation Act). 1996. *Public Law 104-193*. [Online]. Available: http://wdr.doleta.gov/readroom/legislation/pdf/104-193.pdf [accessed January 24, 2007].

Pryor JE, Thompson JM, Robinson E, Clark PM, Becroft DM, Pattison NS, Galvish N, Wild CJ, Mitchell EA. 2003. Stress and lack of social support as risk factors for small-for-gestational-age birth. *Acta Paediatrica* 92(1):62-64.

Quinlivan JA, Archer MA, Evans SF, Newnham JP, Dunlop SA. 2000. Fetal sciatic nerve growth is delayed following repeated maternal injections of corticosteroid in sheep. *Journal of Perinatal Medicine* 28(1):26-33.

Quinn GE, Dobson V, Kivlin J, Kaufman LM, Repka MX, Reynolds JD, Gordon RA, Hardy RJ, Tung B, Stone RA. 1998. Prevalence of myopia between 3 months and 5 1/4 years in preterm infants with and without retinopathy of prematurity. *Ophthalmology* 105(7): 1292-1300.

Quinn GE, Dobson V, Saigal S, Phelps DL, Hardy RJ, Tung B, Summers CG, Palmer EA. 2004. Health-related quality of life at age 10 years in very low-birth-weight children with and without threshold retinopathy of prematurity. *Archives of Ophthalmology* 122(11): 1659-1666.

Raatikainen K, Heiskanen N, Heinonen S. 2005. Marriage still protects pregnancy. *BJOG: An International Journal of Obstetrics and Gynaecology* 112(10):1411-1416.

Ragusa A, De Carolis C, Dal Lago A, Miriello D, Ruggiero G, Brucato A, Pisoni MP, Muscara M, Merati R, Maccario L, Nobili M. 2004. Progesterone supplement in pregnancy: An immunologic therapy? *Lupus* 13(9):639-642.

Raju TNK. 1995. Low birth weight and fetal origins of coronary heart disease: A meta analysis. *Perinatology* 1:243-249.

Raju TNK, Ariagno RL, Higgins R, Van Marter LJ. 2005. Research in neonatology for the 21st century: Executive summary of the National Institute of Child Health and Human Development-American Academy of Pediatrics Workshop. Part i: Academic issues. *Pediatrics* 115(2):468-474.

Ramey SL, Ramey CT. 1999. Early experience and early intervention for children "at risk" for developmental delay and mental retardation. *Mental Retardation and Developmental Disabilities Research Reviews* 5(1):1-10.

Ramey CT, Bryant DM, Wasik BH, Sparling JJ, Fendt KH, La Vange LM. 1992. Infant Health and Development Program for low birth weight, premature infants: Program elements, family participation, and child intelligence. *Pediatrics* 89(3 Suppl):454-465.

Randell SH, Mercer RR, Young SL. 1989. Postnatal growth of pulmonary acini and alveoli in normal and oxygen-exposed rats studied by serial section reconstructions. *American Journal of Anatomy* 186:55-68.

Rasmussen SA, Moore CA, Paulozzi LJ, Rhoenhiser EP. 2001. Risk for birth defects among premature infants: A population-based study. *Journal of Pediatrics* 138:668-673.

Ratliff-Schaub K, Hunt CE, Crowell D, Golub H, Smok-Pearsall S, Palmer P, Schafer S, Bak S, Cantey-Kiser J, O'Bell R. 2001. Relationship between infant sleep position and motor development in preterm infants. *Journal of Developmental and Behavioral Pediatrics* 22(5):293-299.

Rauh V, Culhane JF. 2001. Stress and infection: The contribution of objective conditions and subjective experiences. *Health Psychology* 55(4):220.

Rawlings EE, Moore BA. 1970. The accuracy of methods of calculating the expected date of delivery for use in the diagnosis of postmaturity. *American Journal of Obstetrics and Gynecology* 106(5):676-679.

Rawlings JS, Rawlings VB, Read JA.1995. Prevalence of low birth weight and preterm delivery in relation to the interval between pregnancies among white and black women. *New England Journal of Medicine* 332:69-74.

Rayburn WF, Wilson EA. 1980. Coital activity and premature delivery. *American Journal of Obstetrics and Gynecology* 137(8):972-974.

Read JS, Klebanoff MA. 1993. Sexual intercourse during pregnancy and preterm delivery: Effects of vaginal microorganisms. *American Journal of Obstetrics and Gynecology* 168(2):514-519.

Reagan PB, Salsberry PJ. 2005. Race and ethnic differences in determinants of preterm birth in the USA: Broadening the social context. *Social Science and Medicine* 60(10):2217-2228.

Reeb KG, Graham AV, Zyzanski SJ, Kitson GC. 1987. Predicting low birthweight and complicated labor in urban black women: A biopsychosocial perspective. *Social Science Medicine* 25(12):1321-1327.

Reiner AP, Ziv E, Lind DL, Nievergelt CM, Schork NJ, Cummings SR, Phong A, Burchard EG, Harris TB, Psaty BM, Kwok PY. 2005. Population structure, admixture, and aging-related phenotypes in African American adults: The Cardiovascular Health Study. *American Journal of Human Genetics* 76(3):463-477.

Repka MX. 2002. Ophthalmological problems of the premature infant. *Mental Retardation and Developmental Disabilities Research Reviews* 8(4):249-257.

Repka MX, Summers CG, Palmer EA, Dobson V, Tung B, Davis B. 1998. The incidence of ophthalmologic interventions in children with birth weights less than 1251 grams: Results through 5 1/2 years. *Ophthalmology* 105(9):1621-1627.

Repka MX, Palmer EA, Tung B. 2000. Involution of retinopathy of prematurity. *Archives of Ophthalmology* 118(5):645-649.

Resnick MB, Gueorguieva RV, Carter RL, Ariet M, Sun Y, Roth J, Bucciarelli RL, Curran JS, Mahan CS. 1999. The impact of low birth weight, perinatal conditions, and sociodemographic factors on educational outcome in kindergarten. *Pediatrics* 104(6): e74-e84.

Restrepo M, Munoz N, Day NE, Parra JE, de Romero L, Nguyen-Dinh X. 1990. Prevalence of adverse reproductive outcomes in a population occupationally exposed to pesticides in Colombia. *Scandinavian Journal of Work, Environment, and Health* 16:232-238.

Revich B, Aksel E, Ushakova T, Ivanova I, Zhuchenko N, Klyuev N, Brodsky B, Sotskov Y. 2001. Dioxin exposure and public health in Chapaevsk, Russia. *Chemosphere* 43: 951-966.

Reynolds AJ, Temple JA, Robertson DL, Mann EA. 2001. Long-term effects of an early childhood intervention on educational achievement and juvenile arrest: A 15-year follow-up of low-income children in public schools. *JAMA* 285(18):2339-2346.

Reynolds MASL, Martin JA, Jeng G, Macaluso M. 2003. Trends in multiple births conceived using assisted reproductive technology, United States 1997-2000. *Pediatrics* 111:1159-1162.

Ribas-Fito N, Sala M, Cardo E, Mazon C, De Muga ME, Verdu A, Marco E, Grimalt JO, Sunyer J. 2002. Association of hexachlorobenzene and other organochlorine compounds with anthropometric measures at birth. *Pediatrics Research* 52:163-167.

Richardson DK, Phibbs CS, Gray JE, McCormick MC, Workman-Daniels K, Goldmann DA. 1993. Birth weight and illness severity: Independent predictors of neonatal mortality. *Pediatrics* 91(5 I):969-975.

Richardson DK, Tarnow-Mordi WO, Escobar GJ. 1998. Neonatal risk scoring systems. Can they predict mortality and morbididty? *Clinical Perinatology* 25:591-611.

Richardson DK, Tarnow-Mordi WO, Lee SK. 1999a. Risk adjustment for quality improvement. *Pediatrics* 103(1):e255.

Richardson DK, Shah BL, Frantz ID, Bednarek F, Rubin LP, McCormick MC. 1999b. Perinatal risk and severity of illness in newborns at 6 neonatal intensive care units. *American Journal of Public Health* 89:511-516.

Richardson DK, Zupancic JAF, Escobar GJ, Roberts RH, Coleman-Phox K, McCormick MC. 2003. The Moderately Preterm Infant Project: Interinstitutional practice variation. *Pediatrics Research* 53:382A.

Rich-Edwards JW, Grizzard TA. 2005. Psychosocial stress and neuroendocrine mechanisms in preterm delivery. *American Journal of Obstetrics and Gynecology* 192(5 Suppl):S30-S35.

Rich-Edwards JW, Stampfer MJ, Manson JE, Rosner B, Hankinson SE, Colditz GA, Willett WC, Hennekens CH. 1997. Birth weight and risk of cardiovascular disease in a cohort of women followed up since 1976. *British Medical Journal* 315(7105):396-400.

Rich-Edwards J, Krieger N, Majzoub J, Zierler S, Lieberman E, Gillman M. 2001. Maternal experiences of racism and violence as predictors of preterm birth: Rationale and study design. *Paediatric and Perinatal Epidemiology* 15(Suppl 2):124-135.

Rickards AL, Kitchen WH, Doyle LW, Kelly EA. 1989. Correction of developmental and intelligence test scores for premature birth. *Australian Paediatric Journal* 25(3):127-129.

Ricketts SA, Murray EK, Schwalberg R. 2005. Reducing low birthweight by resolving risks: Results from Colorado's prenatal plus program. *American Journal of Public Health* 95(11):1952-1957.

Riggs MA, Klebanoff MA. 2004. Treatment of vaginal infections to prevent preterm birth: A meta-analysis. *Clinical Obstetrics and Gynecology* 47:796-807.

Ringer SA, Richardson DK, Sacher RA, Keszler M, Churchill WH. 1998. Variations in transfusion practice in neonatal intensive care. *Pediatrics* 101:194-200.

Rini CK, Dunkel-Schetter C, Wadhwa PD, Sandman CA. 1999. Psychological adaptation and birth outcomes: The role of personal resources, stress, and sociocultural context in pregnancy. *Health Psychology* 18(4):333-345.

Ritz B, Yu F, Chapa G, Fruin S. 2000. Effect of air pollution on preterm birth among children born in Southern California between 1989 and 1993. *Epidemiology* 11:502-511.

Rivers A, Caron B, Hack M. 1987. Experience of families with very low birthweight children with neurologic sequelae. *Clinical Pediatrics* 26(5):223-230.

Robert SA. 1999. Socioeconomic position and health: The independent contribution of community socioeconomic context. *Annual Review of Sociology* 25:489-516.

Roberts AK, Monzon-Bordonaba F, Van Deerlin PG, Holder J, Macones GA, Morgan MA, Strauss III JF, Parry S. 1999. Association of polymorphism within the promoter of the tumor necrosis factor alpha gene with increased risk of preterm premature rupture of the fetal membranes. *American Journal of Obstetrics and Gynecology* 180(5):1297-1302.

Roberts EM. 1997. Neighborhood social environments and the distribution of low birthweight in Chicago. *American Journal of Public Health* 87(4):597-603.

Robertson A, Cooper-Peel C, Vos P. 1998. Peak noise distribution in the neonatal intensive care nursery. *Journal of Perinatology* 18(5):361-364.

Robinson R. 1966. Assessment of gestational age by neurological examination. *Archives of Disease in Childhood* 41:437-447.

Rodriguez A, Bohlin G. 2005. Are maternal smoking and stress during pregnancy related to ADHD symptoms in children? *Journal of Child Psychology and Psychiatry and Allied Disciplines* 46(3):246-254.

Rodriguez C, Regidor E, Gutierrez-Fisac JL. 1995. Low birth weight in Spain associated with socidemographic factors. *Journal of Epidemiology and Community Health* 49(1):38-42.

Roesch SC, Dunkel Schetter C, Woo G, Hobel CJ. 2004. Modeling the types and timing of stress in pregnancy. *Anxiety, Stress, and Coping* 17(1):87-102.

Rogers B, Msall M, Owens T, Guernsey K, Brody A, Buck G, Hudak M. 1994. Cystic periventricular leukomalacia and type of cerebral palsy in preterm infants. *Journal of Pediatrics* 125(1):S1-S8.

Rogowski J. 1998. Cost-effectiveness of care for very low birth weight infants. *Pediatrics* 102:35-43.

Rogowski J. 1999. Measuring the cost of neonatal and perinatal care. *Pediatrics* 103(1 Suppl E):329-335.

Rogowski J. 2003. Using economic information in a quality improvement collaborative. *Pediatrics* 111:411-418.

Rogowski J, Horbar J, Staiger D, Kenny M, Carpenter J, Geppert. 2004a. Indirect versus direct hospital quality indicators for very-low-birth weight infants. *JAMA* 291(2): 202-209.

Rogowski J, Staiger D, Horbar J. 2004b. Variations in the quality of care for very low birthweight infants: Implications for policy. *Health Affairs* 88-97.

Rolschau J, Kristoffersen K, Ulrich M, Grinsted P, Schaumburg E, Foged N. 1999. The influence of folic acid supplement on the outcome of pregnancies in the county of Funen in Denmark. I. *European Journal of Obstetrics Gynecology and Reproductive Biology* 87(2):105-110.

Romero R, Oyarzun E, Mazor M, Sirtori M, Hobbins JC, Bracken M. 1989. Meta-analysis of the relationship between asymptomatic bacteriuria and preterm delivery/low birth weight. *Obstetrics and Gynecology* 73(4):576-582 .

Romero R, Avila C, Brekus CA, Morotti R. 1991. The role of systemic and intrauterine infection in preterm parturition. *Annals of New York Academy Sciences* 622:355-375.

Romero R, Mazor M, Munoz H, Gomez R, Galasso M, Sherer DM. 1994. The preterm labor syndrome. *Annals of the New York Academy of Sciences* 734:414-429.

Romero R, Sibai BM, Sanchez-Ramos L. 2000. An oxytocin receptor antagonist (atosiban) in the treatment of preterm labor: A randomized, double-blind, placebo-controlled trial with tocolytic rescue. *American Journal of Obstetrics and Gynecology* 182(5):1173-1183.

Romero R, Kuivaniemi H, Tromp G, Olson JM. 2002. The design, execution, and interpretation of genetic association studies to decipher complex diseases. *American Journal of Obstetrics and Gynecology* 187(5):1299-1312.

Romero R, Espinoza J, Mazor M, Chaiworapongsa T. 2004a. The preterm parturition syndrome. In: Critchley H, Bennett P, Thornton S eds. *Preterm Birth*. London, UK: RCOG Press. Pp. 28-60.

Romero R, Espinoza J, Mazor M. 2004b. Can endometrial infection/inflammation explain implantation failure, spontaneous abortion, and preterm birth after in vitro fertilization? *Fertility and Sterility* 82:779-804.

Romero R, Erez O, Espinoza J. 2005. Intrauterine infection, preterm labor, and cytokines. *Journal of the Society for Gynecologic Investigation* 12463-12465.

Rose SA, Jankowski JJ, Feldman JF, Van Rossem R. 2005. Pathways from prematurity and infant abilities to later cognition. *Child Development* 76(6):1172-1184.

Rosen T, Kuczynski E, O'Neill LM, Funai EF, Lockwood CJ. 2001. Plasma levels of thrombin-antithrombin complexes predict preterm premature rupture of the fetal membranes. *Journal of Maternal and Fetal Medicine* 10:297-300.

Rosen T, Schatz F, Kuczynski E, Lam H, Koo AB, Lockwood CJ. 2002. Thrombin-enhanced matrix metalloproteinase-1 expression: A mechanism linking placental abruption with premature rupture of the membranes. *Journal of Maternal and Fetal Neonatal Medicine* 11:11-17.

Rosenbaum S. 2002. Medicaid. *New England Journal of Medicine* 346:635-640.

Rosenbaum P, Saigal S. 1996. Measuring health-related quality of life in pediatric populations: Conceptual issues. In: Spilker B ed. *Quality of Life and Pharmacoeconomics in Clinical Trials,* 2nd edition. Philadelphia, PA: Lippencott-Raven Publishers. Pp. 785-791.

Rosenberg L. 1965. *Society and the Adolescent Self-Image* Princeton, NJ: Princeton University Press.

Rosenberg AA, Murdaugh E, White CW. 1989. The role of oxygen free radicals in post-asphyxia cerebral hypoperfusion in newborn lambs. *Pediatrics Research* 26:215-219.

Rosenstein IJ, Morgan DJ, Lamont RF, Sheehan M, Dore CJ, Hay PE, Taylor-Robinson D. 2000. Effect of intravaginal clindamycin cream on pregnancy outcome and on abnormal vaginal microbial flora of pregnant women. *Infectious Diseases in Obstetrics and Gynecology* 8(3-4):158-165.

Rossavik IK, Fishburne JI. 1989. Conceptional age, menstrual age, and ultrasound age: A second-trimester comparison of pregnancies of known conception date with pregnancies dated from the last menstrual period. *Obstetrics and Gynecology* 73(2):243-249.

Rothberg AD, Lits B. 1991. Psychosocial support for maternal stress during pregnancy: Effect on birth weight. *American Journal of Obstetrics and Gynecology* 165(2):403-407.

Rothman, Naholder S, Caporaso NE, Garcia-Closas M, Buetow K, Fraumeni JF . 2001. The use of common genetic polymorphisms to enhance the epidemiologic study of environmental carcinogens. *Acta Biochimica et Biophysica* 147(2):C1-C10.

Rotmensch S, Liberati M, Vishne TH, Celentano C, Ben-Rafael Z, Bellati U. 1999. The effect of betamethasone and dexamethasone on fetal heart rate patterns and biophysical activities. A prospective randomized trial. *Acta Obstetricia et Gynecologica Scandinavica* 78(6):493-500.

Rowland AS, Baird DD, Long S, Wegienka G, Harlow SD, Alavanja M, Sandler DP. 2002. Influence of medical conditions and lifestyle factors on the menstrual cycle. *Epidemiology* 13(6):668-674.

Rowley DL. 1994. Research issues in the study of very low birthweight and preterm delivery among African-American women. *Journal of the National Medical Association* 86(10): 761-764.

Rowley DL. 2001. Closing the gap, opening the process: Why study social contributors to preterm delivery among black women. *Maternal and Child Health Journal* 5(2):71-74.

Rowley DL, Hogue CJ, Blackmore CA, Ferre CD, Hatfield-Timajchy K, Branch P, Atrash HK. 1993. Preterm delivery among African-American women: A research strategy. *American Journal of Preventive Medicine* 9(6 Suppl):1-6.

Rumbold A, Crowther CA. 2005. Vitamin C supplementation in pregnancy. *Cochrane Database of Systematic Reviews* 4.

Rush D, Stein Z, Susser M. 1980. A randomized controlled trial of prenatal nutritional supplementation in New York City. *Pediatrics* 65(4):683-697.

Russell R, Green N, Steiner C, Meikle S, Poschman K, Potetz L, Davidoff M, Damus K, Petrini G. 2005. *The National Bill for Hospitalizations of Premature Infants in the United States, Working Paper.* Washington, DC: March of Dimes.

Rust OA, Atlas RA, Reed J, et al. 2001. Revisiting the short cervix detected by transvaginal ultrasound in the second trimester; why cerclage therapy may not help. *American Journal of Obstetrics and Gynecology* 185:1098-1105.

Sable MR, Wilkinson DS. 2000. Impact of perceived stress, major life events and pregnancy attitudes on low birth weight. *Family Planning Perspectives* 32(6):288-294.

Sadler L, Saftlas A, Wang W, Exeter M, Whittaker J. 2004. Treament for cervical intraepithelial neoplasia and risk of preterm delivery. *JAMA* 291(17):2100-2106.

Sagiv SK, Mendola P, Loomis D, Herring AH, Neas LM, Savitz DA, Poole C. 2005. A time-series analysis of air pollution and preterm birth in Pennsylvania, 1997-2001. *Environmental Health Perspectives* 113:602-606.

Sagrestano LM, Feldman P, Rini CK, Woo G, Dunkel-Schetter C. 1999. Ethnicity and social support during pregnancy. *American Journal of Community Psychology* 27(6):869-898.

Saigal S. 2000. Follow-up of very low birthweight babies to adolescence. *Seminars in Neonatology* 5(2):107-118.

Saigal S, Watts J, Campbell D. 1986. Randomized clinical trial of an oscillating air mattress in preterm infants: Effect on apnea, growth, and development. *Journal of Pediatrics* 109(5):857-864.

Saigal S, Rosenbaum P, Hattersley B, Milner R. 1989. Decreased disability rate among 3-year-old survivors weighing 501 to 1000 grams at birth and born to residents of a geographically defined region from 1981 to 1984 compared with 1977 to 1980. *Journal of Pediatrics* 114(5):839-846.

Saigal S, Rosenbaum PL, Szatmari P, Campbell D. 1991. Learning disabilities and school problems in a regional cohort of extremely low birth weight (<1000 g) children: A comparison with term controls. *Journal of Developmental and Behavioral Pediatrics* 12(5): 294-300.

Saigal S, Rosenbaum P, Stoskopf B, Hoult L, Furlong W, Feeney D, Burrows E, Torrance G. 1994a. Comprehensive assessment of the health status of extremely low birth weight children at eight years of age: Comparison with a reference group. *Journal of Pediatrics* 125(3):411-417.

Saigal S, Feeny D, Furlong W, Rosenbaum P, Burrows E, Torrance G. 1994b. Comparison of the health-related quality of life of extremely low birth weight children and a reference group of children at age eight years. *Journal of Pediatrics* 125:418-425.

Saigal S, Feeny D, Rosenbaum P, Furlong W, Burrows E, Stoskopf B. 1996. Self-perceived health status and health-related quality of life of extremely low-birth-weight infants at adolescence. *JAMA* 276(6):453-459.

Saigal S, Stoskopf BL, Feeny D, Furlong W, Burrows E, Rosenbaum PL, Hoult L. 1999. Differences in preferences for neonatal outcomes among health care professionals, parents, and adolescents. *JAMA* 281(21):1991-1997.

Saigal S, Burrows E, Stoskopf BL, Rosenbaum PL, Streiner D. 2000a. Impact of extreme prematurity on families of adolescent children. *Journal of Pediatrics* 137(5):701-706.

Saigal S, Rosenbaum PL, Feeny D, Burrows E, Furlong W, Stoskopf BL, Hoult L. 2000b. Parental perspectives of the health status and health-related quality of life of teen-aged children who were extremely low birth weight and term controls. *Pediatrics* 105(3): 569-574.

Saigal S, Hoult LA, Streiner DL, Stoskopf BL, Rosenbaum PL. 2000c. School difficulties at adolescence in a regional cohort of children who were extremely low birth weight. *Pediatrics* 105(2):325-331.

Saigal S, Stoskopf BL, Streiner DL, Burrows E. 2001. Physical growth and current health status of infants who were extremely low birth weight and controls at adolescence. *Pediatrics* 108(2):407-415.

Saigal S, Rosenbaum P, Stoskopf B, Hoult L, Furlong W, Feeny D, Hagan R. 2005a. Development, reliability and validity of a new measure of overall health for pre-school children. *Quality of Life Research* 14(1):243-257.

Saigal S, Stoskopf B, Pinelli J, Boyle M, Streiner D, Hoult L, Goddeeris J. 2005b. Health status, health care utilization and physical ability of former extremely low birthweight (ELBW) and normal birthweight (NBW) infants at young adulthood (YA). *PAS Reporter* 57:1597.

Saigal S, Stoskopf B, Streiner D, Boyle M, Pinelli J, Paneth N, Goddeeris J. 2006a. Transition of extremely low-birth-weight infants from adolescence to young adulthood: Comparison with normal birth-weight controls. *JAMA* 295(6):667-675.

Saigal S, Stoskopf B, Pinelli J, Streiner D, Hoult L, Paneth N, Goddeeris J. 2006b. Self-perceived health-related quality of life of former extremely low birthweight infants at young adulthood. *Pediatrics* 118(3):1140-1148.

Saint-Anne Dargassies S. 1977. *Neurological Development of the Full-Term and Premature Neonate.* Amsterdam, the Netherlands: Elsevier/North Holland Biomedical Press.

Sakai M, Shiozaki A, Tabata M, Sasaki Y, Yoneda S, Arai T, Kato K, Yamakawa Y, Saito S. 2006. Evaluation of effectiveness of prophylactic cerclage of a short cervix according to interleukin-8 in cervical mucus. *American Journal of Obstetrics and Gynecology* 194(1): 14-19.

Salokorpi T, Rautio T, Sajaniemi N, Serenius-Sirve S, Tuomi H, Von Wendt L. 2001. Neurological development up to the age of four years of extremely low birthweight infants born in Southern Finland in 1991-1994 . *Acta Paediatrica, International Journal of Paediatrics* 90(2):218-221.

Saltvedt S, Almstrom H, Kublickas M, Reilly M, Valentin L, Grunewald C. 2004. Ultrasound dating at 12-14 or 15-20 weeks of gestation? A prospective cross-validation of established dating formulae in a population of in-vitro fertilized pregnancies randomized to early or late dating scan. *Ultrasound in Obstetrics and Gynecology* 24(1):42-50.

Samuelson JL, Buehler JW, Norris D, Sadek R. 2002. Maternal characteristics associated with place of delivery and neonatal mortality rates among very-low-birthweight infants, Georgia. *Paediatric and Perinatal Epidemiology* 16(4):305-313.

Sanchez PJ, Ahmed A. 2005. Toxoplasmosis, syphilis, malaria, and tuberculosis. In: Taeusch HW, Ballard RA, Gleason CA eds. *Avery's Diseases of the Newborn*, 8th edition. Philadelphia, PA: Elsevier Saunders. Pp. 530-550.

Sanchez-Ramos L, Kaunitz M, Gaudier FL, et al. 1999. Efficacy of maintenance therapy after acute tocolysis: A meta-analysis. *American Journal of Obstetrics and Gynecology* 181:484-490.

Sanchez-Ramos L, Kaunitz AM, Delke I. 2005. Progestational agents to prevent preterm birth: A meta-analysis of randomized controlled trials. *Obstetrics and Gynecology* 10(5): 273-279.

Sanders M, Allen M, Alexander GR, Yankowitz J, Graeber J, Jonson TRB, Repka MX. 1991. Gestational age assessment in preterm neonates weighing less than 1500 grams. *Pediatrics* 88(3):542-546.

Sanders MR, Donohue PK, Oberdorf MA, Rosenkrantz TS, Allen MC. 1998. Impact of the perception of viability on resource allocation in the neonatal intensive care unit. *Journal of Perinatology* 18(5):347-351.

Sanjose S, Roman E, Beral V. 1991. Low birthweight and preterm delivery, Scotland, 1981-1984: Effect of parents' occupation. *Lancet* 338(8764):428-431.

Sankaran K, Chiel LY, Walker R, Seshia M, Ohlsson A, the Canadian Neonatal Network. 2002. Variations in mortality rates among Canadian neonatal intensive care units. *Canadian Medical Association Journal* 166:173-178.

Sarason BR, Shearin EN, Pierce GR, Sarason IG. 1987. Interrelations of social support measures: Theoretical and practical implications. *Journal of Personality and Social Psychology* 52:813-832.

Sarnyai Z. 1998. Neurobiology of stress and cocaine addiction. Studies on corticotropin-releasing factor in rats, monkeys, and humans. *Annals of the New York Academy of Sciences* 851:371-387.

Satin AJ, Leveno KJ, Sherman ML, Reedy NJ, Lowe TW, McIntire DD. 1994. Maternal youth and pregnancy outcomes: Middle school versus high school age groups compared with women beyond the teen years. *American Journal of Obstetrics and Gynecology* 171(1): 184-187.

Saugstad OD. 1990. Oxygen toxicity in the neonatal period. *Acta Paediatrica Scandinavia* 79:881-892.

Saugstad OD. 2005. Oxygen for newborns: How much is too much? *Journal of Perinatology* 25(Suppl 2):S45-S49.

Saurel-Cubizolles MJ, Kaminski M. 1986. Work in pregnancy: Its evolving relationship with perinatal outcome. *Social Science and Medicine* 22(4):431-442.

Saurel-Cubizolles MJ, Subtil D, Kaminski M. 1991. Is preterm delivery still related to physical working conditions in pregnancy? *Journal of Epidemiology and Community Health* 45(1):29-34.

Saurel-Cubizolles MJ, Zeitlin J, Lelong N, Papiernik E, Di Renzo GC, Breart G. 2004. Employment, working conditions, and preterm birth: Results from the Europop case-control survey. *Journal of Epidemiology and Community Health* 58(5):395-401.

Sauve RS, Robertson C, Etches P, Byrne PJ, Dayer-Zamora V. 1998. Before viability: A geographically based outcome study of infants weighing 500 grams or less at birth. *Pediatrics* 101(3 I):438-445.

Savitz DA, Pastore LM. 1999. Causes of prematurity. In: McCormick MC, Siegel JE eds. *Prenatal Care: Effectiveness and Implementation.* Cambridge, UK: Cambridge University Press. Pp. 63-104.

Savitz DA, Whelan EA, Rowland AS, Kleckner RC. 1990. Maternal employment and reproductive risk factors. *American Journal of Epidemiology* 132(5):933-945.

Savitz, DA, Dole N, Terry, JW, Zhou H, Thorp JM. 2001. Smoking and pregnancy outcome among African-American and White women in Central North Carolina. *Epidemiology* 12:636-642.

Savitz DA, Henderson L, Dole N, Herring A, Wilkins DG, Rollins D, Thorp JM Jr. 2002a. Indicators of cocaine exposure and preterm birth. *Obstetrics and Gynecology* 99: 458-465.

Savitz DA, Terry JW Jr., Dole N, Thorp JM Jr., Maria Siega-Riz A, Herring AH. 2002b. Comparison of pregnancy dating by last menstrual period, ultrasound scanning, and their combination. *American Journal of Obstetrics and Gynecology* 187(6):1660-1666.

Savitz DA, Dole N, Herring AH, Kaczor D, Murphy J, Siega-Riz AM, Thorp JM Jr., MacDonald TL. 2005. Should spontaneous and medically indicated preterm births be separated for studying aetiology? *Paediatric and Perinatal Epidemiology* 19(2):97-105.

Sawicki G, Dakour J, Morrish DW. 2003. Functional proteomics of neurokinin B in the placenta indicates a novel role in regulating cytotrophoblast antioxidant defences. *Proteomics* 3(10):2044-2051.

Saxena MC, Siddiqui MK, Bhargava AK, Seth TD, Krishnamurti CR, Kutty D. 1980. Role of chlorinated hydrocarbon pesticides in abortions and premature labour. *Toxicology* 17:323-331.

Saxena MC, Siddiqui MK, Seth TD, Krishna Murti CR, Bhargava AK, Kutty D. 1981. Organochlorine pesticides in specimens from women undergoing spontaneous abortion, premature of full-term delivery. *Journal of Analytical Toxicology* 5:6-9.

Sayle AE, Savitz DA, Williams JF. 2003. Accuracy of reporting of sexual activity during late pregnancy. *Paediatric and Perinatal Epidemiology* 17(2):143-147.

Schaid DJ. 1999. Case-parents design for gene-environment interaction. *Genetic Epidemiology* 16(3):261-273.

Schaid DJ, Sommer SS. 1993. Genotype relative risks: Methods for design and analysis of candidate-gene association studies. *American Journal of Human Genetics* 53(5):1114-1126.

Schaid DJ, Rowland CM, Tines DE, Jacobson RM, Poland GA. 2002. Score tests for association between traits and haplotypes when linkage phase is ambiguous. *American Journal of Human Genetics* 70:425-434.

Schendel DE, Berg CJ, Yeargin-Allsopp M, Boyle CA, Decoufle P. 1996. Prenatal magnesium sulfate exposure and the risk for cerebral palsy or mental retardation among very low-birth-weight children aged 3 to 5 years. *JAMA* 276(22):1805-1810.

Scherjon SA, Kok JH, Oosting H, Wolf H, Zondervan HA. 1992. Fetal and neonatal cerebral circulation: A pulsed Doppler study. *Journal of Perinatal Medicine* 20(1):79-82.

Scherjon SA, Smolders-DeHaas H, Kok JH, Zondervan HA. 1993. The "brain-sparing" effect: Antenatal cerebral Doppler findings in relation to neurologic outcome in very preterm infants. *American Journal of Obstetrics and Gynecology* 169(1):169-175.

Scherjon S, Briët J, Oosting H, Kok J. 2000. The discrepancy between maturation of visual-evoked potentials and cognitive outcome at five years in very preterm infants with and without hemodynamic signs of fetal brain-sparing. *Pediatrics* 105(2):385-391.

Schieve LA, Cogswell ME, Scanlon KS, Perry G, Ferre C, Blackmore-Prince C, Yu SM, Rosenberg D. 2000. Prepregnancy body mass index and pregnancy weight gain: Associations with preterm delivery. *Obstetrics and Gynecology* 96(2):194-200.

Schieve LA, Rasmussen SA, Buck GM, Schendel DE, Reynolds MA, Wright VC. 2004. Are children born after assisted reproductive technology at increased risk for adverse health outcomes? *Obstetrics and Gynecology* 103(6):1154-1163.

Schlesinger ER. 1973. Neonatal intensive care: Planning for services and outcomes following care. *Journal of Pediatrics* 82(6):916-920.

Schlesinger M, Kornesbusch K. 1990. The failure of prenatal care policy for the poor. *Health Affairs* 91-111.

Schmidt B, Asztalos EV, Roberts RS, Robertson CMT, Sauve RS, Whitfield MF. 2003. Impact of bronchopulmonary dysplasia, brain injury, and severe retinopathy on the outcome of extremely low-birth-weight infants at 18 months: Results from the Trial of Indomethacin Prophylaxis in Preterms. *JAMA* (9):1124-1129.

Schmidt M, Sangild PT, Blum JW, Andersen JB, Greve T. 2004. Combined acth and glucocorticoid treatment improves survival and organ maturation in premature newborn calves. *Theriogenology* 61(9):1729-1744.

Schmitt SK, Sneed L, Phibbs CS. 2006. Costs of newborn care in California: A population-based study. *Pediatrics* 117:154-160.

Schneider ML, Moore CF, Kraemer GW, Roberts AD, DeJesus OT. 2002. The impact of prenatal stress, fetal alcohol exposure, or both on development: Perspectives from a primate model. *Psychoneuroendocrinology* 27(1-2):285-298.

Schoendorf KC, Hogue CJR, Kleinman JC, Rowley D. 1992. Mortality among infants of black as compared with white college-educated parents. *New England Journal of Medicine* 326(23):1522-1526.

Scholl TO, Johnson WG. 2000. Folic acid: Influence on the outcome of pregnancy. *American Journal of Clinical Nutrition* 71(5 Suppl):1295S-1303S.

Scholl TO, Hediger ML, Huang J, Johnson FE, Smith W, Ances IG. 1992. Young maternal age and parity influences on pregnancy outcome. *Annals of Epidemiology* 2(5):565-575.

Scholl TO, Hediger ML, Belsky DH. 1994. Prenatal care and maternal health during adolescent pregnancy: A review and meta-analysis. *Journal of Adolescent Health* 15(6): 444-456.

Scholl TO, Hediger ML, Schall JI, Khoo C-S, Fischer RL. 1996. Erratum: Dietary and serum folate: Their influence on the outcome of pregnancy. *American Journal of Clinical Nutrition* 64(6):984.

Schulkin J. 1999. Corticotropin-releasing hormone signals adversity in both the placenta and the brain: Regulation by glucocorticoids and allostatic overload. *Journal of Endocrinology* 161(3):349-356.

Schulte HM, Weisner D, Allolio B. 1990. The corticotropin releasing hormone test in late pregnancy: Lack of an adrenocorticotropin and cortisol response. *Clinical Endocrinology* 33:99-106.

Schultheiss TM, Xydas S, Lassar AB. 1995. Induction of avian cardiac myogenesis by anterior endoderm. *Development* 121(12):4203-4214.

Scott SM, Watterberg KL. 1995. Effect of gestational age, postnatal age, and illness on plasma cortisol concentrations in premature infants. *Pediatric Research* 37(1):112-116.

Sebire NJ, Jolly M, Harris JP, Wadsworth J, Joffe M, Beard RW, Regan L, Robinson S. 2001. Maternal obesity and pregnancy outcome: A study of 287,213 pregnancies in London. *International Journal of Obesity* 25(8):1175-1182.

Senat MV, Minoui S, Multon O, Fernandez H, Frydman R, Ville Y. 1998. Effect of dexamethasone and betamethasone on fetal heart rate variability in preterm labour: A randomised study. *British Journal of Obstetrics and Gynaecology* 105(7):749-755.

Serdula M, Williamson DF, Kendrick JS, Anda RF, Byers T. 1991. Trends in alcohol consumption by pregnant women. 1985 through 1988. *JAMA* 265(7):876-879.

Shaddish WR, Cook TD, Campbell DT. 2002. *Experimental and Quasi Experimental Designs for Generalized Causal Inference*. Boston, MA: Houghton Mifflin.

Shah S, Ohlsson A. 2006. Ibuprofen for the prevention of patent ductus arteriosus in preterm and/or low birth weight infants. *Cochrane Review*s 1.

Shah P, Shah V. 2004. Arginine supplementation for prevention of necrotising enterocolitis in preterm infants. *Cochrane Database of Systematic Reviews (Online: Update Software)* 4.

Shah V, Ohlsson A, Halliday HL, Dunn, MS. 2002. Early administration of inhaled corticosteroids for preventing chronic lung disease in ventilated very low birth weight preterm neonates. *Cochrane Review*s 3.

Shalev B, Farr AK, Repka MX. 2001. Randomized comparison of diode laser photocoagulation versus cryotherapy for threshold retinopathy of prematurity: Seven-year outcome. *American Journal of Ophthalmology* 132(1):76-80.

Shankar R, Gude N, Cullinane F, Brennecke S, Purcell AW, Moses EK. 2005. An emerging role for comprehensive proteome analysis in human pregnancy research. *Reproduction* 129(6):685-696.

Shankaran S, Papile L-A, Wright LL, Ehrenkranz RA, Mele L, Lemons JA, Korones SB, Stevenson DK, Donovan EF, Stoll BJ, Fanaroff AA, Oh W, Verter J, Taylor GA, Seibert J, DiPietro M. 1997. The effect of antenatal phenobarbital therapy on neonatal intracranial hemorrhage in preterm infants. *New England Journal of Medicine* 337(7):466-471.

Shankaran S, Papile L-A, Wright LL, Ehrenkranz RA, Mele L, Lemons JA, Korones SB, Stevenson DK, Donovan EF, Stoll BJ, Fanaroff AA, Oh W, Verter J. 2002. Neurodevelopmental outcome of premature infants after antenatal phenobarbital exposure. *American Journal of Obstetrics and Gynecology* 187(1):171-177.

Shaw GM. 2003. Strenuous work, nutrition and adverse pregnancy outcomes: A brief review. *Journal of Nutrition* 133(5):1718S-1721S.

Shaw GM, Carmichael SL, Nelson V, Selvin S, Schaffer DM. 2004. Occurrence of low birthweight and preterm delivery among California infants before and after compulsory food fortification with folic acid. *Public Health Reports* 119(2):170-173.

Shennan A, Crawshaw S, Briley A, Hawken J, Seed P, Jones G, Poston LA. 2006. Randomised controlled trial of metronidazole for the prevention of preterm birth in women positive for cervicovaginal fetal fibronectin: The PREMET Study. *BJOG: An International Journal of Obstetrics and Gynaecology* 113:65-74.

Shepard PM. 1994. Issues of community empowerment. *Fordham Urban Law Journal* 21(3):739-755.

Shevell T, Malone FD, Vidaver J, Porter TF, Luthy DA, Comstock CH, Hankins GD, Eddleman K, Dolan S, Dugoff L, Craigo S, Timor IE, Carr SR, Wolfe HM, Bianchi DW, D'Alton ME. 2005. Assisted reproductive technology and pregnancy outcome. *Obstetrics and Gynecology* 106(5 I):1039-1045.

Shi MM. 2002. Technologies for individual genotyping: Detection of genetic polymorphisms in drug targets and disease genes. *American Journal of PharmacoGenomics* 2(3): 197-205.

Shinwell ES, Karplus M, Reich D, Weintraub Z, Blazer S, Bader D, Yurman S, Dolfin T, Kogan A, Dollberg S, Arbel E, Goldberg M, Gur I, Naor N, Sirota L, Mogilner S, Zaritsky A, Barak M, Gottfried E. 2000. Early postnatal dexamethasone treatment and increased incidence of cerebral palsy. *Archives of Disease in Childhood: Fetal and Neonatal Edition* 83(3):F177-F181.

Shiono PH, Klebanoff MA, Nugent RP, Cotch MF, Wilkins DG, Rollins DE, Carey JC, Behrman RE. 1995. The impact of cocaine and marijuana use on low birth weight and preterm birth: A multicenter study. *American Journal of Obstetrics and Gynecology* 172(1):19-27.

Shiono PH, Rauh VA, Park M, Lederman SA, Zuskar D. 1997. Ethnic differences in birthweight: The role of lifestyle and other factors. *American Journal of Public Health* 87(5):787-793.

Shortell SM, Zimmerman JE, Rousseau DM, Gillies RR, Wagner DP, Draper EA, Knaus WA, Duffy J. 1994. The performance of intensive care units: Does good management make a difference? *Medical Care* 32(5):508-525.

Shubert P, Diss E, and Iams JD. 1992. Etiology of preterm premature rupture of membranes. *Obstetrics and Gynecology Clinics of North America* 19:251-263.

Shukla H, Atakent YS, Ferrara A, Topsis J, Antoine C. 1987. Postnatal overestimation of gestational age in preterm infants. *American Journal of Diseases of Children* 141(10): 1106-1107.

Shults RA, Arndt V, Olshan AF, Martin CF, Royce RA. 1999. Effects of short interpregnancy intervals on small-for-gestational age and preterm births. *Epidemiology* 10:250-254.

Shumway J, O'Campo P, Gielen A, Witter FR, Khouzami AN, Blakemore KJ. 1999. Preterm labor, placental abruption, and premature rupture of membranes in relation to maternal violence or verbal abuse. *Journal of Maternal and Fetal Medicine* 8(3):76-80.

Siega-Riz AM, Adair LS, Hobel CJ. 1994. Institute of Medicine maternal weight gain recommendations and pregnancy outcome in a predominantly Hispanic population. *Obstetrics and Gynecology* 84:565-73.

Siega-Riz AM, Adair LS, Hobel CJ. 1996. Maternal underweight status and inadequate rate of weight gain during the third trimester of pregnancy increases the risk of preterm delivery. *Journal of Nutrition* 126(1):146-153.

Siega-Riz AM, Promislow JH, Savitz DA, Thorp JM Jr, McDonald T. 2003. Vitamin C intake and the risk of preterm delivery. *American Journal of Obstetrics and Gynecology* 189:519-525.

Siega-Riz AM, Savitz DA, Zeisel SH, Thorp JM, Herring A. 2004. Second trimester folate status and preterm birth. *American Journal of Obstetrics and Gynecology* 191:1851-1857.

Silbergeld EK, Patrick TE. 2005. Environmental exposures, toxicologic mechanisms, and adverse pregnancy outcomes. *American Journal of Obstetrics and Gynecology* 192: S11-S21.

Silva MJ, Barr DB, Reidy JA, Malek NA, Hodge CC, Caudill SP, Brock JW, Needham LL, Calafat AM. 2004. Urinary levels of seven phthalate metabolites in the U.S. population from the National Health and Nutrition Examination Survey (NHANES) 1999-2000. *Environmental Health Perspectives* 112(3):331-338.

Silverman WA. 1980. *Retrolental Fibroplasia: A Modern Parable. Monographs in Neonatology.* New York: Grune and Stratton.

Silverman WA. 1998. *Where's the Evidence? Debates in Modern Medicine.* Oxford, UK: Oxford University Press.

Simhan HN, Krohn MA, Roberts JM, Zeevi A, Caritis SN. 2003. Interleukin-6 promoter -174 polymorphism and spontaneous preterm birth. *American Journal of Obstetrics and Gynecology* 189(4):915-918.

Singer LT, Fulton S, Davillier M, Koshy D Salvator A, Baley JE. 2003. Effects of infant risk status and maternal psychological distress on maternal-infant interactions during the first year of life. *Journal of Developmental and Behavioral Pediatrics* 24(4):233-241.

Singer LTP, Salvator AM, Guo SP, Collin MM, Lilien LM, Baley JM. 1999. Maternal psychological distress and parenting stress after the birth of a very low-birth-weight infant. *JAMA* 281(9):799-805.

Singhal A, Fewtrell M, Cole TJ, Lucas A. 2003a. Low nutrient intake and early growth for later insulin resistance in adolescents born preterm. *Lancet* 361(9363):1089-1097.

Singhal A, Wells J, Cole TJ, Fewtrell M, Lucas A. 2003b. Programming of lean body mass: A link between birth weight, obesity, and cardiovascular disease? *American Journal of Clinical Nutrition* 77(3):726-730.

Singhal A, Cole TJ, Fewtrell M, Deanfield J, Lucas A. 2004. Is slower early growth beneficial for long-term cardiovascular health? *Circulation* 109(9):1108-1113.

Slattery MM, Morrison JJ. 2002. Preterm delivery. *Lancet* 360(9344):1489-1497.

Smaill F. 2001. Antibiotics for asymptomatic bacteriuria in pregnancy. *Cochrane Database of Systematic Reviews* 2.

Smith D, Hernandez-Avila M, Tellez-Rojo MM, Mercado A, Hu H. 2002. The relationship between lead in plasma and whole blood in women. *Environmental Health Perspectives* 110:263-268.

Smith GC, Pell JP, Dobbie R. 2003. Interpregnancy interval and risk of preterm birth and neonatal death: Retrospective cohort study. *British Medical Journal* 327:9.

Smith GN, Walker MC, McGrath MJ. 1999. Randomised, double-blind, placebo controlled pilot study assessing nitroglycerin as a tocolytic. *British Journal of Obstetrics and Gynaecology* 106:736-739.

Smith R, Mesiano S, McGrath S. 2002. Hormone trajectories leading to human birth. *Regulatory Peptides* 108:195-264.

Smith VC, Zupancic JAF, McCormick MC, Croen LA, Greene J, Escobar GJ, Richardson DK. 2005. Trends in severe bronchopulmonary dysplasia rates between 1994 and 2002. *Journal of Pediatrics* 146(4):469-473.

So, T. 1993. The role of matrix metalloproteinases for premature rupture of membranes. *Nippon Sanka Fujinka Gakkai Zasshi* 45:227-233.

Sola A, Wen T-C, Hamrick SEG, Ferriero DM. 2005. Potential for protection and repair following injury to the developing brain: A role for erythropoietin? *Pediatrics Research* 57(5 Pt 2):110R-117R.

Soll RF. 2002a. Prophylactic synthetic surfactant for preventing morbidity and mortality in preterm infants. *Cochrane Reviews* 3.

Soll RF. 2002b Prophylactic natural surfactant for preventing morbidity and mortality in preterm infants. *Cochrane Reviews* 3.

Soll RF. 2002c. Synthetic surfactant for respiratory distress syndrome in preterm infants. *Cochrane Reviews* 3.

Soll RF, Morley C. 2001. Prophylactic versus selective use of surfactant for preventing morbidity and mortality in preterm infants. *Cochrane Reviews* 2.

Sommerfelt K, Pedersen S, Ellertsen B, Markestad T. 1996. Transient dystonia in non-handicapped low-birthweight infants and later neurodevelopment. *Acta Paediatrica, International Journal of Paediatrics* 85(12):1445-1449.

Sooranna SR, Lee Y, Kim LU, Mohan AR. Bennett PR, Johnson MR. 2004. Mechanical stretch activates type 2 cyclooxygenase via activator protein-1 transcription factor in human myometrial cells. *Molecular Human Reproduction* 10:109-113.

Sooranna SR, Engineer N, Loudon JA, Terzidou V, Bennett PR, Johnson MR. 2005. The mitogen-activated protein kinase dependent expression of prostaglandin H synthase-2 and interleukin-8 messenger ribonucleic acid by myometrial cells: The differential effect of stretch and interleukin-1b. *Journal of Clinical Endocrinology and Metabolism* 90: 3517-3527.

Sosa C, Althabe F, Belizn J, Bergel E. 2004. Bed rest in singleton pregnancies for preventing preterm birth. *Cochrane Database of Systematic Reviews* 1.

Spellacy WN, Buhi WC. 1972. Amniotic fluid lecithin-sphingomyelin ratio as an index of fetal maturity. *Obstetrics and Gynecology* 39(6):852-860.

Spencer B, Thomas H, Morris J. 1989. A randomized controlled trial of the provision of a social support service during pregnancy: The South Manchester Family Worker Project. *British Journal of Obstetrics and Gynaecology* 96(3):281-288.

Spielman RS, McGinnis RE, Ewens WJ. 1993. Transmission test for linkage disequilibrium: The insulin gene region and insulin-dependent diabetes mellitus (IDDM). *American Journal of Human Genetics* 52(3):506-516.

Spinello A, Nicola S, Piazzi G, Ghazol K, Colonna L, Baltar G. 1994. Epidemiological correlates of preterm premature rupture of membranes. *International Journal of Gynecology and Obstetrics* 47(1):7-15.

Spinnato JA, Sibai BM, Shaver DC, Anderson GD. 1984. Inaccuracy of Dubowitz gestational age in low birth weight infants. *Obstetrics and Gynecology* 63(4):491-495.

Spohr HL, Willms J, Steinhausen HC. 1993. Prenatal alcohol exposure and long-term developmental consequences. *Lancet* 341:907-910.

Spong C, Meis PJ, Thom EA, et al. 2005. Progesterone for prevention of recurrent preterm birth: Impact of gestational age at previous delivery. *American Journal of Obstetrics and Gynecology* 193:1127-11131.

Sram RJ, Benes I, Binkova B, Dejmek J, Horstman D, Kotesovec F, Otto D, Perreault SD, Rubes J, Selevan SG, Skalik I, Stevens RK, Lewtas J. 1996. Teplice program—the impact of air pollution on human health. *Environmental Health Perspectives* 104(Suppl 4): 699-714.

Sram RJ, Binkova B, Dejmek J, Bobak M. 2005. Ambient air pollution and pregnancy outcomes: A review of the literature. *Environmental Health Perspectives* 113:375-382.

Sreenan C, Etches PC, Demianczuk N, Robertson CMT. 2001. Isolated mental developmental delay in very low birth weight infants: Association with prolonged doxapram therapy for apnea. *Journal of Pediatrics* 139(6):832-837.

SSA (U.S. Social Security Administration). 2005a. *Children Receiving SSI, 2004.* [Online]. Available: http://www.ssa.gov/policy/docs/statcomps/ssi_children/2004/ [accessed January 30, 2006].

SSA. 2005b. *Supplemental Security Income.* [Online]. Available: http://www.ssa.gov/notices/ supplemental-security-income/ [accessed January 30, 2006].

SSA. 2005c. *Title XVI Only Disabled Child Claims Applications Filed 1995-2004. Title XVI Disability Research File.* Obtained from the SSA Office of Disability Programs.

SSA. 2005d. *FY 2006 Budget Appendix.* [Online]. Available: http://www.ssa.gov/budget/ app06.pdf [accessed May 10, 2006].

Stancil TR, Hertz-Picciotto I, Schramm M, Watt-Morse M. 2000. Stress and pregnancy among African-American women. *Paediatric and Perinatal Epidemiology* 14(2):127-135.

Stanley FJ, Watson L. 1992. Trends in perinatal mortality and cerebral palsy in Western Australia, 1967 to 1985. *British Medical Journal* 304(6843):1658-1663.

Stanley FJ, Blair E, Alberman E. 2000. Cerebral palsies: Epidemiology and causal pathways. *Clinics in Developmental Medicine* 151.

Stark AR, Carlo WA, Tyson JE, Papile L-A, Wright LL, Shankaran S, Donovan EF, Oh W, Bauer CR, Saha S, Poole WK, Stoll BJ. 2001. Adverse effects of early dexamethasone treatment in extremely-low-birth-weight infants. *New England Journal of Medicine* 344(2):95-101.

Starr A, Amlie RN, Martin WH, Sanders S. 1977. Development of auditory function in newborn infants revealed by auditory brainstem potentials. *Pediatrics* 60(6):831-839.

Steer RA, Scholl TO, Hediger ML, Fischer RL. 1992. Self-reported depression and negative pregnancy outcomes. *Journal of Clinical Epidemiology* 45(10):1093-1099.

Stein A, Campbell EA, Day A, Mcpherson K, Cooper PJ. 1987. Social adversity, low birth weight, and preterm delivery. *British Medical Journal (Clinical Research Edition)* 295(6593):291-293.

Stein JA, Lu MC, Gelberg L. 2000. Severity of homelessness and adverse birth outcomes. *Health Psychology* 19(6):524-534.

Stephenson C, Lockwood C, Ma Y, Guller S. 2005. Thrombin-dependent regulation of matrix metalloproteinase (MMP-9) levels in human fetal membranes. *Journal of Maternal–Fetal and Neonatal Medicine* 18(1):17-22.

Sternfeld B. 1997. Physical activity and pregnancy outcome. Review and recommendations. *Sports Medicine* 23(1):33-47.

Stevens B, Ohlsson A. 2000. Sucrose for analgesia in newborn infants undergoing painful procedures. *Cochrane Database of Systematic Reviews (Online: Update Software)* 2.

Stevens B, Yamada J, Ohlsson A. 2004. Sucrose for analgesia in newborn infants undergoing painful procedures. *Cochrane Database of Systematic Reviews (Online: Update Software)* 3.

Stevens B, Yamada J, Beyene J, Gibbins S, Petryshen P, Stinson J, Narciso J. 2005. Consistent management of repeated procedural pain with sucrose in preterm neonates: Is it effective and safe for repeated use over time? *Clinical Journal of Pain* 21(6):543-548.

Stevens TP, Blennow M, Soll RF. 2002. Early surfactant administration with brief ventilation vs. selective surfactant and continued mechanical ventilation for preterm infants with or at risk for rds. *Cochrane Database of Systematic Reviews (Online: Update Software)* 2.

Stevenson DK, Wong RJ, Vreman HJ. 2005. Reduction in hospital readmission rates for hyperbilirubinemia is associated with use of transcutaneous bilirubin measurements. *Clinical Chemistry* 51(3):481-482.

Stewart A, Pezzani-Goldsmith N. 1994. *The Newborn Infant. One Brain for Life.* Paris, France: Les Editions INSERM.

Stewart JD, Gonzalez CL,Christensen HD, et al. 1997. Impact of multiple antenatal doses of betamethasone on growth and development of mice offspring. *American Journal of Obstetrics and Gynecology* 177(5):1138-1144.

Stjernqvist KM. 1992. Extremely low birthweight infants less than 901g: Impact on the family during the first year. *Scandinavian Journal of Social Medicine* 20(4):226-233.

Stjernqvist K, Svenningsen NW. 1995. Extremely low-birth-weight infants less than 901 g: Development and behaviour after 4 years of life. *Acta Paediatrica, International Journal of Paediatrics* 84(5):500-506.

St John EB, Carlo WA. 2003. Respiratory distress syndrome in VLBW infants: Changes in management and outcomes observed by the NICHD Neonatal Research Network. *Seminars in Perinatology* 27:288-292.

Stoll BJ, Gordon T, Korones SB, Shankaran S, Tyson JE, Bauer CR, Fanaroff AA, Lemons JA, Donovan EF, Oh W, Stevenson DK, Ehrenkranz RA, Papile L-A, Verter J, Wright LL. 1996. Late-onset sepsis in very low birth weight neonates: A report from the national institute of child health and human development neonatal research network. *Journal of Pediatrics* 129(1):63-71.

Stoll BJM, Hansen NIM, Adams-Chapman IM, Fanaroff AAM, Hintz SRM, Vohr BM, Higgins RDM, for the National Institute of Child Health and Human Development Neonatal Research Network. 2004. Neurodevelopmental and growth impairment among extremely low-birth-weight infants with neonatal infection. *JAMA* 292(19):2357-2365.

STOP-ROP (Supplemental Therapeutic Oxygen for Prethreshold Retinopathy of Prematurity). 2000. STOP-ROP, a randomized, controlled trial. I: Primary outcomes. *Pediatrics* 105(2):295-310.

Strauss RS. 2000. Adult functional outcome of those born small for gestational age: Twenty-six-year follow-up of the 1970 British Birth Cohort. *JAMA* 283(5):625-632.

Stromme P, Hagberg G. 2000. Aetiology in severe and mild mental retardation: A population-based study of Norwegian children. *Developmental Medicine and Child Neurology* 42(2):76-86.

Super M, Heese HDV, MacKenzie D, Dempster WS, Plessis JD, Ferreira JJ. 1981. An epidemiological study of well-water nitrates in a group of south west african/namibian infants. *Water Research* 15:1265-1270.

Susser M, Susser E. 1996. Choosing a future for epidemiology: II. From black box to Chinese boxes and ecoepidemiology. *American Journal of Public Health* 86:674-677.

Symington A, Pinelli J. 2006. Developmental care for promoting development and preventing morbidity in preterm infants. *Cochrane Reviews* 1.

Synnes AR, Chien LY, Peliowski A, Baboolal R, Lee SK and the Canadian NICU Network. 2001. Variation in intraventricular hemorrhage incident rates among Canadian intensive care units. *Journal of Pediatrics* 138:525-531.

Szatmari P, Saigal S, Rosenbaum P, Campbell D, King S. 1990. Psychiatric disorders at five years among children with birthweights <1000 g: A regional perspective. *Developmental Medicine and Child Neurology* 32(11):954-962.

Szekeres-Bartho J. 2002. Immunological relationship between the mother and the fetus. *International Reviews of Immunology* 21:471-495.

Szymonowicz W, Walker AM, Yu YV, Stewart ML, Cannata J, Cussen L. 1990. Regional cerebral blood flow after hemorrhagic hypotension in the preterm, near-term, and newborn lamb. *Pediatrics Research* 28:361-366.

Taeusch HW, Ballard RA, Gleason CA eds. 2005. *Avery's Diseases of the Newborn*, 8th edition. Philadelphia, PA: Elsevier Saunders.

Taffel S. 1980. Factors associated with low birth weight. United States, 1976. *Vital and Health Statistics. Series 21, Data from the National Vital Statistics System* (37):1-37.

Taipale P, Hiilesmaa V. 1998. Sonographic measurement of uterine cervix at 18-22 weeks' gestation and the risk of preterm delivery. *Obstetrics and Gynecology* 92(6):902-907.

Tasi HJ, Kho JY, Shaikh N, Choudhry S, Naqvi M, Navarro D, Matallana H, Castro R, Lilly CM, Watson HG, Meade K, LeNoir M, Thyne S, Ziv E, Burchard EG. 2006. Admixture-matched case-control study: A practical approach for genetic association studies in admixed populations. *Human Genetics* 118:626-639.

Taylor ES. 1985. Discussion of Main DM, Gabbe SG, Richardson D et al. *American Journal of Obstetrics and Gynecology* 151:892.

Taylor HG, Hack M, Klein NK. 1998. Attention deficits in children with <750 gm birth weight. *Child Neuropsychology* 4(1):21-34.

Taylor HG, Klein N, Minich NM, Hack M. 2000. Middle-school-age outcomes in children with very low birthweight. *Child Development* 71(6):1495-1511.

Taylor HG, Klein N, Minich NM, Hack M. 2001. Long-term family outcomes for children with very low birth weights. *Archives of Pediatrics and Adolescent Medicine* 155(2):155-161.

Taylor PR, Lawrence CE, Hwang HL, Paulson AS. 1984. Polychlorinated biphenyls: Influence on birthweight and gestation. *American Journal of Public Health* 74:1153-1154.

Taylor PR, Stelma JM, Lawrence CE. 1989. The relation of polychlorinated biphenyls to birth weight and gestational age in the offspring of occupationally exposed mothers. *American Journal of Epidemiology* 129:395-406.

Taylor SE. 2006. Social support. In: Friedman HS, Silver RC eds. *Oxford Handbook of Health Psychology*. New York: Oxford University Press.

Taylor SE, Repetti RL. 1997. Health psychology: What is an unhealthy environment and how does it get under the skin? *Annual Review of Psychology* 48:411-447.

Teixeira JM, Fisk NM, Glover V. 1999. Association between maternal anxiety in pregnancy and increased uterine artery resistance index: Cohort based study. *British Medical Journal* 318(7177):153-157.

Teramo K, Hallman M, Raivio KO. 1980. Maternal glucocorticoid in unplanned premature labor. Controlled study on the effects of betamethasone phosphate on the phospholipids of the gastric aspirate and on the adrenal cortical function of the newborn infant. *Pediatrics Research* 14:326-329.

Terrone DA, Smith LG Jr., Wolf EJ, Uzbay LA, Sun S, Miller RC. 1997. Neonatal effects and serum cortisol levels after multiple courses of maternal corticosteroids. *Obstetrics and Gynecology* 90(5):819-823.

Terrone DA, Rinehart BK, Rhodes PG, Roberts WE, Miller RC, Martin Jr. JN, Moawad AH, Carpenter RJ, Hill WC, Wagner A. 1999. Multiple courses of betamethasone to enhance fetal lung maturation do not suppress neonatal adrenal response. *American Journal of Obstetrics and Gynecology* 180(6 I):1349-1353.

Terzidoo V, Sooranna SR, Kim LU, Thorton S, Bennett PR, Johnson MR. 2005. Mechanical stretch up-regulates the human oxytocin receptor in primary human uterine myocytes. *Journal of Clinical Endocrinology Metabolism* 90:237-246.

Therien JM, Worwa CT, Mattia FR, deRegnier R-AO. 2004. Altered pathways for auditory discrimination and recognition memory in preterm infants. *Developmental Medicine and Child Neurology* 46(12):816-824.

Theunissen NCM, Veen S, Fekkes M, Koopman HM, Zwinderman K. 2001. Quality of life in preschool children born preterm. *Developmental Medicine and Child Neurology* 43: 460-465.

Thibeault DW, Mabry S, Rezaiekhaligh M. 1990. Neonatal pulmonary oxygen toxicity in the rat and lung changes. *Pediatric Pulmonology* 9:96-108.

Thibeault DW, Mabry SM, Ekekezie I, Truog WE. 2000. Lung elastic tissue maturation and perturbations during the evolution of chronic lung disease. *Pediatrics* 106:1452.

Thoits PA. 1995. Stress, coping, and social support processes: Where are we? What next? *Journal of Health and Social Behavior* Spec No:53-79.

Thoman EB, Ingersoll EW, Acebo C. 1991. Premature infants seek rhythmic stimulation, and the experience facilitates neurobehavioral development. *Journal of Developmental and Behavioral Pediatrics* 12(1):11-18.

Thomas M, Greenough A, Morton M. 2003. Prolonged ventilation and intact survival in very low birth weight infants. *European Journal of Pediatrics* 162(2):65-67.

Thome UH, Carlo WA. 2002. Permissive hypercapnia. *Seminars in Neonatology* 7(5): 409-419.

Thorp JA, Gaston L, Caspers DR, Pal ML. 1995. Current concepts and controversies in the use of vitamin K. *Drugs* 49(3):376-387.

Thurin A, Hausken J, Hillensjo T, Jablonowska B, Pinborg A, Strandell A, Bergh C. 2004. Elective single-embryo transfer versus double-embryo transfer in in vitro fertilization. *New England Journal of Medicine* 351(23):2392-2402.

Tideman E, Ley D, Bjerre I, Forslund M. 2001. Longitudinal follow-up of children born preterm: Somatic and mental health, self-esteem and quality of life at age 19. *Early Human Development* 61(2):97-110.

Tilford JM, Robbins JM, Hobbes CA. 2001. Improving estimates of caregiver time cost and family impact associated with birth defects. *Teratology* 64:S37-S41.

Timor-Tritsch IE, Farine D, Rosen MG. 1988. A close look at early embryonic development with the high-frequency transvaginal transducer. *American Journal of Obstetrics and Gynecology* 159(3):676-681.

Tin W. 2002. Oxygen therapy: 50 years of uncertainty. *Pediatrics* 110(3):615-616.

Tin W, Wariyar U. 2002. Giving small babies oxygen: 50 years of uncertainty. *Seminars in Neonatology* 7(5):361-367.

To MS, Alfirevic Z, Heath VCF, Cicero S, Cacho AM, Williamson PR, Nicolaides KH. 2004. Cervical cerclage for prevention of preterm delivery in women with short cervix: Randomised controlled trial. *Lancet* 363(9424):1849-1853.

Tommiska V, Heinonen K, Kero P, Pokela M-L, Tammela O, Jarvenpaa A-L, Salokorpi T, Virtanen M, Fellman V, Marlow N. 2003. A national two year follow up study of extremely low birthweight infants born in 1996-1997. *Archives of Disease in Childhood: Fetal and Neonatal Edition* 88(1): F29-F35.

Torday JS, Rehan VK. 2003. Testing for fetal lung maturation: A biochemical "window" to the developing fetus. *Clinics in Laboratory Medicine* 23(2):361-383.

Torrance GW, Furlong W, Feeny D, Boyle M. 1995. Multi-attribute preference functions. Health utilities index. *PharmacoEconomics* 7:503-520.

Torres-Sanchez LE, Berkowitz G, Lopez-Carrillo L, Torres-Arreola L, Rios C, Lopez-Cervantes M. 1999. Intrauterine lead exposure and preterm birth. *Environmental Research* 81(4): 297-301.

Tourangeau AE, Cranley LA, Jeffs L. 2006. Impact of nursing on hospital patient mortality: A focused review and related policy implications. *Quality and Safety in Health Care* 15(1):4-8.

Towers CV, Bonebrake R, Padilla G, Rumney P. 2000. The effect of transport on the rate of severe intraventricular hemorrhage in very low birth weight infants. *Obstetrics and Gynecology* 95(2):291-295.

Treloar SA, Macones GA, Mitchell LE, Martin NG. 2000. Genetic influences on premature parturition in an Australian twin sample. *Twin Research* 3(2):80-82.

Tsai SS, Yu HS, Liu CC, Yang CY. 2003. Increased incidence of preterm delivery in mothers residing in an industrialized area in Taiwan. *Journal of Toxicology and Environmental Health* A(66):987-994.

Tsai SS, Chen CC, Hsieh HJ, Chang CC, Yang CY. 2006. Air pollution and postneonatal mortality in a tropical city: Kaohsiung, Taiwan. *Inhalation Toxicology* 18(3):185-189.

Tsuji M, Saul JP, du Plessis A, Eichenwald E, Sobh J, Crocker R, Volpe JJ. 2000. Cerebral intravascular oxygenation correlates with mean arterial pressure in critically ill premature infants. *Pediatrics* 106:625-632.

Tudehope DI, Burns YR, Gray PH, Mohay HA, O'Callaghan MJ, Rogers YM. 1995. Changing patterns of survival and outcome at 4 years of children who weighed 500-999 g at birth. *Journal of Paediatrics and Child Health* 31(5):451-456.

Tuntiseranee P, Geater A, Chongsuvivatwong V, Kor-anantakul O. 1998. The effect of heavy maternal workload on fetal growth retardation and preterm delivery a study among southern Thai women. *Journal of Occupational and Environmental Medicine* 40(11):1013-1021.

Turner RJ, Grindstaff CF, Phillips N. 1990. Social support and outcome in teenage pregnancy. *Journal of Health and Social Behavior* 31(1):43-57.

Tuthill RW, Giusti RA, Moore GS, Calabrese EJ. 1982. Health effects among newborns after prenatal exposure to cio2-disinfected drinking water. *Environmental Health Perspectives* 46:39-45.

Tyson JE, Kennedy K, Broyles S, Rosenfeld CR. 1995. The small for gestational age infant: Accelerated or delayed pulmonary maturation? Increased or decreased survival? *Pediatrics* 95(4):534-538.

Tyson JE, Younes N, Verter J, Wright LL. 1996. Viability, morbidity, and resource use among newborns of 501- to 800-g birth weight. *JAMA* 276(20):1645-1651.

Ugwumadu A, Manyonda I, Reid F, Hay P. 2003. Effect of early oral clindamycin on late miscarriage and preterm delivery in asymptomatic women with abnormal vaginal flora and bacterial vaginosis: A randomised controlled trial. *Lancet* 361:983-988.

Umbach DM. 2000. Invited commentary: On studying the joint effects of candidate genes and exposures. *American Journal of Epidemiology* 152(8):701-703.

UNICEF, WHO (United Nations Children's Fund, World Health Organization). 2004. *Low Birthweight: Country, Regional, and Global Estimates.* New York: United Nations Children's Fund.

Usher R, McLean F. 1969. Intrauterine growth of live-born Caucasian infants at sea level: Standards obtained from measurements in 7 dimensions of infants born between 25 and 44 weeks of gestation. *Journal of Pediatrics* 74(6):901-910.

Uthaya S, Thomas EL, Hamilton G, Doré CJ, Bell J, Modi N. 2005. Altered adiposity after extremely preterm birth. *Pediatric Research* 57(2):211-215.

Vadillo-Ortega F, Sadowsky D, Haluska G, Hernandez-Guerrero C, Guevara-Silva R, Gravett MG, Novy MJ. 2002. Identification of matrix metalloproteinase-9 in amniotic fluid and amniochorion in spontaneous labor and after experimental intrauterine infection or interleukin1B infusion in pregnant rhesus monkeys. *American Journal of Obstetrics and Gynecology* 186:128-138.

Vamvakas EC, Strauss RG. 2001. Meta-analysis of controlled clinical trials studying the efficacy of rHuEPO in reducing blood transfusions in the anemia of prematurity. *Transfusion* 41(3):406-415.

Van Den Bergh BRH, Marcoen A. 2004. High antenatal maternal anxiety is related to ADHD symptoms, externalizing problems, and anxiety in 8- and 9-year-olds. *Child Development* 75(4):1085-1097.

Van Den Bergh BRH, Mennes M, Oosterlaan J, Stevens V, Stiers P, Marcoen A, Lagae L. 2005. High antenatal maternal anxiety is related to impulsivity during performance on cognitive tasks in 14- and 15-year-olds. *Neuroscience and Biobehavioral Reviews* 29(2):259-269.

Van Den Hout BM, Stiers P, Haers M, Van Der Schouw YT, Eken P, Vandenbussche E, Van Nieuwenhuizen O, De Vries LS. 2000. Relation between visual perceptual impairment and neonatal ultrasound diagnosis of haemorrhagic ischaemic brain lesions in 5-year-old children. *Developmental Medicine and Child Neurology* 42(6):376-386.

Vander JF, Handa J, McNamara JA, Trese M, Spencer R, Repka MX, Rubsamen P, Li H, Morse LS, Tasman WS, Flynn JT. 1997. Early treatment of posterior retinopathy of prematurity: A controlled trial. *Ophthalmology* 104(11):1731-1736.

Van Dijk M, Mulders J, Poutsma A, Konst AA, Lachmeijer AM, Dekker GA, Blankenstein MA, Oudejans CBM. 2005. Maternal segregation of the Dutch preeclampsia locus at 10q22 with a new member of the winged helix gene family. *Nature Genetics* 37:514-519.

Van Meurs KP, Wright LL, Ehrenkranz RA, Lemons JA, Bethany Ball M, Kenneth Poole W, Perritt R, Higgins RD, Oh W, Hudak ML, Laptook AR, Shankaran S, Finer NN, Carlo WA, Kennedy KA, Fridriksson JH, Steinhorn RH, Sokol GM, Ganesh Konduri G, Aschner JL, Stoll BJ, D'Angio CT, Stevenson DK. 2005. Inhaled nitric oxide for premature infants with severe respiratory failure. *New England Journal of Medicine* 353(1):13-22.

Van Voorhis BJ. 2006. Outcomes from assisted reproductive technology. *Obstetrics and Gynecology* 107:183-200.

Van Wassenaer AG, Briët JM, Van Baar A, Smit BJ, Tamminga P, De Vijlder JJM, Kok JH. 2002. Free thyroxine levels during the first weeks of life and neurodevelopmental outcome until the age of 5 years in very preterm infants. *Pediatrics* 110(3):534-539.

Varma R, Gupta JK. 2006. Antibiotic treatment of bacterial vaginosis in pregnancy: Multiple meta-analyses and dilemmas in interpretation. *European Journal of Obstetrics, Gynecology, and Reproductive Biology* 124:10-14.

Varner MW, Esplin MS. 2005. Current understanding of genetic factors in preterm birth. *BJOG: An International Journal of Obstetrics and Gynaecology* 112(s1):28-31.

Vaucher YE. 2002. Bronchopulmonary dysplasia: An enduring challenge. *Pediatrics in Review/American Academy of Pediatrics* 23(10):349-358.

Veddovi M, Kenny DT, Gibson F, Bowen J, Starte D. 2001. The relationship between depressive symptoms following premature birth, mothers' coping style, and knowledge of infant development. *Journal of Reproductive and Infant Psychology* 19(4):313-323.

Veerappan S, Rosen H, Craelius W, Curcie D, Hiatt M, Hegyi T. 2000. Spectral analysis of heart rate variability in premature infants with feeding bradycardia. *Pediatric Research* 47(5):659-662.

Ventura SJ, Mosher WD, Curtin SC, Abma JC, Henshaw S. 2001. Trends in pregnancy rates for the United States, 1976-97: An update. *National Vital Statistics Reports: From the Centers for Disease Control and Prevention, National Center for Health Statistics, National Vital Statistics System* 49(4):1-9.

Vermeulen GM, Bruinse HW. 1999. Prophylactic administration of clindamycin 2% vaginal cream to reduce the incidence of spontaneous preterm birth in women with an increased recurrence risk: A randomised placebo-controlled double-blind trial. *British Journal of Obstetrics and Gynaecology* 106(7):652-657.

Vickers A, Ohlsson A, Lacy JB, Horsley A. 2004. Massage for promoting growth and development of preterm and/or low birth-weight infants. *Cochrane Database of Systematic Reviews (Online: Update Software)* 2.

The Victorian Infant Collaborative Study Group. 1997. *Journal of Paediatrics and Child Health* 33(3):202-208.

Vigano P, Mangioni S, Pompei F, Chiodo I. 2003. Maternal-conceptus cross talk—a review. *Placenta* 24:S56-S61.

Villanueva CM, Durand G, Coutte MB, Chevrier C, Cordier S. 2005. Atrazine in municipal drinking water and risk of low birth weight, preterm delivery, and small-for-gestational-age status. *Occupational and Environmental Medicine* 62:400-405.

Villar J, Gulmezoglu AM, de Onis M. 1998. Nutritional and antimicrobial interventions to prevent preterm birth: An overview of randomized controlled trials. *Obstetrics and Gynecology Survey* 53:575-585.

Villar J, Merialdi M, Gnlmezoglu AM, Abalos E, Carroli G, Kulier R, De Onis M. 2003a. Characteristics of randomized controlled trials included in systematic reviews of nutritional interventions reporting maternal morbidity, mortality, preterm delivery, intrauterine growth restriction and small for gestational age and birth weight outcomes. *Journal of Nutrition* 133(5 Suppl 1):1632S-1639S.

Villar J, Merialdi M, Gulmezoglu AM, Abalos E, Carroli G, Kulier R, De Oni M. 2003b. Nutritional interventions during pregnancy for the prevention or treatment of maternal morbidity and preterm delivery: An overview of randomized controlled trials. *Journal of Nutrition* 133(5 Suppl 1):1606S-1625S.

Vogel I, Thorsen P, Curry A, Sandager P, Uldbjerg N. 2005. Biomarkers for the prediction of preterm delivery. *Acta Obstetricia et Gynecologica Scandinavica* 84(6):516-525.

Vogler GP, Kozlowski LT. 2002. Differential influence of maternal smoking on infant birth weight: Gene-environment interaction and targeted intervention. *JAMA* 287(2):241-242.

Vohr B. 2004. Follow-up care of high-risk infants. *Pediatrics* 114(5 Suppl 2):1377-1397.

Vohr BR, Coll CTG. 1985. Neurodevelopmental and school performance of very low-birth-weight infants: A seven-year longitudinal study. *Pediatrics* 76(3):345-350.

Vohr BR, Wright LL, Dusick AM, Mele L, Verter J, Steichen JJ, Simon NP, Wilson DC, Broyles S, Bauer CR, Delaney-Black V, Yolton KA, Fleisher BE, Papile L-A, Kaplan MD. 2000. Neurodevelopmental and functional outcomes of extremely low birth weight infants in the National Institute of Child Health and Human Development Neonatal Research Network, 1993-1994. *Pediatrics* 105(6):1216-1226.

Vohr BR, Wright LL, Dusick AM, Perritt R, Poole WK, Tyson JE, Steichen JJ, Bauer CR, Wilson-Costello DE, Mayes LC. 2004. Center differences and outcomes of extremely low birth weight infants. *Pediatrics* 113(4 I):781-789.

Vohr BR, Wright LL, Poole WK, McDonald SA, for the NICHD Neonatal Research Network Follow-up Study. 2005. Neurodevelopmental outcomes of extremely low birth weight infants <32 weeks' gestation between 1993 and 1998. *Pediatrics* 116(3):635-643.

Volpe JJ. 2001. *Neurology of the Newborn*, 4th edition. Philadelphia, PA: WB Saunders. Pp. 217-497.

Von Korff M, Koepsell T, Curry S, Diehr P. 1992. Multilevel analysis in epidemiologic research on health behaviors and outcomes. *American Journal of Epidemiology* 135(10): 1077-1082.

Vuadens F, Benay C, Crettaz D, Gallot D, Sapin V, Schneider P, Bienvenut WV, Lemery D, Quadroni M, Dastugue B, Tissot JD. 2003. Identification of biologic markers of the premature rupture of fetal membranes: Proteomic approach. *Proteomics* 3(8):1521-1525.

Wacholder S, Rothman N, Caporaso N. 2000. Population stratification in epidemiologic studies of common genetic variants and cancer: Quantification of bias. *Journal of the National Cancer Institute* 92(14):1151-1158.

Wada K, Jobe AH, Ikegami M. 1997. Tidal volume effects on surfactant treatment responses with the initiation of ventilation in preterm lambs. *Journal of Applied Physiology* 83:1054-1061.

Wadhwa PD, Sandman CA, Porto M, Dunkel-Schetter C, Garite TJ. 1993. The association between prenatal stress and infant birth weight and gestational age at birth: A prospective investigation. *American Journal of Obstetrics and Gynecology* 169(4):858-865.

Wadhwa PD, Dunkel-Schetter C, Chicz-DeMet A, Porto M, Sandman CA. 1996. Prenatal psychosocial factors and the neuroendocrine axis in human pregnancy. *Psychosomatic Medicine* 58(5):432-446.

Wadhwa PD, Culhane JF, Rauh V, Barve SS. 2001. Stress and preterm birth: Neuroendocrine, immune/inflammatory, and vascular mechanisms. *Maternal and Child Health Journal* 5(2):119-125.

Waitzman NJ, Scheffler RM, Romano PS. 1996. *The Costs of Birth Defects: The Value of Prevention*. Lanham, MD: University Press of America.

Waldron I, Hughes ME, Brooks TL. 1996. Marriage protection and marriage selection-prospective evidence for reciprocal effects of marital status and health. *Social Science and Medicine* 43(1):113-123.

Waller DK, Spears WD, Gu Y, Cunningham GC. 2000. Assessing number-specific error in the recall of onset of last menstrual period. *Paediatric and Perinatal Epidemiology* 14(3): 263-267.

Walsh MC, Szefler S, Davis J, Allen M, Van Marter L, Abman S, Blackmon L, Jobe A. 2006. Summary proceedings from the bronchopulmonary dysplasia group. *Pediatrics* 117(3): S52-S56.

Walsh-Sukys M, Reitenbach A, Hudson-Barr D, DePompei P. 2001. Reducing light and sound in the neonatal intensive care unit: An evaluation of patient safety, staff satisfaction and costs. *Journal of Perinatology* 21(4):230-235.

Walther FJ, Den Ouden AL, Verloove-Vanhorick SP. 2000. Looking back in time: Outcome of a national cohort of very preterm infants born in The Netherlands in 1983. *Early Human Development* 59(3):175-191.

Wang H, Parry S, Macones G, Sammel MD, Ferrand PE, Kuivaniemi H, Tromp G, Halder I, Shriver MD, Romero R, Strauss JF III. 2004. Functionally significant SNP MMP8 promoter haplotypes and preterm premature rupture of membranes (PPROM). *Human Molecular Genetics* 13(21):2659-2669.

Wang ML, Dorer DJ, Fleming MP, Catlin EA. 2004. Clinical outcomes of near-term infants. *Pediatrics* 114(2 I):372-376.

Wang TH, Chang YL, Peng HH, Wang ST, Lu HM, Teng SH, Chang SD. 2005. Rapid detection of fetal aneuploidy using proteomics approaches on amniotic fluid supernatant. *Prenatal Diagnosis* 25(7):559-566.

Wang X, Zuckerman B, Coffman GA, Corwin MJ. 1995. Familial aggregation of low birth weight among whites and blacks in the United States. *New England Journal of Medicine* 333(26):1744-1749.

Wang X, Chen D, Niu T, Wang Z,Wang L, Ryan L, Smith T, Christiani DC, Zuckerman B, Xu X. 2000. Genetic susceptibility to benzene and shortened gestation: Evidence of gene-environment interaction. *American Journal of Epidemiology* 152:693-700.

Wang X, Zuckerman B, Pearson C, Kaufman G, Chen C, Wang G, Niu T, Wise PH, Bauchner H, Xu X. 2002. Maternal cigarette smoking, metabolic gene polymorphism, and infant birth weight. *JAMA* 287(2):195-202.

Wang Y, Wysocka J, Perlin JR, Leonelli L, Allis CD, Coonrod SA. 2004. Linking covalent histone modifications to epigenetics: The rigidity and plasticity of the marks. *Cold Spring Harbor Symposia on Quantitative Biology* 69:161-169.

Wapner RJ for the NICHF MFMU Network. 2003. A randomized controlled trial of single vs. weekly courses of corticosteroids. *American Journal of Obstetrics and Gynecology* 189:S56 (SMFM abstract 2).

Wapner RJ for the NICHD MFMU Network. 2005. Maternal and fetal adrenal function following single and repeat courses of antenatal corticosteroids. *American Journal of Obstetrics and Gynecology* 193:S5 (SMFM abstract 10).

Ware J, Taeusch HW, Soll RF, McCormick MC. 1990. Health and developmental outcomes of a surfactant controlled trial: Follow-up at 2 years. *Pediatrics* 85(6):1103-1107.

Wariyar U, Tin W, Hey E. 1997. Gestational assessment assessed. *Archives of Disease in Childhood: Fetal and Neonatal Edition* 77(3):F216-F220.

Warren WB, Timor-Tritsch I, Peisner DB, Raju S, Rosen MG. 1989. Dating the early pregnancy by sequential appearance of embryonic structures. *American Journal of Obstetrics and Gynecology* 161(3):747-753.

Warshaw JB. 1985. Intrauterine growth retardation: Adaptation or pathology? *Pediatrics* 76(6):998-999.

Wassermann M, Ron M, Bercovici B, Wassermann D, Cucos S, Pines A. 1982. Premature delivery and organochlorine compounds: Polychlorinated biphenyls and some organochlorine insecticides. *Environmental Research* 28:106-112.

Wathes DC, Porter DG. 1982. Effect of uterine distension and oestrogen treatment on gap junction formation in the myometrium of the rat. *Journal of Reproduction and Fertility* 65:497-505.

Watterberg KL, Gerdes JS, Gifford KL, Lin H-M. 1999. Prophylaxis against early adrenal insufficiency to prevent chronic lung disease in premature infants. *Pediatrics* 104(6):1258-1263.

Weaver VM, Buckley TJ, Groopman JD. 1998. Approaches to environmental exposure assessment in children. *Environmental Health Perspectives* 106(Suppl 3):827-832.

Weiler HA, Yuen CK, Seshia MM. 2002. Growth and bone mineralization of young adults weighing less than 1500 g at birth. *Early Human Development* 67(1-2):101-112.

Wells DA, Gillies D, Fitzgerald DA. 2005. Positioning for acute respiratory distress in hospitalised infants and children. *Cochrane Database of Systematic Reviews (Online: Update Software)* 2.

Wellstone P, Farrell J, McDonald A. 1999, August 3.Wellstone challenges White House assertion of welfare reform "success story"; cites disturbing evidence of childhood poverty and hunger, dearth of information on former recipients [press release].

Wen SW, Goldenberg RL, Cutter GR, Hoffman HJ, Cliver SP. 1990. Intrauterine growth retardation and preterm delivery: Prenatal risk factors in an indigent population. *American Journal of Obstetrics and Gynecology* 162(1):213-218.

Wen SW, Demissie K, Yang Q, Walker MC. 2004. Maternal morbidity and obstetric complications in triplet pregnancies and quadruplet and higher-order multiple pregnancies. *American Journal of Obstetrics and Gynecology* 191(1):254-258.

Wenstrom KD, Andrews WW, Tamura T, Dubard MB, Johnston KE, Hemstreet GP. 1996. Elevated amniotic fluid interleukin-6 levels at genetic amniocentesis predict subsequent pregnancy loss. *American Journal of Obstetrics and Gynecology* 175:830-833.

Wenstrom KD, Weiner CP, Merrill D, Niebyl J. 1997. A placebo-controlled randomized trial of the terbutaline pump for prevention of preterm delivery. *American Journal of Perinatology* 14(2):87-91.

West SG, Aiken LS. 1997. Toward understanding individual effects in multicomponent prevention programs: Design and analysis strategies. In: Bryant K, Windle M, West S eds. *The Science of Prevention: Methodological Advances from Alcohol and Substance Abuse Research*. Washington, DC: American Psychological Association. Pp. 167-209.

White KR. 2003. The current status of EHDI programs in the United States. *Mental Retardation and Developmental Disabilities Research Reviews* 9(2):79-88.

Whitehead N, Hill HA, Brogan DJ, Blackmore-Prince C. 2002. Exploration of threshold analysis in the relation between stressful life events and preterm delivery. *American Journal of Epidemiology* 155(2):117-124.

Whitehead NS, Brogan DJ, Blackmore-Prince C, Hill HA. 2003. Correlates of experiencing life events just before or during pregnancy. *Journal of Psychosomatic Obstetrics and Gynaecology* 24:77-86.

Whitelaw A. 2001. Intraventricular streptokinase after intraventricular hemorrhage in newborn infants. *Cochrane Database of Systematic Reviews (Online: Update Software)* 1.

Whitelaw A, Kennedy CR, Brion LP. 2001. Diuretic therapy for newborn infants with posthemorrhagic ventricular dilatation. *Cochrane Database of Systematic Reviews* 2.

Whitfield MF, Grunau RVE, Holsti L. 1997. Extremely premature (<800 g) schoolchildren: Multiple areas of hidden disability. *Archives of Disease in Childhood: Fetal and Neonatal Edition* 77(2):F85-F90.

Wideman GL, Baird GH, Bolding OT. 1964. Ascorbic acid deficiency and premature rupture of fetal membranes. *American Journal of Obstetrics and Gynecology* 88:592-595.

Wijnberger LDE, Huisjes AJM, Voorbij HAM, Franx A, Bruinse HW, Mol BWJ. 2001. The accuracy of lamellar body count and lecithin/sphingomyelin ratio in the prediction of neonatal respiratory distress syndrome: A meta-analysis. *BJOG: An International Journal of Obstetrics and Gynaecology* 108(6):583-588.

Wilhelm M, Ritz B. 2003. Residential proximity to traffic and adverse birth outcomes in Los Angeles County, California, 1994-1996. *Environmental Health Perspectives* 111: 207-216.

Wilhelm M, Ritz B. 2005. Local variations in CO and particulate air pollution and adverse birth outcomes in Los Angeles County, California, USA. *Environmental Health Perspectives* 113:1212-1221.

Wilkerson DS, Volpe AG, Dean RS, Titus JB. 2002. Perinatal complications as predictors of infantile autism. *International Journal of Neuroscience* 112(9):1085-1098.

Wilkins R, Sherman GJ, Best PA. 1991. Birth outcomes and infant mortality by income in urban Canada, 1986. *Health Reports/Statistics Canada, Canadian Centre for Health Information=Rapports sur la sante/Statistique Canada, Centre canadien d'information sur la sante* 3(1):7-31.

Willet K, Jobe A, Ikegami M, Newnham J, Brennan S, SLY PD. 2000. Antenatal endotoxin and glucocorticoid effects on lung morphometry in preterm lambs. *Pediatrics Research* 48:782.

Willet KE, Jobe AH, Ikegami M, Kovar J, Sly PD. 2001. Lung morphometry after repetitive antenatal glucocorticoid treatment in preterm sheep. *American Journal of Respiratory and Critical Care Medicine* 163:1437-1443.

Williams G, Oliver JM, Allard A, Sears L. 2003. Autism and associated medical and familial factors: A case control study. *Journal of Developmental and Physical Disabilities* 15(4):335-349.

Willis WO, de Peyster A, Molgaard CA, Walker C, MacKendrick T. 1993. Pregnancy outcome among women exposed to pesticides through work or residence in an agricultural area. *Journal of Occupational Medicine* 35:943-949.

Wilson WJ. 1987. *The Truly Disadvantaged: The Inner City, the Underclass, and Public Policy.* Chicago, IL: The University of Chicago Press.

Wilson-Costello D, Friedman H, Minich N, Fanaroff AA, Hack M. 2005. Improved survival rates with increased neurodevelopmental disability for extremely low birth weight infants in the 1990s. *Pediatrics* 115(4):997-1003.

Windham GC, Hopkins B, Fenster L, Swan SH. 2000. Prenatal active or passive tobacco smoke exposure and the risk of preterm delivery or low birth weight. *Epidemiology* 11:427-433.

Wisborg K, Henriksen TB, Hedegaard M, Secher NJ. 1996. Smoking during pregnancy and preterm birth. *British Journal of Obstetrics and Gynaecology* 103:800-805.

Wise P. 2003. The anatomy of a disparity in infant mortality. *Annual Review of Public Health* 24:341-362.

Wisser J, Dirschedl P. 1994. Embryonic heart rate in dated human embryos. *Early Human Development* 37(2):107-115.

Wisser J, Dirschedl P, Krone S. 2003. Estimation of gestational age by transvaginal sonographic measurement of greatest embryonic length in dated human embryos. *Ultrasound in Obstetrics and Gynecology* 4(6):457-462.

Wolke D. 1998. Psychological development of prematurely born children. *Archives of Disease in Childhood* 78(6):567-570.

Wong AH, Gottesman, II, Petronis A. 2005. Phenotypic differences in genetically identical organisms: The epigenetic perspective. *Human Molecular Genetics* 2005:15.

Woo GM. 1997. Daily demands during pregnancy, gestational age, and birthweight: Reviewing physical and psychological demands in employment and non-employment contexts. *Annals of Behavioral Medicine* 19(4):385-398.

Wood NS, Marlow N, Costeloe K, Gibson AT, Wilkinson AR, the EPICure Study Group. 2000. Neurologic and developmental disability after extremely preterm birth. *New England Journal of Medicine* 343(6):378-384.

Wood NS, Costeloe K, Gibson AT, Hennessy EM, Marlow N, Wilkinson AR. 2005. The EPICure study: Associations and entecedents of neurological and developmental disability at the 30 months of age following extremely preterm birth. *Archives of Disease in Childhood: Fetal and Neonatal Edition* 90(2):F134-F140.

Woodgate PG, Davies MW. 2001. Permissive hypercapnia for the prevention of morbidity and mortality in mechanically ventilated newborn infants. *Cochrane Database of Systematic Reviews (Online: Update Software)* 2.

Woodruff TJ, Parker JD, Kyle AD, Schoendorf KC. 2003. Disparities in exposure to air pollution during pregnancy. *Environmental Health Perspectives* 111:942-946.

WHO (World Health Organization). 1958. *Constitution of the WHO.* Annex 1, Geneva, Switzerland: WHO.

WHO. 1995. Maternal anthropometry and pregnancy outcomes: A WHO collaborative study. *Bulletin of the World Health Organization* 73 Supp.:1-98.

Wright JM, Schwartz J, Dockery DW. 2003. Effect of trihalomethane exposure on fetal development. *Occupational Environmental Medicine* 60:173-180.

Wright JM, Schwartz J, Dockery DW. 2004. The effect of disinfection by-products and mutagenic activity on birth weight and gestational duration. *Environmental Health Perspectives* 112:920-925.

Wu YW, Colford JM Jr. 2000. Chorioamnionitis as a risk factor for cerebral palsy: A meta-analysis. *JAMA* 284(11):1417-1424.

Xiong X, Buekens P, Fraser WD, Beck J, Offenbacher S. 2005. Periodontal disease and adverse pregnancy outcomes: A systematic review. *BJOG: An International Journal of Obstetrics and Gynaecology* 113:135-143.

Xu X, Ding M, Li B, Christiani DC. 1994. Association of rotating shiftwork with preterm births and low birth weight among never smoking women textile workers in China. *Occupational and Environmental Medicine* 51(7):470-474.

Xu X, Ding H, Wang X. 1995. Acute effects of total suspended particles and sulfur dioxides on preterm delivery: A community-based cohort study. *Archives of Environmental Health* 50:407-415.

Xu Y, Cook TJ, Knipp GT. 2005. Effects of Di-(2-Ethylhexyl)-Phthalate (DEHP) and its metabolites on fatty acid homeostasis regulating proteins in rat placental HRP-1 trophoblast cells. *Toxicological Sciences* 84(2):287-300.

Xue WC, Chan KY, Feng HC, Chiu PM, Ngan HY, Tsao SW, Cheung ANY. 2004. Promoter hypermethylation of multiple genes in hydatidiform mole and choriocarcinoma. *Journal of Molecular Diagnostics* 6:326-334.

Yallampalli C, Dong YL, Gangula PR, Fang L. 1998. Role and regulation of nitric oxide in the uterus during pregnancy and parturition. *Journal of the Society for Gynecologic Investigation* 5:58-67.

Yang CY, Cheng BH, Tsai SS, Wu TN, Lin MC, Lin KC. 2000. Association between chlorination of drinking water and adverse pregnancy outcome in Taiwan. *Environmental Health Perspectives* 108:765-768.

Yang CY, Cheng BH, Hsu TY, Chuang HY, Wu TN, Chen PC. 2002a. Association between petrochemical air pollution and adverse pregnancy outcomes in Taiwan. *Archives of Environmental Health* 57:461-465.

Yang CY, Chiu HF, Tsai SS, Chang CC, Chuang HY. 2002b. Increased risk of preterm delivery in areas with cancer mortality problems from petrochemical complexes. *Environmental Research* 89:195-200.

Yang CY, Chang CC, Chuang HY, Ho CK, Wu TN, Tsai SS. 2003a. Evidence for increased risks of preterm delivery in a population residing near a freeway in Taiwan. *Archives of Environmental Health* 58:649-654.

Yang CY, Chang CC, Tsai SS, Chuang HY, Ho CK, Wu TN. 2003b. Arsenic in drinking water and adverse pregnancy outcome in an arseniasis-endemic area in northeastern Taiwan. *Environmental Research* 91:29-34.

Yang CY, Chang CC, Chuang HY, Ho CK, Wu TN, Chang PY. 2004a. Increased risk of preterm delivery among people living near the three oil refineries in Taiwan. *Environmental International* 30:337-342.

Yang H, Kramer MS, Platt RW, Blondel B, Bréart G, Morin I, Wilkins R, Usher R. 2002c. How does early ultrasound scan estimation of gestational age lead to higher rates of preterm birth? *American Journal of Obstetrics and Gynecology* 186(3):433-437.

Yang J, Hartmann KE, Savitz DA, Herring AH, Dole N, Olshan AF, Thorp JM Jr. 2004b. Vaginal bleeding during pregnancy and preterm birth. *American Journal of Epidemiology* 106:118-125.

Yeast JD, Poskin M, Stockbauer JW, Shaffer S. 1998. Changing patterns in regionalization of perinatal care and the impact on neonatal mortality. *American Journal of Obstetrics and Gynecology* 178(1 I):131-135.

Yeh TF, Lin YJ, Huang CC, Chen YJ, Lin CH, Lin HC, Hsieh WS, Lien YJ. 1998. Early dexamethasone therapy in preterm infants: A follow-up study. *Pediatrics* 101(5).

Yen IH, Kaplan GA. 1999. Neighborhood social environment and risk of death: Multilevel evidence from the Alameda County Study. *American Journal of Epidemiology* 149(10): 898-907.

Yen IH, Syme SL. 1999. The social environment and health: A discussion of the epidemiologic literature. *Annual Review of Public Health* 20:287-308.

Yoder BA, Siler-Khodr T, Winter VT, Coalson JJ. 2000. High-frequency oscillatory ventilation: Effects on lung function, mechanics, and airway cytokines in the immature baboon model for neonatal chronic lung disease. *American Journal of Respiratory and Critical Care Medicine* 162:1867-1876.

Yoon BH, Romero R, Yang SH, Jun JK, Kim I-O, Choi JH. 1996. Interleukin-6 concentrations in umbilical cord plasma are elevated in neonates with white matter lesions associated with periventricular leukomalacia. *American Journal of Obstetrics and Gynecology* 174:1433-1440.

Yoon BH, Jun JK, Romero R, Park KH, Gomez R, Choi JH. 1997a. Amniotic fluid inflammatory cytokines (interleukin-6, interleukin-1b, and tumor necrosis factor-a), neonatal brain white matter lesions, and cerebral palsy. *American Journal of Obstetrics and Gynecology* 177:19-26.

Yoon BH, Romero R, Kim CJ, Koo JN, Choe G, Syn HC. 1997b. High expression of tumor necrosis factor-a and interleukin-6 in periventricular leukomalacia. *American Journal of Obstetrics and Gynecology* 177:406-411.

Yoon BH, Kim CJ, Romero R, Jun JK, Park KH, Choi ST. 1997c. Experimentally-induced intrauterine infection causes fetal brain white matter lesions in rabbits. *American Journal of Obstetrics and Gynecology* 177:797-802.

Yoon BH, Romero R, Jun JK, Maymon E, Gomez R, Mazor M, Park JS. 1998. An increase in fetal plasma cortisol but not dehydroepiandrosterone sulfate is followed by the onset of preterm labor in patients with preterm premature rupture of the membranes. *American Journal of Obstetrics and Gynecology* 179:1107-1114.

Yoshikawa H. 1995. Long-term effects of early childhood programs on social outcomes and delinquency. *Future of Children* 5(3):51-75.

Yoshinaga-Itano C. 2000. Successful outcomes for deaf and hard-of-hearing children. *Seminars in Hearing* 21(4):309-326.

Yoshioka H, Goma H, Nioka S, Ochi M, Mikaye H, Zaman A, Masumura M, Sawada T, Chance B. 1994. Bilateral carotid artery occlusion causes periventricular leukomalacia in neonatal dogs. *Brain Research: Developmental Brain Research* 78(2):273-278.

Yost NP, Owen J, Berghella V, MacPherson C, Swain M, Dildy GA III, Miodovnik M, Langer O, Sibai B. 2004. Second-trimester cervical sonography: Features other than cervical length to predict spontaneous preterm birth. *Obstetrics and Gynecology* 103(3): 457-462.

Young RSK, Yagel SK, Twofighi J. 1983. Systemic and neuropathic effects of E. coli endotoxin in neonatal dogs. *Pediatrics Research* 17:349-353.

Yue X, Mehmet H, Penrice J, Cooper C, Cady E, Wyatt JS, Reynolds EO, Edwards AD, Quier MV. 1997. Apoptosis and necrosis in the newborn piglet brain following transient cerebral hypoxia-ischemia. *Neuropathology and Applied Neurobiology* 23:16-25.

Zachman RD, Bauer CR, Boehm J, Korones SB, Rigatto H, Rao AV. 1988. Effect of antenatal dexamethasone on neonatal leukocyte count. *Journal of Perinatology* 8(2):111-113.

Zahr LK, de Traversay J. 1995. Premature infant responses to noise reduction by earmuffs: Effects on behavioral and physiologic measures. *Journal of Perinatology: Official Journal of the California Perinatal Association* 15(6):448-455.

Zambrana RE, Dunkel-Schetter C, Collins NL, Scrimshaw SC. 1999. Mediators of ethnic-associated differences in infant birth weight. *Journal of Urban Health* 76(1):102-116.

Zeitlin JA, Saurel-Cubizolles M-J, Ancel P-Y, Di Renzo GC, Bréart G, Papiernik E, Patel N, Saurel-Cubizolles MJ, Taylor D, Todini S, Kudela M, Vetr M, Heikkilä A, Erkkola R, Forström J, Lucidarme P, Tafforeau J, Knnzel W, Herrero-Garcia J, Dudenhausen J, Henrich W, Antsaklis A., Haritatos G, Kovacs L, Nyari T, Bartfai G, O'Herlihy C, Murphy J, Stewart H, Bruschettini PL, Moscioni P, Cosmi E, Spinelli A, Serena D, Breborowicz GH, Anholcer A, Stamatian F, Mikhailov AV, Pajntar M, Pirc M, Verdenik I, Escribà-Aguir V, Carrera JM, Marsal K, Stale H, Buitendijk S, Van der Pal K, Van Geijn H, Gökmen O, Gnler C, Caglar T, Owen P. 2002. Marital status, cohabitation, and the risk of preterm birth in Europe: Where births outside marriage are common and uncommon. *Paediatric and Perinatal Epidemiology* 16(2):124-130.

Zeltner TB, Burri PH. 1987. The postnatal development and growth of the human lung. II. Morphology. *Respiratory Physiology* 67:269.

Zhang YL, Zhao YC, Wang JX, Zhu HD, Liu QF, Fan YG, Wang NF, Zhao JH, Liu HS, Ou-Yang L, Liu AP, Fan TQ. 2004. Effect of environmental exposure to cadmium on pregnancy outcome and fetal growth: A study on healthy pregnant women in China. *Journal of Environmental Science and Health. Part A, Toxic/Hazardous Substances and Environmental Engineering* 39:2507-2515.

Zhu BP, Le T. 2003. Effect of interpregnancy interval on infant low birth weight: A retrospective cohort study using the Michigan Maternally Linked Birth Database. *Maternal and Child Health Journal* 7:169-178.

Zhu BP, Haines KM, Le T, McGrath-Miller K, Boulton ML. 2001. Effect of the interval between pregnancies on perinatal outcomes among white and black women. *American Journal of Obstetrics and Gynecology*. 185:1403-1410.

Zoban P, Cerny M. 2003. Immature lung and acute lung injury. *Physiology Research* 52: 507-516.

Zuckerman BS, Beardslee WR. 1987. Maternal depression: A concern for pediatricians. *Pediatrics* 79:110-117.

Zupancic JA. 2006. A systematic review of costs associated with prematurity. Institute of Medicine, Committee on Understanding Premature Birth and Assuring Healthy Outcomes.

A

Data Sources and Methods

The Committee on Understanding Premature Birth and Assuring Healthy Outcomes was asked to evaluate the state of the science on the causes and consequences of preterm birth. The committee assessed the various factors contributing to preterm birth; reviewed the economic, medical, social, psychological, and educational outcomes for children and families; addressed research gaps and needs; and explored changes in health policies.

To provide a comprehensive response to the study charge, the committee examined data from a variety of sources. These data sources included a review of recent scientific literature, public input through a series of workshops, and commissioned papers on selected topics. The study was conducted over a 21-month period.

DESCRIPTION OF THE STUDY COMMITTEE

A study committee composed of 17 members was assembled to assess the available data and make recommendations. The committee membership included individuals with expertise in obstetrics and gynecology, pediatrics, environmental health, epidemiology, psychology, economics, genetics, and public health. The committee convened for six 2-day meetings in March 2005, June 2005, August 2005, October 2005, December 2005, and January 2006.

LITERATURE REVIEW

Three strategies were combined to identify literature in support of the committee's charge. First, a search on the EMBASE and Medline databases was conducted to obtain articles from peer-reviewed journals. The searches focused on preterm birth and low birth weight, including their genetic, behavioral, biological, and environmental causes, as well as their economic, educational, health, and family consequences. Second, the reports of federal agencies, such as the National Institutes of Health and the Centers for Disease Control and Prevention, relevant to preterm birth and low birth weight were also gathered. Finally, committee members and workshop participants submitted articles and reports on those topics. The resulting database included more than 800 articles and reports.

COMMISSIONED PAPERS

The study committee commissioned three papers intended to provide in-depth information on selected topics, beyond the independent analysis of the literature conducted by the committee. The topics of these papers included geographic variations in rates of preterm birth, prematurity-related ethical issues, and the economic costs associated with preterm birth. The members of the committee determined the topics and the authors of the papers. These papers were not intended to serve as substitutes for the committee's own review and analysis of the literature. The committee independently deliberated on these topics before it received the drafts of the papers.

PUBLIC WORKSHOPS

The committee hosted three public workshops to gain additional information on specific aspects of the study charge. These workshops were held in conjunction with the March, June, and August meetings. The study committee determined the topics and the speakers.

The first workshop was intended to provide an overview of key issues in the area of preterm birth and to discuss the committee's charge. Content focused on the biological pathways associated with preterm birth, as well as the educational, economic, and family consequences. Additionally, representatives from the study's sponsors were invited to discuss the charge to the committee. The second workshop focused on the role of maternal conditions, such as infection, inflammation, and preeclampsia in preterm birth; the epidemiology of preterm birth; public policies that may address the problem of preterm birth; controversial issues in the care of preterm infants; and racial disparities in the rates of preterm birth. The third and final workshop focused on barriers to clinical research. Specifically, presenters addressed issues related to the current state of the workforce, key issues in career development, ethics and liability issues in research, funding of research, drug development research, and the leadership required for the development of research capacity within departments of obstetrics and gynecology. Each workshop was open to the public; and individuals were invited to present information to the committee, discuss their presentations, and address inquiries from the committee. The agendas of these workshops, including the names of the workshop participants, are included in Boxes A-1 through A-3.

BOX A-1

Institute of Medicine
Committee on Understanding Premature Birth and
Assuring Healthy Outcomes

The National Academies Building
2100 C Street, NW
Washington, D.C.
Room 150

AGENDA
Wednesday March 30, 2005

12:30 p.m.   **WELCOME AND INTRODUCTIONS**
Richard E. Behrman, M.D.
Chair, Committee on Understanding Premature Birth and
Assuring Healthy Outcomes

OVERVIEW OF KEY ISSUES

12:45 p.m.   Pathogenesis of Prematurity
Charles J. Lockwood, M.D.
Chair, Department of Obstetrics and Gynecology
Yale School of Medicine

1:15 p.m.   Discussion

1:30 p.m.   Educational and Family Sequelae of Prematurity: Findings
from Naturalistic and Experimental Studies
Sharon Landesman Ramey, Ph.D.
Professor, School of Nursing and Health Studies
Georgetown University

1:50 p.m.   Economic Consequences of Prematurity
Scott Grosse, Ph.D.
Senior Health Economist, National Center for Birth
    Defects and Developmental Disabilities
Centers for Disease Control and Prevention

2:10 p.m. Impact of Prematurity: A Parent Perspective
Kathy Paz
President and Founder
Preemies Today

2:30 p.m. Discussion

3:00 p.m. BREAK

3:15 p.m. **DELIVERY OF STUDY CHARGE**
Duane Alexander, M.D.
Director, National Institute of Child Health and Human
    Development
National Institutes of Health

Scott Grosse, Ph.D.
Senior Health Economist, National Center for Birth
Defects and Developmental Disabilities

Eve M. Lackritz, M.D.
Chief, Maternal and Infant Health Branch, Division of
    Reproductive Health, National Center for Chronic
    Disease Prevention and Health Promotion
Centers for Disease Control and Prevention

3:45 p.m. **DISCUSSION OF STUDY CHARGE**
Richard Schwarz, M.D.
Vice Chair of Obstetrics and Gynecology
Maimonides Medical Center

Michael Katz, M.D.
Senior Vice President for Research and Global Programs
March of Dimes Birth Defects Foundation

Enriqueta C. Bond, Ph.D.
President
The Burroughs Wellcome Fund

continued

BOX A-1 Continued

Ann Koontz, C.N.M., Dr.P.H.
Associate Director, Division of Perinatal Systems and
   Women's Health
Maternal and Child Health Bureau, Health Resources and
   Services Administration

Loretta Finnegan, M.D.
Medical Advisor for the Director, Office of Research on
   Women's Health
National Institutes of Health

Debra Hawks, M.P.H.
Director, Practice Activities
American College of Obstetricians and Gynecologists

Sean Tipton
Director of Public Affairs
American Society for Reproductive Medicine

Arnold Cohen, M.D.
Chairman, Department of Obstetrics and Gynecology,
   Albert Einstein Medical Center
Society for Maternal-Fetal Medicine

5:15 p.m.   **ADJOURN**

BOX A-2

Institute of Medicine
Committee on Understanding Premature Birth and Assuring
Healthy Outcomes
The National Academies Building
2100 C Street, NW
Washington, D.C.
Room 180

AGENDA
Wednesday, June 22, 2005

7:30 a.m.   **WELCOME AND INTRODUCTIONS**
Richard E. Behrman, M.D.
Chair, Committee on Understanding Premature Birth and
Assuring Healthy Outcomes

7:45 a.m.   **THE ROLE OF INFECTION AND INFLAMMATION IN
PREMATURE BIRTH**

Prenatal Infection and Inflammation
Robert Goldenberg, M.D.
Department of Obstetrics and Gynecology
University of Alabama at Birmingham

8:30 a.m.   Discussion

8:45 a.m.   Antenatal and Postnatal Inflammation Effects on the
Preterm Lung
Alan Jobe, M.D., Ph.D.
Department of Pediatrics
Cincinnati Children's Hospital Medical Center

9:05 a.m.   Inflammation and Perinatal Brain Damage
Michael O'Shea, M.D., M.P.H.
Department of Pediatrics
Wake Forest University School of Medicine

9:25 a.m.   Discussion

10:00 a.m. BREAK

continued

BOX A-2 Continued

10:15 a.m. **Preeclampsia: Maternal/Fetal Mortality and Morbidity**
John Hauth, M.D.
Department of Obstetrics and Gynecology
University of Alabama School of Medicine

10:45 a.m. Discussion

11:15 a.m. **EPIDEMIOLOGY OF PRETERM BIRTH**
Michael Kramer, M.D.
Departments of Pediatrics and Epidemiology and
  Biostatistics
McGill University

12:00 a.m. Discussion

12:30 p.m. LUNCH

1:30 p.m. **OVERVIEW OF POLICIES RELATING TO PRETERM DELIVERY**
Wendy Chavkin, M.D., M.P.H.
Department of Population and Family Health
Columbia University's Mailman School of Public Health

2:00 p.m. Discussion

2:15 p.m.   **CONTROVERSIAL ISSUES IN NEONATAL CARE**
F. Sessions Cole, M.D.
Department of Pediatrics
Washington University School of Medicine

Jerold F. Lucey, M.D.
Department of Pediatrics
University of Vermont College of Medicine

Robert M. Nelson, M.D., Ph.D.
Department of Anesthesia and Critical Care Medicine
The Children's Hospital of Philadelphia

4:00 p.m.   **ADJOURN—Reception**

Thursday, June 23, 2005
Room 180

8:30 a.m.   **Racial Disparities in Preterm Delivery:**
Health Care and Research Issues
Carol Rowland Hogue, Ph.D., M.P.H.
Department of Epidemiology
Emory University School of Public Health

9:30 a.m.   **ADJOURN**

BOX A-3

Institute of Medicine
Committee on Understanding Premature Birth and Assuring Healthy Outcomes

Keck Center of the National Academies
500 Fifth Street, NW
Washington, D.C.
Room 100

Public Workshop on Barriers to Clinical Research Related to Premature Birth
Wednesday, August 10, 2005

8:30 a.m. **Welcome and Introductions**
Richard Behrman, M.D., J.D.
Chair, Committee on Understanding Premature Birth and Assuring Healthy Outcomes

8:45 a.m. **Nurse-Midwife Workforce**
Kerri Durnell Schuiling, Ph.D., C.N.M, F.A.C.N.M.
Professor and Associate Dean for Nursing Education
Northern Michigan University
Senior Staff Researcher, American College of Nurse-Midwives

9:00 a.m. Discussion

9:15 a.m. **Career Development**
Jerome F. Strauss III, M.D., Ph.D.
Professor and Director, Center for Research on Reproduction and Women's Health
University of Pennsylvania Medical Center

9:30 a.m. *Diane Magrane, M.D.*
Associate Vice President, Faculty Development and Leadership Programs
Association of American Medical Colleges

9:45 a.m. Discussion

10:15 a.m. BREAK

10:30 a.m. **Funding of Research on Premature Birth**
John V. Ilekis, Ph.D.
Health Scientist Administrator, Pregnancy and
  Perinatology Branch
Center for Developmental Biology and Perinatal Medicine
National Institutes of Health
National Institute of Child Health and Development

10:50 a.m. *William Callaghan, M.D., M.P.H.*
Senior Scientist, Maternal and Infant Health Branch
Division of Reproductive Health
National Center for Chronic Disease Prevention and
  Health Promotion
Centers for Disease Control and Prevention

11:05 a.m. *Enriqueta C. Bond, Ph.D.*
President
Burroughs Wellcome Fund

11:20 a.m. *Nancy Green, M.D.*
Medical Director
March of Dimes

11:35 a.m. Discussion

1:00 p.m. **Ethical and Liability Issues in Reproductive Research**
Robert M. Nelson, M.D., Ph.D.
Associate Professor of Anesthesiology and Critical Care
University of Pennsylvania School of Medicine
The Children's Hospital of Philadelphia

1:10 p.m. *Robert Goldenberg, M.D.*
Professor of Obstetrics and Gynecology
University of Alabama at Birmingham

1:20 p.m. *John M. Gibbons, Jr., M.D.*
Professor of Obstetrics and Gynecology
University of Connecticut School of Medicine
Past President, American College of Obstetricians and
  Gynecologist

continued

BOX A-3 Continued

1:30 p.m.   Discussion

2:00 p.m.   **Training Required for Future Reproductive Research**
             Sudhansu K. Dey, Ph.D.
             Professor, Department of Pediatrics, Departments of Cell
                and Developmental Biology and Pharmacology
             Vanderbilt University

2:15 p.m.   *Jeff Reese, M.D.*
             Associate Professor, Department of Pediatrics
             Vanderbilt University

2:30 p.m.   Discussion

3:00 p.m.   *Theodore M. Danoff, M.D., Ph.D*
             Director, Discovery Medicine
             Hypertension, PTL, Renal and Thrombosis Disease Area
             Glaxo Smith Kline

3:15 p.m.   Discussion

3:35 p.m.   BREAK

3:50 p.m.   *Robert Goldenberg, M.D.*
             Professor, Department of Obstetrics and Gynecology
             University of Alabama at Birmingham

             Jerome F. Strauss III, M.D., Ph.D.
             Professor and Director, Center for Research on
             Reproduction and Women's Health
             University of Pennsylvania Medical Center

Linda J. Heffner, M.D., Ph.D.
Professor and Chair, Department of Obstetrics and
Gynecology
Boston University Medical Center

David Eschenbach, M.D.
Professor and Chair, Department of Obstetrics and
Gynecology
University of Washington

Garland D. Anderson, M.D.
Professor and Chair, Department of Obstetrics and
Gynecology
University of Texas Medical Branch

Katherine E. Hartmann, M.D., Ph.D.
Director, Center for Women's Health Research
University of North Carolina

4:45 p.m.   Discussion

5:30 p.m.   **Adjourn**

**Thursday, August 11, 2005
Room 110**

9:00 a.m.   **Economic Costs of Premature Birth**
Stavros Petrou, M.Phil., Ph.D.
National Perinatal Epidemiology Unit
University of Oxford

10:30 a.m.   **Adjourn**

B

Prematurity at Birth: Determinants, Consequences, and Geographic Variation

Greg R. Alexander[1]

Throughout the latter half of the 20th century, infant mortality rates have continued to decline in the United States (1–6). The ongoing reduction in the risk of an infant death has largely been driven by improvements in birth weight- and gestational age-specific infant mortality rates stemming from advancements in intensive medical care services and technology (6–8). However, as the decline in infant mortality rates has tapered off in recent years and has reversed in some states, growing concerns about the direction of future trends in U.S. infant mortality rates have emerged (9). These concerns are heightened by the simultaneous increases in low birth weight and preterm birth rates that have been observed for over 2 decades in the United States and elsewhere (3, 8, 10–14). As it is unclear if yet another technological breakthrough in high-risk medical services will emerge to drive further reductions in infant death rates, the need to prevent premature births has been increasingly voiced and has become paramount (4, 15).

The importance of reducing the risk of low birth weight and preterm birth has long been recognized if for no other reason than that the health care costs associated with an extremely small or early birth are many times higher than those of infants of normal weight (16, 17). Lowering the risk of infant mortality through reductions in high-risk preterm births would likely be much more cost-effective than the current reliance on improving their

[1]Greg R. Alexander, M.P.H., Sc.D., Colleges of Medicine and Public Health, University of South Florida, Tampa.

survival with high-risk intensive care services after they are born (17–19). Beyond the elevated health care costs of newborn premature infants, however, those born preterm have an appreciable risk of long-term neurological impairment and developmental delay (20–22). The ongoing medical and support service needs of these infants and their families add to the overall health care system cost burden over time and emphasize the continuing health and developmental problems that some preterm infants face. Finally, the high preterm birth rates in the United States have been identified as a major contributor to this nation's relatively poor ranking in infant mortality among other developed countries (23). Although low birth weight has often received greater attention than preterm birth as the leading factor underlying poor pregnancy outcomes in the United States, it has been recognized that to successfully address these problems, the "key goal is prevention of preterm birth" (23).

Policy makers and the public need to be kept informed of the rapid developments in research and their implications for clinical practice and public programs and policies. Because of the continuing problem that premature birth poses in the United States and other countries, as well as the rapid and ongoing developments in research in this area, there has been a recognized need for periodic forums, reports, and public investigative committees that would increase knowledge and awareness of evolving strategies for the prevention of preterm birth. In 1985, the Institute of Medicine released the report of its Committee to Study the Prevention of Low Birth Weight (24). That report addressed the epidemiology of low birth weight and assessed preventive approaches for cost and effectiveness. That same year, Émile Papiernik, an international French innovator and leader in prematurity research, organized a conference in Evian, France, entitled Prevention of Preterm Birth: New Goals and New Practices in Prenatal Care. That conference focused on reducing the risk of preterm labor and delivery and offered participants an opportunity to disclose their latest research findings (25). A follow-up to the 1985 Evian conference was held in the United States in 1988. That conference, Advances in the Prevention of Low Birth Weight, was hosted by H. Berendes, S. Kessel, and S. Yaffe and focused on the results of clinical trials and community-based interventions aimed at reducing low birth weight (25). Yet another follow-up to those conferences, The International Conference on Preterm Birth: Etiology, Mechanisms and Prevention, was held in 1997 (26). That conference was also developed to provide an overview of studies in preterm birth research, a review of risk factors and potential etiologic pathways, and an assessment of the then current intervention and prevention strategies.

Other reports, conferences, and national efforts, including the current Prematurity Campaign of the National March of Dimes, have been developed over the last 2 decades to address the widely perceived problem of increasing rates of low birth weight and preterm births in the United States (19). For the most part, the continued and still current consensus of all of these forums and their related reports is that the proposed interventions do not work (27–30). Although major advances have occurred in the area of preterm birth research and related perinatal and maternal-infant medical care, preterm birth rates have continued to climb. despite these developments and intervention efforts (10, 28). New social trends, including changes in the rate of multiple births, the use of assisted reproductive technology (ART), the increasing average maternal age, the proportion of married mothers, the early use of prenatal care, etc., have accompanied this increase in preterm birth rates (10). This complex array of social and medical care developments and the intractability of the present preterm birth trends necessitate the ongoing and heightened attention of health researchers, health care providers, public health practitioners, and policy makers. The impact on families is plainly too great (ranging from the risk of an infant death to long-term developmental delays and impairment), and the costs (both financial and emotional) are too high to ignore or simply accept.

DEFINITION AND MEASUREMENT OF PREMATURITY

Defining and Conceptualizing Preterm Birth

The definition of prematurity has evolved in the literature of the last century. Initially used to designate an infant born too early or too small, it was often defined by the use of either birth weight or gestational age (31). As birth weight is more reliably measured than gestational age, low birth weight (a birth weight of <2,500 grams) was the more obvious choice to delineate a premature birth. Nevertheless, being born too small is conceptually and, in some cases, etiologically distinct from being born too early. Low birth weight may result from an early birth but also from fetal growth restriction, i.e., being small for a given gestational age. As the etiologies of these distinct types of low birth weight deliveries are different, it became more widely accepted to separate prematurity into two categories, i.e., either low birth weight or preterm. By current convention, "preterm" now refers to an early delivery and is defined by gestational age. "Low birth weight" refers to the weight of the infant at delivery. Relatedly, fetal growth refers to the birth weight of the infant for a specific gestational age. Small-for-gestational age (SGA), usually defined as less than the 10th percentile of birth weight for gestational age, is a commonly used indicator of fetal growth restriction. As illustrated in Figure B-1, these indicators may overlap; i.e., a low birth weight infant may often be preterm and SGA. They are not interchangeable, however, as each has distinct etiologies and risk factors (32, 33). Among low birth weight infants, approximately two-thirds

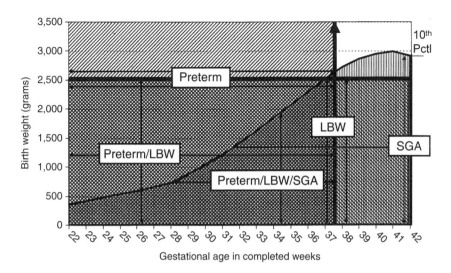

FIGURE B-1 Comparison of preterm (<37 weeks of gestation), low birth weight (<2,500 grams), and SGA (less than the 10th percentile of birth weight). Source: 1985–1988 and 1995–2000 Birth Cohort Linked Birth/Infant death Data Set, CD-ROM Series 20, USDHHS, CDCP, NCHS; 1980–2000 Natality Data Set, CD-ROM Series 21, USDHHS, CDCP, NCHS.

are born preterm, whereas less than 20 percent of SGA age infants are born preterm.

Typically, preterm birth is defined as a delivery or birth at a gestational age less than 37 weeks. Other commonly used subcategories of preterm birth have been established and delineate moderately preterm (birth at 33 to 36 weeks of gestation), very preterm (birth at <33 weeks of gestation), and extremely preterm (birth at ≤28 weeks of gestation). Table B-1 provides recent data on all live births to U.S. resident mothers for various gestational age and preterm categories.

Preterm birth is an outcome defined by a single end point, i.e., being born before an established gestational age (37 weeks). Fundamentally, infants born preterm are assumed to have a certain added risk of death, disease, and disability compared with the risk for normal-term infants. However, although preterm births may be grouped together on the basis of having a higher risk of adverse outcomes, several distinct clinical categories of preterm delivery have been identified (34, 35). Preterm births have been classified into three separate subgroups according to clinical presentation:

• Births occurring after spontaneous premature labor, related to premature contractions (50% of cases)

TABLE B-1 Gestational Ages of Live Births in
the United States, 1995 to 2000

Gestational Age Category (Weeks of Gestation)	Percentage of Births
% Extremely Preterm (≤28)	0.8
% Very Preterm (≤32)	2.2
% Moderate Preterm (33-36)	8.9
% Preterm (<37)	11.2
% Preterm (37-41)	81.9
% Postterm (42+)	7.0

SOURCE: 1995–2000 Birth Cohort Linked Birth/Infant death
Data Set, CD-ROM Series 20, USDHHS, CDCP, NCHS; 1980–
2000 Natality Data Set, CD-ROM Series 21, USDHHS, CDCP,
NCHS.

- Spontaneous rupture of the membranes (roughly 30 percent of cases)
- Indicated delivery of a premature infant for the benefit of either the infant or the mother (about 20 percent of cases) (36, 37)

Although preterm birth may be defined as a delivery before what is considered the normal length of gestation, preterm birth is recognized as stemming from several pathways (e.g., infections and fetal growth restriction) that may operate separately or that may interact with one another. In essence, preterm birth is not a single entity but is the result of one or more causal processes, each of which may result in a similar event: being born too soon.

Although the subclassification of preterm birth by clinical presentation is a step toward separating preterm deliveries into more homogeneous subgroups, there continues to be ongoing discussion regarding whether the widely used three-category classification truly defines separate preterm entities. The accurate classification of preterm birth subgroups is an important step toward establishing risk factors and ensuring that interventions are targeted at those who are truly at risk. To the extent that the components of an intervention are focused on a specific etiologic pathway for preterm birth but targeted broadly to all individuals at risk for preterm birth in general, the intervention may well appear to lack efficacy. Moreover, risk factors and predeterminants may differ by preterm subgroup, further hindering research in establishing separate and distinct categories of preterm birth. Some researchers suggest combining spontaneous premature labor (contractions) and spontaneous rupture of the membranes, and it has been noted that the risk factors for these categories are somewhat similar

(34). Because of these findings, which suggest that spontaneous rupture of membranes and spontaneous labor are the result of similar processes, there is an argument for combining these back together into one group. However, some researchers further suggest that there is more etiologic overlap between spontaneous and indicated preterm birth than was first suspected (34). For example, maternal hypertension and fetal intrauterine growth restriction are indications for preterm delivery and are also suspected to be risk factors for spontaneous preterm birth (34).

Notwithstanding the ongoing debates and developments about pathways, the value of identifying the distinct etiologic pathways that lead to preterm birth is evident. Limitations to the conceptualization of preterm birth and its various subtypes decidedly hinder the advancement of our understanding of the causes and prevention of preterm birth. The research results of the investigation of poorly defined preterm etiologic categories may prove misleading despite impressive statistical findings. The ongoing refinement of a better conceptualization of preterm birth and the articulation of its numerous etiologic pathways are essential for improving research on the prevention of preterm birth.

Measurement of Gestational Age

Over and above the classification of preterm etiologic subcategories, the basic determination of whether a delivery was "too soon" depends on the measurement of gestational age. An accurate estimate of gestational age is essential, not just for research on preterm birth but also for the management of the pregnancy and newborn infants (38, 39). Gestational age is a proxy for the extent of fetal development and the fetus's readiness for birth. As an indicator of the maturity of a newborn, gestational age is closely associated with the newborn's chances for survival and the likelihood that the infant will develop complications as a neonate. Moreover, knowledge of gestational age is necessary for interpreting the results of a preterm infant's neurodevelopmental examination and for assessing the infant's developmental progress.

Gestational age is used for a variety of statistical indicators that gauge the health status of populations and assess the need for interventions (39). Hence, the percentages of infants born preterm and very preterm may reflect the prevalence of a variety of population-specific perturbations, including infection, psychosocial and physical stresses, poor nutrition, and substance abuse. The percentages of infants born SGA, based on percentiles of birth weight for gestational age, are used to provide some indication of nutritional deficits during pregnancy. Lastly, gestational age is used in conjunction with the month that prenatal care began and the number of prenatal care visits to calculate indices of adequacy of prenatal care utilization. These gestational age–based health status and health care utilization indices are useful on a population level to ensure that service needs are met, target services to at-risk populations, and evaluate the efficacies of those interventions.

Gestational age has typically been defined as the length of time from the date of the last normal menses to the date of birth (40, 41). This definition may overestimate the actual duration of pregnancy by approximately 2 weeks, which is the average interval from the beginning of the last menstrual cycle to the point of conception. The definition of gestational age, based on the last menstrual period (LMP), has several limitations (42–46). There is wide individual variability (i.e., ~7 to 25 days) in the interval between the onset of the LMP and the date of conception. Errors in correctly recalling the date of LMP may occur because of irregular menses and bleeding early in pregnancy. Approximately 20 percent of live birth certificates in the United States have been reported to have a missing or incomplete date of LMP, and greater proportions of missing or implausible dates of LMP have been reported for women of lower socioeconomic status, who by virtue of their higher rates of preterm delivery and the delivery of infants who are SGA often have the greatest medical need for an accurate estimate of gestational age.

The interval between the date of LMP and the date of birth has served as the "gold standard" for determining the gestational age of the infant and, as such, has been used in studies for validation of alternative gestational age estimation methods (47). Studies of the validity and reliability of alternative gestational age measures are needed to assess the degree to which the alternative measures consistently predict, agree with, or are correlated with the selected gold standard measure across the full range of gestational age values. These studies may further look for evidence of any systematic biases that might stem from examination procedures or study population characteristics. Because of the widely recognized limitations to the estimation of gestational age by LMP, a number of alternative prenatal and postnatal approaches to the determination of gestational age have been developed (47–49). Table B-2 provides a list of prenatal measures for estimating gestational age and further indicates the specific focus of the measures (39).

Obstetric measures of fetal heart tones, quickening, and uterine fundal growth have often been used to confirm gestational age on the basis of LMP but are limited because of wide individual variability, confounding variables (e.g., polyhydramnios), and the requirement of an early initiation of prenatal care (39). Many view early prenatal ultrasound (e.g., in the first trimester or early in the second trimester) as the new gold standard for validation of new gestational age measures, even though ultrasound methods were originally validated with LMP as the gold standard. Ultrasound estimates of gestational age are based on different measures of fetal size

TABLE B-2 Prenatal Methods for Determining Gestational Age

Method	Focus of Measure
Last menstrual period[a]	pregnancy duration
Fetal heart tones[b]	physical and neurological maturity
Quickening[b]	physical and neurological maturity
Uterus at umbilicus[b]	fetal size
Uterine fundal height[b]	fetal size
Presence of embryo sac[c]	fetal size
Crown-rump length[d]	fetal size
Head circumference[d]	fetal size
Biparietal diameter[d]	fetal size
Femur length[d]	fetal size
Sacral length	fetal size
Foot length	fetal size
Jaw size	fetal size
Chest diameter	fetal size
Abdominal Circumference[e]	fetal size

[a]Traditional measure of gestational age duration commonly used in population-based, public health studies that use vital records.
[b]Typically monitored by obstetricians during prenatal care visits.
[c]More recently developed ultrasound measure for clinical use.
[d]Commonly used ultrasound measures for estimation of gestational age.
[e]More typically used to assess adequacy of growth for gestational age.

(e.g., crown-rump length; biparietal diameter; femur length; sacral length; foot length; jaw size; and abdominal, chest, and head circumference) and are the most accurate early in gestation. As the pregnancy progresses beyond the second trimester, there is more individual variation in normal fetal growth increases, and variations in fetal growth are decidedly influenced by individual and environmental factors, including uteroplacental insufficiency, maternal exposure to drugs or toxins, and congenital infections.

Although many pregnant women in the United States may receive an ultrasound, far fewer receive an ultrasound early enough to obtain the most reliable estimate of gestational age. Minority and impoverished women, who often face barriers to access to prenatal care services, may be less likely to obtain an early ultrasound. As such, ultrasound-based gestational age estimates may be less accurate for these groups. Furthermore, ultrasound is not universally available, particularly in less developed countries. Finally, the quality of the ultrasound equipment and the level of training of the ultrasound technicians may vary across sites of care, and the reference populations used to validate the various ultrasound measures may differ.

Because accurate prenatal estimates of gestational age are not universally available, postnatal assessments of gestational age have also been developed (39). Examining the physical and neurological characteristics of the

TABLE B-3 Postnatal Methods for Determining Gestational Age

Method	Focus of Measure
Birth weight[a]	infant size
Head circumference	infant size
Foot length	infant size
Crown-heel length	infant size
Dubowitz[b]	physical and neurological maturity
Ballard[c]	physical and neurological maturity
Revised Ballard[d]	physical and neurological maturity
Lens vessels[d]	physical maturity
Cranial ultrasound	physical and neurological maturity
Nerve conduction velocities	physical and neurological maturity

[a]Still used as a gross indicator of gestational age, although limitations are widely known. Birth weight is more typically used to assess the adequacy of growth for gestational age and as a research method to impute missing gestational age values and to identify grossly inaccurate gestational age values

[b]Because of a preference for the Ballard measure, this measure may have limited use in the United States.

[c]Probably the most commonly used means of estimating the gestational ages of newborns in the United States.

[d]Applicable only to a limited range of gestational ages.

newborn, Dubowitz and coworkers devised a scoring system to estimate gestational age (47). It was later revised and shortened by Ballard and colleagues (48, 49), and other postnatal methods of determining gestational age have also been developed. Concerns have been raised regarding the accuracy of these approaches, particularly for preterm and very preterm infants (43). Among these concerns is their ability to be universally applied to various subpopulations, including different racial groups (50). Table B-3 details the postnatal approaches to the determination of gestational age (39). The specific trait being measured by each gestational age estimation method, e.g., pregnancy duration, fetal size, or physical and neurological maturity, is also provided.

There are distinct conceptual differences among the alternative strategies for estimating gestational age, and these differences have implications for research on preterm birth and international comparisons of the percentages of infants born preterm. Gestational age based on LMP is a direct measure of the duration of the pregnancy and is thus a unit-of-time measure. Many of the prenatal measures of gestational age (uterine fundal height and ultrasound) and the newborn measures of gestational age (birth weight, length, head circumference, and foot length) are direct measures of fetal or infant size, and these use the extent of fetal growth as an indirect measure of the duration of gestation. The remaining postnatal measures (e.g., the

Dubowitz score, the Ballard score, lens vessels, nerve conduction velocities, and cranial size by ultrasound) evaluate different aspects of infant maturity by using physical or neurological milestones that are typically observed by a certain gestational age. All of the alternative measures of gestational age translate their findings to the same scale as gestational age from LMP (20 to 44 weeks of gestation), even though "weeks" is strictly a measure of duration of time. Although these measures are highly correlated, they are not the same. Their absolute agreement may vary across the range of gestational ages. To the extent that different populations use different gestational age estimates, either separately or in combination, direct comparisons of preterm birth rates are compromised.

Underpinning these indirect measures of the duration of gestational age are three assumptions: (a) that the extent of normal growth and maturation observed occurs in most infants at a similar point in time in each pregnancy, (b) that the normal rate of intrauterine growth and maturation is about the same, and (c) that readiness for birth is a direct function of time in utero. Although pregnancy duration, fetal size, and newborn physical and neurological maturation are clearly associated with one another and, furthermore, are associated with infant morbidity and mortality, it must be emphasized that all of these gestational age estimation measures are attempting to define operationally variations in the underlying biological conditions that correspond to an optimal point of readiness for birth. This relationship between the duration of pregnancy, the extent of fetal size, the degree of physical and neurological maturation, and the readiness for birth may well vary among populations and may be influenced by a variety of factors. As such, the validity of these gestational age measures, as indicators of readiness for birth, is based on a set of assumptions that have proven more tenuous as our medical technology has extended the limits of viability to the extremes of gestational age.

There is growing evidence in the literature that these alternative measures of gestational age do not correspond with one another to the extent once believed, even within the basic prenatal and postnatal categories. Some gestational age measures may tend to underestimate the gestational age and others may tend to overestimate it, and this may vary by gestational age (42, 43). Furthermore, some measures may not provide consistently valid estimates for specific subgroups (43). Herein lie the concerns for research on preterm birth. Studies that change their means of measuring gestational age during the course of the investigation may uncover trends in the rate or incidence of preterm birth that merely reflect the change in measurement approach. Such biased results may provide inaccurate assessments of the impacts of interventions. Other studies that use different gestational age measures more frequently for some population subgroups, or geographic areas than others may artificially inflate or deflate the preterm birth rates for those comparison groups. This may lead to the inaccurate determination of cases of preterm birth and a biased establishment of risk characteristics and high-risk areas. As indicated earlier, this represents a major concern for international comparisons of preterm birth rates.

Epidemiological studies of preterm birth in large populations, which often use vital records, typically rely on LMP or, more recently, LMP and the clinical estimate as reported on the birth certificate to define gestational age. It is these studies that have typically established current national trends and international comparisons in preterm birth rates. Meanwhile, clinical studies may more typically have access to early ultrasound data, although the study populations selected may be less representative of the larger population at risk of preterm birth. These measurement issues hinder comparisons among study findings, limit the interpretation and generalizability of the results, and persist as an ever lurking potential bias to research on preterm birth.

TRENDS, VARIABILITY, AND RISK

Trends

During the last 2 decades of the 20th century, preterm birth rates in the United States exhibited a steady increase. As depicted in Figure B-2, an approximately 30 percent increase was observed for both the preterm birth and the very preterm birth rates between 1980 and 2000.

Furthermore, examination of the gestational age distribution during the latter part of this period reveals a slight decrease in mean gestational age from 39.2 weeks for 1985 to 1988 to 38.8 weeks for 1995 to 2000. Additionally, there is an overall shift in the distribution, resulting in a great proportion of preterm births and a decrease in postterm births (42-plus weeks of gestation). These patterns are illustrated in Figure B-3, which displays the gestational age distributions of live births to U.S. resident mothers, using data from the NCHS linked live birth infant death cohort files.

For the two time periods portrayed in Figure B-3, Table B-4 provides the proportion of births for the various preterm birth categories. Between 1985–1988 and 1995–2000, the proportion of preterm birth rose approximately 15 percent.

These increasing trends in preterm delivery have not been consistent among racial groups in the United States. Figure B-4 provides trends in the percentages of preterm and very preterm births for whites and African Americans on the basis of the reported race of the mother. Although a steady increase in these rates is evident for whites, this temporal pattern is not evident for African Americans. This divergence in trends in the rates of preterm delivery has been the subject of investigation (8, 51). Differential

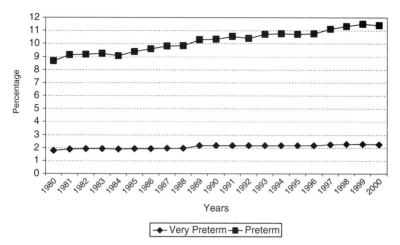

FIGURE B-2 Trends in maturity: percentages of deliveries to U.S. resident mothers by preterm birth category, 1980 to 2000. A change certificates. Source: 1985–1988 and 1995–2000 Birth Cohort Linked Birth/Infant death Data Set, CD-ROM Series 20, USDHHS, CDCP, NCHS; 1980–2000 Natality Data Set, CD-ROM Series in reporting of some variables occurred starting with 1989 birth 21, USDHHS, CDCP, NCHS.
NOTE: Change in reporting for some variables with 1989 certificate.

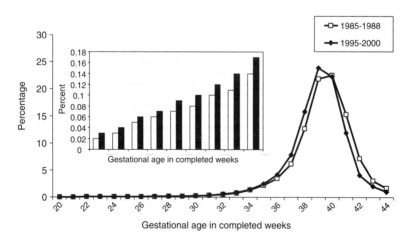

FIGURE B-3 Gestational age distributions,1985 to 1988 and 1995 to 2000. Source: 1985–1988 and 1995–2000 Birth Cohort Linked Birth/Infant death Data Set, CD-ROM Series 20, USDHHS, CDCP, NCHS; 1980–2000 Natality Data Set, CD-ROM Series 21, USDHHS, CDCP, NCHS.

TABLE B-4 Gestational Ages of Live Births in the United States, 1985–1988 and 1995–2000

	Percentages of Births	
Gestational Age Categories	1985–1988	1995–2000
% Extremely Preterm (≤28 wks)	0.66	0.82
% Very Preterm (≤2 wks)	1.9	2.2
% Moderate Preterm (33–36 wks)	7.7	8.9
%Preterm (<37 wks)	9.7	11.2
%Preterm (37–41 wks)	78.5	81.9
%Postterm (42+ wks)	11.9	7.0

SOURCE: 1985–1988 and 1995–2000 Birth Cohort Linked Birth/Infant death Data Set, CD-ROM Series 20, USDHHS, CDCP, NCHS; 1980–2000 Natality Data Set, CD-ROM Series 21, USDHHS, CDCP, NCHS.

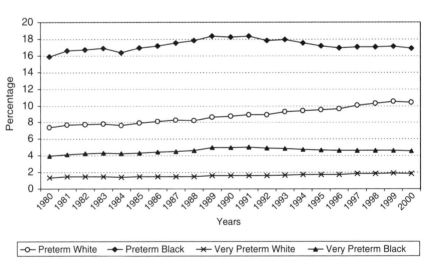

FIGURE B-4 Trends in maturity: percentages of preterm and very preterm births among whites and African Americans, 1980 to 2000. A change in reporting of some variables occurred starting with 1989 birth certificates. Source: 1985–1988 and 1995–2000 Birth Cohort Linked Birth/Infant death Data Set, CD-ROM Series 20, USDHHS, CDCP, NCHS; 1980–2000 Natality Data Set, CD-ROM Series 21, USDHHS, CDCP, NCHS.
NOTE: Change in reporting for some variables with 1989 certificate.

changes in the proportion of white multiple births and the proportions of births among older and unmarried mothers are potential contributors to these dissimilar trends in prematurity, as are changes in racial disparities in vital record reporting practices, e.g., more complete reporting of extremely preterm deliveries. Differentials in the measurement of gestational age among these groups may also be involved.

Geographic Variability

Considerable geographic variability in very preterm and preterm rates is evident in the U.S. As shown in Figures B-5a and B-5b, higher preterm and very preterm rates are evident in the southeastern states. While the racial composition of states may partly underlie the observed geographic pattern, other factors are likely to be involved. Recent investigations have established that prevailing national trends in preterm births are not applicable to each dtate and there is considerable state heterogeneity in both preterm rates and trends in preterm rates by racial groups, potentially reflecting reporting issues and other demographic, economic, social risk, and health care delivery and financing factors.

Sociodemographic Variability

Racial and ethnic variations in gestational age and preterm birth percentages have long been observed (3, 7, 9). Figure B-6 presents the percent gestational age distribution for whites, African Americans, Japanese, Asian Indian, and Samoan births, all to U.S. resident mothers. Although the mode is similar for each group, important differences are evident in the very preterm tail, with African Americans exhibiting the highest proportion of very preterm births (Figure B-7).

Geographic variations in preterm and very preterm birth rates are also observed within each major racial group (Figures B-8a to B-8d). For whites, higher percentages of preterm and very preterm births are seen from Texas through the Appalachian States. Higher percentages of very preterm births for African Americans are also noted for the mid-Atlantic states and the midwestern states of Illinois and Michigan.

Differences in gestational age distributions have been noted by maternal disease group. As depicted in Figure B-9, which displays data for the infants of white mothers only, the preterm tails of the gestational age distributions of births of hypertensive and diabetic mothers tend to be elevated, indicating higher proportions of infants born preterm. Gestational age information is also provided for the infants of white mothers who smoke. Although the impact of smoking appears to be modest, a higher percentage of very preterm births is still evident among women who smoke.

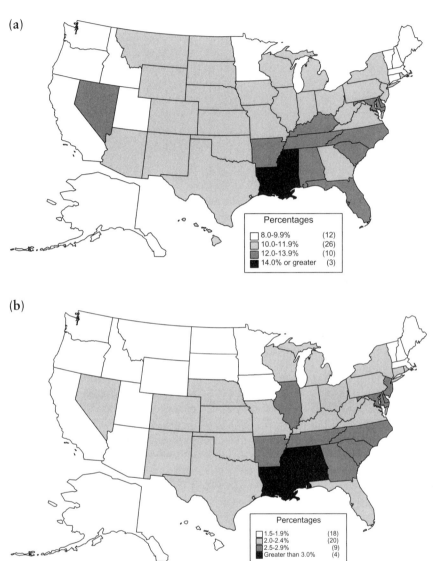

FIGURES B-5 Percentages of preterm (a) and very preterm (b) deliveries by state, 1995 to 2000. Values in parentheses are numbers of states. Source: 1995–2000 Birth Cohort Linked Birth/Infant death Data Set, CD-ROM Series 20, USDHHS, CDCP, NCHS; 1980–2000 Natality Data Set, CD-ROM Series 21, USDHHS, CDCP, NCHS.

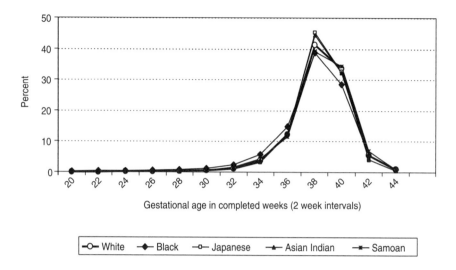

FIGURE B-6 Gestational age distribution of live births by race, United States, 1999 and 2000. Source: 1995–2000 Birth Cohort Linked Birth/Infant death Data Set, CD-ROM Series 20, USDHHS, CDCP, NCHS; 1980–2000 Natality Data Set, CD-ROM Series 21, USDHHS, CDCP, NCHS.

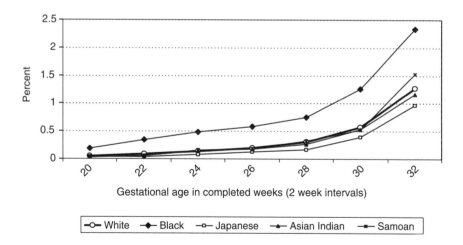

FIGURE B-7 Gestational age distribution of live births by race (20–32 weeks gestation), United States, 1999 and 2000. Source: 1995–2000 Birth Cohort Linked Birth/Infant death Data Set, CD-ROM Series 20, USDHHS, CDCP, NCHS; 1980–2000 Natality Data Set, CD-ROM Series 21, USDHHS, CDCP, NCHS.

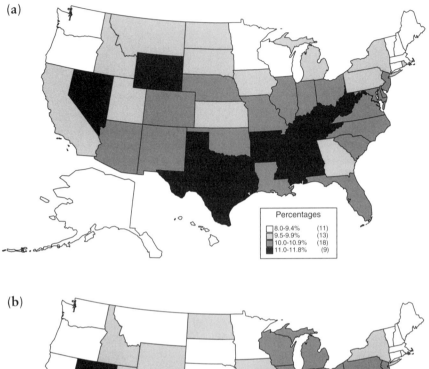

FIGURE B-8 Percentages of preterm and very preterm deliveries by race, 1995 to 2000: (a) preterm deliveries for whites; (b) preterm deliveries for African Americans; (c) very preterm deliveries for whites; (d) very preterm deliveries for African Ameri-

(c)

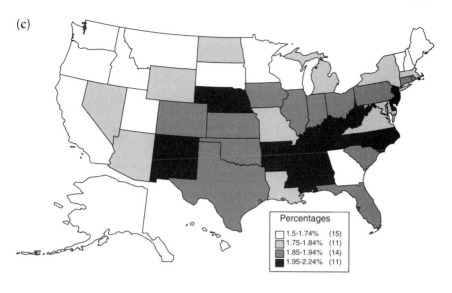

(d)

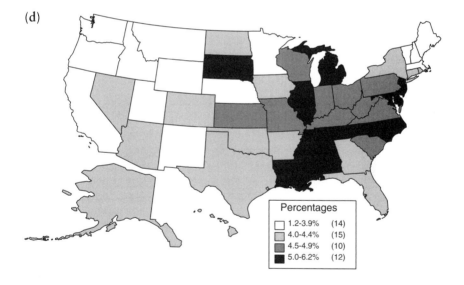

cans. Values in parentheses are numbers of states. Source: 1995–2000 Birth Cohort
Linked Birth/Infant death Data Set, CD-ROM Series 20, USDHHS, CDCP, NCHS;
1980–2000 Natality Data Set, CD-ROM Series 21, USDHHS, CDCP, NCHS.

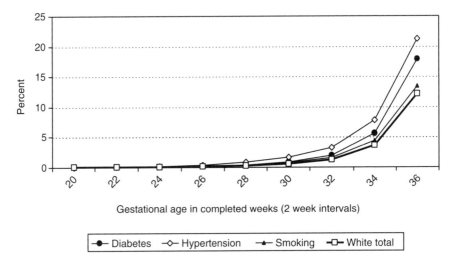

Gestational age in completed weeks (2 week intervals)

—●— Diabetes —◇— Hypertension —▲— Smoking —□— White total

FIGURE B-9 Gestational age distribution of live births among white mothers by maternal disease group (diabetes, hypertension, and smoking), United States, 1999 and 2000. Source: 1995–2000 Birth Cohort Linked Birth/Infant death Data Set, CD-ROM Series 20, USDHHS, CDCP, NCHS; 1980–2000 Natality Data Set, CD-ROM Series 21, USDHHS, CDCP, NCHS.

Gestational ages vary markedly when multiple births are involved (52). The entire gestational age distribution for triplets and twins is shifted toward the preterm tail, and the average gestational age of these multiple births is 2 to 4 weeks shorter than that of singleton births (Figure B-10). The increasing trend in multiple births has been identified as a possible major contributor to the concurrent rise in preterm birth rates and has been related to changes in the use of ART (53).

Variations in gestational age by mode of delivery have also been noted (Figure B-11). Higher percentages of preterm and very preterm deliveries than term deliveries are found to be performed by cesarean section. Although trends in the use of cesarean section have varied over the last 2 decades, there has been a general increase in the use of cesarean section for the delivery of preterm and low birth weight infants (54).

A comparison of the very preterm tail of the gestational age distribution of extremely low-risk mothers (defined as women who are married and aged 20 to 34 years; have 13 or more years of education; are multiparous with average parity for age; and have adequate prenatal care utilization; vaginal delivery; and no reports of medical risk factors, tobacco use, or alcohol use during pregnancy) with all other mothers reveals marked differ-

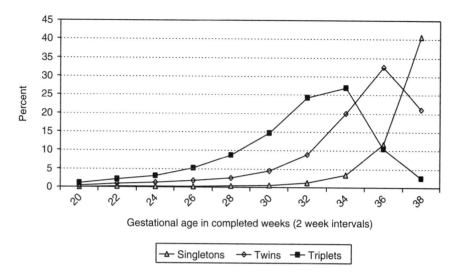

Gestational age in completed weeks (2 week intervals)

—△— Singletons —◇— Twins —■— Triplets

FIGURE B-10 Gestational age distribution of live births by multiple births, United States, 1996 to 2000. Source: 1995–2000 Birth Cohort Linked Birth/Infant death Data Set, CD-ROM Series 20, USDHHS, CDCP, NCHS; 1980–2000 Natality Data Set, CD-ROM Series 21, USDHHS, CDCP, NCHS.

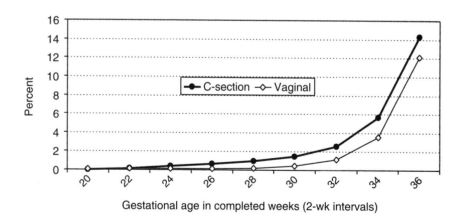

Gestational age in completed weeks (2-wk intervals)

FIGURE B-11 Gestational age distribution of live births by mode of delivery, United States, 1999 and 2000 (C-section indicates delivery by cesarean section). Source: 1995–2000 Birth Cohort Linked Birth/Infant death Data Set, CD-ROM Series 20, USDHHS, CDCP, NCHS; 1980–2000 Natality Data Set, CD-ROM Series 21, USDHHS, CDCP, NCHS.

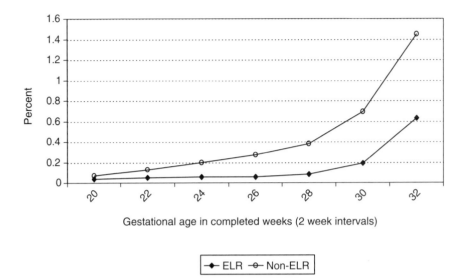

Gestational age in completed weeks (2 week intervals)

[—◆— ELR —ᴏ— Non-ELR]

FIGURE B-12 Gestational age distribution of live births for extremely low-risk (ELR) mothers, United States, 1996 to 2000. Source: 1995–2000 Birth Cohort Linked Birth/Infant death Data Set, CD-ROM Series 20, USDHHS, CDCP, NCHS; 1980–2000 Natality Data Set, CD-ROM Series 21, USDHHS, CDCP, NCHS.

ences in the risk of preterm birth (Figure B-12). A nearly threefold difference in the very preterm birth rates is observed for these two groups.

Risk

The numerous efforts to prevent preterm birth have had little success (28–30, 55, 56). Moreover, there has been only modest success in accurately identifying women at risk for preterm birth, although quite a number of risk factors have been identified (24). Unfortunately, many of the better-established and more-predictive risk factors are either immutable in the current pregnancy or, because of our present state of knowledge, pose significant challenges for either prevention or effective intervention. These risk factors are detailed in Table B-5 and include those that predate the pregnancy, e.g., a previous low birth weight or preterm delivery, multiple second-trimester abortions, maternal stature and body mass, and a history of infertility. Placental abnormalities, cervical or uterine anomalies, and preeclampsia are additional medical risk factors for prematurity that cannot be readily prevented. Finally, intrauterine infection remains in this category as

TABLE B-5 Immutable Medical Risk Factors Associated with Preterm Birth

Previous low birth weight or preterm delivery
Multiple 2nd trimester spontaneous abortion
Prior first trimester induced abortion
Familial and intergenerational factors
History of infertility
Nulliparity
Placental abnormalities
Cervical and uterine anomalies
Gestational bleeding
Intrauterine growth restriction
In utero diethylstilbestrol exposure
Multiple gestations
Infant sex
Short stature
Low prepregnancy weight/low body mass index
Urogenital infections
Preeclampsia

research on the efficacy of antibiotic therapy for the prevention of preterm delivery from these infections continues.

Demographic risks associated with preterm delivery include African American race, single marital status, low socioeconomic status, maternal age, and others (Table B-6). Although demographic factors cannot cause the premature expulsion of a fetus, these factors may antagonize some other risk factor(s).

Social, behavioral, stress, and maternal psychological factors have frequently been linked to pregnancy outcomes; and chronic stress has been related to low socioeconomic status (57–66). There have been difficulties in measuring the amount of stress caused by life events, but consistent associations between perceived stress and preterm birth have been reported.

TABLE B-6 Demographic Risk Factors Associated with Preterm Birth

Race/ethnicity
Single Marital Status
Low Socioeconomic status
Seasonality of pregnancy and birth
Maternal Age
Employment-related physical activity
Occupational exposures
Environment exposures

TABLE B-7 Possibly Mutable Risk Factors
Associated with Preterm Birth

No or inadequate prenatal care usage
Cigarette smoking
Use of marijuana and other illicit drugs
Cocaine use
Alcohol consumption
Caffeine intake
Maternal weight gain
Dietary intake
Sexual activity during late pregnancy
Leisure-time physical activities

Chronic stressors may include financial insecurities, poor and crowded living conditions, unemployment, stressful working conditions, domestic violence, and unsatisfying marital relationships. Many of these risk factors are multifactorial and are deeply intertwined with social class, culture, race, and ethnicity. Continued research in the area of stress and its relationship to preterm birth is needed to determine the capacity for the prevention of preterm birth through the alleviation of stress. Essential to the development of successful interventions in this area is the elucidation of the biological pathways by which stressors influence preterm labor and the identification of biological markers that are more specific indicators of risk than the current measures of demographics and socioeconomic status.

Although it is often difficult to modify risk factors, a number of maternal behavioral risk factors for preterm delivery have been identified and are potentially mutable (Table B-7). Among those that can be targeted for the prevention of preterm birth include cigarette smoking, prenatal care utilization, and illicit drug use. Illicit drug use during pregnancy has been associated with a more than twofold increased risk of preterm premature rupture of membranes. However, the proportion of the pregnant population engaged in illicit drug use may be small, and to the extent that intervention efforts are effective in preventing drug use during pregnancy, the potentially attainable decrease in overall preterm birth rates from such interventions may be quite modest.

Table B-8 details risk factors for preterm birth by four time periods (1980 to 1984, 1985 to 1989, 1990 to 1994, and 1995 to 1999). The risk factors include the age of the mother, level of maternal education achieved, marital status, parity, maternal race, maternal nativity status, maternal complications of diabetes and hypertension, maternal smoking, and multiple births. For each risk factor, the table provides the percentage of births with the characteristic, the percentage of preterm births with the characteristic, and the percentage of preterm births among all births with the characteristic. Odds ratios (ORs) are derived from a logistic regression by using preterm birth as the outcome variable. The attributable risk (AR) fraction is also indicated. The increasing role of multiple births in the increasing rates of preterm birth in the United States are evident from the data in Table B-8, with nearly 15 percent of preterm births being either twins or higher-order multiple births. The numbers of births to older mothers are also observed to be increasing, and the risk of a preterm birth is noted to rise with advancing maternal age (Table B-8 and Figure B-13). Nevertheless, the overall contribution of maternal age to preterm birth rates remains modest in comparison with the contributions of other maternal characteristics, e.g., multiple births and marital status.

Gestational Age–Specific Mortality

Although the rates of preterm birth have been increasing over the last 20 years, infant mortality rates in the United States have continued to decline (10). Despite the occurrence of more high-risk births, the improvement in infant mortality appears to be driven by advancements in survival. As portrayed in Figure B-14, improvements in gestational age–specific infant mortality are evident for each gestational age interval beyond 20 to 21 weeks of gestation between the periods 1985–1988 and 1995–2000. Figure B-15 indicates the percent decline in gestational age–specific mortality between the periods. For births at 24 weeks gestation and greater, a more than 30 percent reduction in mortality risk occurred between the time periods. An approximately 40 percent decrease in infant mortality or better was evident for births at 26 to 31 weeks of gestation. Even births in the range of 22 to 23 weeks of gestation experienced some improvement in survival.

Within each of the well-established gestational age categories (i.e., very preterm, moderately preterm, term, and postterm), infant mortality rates were markedly lower for the 1995–2000 time period (Table B-9).

Geographic variations in infant mortality rates for preterm and very preterm births are provided in Figures B-16 and B-17 for 1995 to 2000 U.S. resident births. Considerable variation in the mortality risk of these high risk infants is apparent. States along the southern Atlantic coast evinced markedly higher mortality rates and for very preterm infants, elevated rates were also observed for several midwestern industrial states. Myriad factors may underlie these variations in the survival of preterm and very preterm births. In addition to differences in rates that may be influenced by gestational age measurement and reporting issues, variations in population risk characteristics may also be involved. Lastly, attributes of the health care system, including availability, access, and quality, may further be associated with these geographic patterns in infant mortality risk.

TABLE B-8 Risk Factors for Preterm Birth

	1980–1984			1985–1989		
	% Total	OR	AR$_{total}$	% Total	OR	AR$_{total}$
	% Among Preterm Births			% Among Preterm Births		
Factor	% Preterm			% Preterm		
Total % Preterm	9.1			9.8		
Age in teens	5.3	1.3	3.9	4.6	1.20	3.2
	8.7	(1.29–		7.6	(1.19–	
	15.8	1.31)^a		16.1	1.21)	
Older age	5.2	1.19	0.3	7.6	1.21	0.4
	5.6	(1.18–		7.9	(1.21–	
	9.7	1.20)		10.2	1.22)	
High level of education	34.3	0.84	–11.9	38.3	0.84	–13.0
	27.4	(0.84–		30.3	(0.83–	
	7.0	0.85)		7.8	0.84)	
Low level of education	19.6	1.26	8.9	18.4	1.21	7.8
	26.1	(1.26–		24.8	(1.21–	
	12.4	1.27)		13.2	1.22)	
Unmarried	19.3	1.42	14.8	24.0	1.43	16.8
	30.7	(1.42–		36.7	(1.42–	
	15.0	1.43)		15.0	1.43)	
Primiparous	42.3	1.10	0.3	41.3	1.08	–0.7
	42.9	(1.10–		40.9	(1.07–	
	9.1	1.11)		9.7	1.08)	
High parity	3.6	1.20	2.1	3.1	1.23	2.1
	5.3	(1.19–		5.2	(1.22–	
	15.0	1.22)		16.3	1.24)	
African-American race	15.6	1.91	14.8	15.8	1.94	15.0
	27.9	(1.91–		28.5	(1.93–	
	16.5	1.92)		17.6	1.95)	
Foreign born	9.9	1.03	0.22	13.1	1.01	–0.2
	10.2	(1.02–		12.9	(1.00–	
	9.2	1.04)		9.6	1.01)	

1990–1994			1995–1999		
% Total	OR	AR_{total}	% Total	OR	AR_{total}
% Among Preterm Births			% Among Preterm Births		
% Preterm			% Preterm		
	10.6			11.1	
5.0	1.21	2.6	4.8	1.17	1.8
7.3	(1.19–		6.5	(1.16–	
15.7	1.23)		15.1	1.17)	
9.9	1.20	0.9	12.6	1.21	1.6
10.7	(1.19–		14.0	(1.20–	
11.3	1.22)		12.4	1.21)	
37.9	0.85	−12.1	45.1	0.87	−9.6
30.7	(0.84–		39.9	(0.86–	
8.4	0.85)		9.8	0.87)	
21.6	1.16	7.0	19.6	1.11	4.2
26.9	(1.15–		22.8	(1.11–	
13.1	1.17)		12.8	1.12)	
30.2	1.35	16.2	32.3	1.23	12.1
41.3	(1.34–		40.5	(1.23–	
14.6	1.36)		13.9	1.24)	
40.6	1.05	−1.8	40.7	1.07	−1.4
39.6	(1.04–		39.8	(1.07–	
10.3	1.06)		10.9	1.08)	
3.8	1.25	2.4	3.3	1.27	1.9
6.0	(1.23–		5.1	(1.26–	
17.4	1.27)		17.0	1.28)	
16.4	1.97	13.8	15.4	1.69	9.8
27.9	(1.95–		23.6	(1.68–	
18.0	1.98)		17.1	1.70)	
17.0	1.04	−1.2	19.3	0.99	−1.5
16.0	(1.03–		17.9	(0.995–	
9.9	1.05)		10.3	1.00)	

continued

TABLE B-8 Continued

	1980–1984			1985–1989		
	% Total	OR	AR_{total}	% Total	OR	AR_{total}
	% Among Preterm Births			% Among Preterm Births		
Factor	% Preterm			% Preterm		
Multiple births	2.0	8.55	7.4	2.2	9.28	8.4
	9.3	(8.48–		10.3	(9.21–	
	41.7	8.62)		45.6	9.34)	
Hypertension	—	—	—	—	—	—
Diabetes	—	—	—	—	—	—
Smoking	—	—	—	—	—	—

Note: Values in parentheses indicate confidence intervals.

Figure B-18 depicts gestational age-specific infant mortality rates for births from 1995 to 2000 among white and African American U.S. resident mothers. At between 26 and 33 weeks of gestation, little difference in infant mortality is evident between the racial groups. This stands in contrast to reports from earlier time periods in the United States in which preterm African American infants were observed to have a survival advantage over white preterm infants (6, 8). At the limit of viability, African American infants continue to have a greater chance of survival. For infants born moderately preterm, term, and postterm, whites exhibit a lower infant mortality rate.

DISCUSSION

The information provided in this paper reveals an ongoing rise in the rate of preterm births in the United States and considerable geographic variation in rates across U.S. states. Furthermore, during this period of increasing preterm birth rates, the mortality risk associated with a preterm

1990–1994			1995–1999		
% Total	OR	AR_{total}	% Total	OR	AR_{total}
% Among Preterm Births			% Among Preterm Births		
% Preterm			% Preterm		
2.5	9.88	9.9	2.9	13.14	12.3
12.1	(9.74–		14.8	(13.06–	
51.6	10.02)		57.1	13.21)	
3.4	1.84	2.9	4.3	2.27	4.7
6/3	(1.81–		8.8	(2.26–	
19.2	1.87)		22.5	2.29)	
2.4	1.28	0.7	2.6	1.37	1.1
3.0	(1.25–		3.6	(1.36–	
13.2	1.31)		15.4	1.38)	
12.4	1.25	3.2	10.7	1.26	2.6
15.2	(1.24–		13.1	(1.25–	
12.9	1.26)		13.6	1.26)	

birth declined. However, marked geographic variations in the rates of survival among infants born preterm were also noted. Finally, racial disparities in the rates of preterm birth continued to be a persistent feature of pregnancy outcome statistics in the United States. Of concern, these racial disparities are increasing (6).

Interpreting these trends and variations in preterm rates presents a difficult task. Over the years, many popular conjectures have emerged to explain these rising rates and have covered a wide range of possibilities, including changes in rates of substance use (e.g., epidemics in cocaine use), alterations in population demographics (e.g., growing numbers of older mothers), advances in medical technology (e.g., the greater use of ART, leading to more multiple births), and developments in medical practice (e.g., a greater willingness of obstetricians and maternal-fetal medicine specialists to intervene and deliver high-risk fetuses earlier in pregnancy because of earlier entry into prenatal care, leading to the earlier identification of high-risk conditions, coupled with the development and availability of therapies, including surfactant and steroids, and perinatal and neonatal care for high-

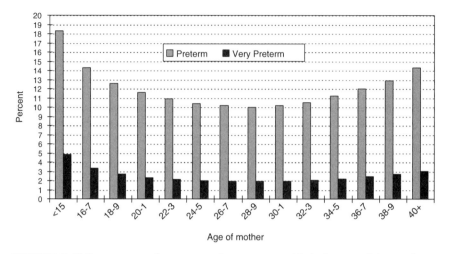

FIGURE B-13 Percentages of preterm and very preterm births by age of the mother, 1995 to 2000. Source: 1985–1988 and 1995–2000 Birth Cohort Linked Birth/ Infant Death Data Set, CD-ROM Series 20, USDHHS, CDCP, NCHS; 1980–2000 Natality Data Set, CD-ROM Series 21, USDHHS, CDCP, NCHS.

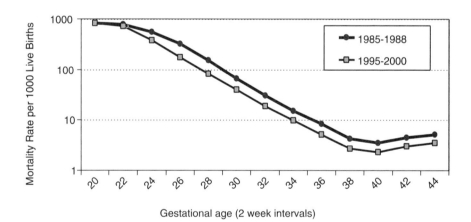

FIGURE B-14 Gestational age-specific infant mortality rates by time period, 1985–1988 and 1995–2000. Source: 1985–1988 and 1995–2000 Birth Cohort Linked Birth/Infant Death Data Set, CD-ROM Series 20, USDHHS, CDCP, NCHS; 1980–2000 Natality Data Set, CD-ROM Series 21, USDHHS, CDCP, NCHS.

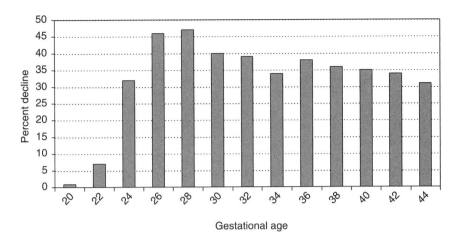

Gestational age

FIGURE B-15 Percent decline in gestational age-specific infant mortality rates between 1985–1988 and 1995–2000. Source: 1985–1988 and 1995–2000 Birth Cohort Linked Birth/Infant Death Data Set, CD-ROM Series 20, USDHHS, CDCP,
NCHS; 1980–2000 Natality Data Set, CD-ROM Series 21, USDHHS, CDCP,
NCHS.

TABLE B-9 Gestational Age Specific Infant Mortality 1985–1988 and
1995–2000

Gestatinal Age Categories (wk of Gestation)	Infant Mortality Rate	
	1985–1988	1995–2000
Very Preterm (<33 wks)	198.9	151.3
Moderately Preterm (33–36 wks)	14.0	8.8
Term (37–41 wks)	4.2	2.7
Postterm (>41 wks)	4.6	3.1

SOURCE: 1985–1988 and 1995–2000 Birth Cohort Linked Birth/Infant Death Data Set, CD-
ROM Series 20, USDHHS, CDCP, NCHS; 1980–2000 Natality Data Set, CD-ROM Series 21,
USDHHS, CDCP, NCHS.

risk births) (10). Preterm birth prevention programs, which often involve
social support and patient education, have also been proposed and implemented but have shown little success (28, 30). Lastly, more prenatal care
has been touted as a solution, even though it has been argued that little is
done in the typical prenatal practice that would prevent preterm birth (26).

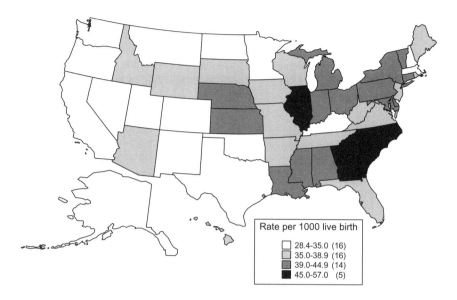

FIGURE B-16 Infant mortality rates among preterm deliveries, by state, 1995 to 2000. Source: 1995–2000 Birth Cohort Linked Birth/Infant death Data Set, CD-ROM Series 20, USDHHS, CDCP, NCHS; 1980–2000 Natality Data Set, CD-ROM Series 21, USDHHS, CDCP, NCHS

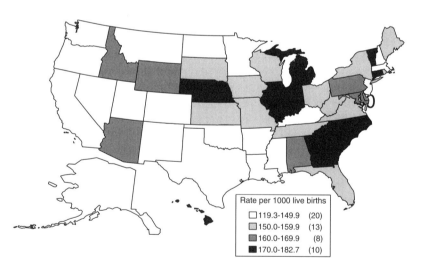

FIGURE B-17 Infant mortality rates among very preterm deliveries, by state, 1995 to 2000. Source: 1995–2000 Birth Cohort Linked Birth/Infant death Data Set, CD-ROM Series 20, USDHHS, CDCP, NCHS; 1980–2000 Natality Data Set, CD-ROM Series 21, USDHHS, CDCP, NCHS.

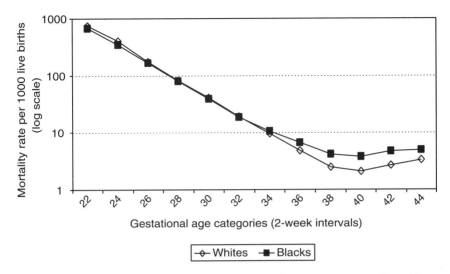

FIGURE B-18 Gestational age-specific infant mortality rates among U.S. resident African Americans and whites, by state, 1995 to 2000. Source: 1995–2000 Birth Cohort Linked Birth/Infant Death Data Set, CD-ROM Series 20, USDHHS, CDCP, NCHS; 1980–2000 Natality Data Set, CD-ROM Series 21, USDHHS, CDCP, NCHS.

Reporting Issues and Their Potential Impact

Most of the proposed "causes" of the trends and geographic variations in preterm birth rates are plausible and may operate individually or in combination. What is unclear is the extent to which each potential determinant is associated with observed variations in preterm birth rates and what other possible factors might also be involved. A typical approach for interpreting changes in preterm birth rates involves a systematic assessment of the likely precursors, starting with data reporting, regulations, procedures, processes, training, quality, completeness, etc. Variations and changes in gestational age measurement approaches and data reporting may substantially influence geographic and temporal comparisons of preterm birth rates. Before consideration of the potential roles of changes in maternal demographic and behavioral characteristics (including the age of the mother, substance use and abuse, and multiple births), social and physical environment factors (including violence, poverty, infections, stress, and environmental hazards), and health care service attributes and practices (involving availability, access, utilization, types, and the content and quality of services and programs), reporting considerations must be addressed.

Several specific reporting issues may affect trends and variations in preterm birth rates. These include changes or differences in:

- the reporting of deliveries of infants weighing <500 grams as either a miscarriage, a fetal death, or a live birth;
- the definition of fetal death involving birth weight and gestational age criteria;
- the measurement of gestational age, e.g., by the use of LMP and clinical estimates; and
- reporting regulations, procedures, processes, training, and quality at hospitals and by state and local jurisdictions.

Geographic Comparisons

Differences in preterm birth rates because of differences in data reporting, validity, accuracy, and completeness are difficult to separate from differences in the high-risk characteristics of the population and environment and the availability of health care and the accessibility and quality of the health care system. As the data included in this appendix have highlighted (Figures B-5a and B-5b, B-8a to B-8d, B-16, and B-17), considerable state variations in preterm birth rates and the survival of infants born preterm are evident. The extent to which population-related and health care system–related risk factors contribute to these variations can be assessed only with a solid understanding of each state's definitions of a live birth, a fetal death, gestational age, and other reporting attributes. As data are typically collected within hospitals within states, state aggregations of information may obscure what might be significant reporting variations among and within hospitals. Hence, in the United States, where there is considerable similarity in vital statistics reporting regulations, data definitions, reporting procedures, and population characteristics, comparisons among states are still made tenuous by the influence of these myriad confounding factors.

The problem of data reporting is magnified at the international level, where substantial differences in the definitions of live births and fetal deaths exist stemming from variations in vital record reporting, laws, and procedures. Infant mortality and low birth weight rates for the United States have repeatedly been indicated to compare poorly with those for other industrialized nations (23, 67). From these data, it is logical to infer that U.S. preterm birth rates are also higher than those in many other countries of similar status, despite potentially higher investments to health care in the United States. The precise delineation of where the United States ranks in preterm delivery is still difficult, as the impacts of different national standards of practice related to the measurement of gestational age are often unclear. For example, it may not be known what measure is typically used to estimate gestational age, e.g., ultrasound or LMP. Some nations may rely on periodic surveys rather than vital records to establish preterm birth rate trends. Hence, observations of marked differences in preterm birth rates between European countries and the United States are fraught with the potential for error. Although there may be an ongoing desire to determine the health care system policies and programs that underlie the preferable preterm birth rates of some nations, such assessments may be flawed and highly speculative if a careful review of potential reporting variations is first performed and then the influences of variations in population and environmental characteristics are taken into account. Often, the confounding effects of these many factors cannot be accurately established to sufficiently assess the contribution of any particular intervention. Currently, the two-fold and greater differences in very preterm birth rates among U.S. states are largely unexplained. Establishing which factors underlie similar or greater international variations poses an even more daunting task.

The difficulty in making relatively unbiased comparisons in preterm birth rates among countries may underscore the paucity of published international reports (23). International comparisons of low birth weight rates have been made available (67). Nevertheless, such reports emphasize that interpreting international comparisons and trends must be made cautiously and typically tend to shy away from speculating on the range of determinants that may underlie the observed differences in rates. Recognizing the limitations of the available data, recent reports indicate that the U.S. low birth weight percentage is above the average for more developed countries (8 versus 7 percent) (67). However, many low birth weight infants are SGA and not preterm, and the proportion of term low birth weight infants could vary markedly by country. As such, the U.S. standing for low birth weight may not provide an unbiased estimate of its preterm birth rate ranking. Nevertheless, given nutritional levels in the United States, it is unlikely that the United States would fare better in a valid ranking of preterm rates. With a current preterm birth rate of approximately 12 percent, a level notably above the preterm birth rates (≤7 percent) reported for several European countries some years ago, it is a reasonable assumption that preterm birth is a serious problem in the United States that has persisted for some time (23).

Understanding the variation in preterm birth rates among states within the United States may be a logical first step that should be taken before an attempt is made to make more global contrasts. For both national and international comparisons, an assessment of the definitions of birth and fetal death and procedures for the reporting of births and fetal deaths are clear starting points. Although some discrepancies in definitions can be taken into account analytically, variations in laws that affect the reporting of preterm births and fetal deaths still remain a challenge. As such work progresses, several documented interventions that have been implemented by other developed countries may well be worth considering simply on the basis of their humane approach to providing services to women and children (68). These include universal health care coverage for women and children and maternal work and parental leave policies.

Racial Disparities

The factors that underlie the growing racial disparities in infant mortality remain open to speculation (50). Clearly, there have been improvements in survival for both the white and the African American populations in the United States over the last few decades (69). The improvement in preterm infant survival probably reflects technological and practice developments in high-risk obstetric, perinatal, and neonatal care (70–76). In the obstetric area, antenatal corticosteroids and intrapartum antibiotics have been linked to reductions in neonatal morbidity and mortality. Advances in neonatal care include high-frequency ventilation, surfactant, and postnatal steroids. Regionalization of high-risk perinatal services facilitates appropriate access to these obstetric and neonatal intensive care services. Nevertheless, whites have experienced greater improvements in survival for both preterm and term infants, thereby closing the racial disparity found for preterm infants (in which African American infants have long had a survival advantage) and widening the disparity for more mature and postmature births (6). It has been postulated that the development and impact of several therapies, e.g., surfactant and steroids, may have differentially benefited preterm white infants, who may be relatively more immature and who are known to be at greater risk of mortality (7, 8, 72, 77).

State variations in the risk of mortality for preterm infants were observed in these data and are largely unexplained. Further investigation is needed to explore how the racial compositions of state populations may partly underlie these variations. With a decreasing racial disparity in the rates of survival of infants born preterm, racial variations in access to tertiary perinatal hospital care may be involved in these observed geographic patterns (78). Although limitations to health care access are typically a concern for more impoverished populations, in some parts of the country, African American women may be more likely than white women to deliver their infants in a tertiary-care center (79). Further investigation will be needed to establish the extent to which racial variations in access to high-risk obstetric and neonatal care exists, has changed over time, and may differ among the states. Although early access to prenatal care does not necessarily have a direct impact on preterm birth rates, early access may facilitate delivery in a risk-appropriate hospital. However, recent investigations of prenatal care use by race groups in the United States have revealed that racial disparities in early, adequate, and intensive use of prenatal care were reduced during the 1990s (80, 81).

SUMMARY

The current levels of preterm delivery rates in the United States represent a significant health care concern. Preterm birth rates continue to rise, and best estimates suggest that they are elevated in relation to those in other industrialized nations (23). Major geographic and racial disparities in preterm birth rates continue to exist, and these variations offer potential opportunities to better understand the population-based risk factors for preterm birth and the impacts of preterm birth prevention programs and policies. Although progress in the delineation of the risk factors and etiologic pathways for preterm birth has been made, much still needs to be done before cost-effective and efficacious prevention strategies can be implemented at the population level. The general ineffectiveness of current interventions for the prevention of preterm delivery has changed little in the last decade. On the plus side, however, the chances for survival of infants born preterm continue to increase. So long as the medical and support services needed are available to assist these infants and their families, this represents a noteworthy achievement. However, concerns have been voiced that our willingness to support accessibility to these services and the availability of these services for these infants may lag behind our drive to improve survival (82).

REFERENCES

1. Centers for Disease Control and Prevention. Infant mortality and low birth weight among black and white infants—United States, 1980–2000. Morb Mortal Wkly Rep 2002; 51:589–592.
2. Carmichael SL, Iyasu S. Changes in the black-white infant mortality gap from 1983 to 1991 in the United States. Am J Prev Med 1998; 15(3):220–227.
3. Demissie K, Rhoads GG, Ananth CV, Alexander GR, Kramer MS, Kogan MD, Joseph KS. Trends in preterm birth and neonatal mortality among blacks and whites in the United States from 1989 to 1997. Am J Epidemiol 2001; 154:307–315.
4. Lee KS, Paneth N, Gartner LM, et al. Neonatal mortality: an analysis of the recent improvement in the United States. Am J Public Health 1980; 70(1):15–21.
5. Philip, AGS. Neonatal mortality rate: is further improvement possible? J Pediatr 1995; 126(3):427–432.
6. Alexander GR, Slay M, Bader D, Kogan M. The increasing racial disparity in infant mortality rates: composition and contributors to recent U.S. trends. In press.
7. Alexander GR, Tompkins ME, Allen MC, et al. Trends and racial differences in birth weight and related survival. Maternal Child Health J 1999; 3(1):71–79.
8. Allen MC, Alexander GR, Tompkins ME, et al. Racial differences in temporal changes in newborn viability and survival by gestational age. Paediatr Perinat Epidemiol 2000; 14:152–158.

9. Centers for Disease Control and Prevention. State Infant Mortality Initiative. Atlanta, GA: Centers for Disease Control and Prevention, 2006.

10. Alexander GR, Slay M. Prematurity at birth: trends, racial disparities, and epidemiology. Mental Retard Dev Dis Res Rev 2002; 8(4):215–220.

11. Centers for Disease Control and Prevention. Preterm singleton births—United States, 1989–1996. Morb Mortal Wkly Rep 1999; 48(9):185–189.

12. Joseph KS, Kramer MS, Marcoux S, et al. Determinants of preterm birth rates in Canada from 1981 through 1994. N Engl J Med 1998; 339:1434–1439.

13. Kramer MS. Preventing preterm birth: are we making progress? Prenatal Neonatal Med 1998; 3:10–12.

14. Sepkowitz S. Why infant very low birth weight rates have failed to decline in the United States vital statistics. Int J Epidemiol 1994; 23(2):321–326.

15. Paneth NS. Technology at birth. Am J Public Health 1990; 80:791–792.

16. Levit EM, Baker LS, Corman H, Shiono PH. The direct cost of low birth weight. Future Child 1995; 5(1):35–56.

17. Rogowski JA. The economics of preterm delivery. Prenatal Neonatal Med 1998; 3: 16–20.

18. Johnston RB, Williams MA, Hogue CJR, et al. Overview: new perspectives on the stubborn challenge of preterm birth. Paediatr Perinat Epidemiol 2001; 15(Suppl 2):3–6.

19. Mattison DR, Damus K, Fiore E, et al. Preterm delivery: a public health perspective. Paediatr Perinat Epidemiol 2001; 15(Suppl 2):7–17.

20. McCormick MC. The contribution of low birth weight to infant mortality and childhood morbidity. N Engl J Med 1985; 312:82–89.

21. Hack M, Taylor HG, Klein N, et al. School-age outcomes in children with birth weights under 750g. N Engl J Med 1994; 331:753–759.

22. Saigal S, Hoult LA, Streiner DL, et al. School difficulties at adolescence in a regional cohort of children who were extremely low birth weight. Pediatrics 2000; 105:325–331.

23. Paneth NS. The problem of low birth weight. Future Child 1995; 5(1):19–34.

24. Institute of Medicine. Preventing Low Birth Weight. Washington, DC: National Academy Press. 1985.

25. Berendes HW, Kessel S, Yaffe S. Advances in the Prevention of Low Birth Weight Proceedings of an International Symposium. Washington, DC: National Center for Education in Maternal and Child Health, 1991.

26. Alexander GR. Preterm birth: etiology, mechanisms, and prevention. Prenatal Neonatal Med 1998; 3(1):3–9.

27. Alexander GR, Howell E. Preventing preterm birth and increasing access to prenatal care: two important but distinct national goals. Am J Prev Med 1997; 13(4):290–291.

28. Alexander GR, Weiss J, Hulsey TC, et al. Preterm birth prevention: an evaluation of programs in the United States. Birth 1991; 18(3):160–169.

29. Goldenberg RL, Rouse DJ. Prevention of premature birth. N Engl J Med 1998; 339(5):313–320.

30. Goldenberg RL, Andrews WW. Intrauterine infection and why preterm prevention programs have failed. Editorial. Am J Public Health 1996; 86:781–783.

31. Silverman WA. Nomenclature for duration of gestation, birth weight and intrauterine growth. Pediatrics 1967; 39:935–939.

32. Kramer MS. Determinants of low birth weight: methodological assessment and meta-analysis. Bull W H O 1987; 65:663–737.

33. Kramer MS. Intrauterine growth and gestational duration determinants. Pediatrics 1987; 80(4):502–511.

34. Klebanoff MA. Conceptualizing categories of preterm birth. Prenatal Neonatal Med 1998; 3:13–15.

35. Klebanoff MA, Shiono PA. Top down, bottom up, and inside out: reflections on preterm birth. Paediatr Perinat Epidemiol 1995; 9:125–129.
36. Tucker JM, Goldenberg RL, Davis RO, et al. Etiologies of preterm birth in an indigent population: is prevention a logical explanation? Obstet Gynecol 1991; 77:343–347.
37. Guinn DA, Goldenberg RL, Hauth CJ, et al. Risk factors for the development of preterm premature rupture of the membranes after arrest of preterm labor. Am J Obstet Gynecol 1995; 173:310–315.
38. Allen MC, Amiel-Tison C, Alexander GR. Measurement of gestational age and maturity. Prenat Neonat Med 1998; 3(1):56–59.
39. Alexander GR, Allen MC. Conceptualization, measurement, and use of gestational age. I. Clinical and public health practice. J Perinatol 1996; 16(2):53–59.
40. Reid J. On the duration of pregnancy in the human female. Lancet 1850; ii:77–81.
41. Treloar AE, Behn BG, Cowan DW. Analysis of the gestational interval. Am J Obstet Gynecol 1967; 99:34–45.
42. Kramer MS, McLean FH, Boyd ME, Usher RH. The validity of gestational age estimation by menstrual dating in term, preterm, and postterm gestations. JAMA 1988; 260:3306–3308.
43. Alexander GR, Tompkins ME, Hulsey TC, Petersen DJ, Mor JM. Discordance between LMP-based and clinically estimated gestational age: implications for research, programs and policy. Public Health Rep 1995; 110(4):395–402.
44. Alexander GR, Tompkins ME, Cornely DA. Gestational age reporting and preterm delivery. Public Health Rep 1990; 105(3):267–275.
45. David RJ. The quality and completeness of birthweight and gestational age data in computerized data files. Am J Public Health 1980; 70:964–973.
46. Gjessing HK, Skjaerven R, Wilcox AJ. Errors in gestational age: evidence of bleeding early in pregnancy. Am J Public Health 1999; 89:213–218.
47. Dubowitz LMS, Dubowitz V, Goldberg C. Clinical assessment of gestational age in the newborn infant. J Pediatr 1970; 77(1):1–10.
48. Ballard JL, Novak KK, Driver M. A simplified score for assessment of fetal maturation of newly born infants. J Pediatr 1979; 95(5 Pt 1):769–774.
49. Ballard PL. Scientific rationale for the use of antenatal glucocorticoids to promote fetal development. Pediatr Rev 2000; 1(5):E83–E90.
50. Papiernik É, Alexander GR. Discrepancy between gestational age and fetal maturity among ethnic groups. In: Chervenak F, ed. Fetus as a Patient. Carnforth, United Kingdom: Parthenon Publishing, 1999.
51. Centers for Disease Control and Prevention. State-specific changes in singleton preterm births among black and white women—United States, 1990 and 1997. Morb Mortal Wkly Rep 2000; 49:837–840.
52. Blondel B, Kogan, MD, Alexander GR, et al. The impact of the increasing number of multiple births on the rates of preterm birth and low birth weight: an international study. Am J Public Health 2002; 92:1323–1330.
53. Centers for Disease Control and Prevention. Contribution of assisted reproductive technology and ovulation-inducing drugs to triplet and higher-order multiple births. United States, 1980–1997. Morb Mortal Wkly Rep 2000; 49:535–539.
54. Centers for Disease Control and Prevention. Births: Final Data for 2003. National Vital Statistics Reports 54(2). Hyattsville, Maryland: National Center for Health Statistics.
55. Goldenberg RL. The prevention of low birth weight and its sequela. Prevent Med 1994; 23:627–631.
56. Copper RL, Goldenberg RL, Creasy RK, et al. A multicenter study of preterm birth weight and gestational age-specific neonatal mortality. Am J Obstet Gynecol 1993; 168(1):78–84.

57. Berkowitz GS, Lapinski RH. Relative and attributable risk estimates for preterm birth. Prenatal Neonatal Med 1998; 3:53–55.

58. Berkowitz GS, Papiernik E. Epidemiology of preterm birth. Epidemiol Rev 1993; 15:414–443.

59. Copper RL, Goldenberg RL, Elder N, et al. The preterm prediction study: maternal stress is associated with spontaneous preterm birth at less than thirty-five weeks' gestation. Am J Obstet Gynecol 1996; 175:1286–1292.

60. Holtzman C, Paneth N, Fisher R, et al. Rethinking the concept of risk factors for preterm delivery: antecedents, markers and mediators. Prenatal Neonatal Med 1998; 3:47–52.

61. Kogan MD, Alexander GR. Social and behavioral factors in preterm birth. Prenat Neonat Med 1998; 3:29–31.

62. Kramer MS, Goulet L, Lydon J, et al. Socio-economic disparities in preterm birth: causal pathways and mechanisms. Paediatr Perinat Epidemiol 2001; 15(Suppl 2):104–123.

63. McCauley J, Kern DE, Kolodner K, et al. The "battering syndrome": prevalence and clinical characteristics of domestic violence in primary care internal medical practices. Ann Intern Med 1995; 123:737–746.

64. Muhajarine N, D'Arcy C. Physical abuse during pregnancy: prevalence and risk factors. Can Med Assoc J 1999; 160:1007–1011.

65. Nordentoft M, Lou HC, Hansen D, et al. Intrauterine growth retardation and premature delivery: the influence of maternal smoking and psychosocial factors. Am J Public Health 1996; 86:347–354.

66. Peacock JL, Bland M, Anderson HR. Preterm delivery: effects of socioeconomic factors, psychological stress, smoking, alcohol, and caffeine. Br Med J 1995; 311:531–536.

67. United Nations Children's Fund and World Health Organization. Low Birthweight: Country, Regional and Global Estimates. New York: United Nations Children's Fund, 2004.

68. DiRenzo GC, Moscioni P, Perazzi A, Papiernik E, Breart G, Saurel-Cubizolles MJ. Social policies in relation to employment and pregnancy in European countries. Prenat Neonat Med 1998; 3(1):147–156.

69. Allen MC, Donohue PK, Dusman AE. The limit of viability: neonatal outcomes of infants born at 22 to 25 weeks gestation. N Engl J Med 1993; 329:1597–1601.

70. Curley AE, Halliday HL. The present status of exogenous surfactant for the newborn. Early Hum Dev 2001; 61(2):67–83.

71. Eichenwald EC, Stark AR. High-frequency ventilation: current status. Pediatr Rev 1999; 20(12):e127–e133.

72. Hamvas A, Wise PH, Yang RK, et al. The influence of the wider use of surfactant therapy on neonatal mortality among blacks and whites. N Engl J Med 1996; 334:1635–1640.

73. Horbar JD, Lucey JF. Evaluation of neonatal intensive care technologies. Future Child 1995; 5(1):139–161.

74. Howell EM, Vert P. Neonatal intensive care and birth weight-specific perinatal mortality in Michigan and Lorraine. Pediatrics 1993; 91(2):464–470.

75. Schwartz RM, Luby AM, Scanlon JW, et al. Effects of surfactant on morbidity, mortality, and resource use in newborn infants weighing 500 to 1500 g. N Engl J Med 1994; 330(21):1476–1480.

76. Thorp JM, Hartmann KE, Berkman ND, et al. Antibiotic therapy for the treatment of preterm labor: a review of the evidence. Am J Obstet Gynecol 2002; 186:587–592.

77. Alexander GR, Kogan M, Bader D, et al. U.S. birth weight-gestational age-specific neonatal mortality: 1995–7 rates for whites, Hispanics and African-Americans. Pediatrics 2003; 111(1):e61–e66.

78. Langkamp DL, Foye HR, Roghmann KJ. Does limited access to NICU services account for higher neonatal mortality rates among blacks? Am J Perinatol 1990; 7(3):227–231.

79. Region IV Network for Data Management and Utilization. Consensus in Region IV: Women and Infant Health Indicators for Planning and Assessment. 2000.

80. Alexander, GR, Kogan MD, Nabukera S. Racial differences in prenatal care use in the United States: are the disparities decreasing? Am J Public Health 2002; 92(12):1970–1975.

81. Kogan MD, Martin J, Alexander GR, et al. The changing pattern of prenatal care utilization in the U.S., 1981–1995: using different prenatal care indices. JAMA 1998; 279(20):1623–1628.

82. Alexander GR, Petersen DJ, Allen MC. Life on the edge: preterm births at the limit of viability—committed to their survival, are we equally committed to their prevention and long-term care? Medicolegal OB/Gyn Newsl 2000; 8(4):1, 18–21.

C

A Review of Ethical Issues Involved in Premature Birth

Gerri R. Baer and Robert M. Nelson[1]

Morning rounds on any day in any academic neonatal intensive care unit (NICU) are likely to involve some reference to an ethical dilemma. Many ethical questions have been defined in the area of premature birth, and many more will arise. Advances in medical technology have allowed neonatologists to provide premature infants mechanical ventilation, intravenous nutrition, and artificial surfactant, but prevention of major complications of prematurity remains elusive. It also appears that a threshold of viability has been reached, before which neonatal technology is of no benefit.

In this paper, we provide a review of the literature describing ethical issues related to premature birth. We focused our initial literature searches on empirical studies and added judicial decisions, commentaries, and ethical analyses to complement the data. There are many ethical issues related to prematurity for which there are no empirical data, and we have commented accordingly.

We first present the literature on decision making, which is one of the most frequently addressed areas in neonatal ethics. We discuss the two main frameworks for decision making in the neonatal period, describe several high-profile court cases, and present the difficulties with achieving informed

[1]G. R. Baer, Department of Pediatrics, The Children's Hospital of Philadelphia and the University of Pennsylvania School of Medicine, Philadelphia. R. M. Nelson, Department of Pediatrics and Department of Anesthesiology and Critical Care, The Children's Hospital of Philadelphia and the University of Pennsylvania School of Medicine, Philadelphia.

consent. Next, we review approaches to conflicts between the autonomy of the pregnant woman and her obligations of beneficence toward the fetus. We then present the current attitudes and practices with respect to the limits of viability.

Next, we present the literature related to ethical issues in end-of-life care, including the practice of withholding or withdrawing life-sustaining medical treatments, pain control and palliative care, the concept of futility, and the differences in end-of-life practices between U.S. physicians and physicians in some parts of Europe. We then examine the literature concerning the economic and social implications of premature birth. Finally, we comment on the inclusion of pregnant women, fetuses, and neonates in research.

ETHICAL ASPECTS OF DECISION MAKING

The predominant ethical paradigm for decision making about the early stages of reproduction (i.e., preventing pregnancy, becoming pregnant, deciding to stay pregnant, and engaging in activities that may help or harm a fetus) focuses on the autonomy of the woman. A transition occurs in midpregnancy, wherein the emphasis on a woman's autonomy is weakened in favor of balancing fetal and maternal "best interests." For some, this shift may be viewed as occurring when either the choice or the opportunity for termination of the pregnancy has passed. This time of transition during pregnancy from a previable to a viable fetus (i.e., 23 to 25 weeks of gestation) can also be viewed as an ethical (and perhaps legal) transition from an individual autonomy-based model of decision making to a negotiated beneficence-based model of decision making. This view, although useful, is perhaps an oversimplification, as fetal interests are often important factors early in pregnancy and maternal autonomy remains influential during the late stages of pregnancy.

The paradigm (in the United States and most Western countries) for proxy decision making for infants and children focuses on a child's "best interest," with the parents or guardians generally viewed as the primary surrogate decision makers for their infants. However, health care professionals play an important role in determining what actions are, in fact, in a child's best interest, leading to a more complex "negotiated" decision-making process. Ethical dilemmas may arise when parents and the medical professionals caring for their infants disagree on the best course of action.

Empirical Data Concerning Proxy Decision Making

Parents largely believe that they do and should take primary responsibility for decisions concerning the limitation or withdrawal of life-sustaining medical treatment (LSMT) from their critically ill infants. The majority of health care professionals believe that parents should not be solely responsible, but also that physicians often make the "final" decision in actuality. The dramatic difference in perceptions may reflect a complex process of shared decision making by use of a "negotiated" model of best interest. We first present data on parental perceptions, followed by data on health care professionals' perceptions and studies that have combined both groups. Most of the following data were collected outside the United States and thus may not reflect the attitudes of families and the practices of physicians in the United States.

Semistructured interviews of parents of infants in NICUs were performed in Scotland by a research team led by Hazel McHaffie. Parents were interviewed about whether any discussion of limitation of their infants' LSMT had occurred. The interviews revealed that 56 percent of the parents thought that they had taken the responsibility for decision making, with three-quarters of those believing that it had been their decision alone and one-quarter believing that the decision had been made in conjunction with the infant's doctors. Eighty-three percent of parents believed that the correct person(s) had made the decision. The authors concluded that parents desire involvement in decision making (1).

An international study group interviewed the parents of surviving very low birth weight (VLBW) infants to examine their perceptions of perinatal counseling and decision making at nine centers in Pacific Rim countries and two centers in San Francisco, California. The majority of subjects were the parents of survivors, as cultural taboos prevented interviewing the parents of deceased infants in most countries. In all countries, more than 90 percent of the parents believed that the physician's opinion was important in decisions regarding resuscitation status. A large majority of the parents in all countries (93 to 100 percent) considered the physician's opinion in decisions regarding resuscitation status. In all locations except Melbourne, Australia, the majority of parents (75 to 86 percent) perceived that there was joint decision making between the physician and the parents. In Melbourne, three-quarters of the parents perceived that the physician made the decision alone. A majority of parents at all sites (62 to 95 percent) preferred the model of joint decision making. In the assessment of antenatal counseling, a majority of the parents at all centers (65 to 90 percent) believed that they understood their infant's prognosis after antenatal counseling. More than three-quarters of all parents thought that the sequelae of their infants' illnesses were better than they had expected. The authors concluded that parents across the Australasian countries make decisions similarly, with importance placed on physician and partner input. They also concluded that parents prefer a joint decision-making approach and believe that it often happens. Finally, parental assessment of the adequacy of antenatal counseling was found to differ by center and by topic (2).

In contrast to many studies showing parental preference for joint decision making, a qualitative interview study from Norway revealed that most
parents believed that the physician should be the one to make the final
decision on an "end-of-life" question but that the decision should be made
with parental involvement. Families emphasized health care professionals'
experience and knowledge, the parents' incapability to make a rational decision, and the parents' need to be taken seriously and listened to (3).

The Scottish research team also performed surveys of health care professionals concerning decision making in the NICU. Analysis of those data
revealed that only 3 percent of physicians and 6 percent of nurses believe
that parents should make the ultimate decision to withhold or withdraw
LSMT. Rather, parents should be involved but should not be solely responsible for decision making (4).

A recent survey of New England neonatologists sought to describe current practices of delivery room decision making and prenatal consultation
at the border of viability. Given a hypothetical scenario of impending delivery of a 23.5- to 24.5-week preterm infant of appropriate weight for gestational age, more than three-quarters of neonatologists believed that they
and the parents should make the final decision together. However, only 40
percent of the neonatologists believed that both parties actually made the
final decision. Half the neonatologists reported that they made these decisions alone, in reality. Regarding their role in perinatal consultations with
parents, 58 percent of the neonatologists believed that their primary role in
discussing resuscitation strategies with parents was providing factual information, in contrast to the 40 percent who believed that their primary role
was assisting the parents in weighing the risks and the benefits of their
resuscitation options. Predictors of shared decision making were believing
that the primary role of the neonatologist was to assist parents in weighing
their options (odds ratio [OR] = 4.1, p = 0.004) and being in practice >10
years (OR = 3.6, p = 0.004). The authors concluded that neonatologists
should continue to incorporate parental preferences and should improve
communication about long-term outcomes and quality-of-life issues with
families to comply with American Academy of Pediatrics (AAP) recommendations on perinatal consultation (5).

In a Canadian survey of parents of extremely low birth weight (ELBW)
survivors, neonatologists, and neonatal nurses, nearly all parents and more
than three-quarters of the health care professionals either agreed or strongly
agreed that the parents should have the final word regarding the initiation
or the limitation of treatment. In contradiction to that finding, the health
care professionals also agreed or strongly agreed nearly 100 percent of the
time that doctors should make the final decision. Parents agreed or strongly
agreed 50 to 75 percent of the time that doctors should make the final
decision. The authors concluded that the physicians polled believed that

they should have more of a role in decision making than the parents wanted to allow them (6).

A comparative case-based qualitative study of decision making was conducted in NICUs in both France and the United States. Over a 2-year period, the investigators interviewed 60 clinicians and 71 parents, as well as conducted a chart review of end-of-life cases. The investigators concluded that the autonomy that parents are thought to have in the United States is not true autonomy, citing findings that the clinicians decide when to broach issues and decision points, that withdrawal is offered only on severely moribund infants who are certain to die, and that neonatologists do not ask parents' permission to continue treatment; rather, they ask parents' permission only to discontinue treatment (7).

The "Best Interests" Standard and Decision Making

The model of collaborative decision making is endorsed by numerous sets of professional guidelines. Many authors have acknowledged that although a collaborative model with emphasis on parental autonomy and values is ideal, it remains difficult to achieve. There is an imbalance of knowledge, control, and expertise in favor of medical professionals, who at times may have a different assessment of an infant's "best interest."

In her commentary on decision making and parental autonomy, McHaffie made the case that parental autonomy was impossible. She argued that (a) physicians may present facts along with guidance toward the recommended medical option; (b) an imbalance of power exists between parent and physician; (c) parents rely on the medical team for facts, and the physician may include or exclude information in an effort to persuade the parents to choose his or her professional recommendation; and (d) physicians may not offer certain options unless they are convinced that the options were the appropriate course of treatment, thus weighting the balance of power in the relationship toward the physician (4).

A group of prominent North American neonatologists, pediatricians, and intensive care physicians convened to review questions regarding decision making at the end of life in ELBW infants. The results of their discussions were published in 1994. Questions were asked regarding the withdrawal of a burdensome treatment in several cases of infants with chronic disease. These physicians concluded that "parents, in consultation with a physician who has provided ongoing care to the child, are in the best position to make the difficult decision to discontinue support." These discussions also shed light on ethical dilemmas, such as the fact that parents' options for withdrawing life-sustaining treatments are subject to their "physicians' practice styles and moral values." The group concluded that "physicians should be careful to separate their personal views . . . from current medical, legal, and moral standards of care for such children" (8).

The AAP Committee on Fetus and Newborn published guidelines in *The Initiation or Withdrawal of Treatment for High-Risk Newborns* and recommended an active role for parents in decision making. However, they state, "physicians should not be forced to undertreat or overtreat an infant if, in their best medical judgment, the treatment is not in compliance with the standard of care for that infant" (9).

Leuthner, in a commentary on the four AAP policy statements related to decision making for premature and/or critically ill newborns, argued that the most appropriate model of "best interest" is a "negotiated" model. That model strongly incorporates parental values as well as the objective medical facts and acknowledges that the moral values of the physician should be respected (10).

Loretta Kopelman, a bioethicist who has written extensively about ethical issues in prematurity, recently proposed a

> negative version of the Best Interests Standard, which applies to incompetent individuals of all ages and (1) instructs decision makers to decide what act(s) [is] in the incompetent individual's immediate and long-term interests and maximize his or her net benefits and minimize net burdens, setting that act(s) as a prima facie duty; (2) presupposes a consensus among reasonable and informed persons of good will about what choices for the incompetent individual are, all things considered, not unacceptable; and (3) determines the scope of the Best Interests Standard in terms of the scope of established moral or legal duties to incompetent individuals" (11).

She defended this version of "best interests," as it allows parents to make choices within ranges of options that are acceptable to "reasonable and informed people of good will and fulfill basic duties." Use of this standard "requires what is reasonable" and "makes room for individualized and compassionate choices that may reflect somewhat different values" (11).

Parental Informed Consent: Legal Precedents

Ethically, physicians have a duty to inform the parents and potential parents of newborns about resuscitation procedures and potential outcomes for their preterm infants as well as to obtain their consent (either implicit or explicit) to proceed with resuscitation and treatment. The process of informing is inherently flawed by the uncertainty of predicting outcomes and is often flawed by the urgency and tension of the potential parents' situation. The question of whether physicians require parental consent to resuscitate premature infants has been addressed in several high-profile court cases.

Although the 1994 *State v. Messenger* case in Michigan supported the right of a parent to refuse LSMT for a 25-week-gestation infant, the more recent *Miller v. HCA* (Texas, 2003) and *Montalvo* (Wisconsin, 2002) cases have restricted the parents' role in resuscitation decisions of an ELBW infant. The *Miller* case held that a physician was not bound by the prior expressed wishes of the parent since the infant could not be evaluated prior to birth. Although the *Miller* infant was resuscitated, the court decision does not compel resuscitation of ELBW infants but allows for professional judgment about "warranted medical treatment."

State v. Messenger (1994) in Michigan affirmed the right of an infant's father to refuse treatment for his child who was born at 25 weeks of gestation. The *Messenger* infant was resuscitated against the expressed wishes of his parents. Once in the NICU, the infant's father, a physician, asked to be alone with his son and disconnected the ventilator so that the infant would expire. Dr. Messenger was charged with manslaughter and tried in a criminal court, where he was acquitted by a jury (12).

The problem of achieving informed consent for resuscitation of premature infants was brought to public attention by the case of *Miller v. HCA* (which was decided in 2003). Sidney Miller was born in 1990, at 23 weeks of gestation and with a body weight of 615 grams. Prior to delivery, the Miller parents had told their obstetrician and the neonatologist that they wanted no heroic measures performed to resuscitate the infant. A hospital administrator incorrectly informed the medical team that the hospital had a policy of resuscitating every infant born weighing at least 500 grams. The neonatologist at the delivery noted that the infant had a heartbeat and cried spontaneously, so he intubated her and began artificial ventilation. At several days of life, Sidney suffered a brain hemorrhage and now lives severely mentally and physically impaired. The Millers sued the hospital for battery and negligence for treating the infant without consent. Initially, the family was awarded $60 million by a jury, but the judgment was overturned by the Texas Court of Appeals. Citing the Texas Natural Death Act, the court ruled that parents could withhold treatment only if their child's medical condition was terminal. In the subsequent appeal to the Texas Supreme Court, it was decided that parental consent was not required for resuscitation, during the "emergent circumstances" of preterm birth. "Sidney could only be properly evaluated when she was born. Any decision . . . made before Sidney's birth . . . would necessarily be based on speculation." Although "best practice is to obtain parental consent before birth to make an evaluation and render 'warranted medical treatment,'" the Court declined "to impose liability [for battery or negligence] . . . solely for providing life-sustaining treatment under emergent circumstances to a new-born infant without that consent" (13).

It should be noted that the absence of a parental right to refuse resuscitation does not imply that a physician is obligated to resuscitate. A physician should still make a professional judgment as to whether resuscitation is medically warranted.

Empirical Data Regarding Informed Consent

Concerns about the challenge of obtaining informed consent for neonatal resuscitation are reinforced by evidence that health care professionals incorrectly estimate survival and disability rates for ELBW infants. Achieving informed consent for procedures and research may also be problematic. One study has shown that parents have difficulty recalling crucial content communicated during the consent process for research. Underestimating survival of preterm infants may also lead to inappropriate obstetrical decision making.

The difficulty in ensuring accurate prenatal counseling was demonstrated in a study from Vermont, which tested health care professionals' estimates of survival before and after an intervention to educate them on current survival data. Obstetricians, neonatologists, nurses, and nurse practitioners were found to underestimate survival rates and overestimate major disability rates for premature infants at various gestational ages. Physicians and nurses underestimated the rates of survival at 23 to 28 weeks gestation, and nurse practitioners underestimated the rates of survival at 23 to 27 weeks gestation. For example, physicians' mean estimate of the rate of survival at 25 weeks gestation (prior to the study intervention) was ~50 percent, although the actual survival rate was closer to 75 percent. Physicians and nurses overestimated disability rates at <26 weeks of gestation, and nurse practitioners overestimated disability rates at <28 weeks gestation. For example, nurse practitioners' mean estimate of major disability at 25 weeks gestation was ~65 percent, whereas the actual disability rate was ~30 percent. The inaccuracy of health professionals' estimations of survival and disability rates decreased after an educational intervention, but the inaccuracies did not completely disappear. The authors concluded that improved education of health care professionals is needed to ensure accurate counseling for families (14).

Obstetricians and family practice physicians who performed deliveries were surveyed in Alabama in 1992 regarding the perceived rates of survival and obstetric practices between 23 and 36 weeks gestation. The respondents significantly underestimated the rates of survival and freedom from handicap for all gestational ages. The respondents reported that they would transfer pregnant women to a perinatal center for management at a mean of 23 weeks gestation, and most would administer steroids for fetal lung maturity at a median earliest gestational age of 25 weeks. However, only half of the respondents would have performed a delivery by cesarean section for fetal distress at 25 weeks gestation, which raised concerns for the authors that underestimation of the rates of survival and survival free of handicap was leading to inappropriate obstetric care. When compared with the authors' study that estimated rates of survival and that had been conducted 10 years earlier, estimates of survival had improved, but perinatal management had not changed adequately to reflect the improved rates of survival (15).

The validity of informed consent obtained in the neonatal period was examined by Ballard et al. In telephone or face-to-face interviews of parents who had consented to enroll their neonates in the NEOPAIN trial, the investigators found that 8 percent of parents had no recollection of the study at all. Of the parents who recalled the study, about two-thirds recalled the purpose of the study. Ninety-five percent of parents who recalled that their infants had entered the study could verbalize potential benefits, but only 5 percent could recall one or more risks. The time interval between the time that they signed the consent and the study interviews did not affect understanding of the NEOPAIN study's purpose, risks, benefits, or voluntary nature. Mothers were more likely than fathers to recall the purpose and benefits of the study, and administration of magnesium sulfate had no effect on the mother's recall. When stringent criteria of informed consent were used (understanding of the purpose, benefits, and risks of the study; understanding the voluntary nature of the study; and freedom from coercion), only 3 percent of the parents met the criteria for giving informed consent. The authors were concerned that the provision of informed consent by parents of ill neonates is not achievable in the current model. They suggested modifications to the process, including emphasis of the presence of risks and an interactive consent process that includes plenty of time for the parents to ask questions (16).

ETHICAL TENSIONS DURING PREGNANCY: BALANCING THE INTERESTS OF THE PREGNANT WOMAN AND HER FETUS

Over the past 2 to 3 decades, multiple paradigms have been proposed for the discussion and resolution of so-called maternal-fetal conflicts. Some authors have proposed that maternal autonomy should be the dominant concern in decision making, whereas others have established the fetus as a patient who should be treated according to the principles of beneficence. A number of cases of court-ordered interventions for pregnant women have received publicity, but these cases are rare. The tension between maternal autonomy and fetal best interest may be seen in decisions about the mode and the location of delivery. For example, a pregnant woman may decide against delivery by cesarean section in the case of fetal distress, yet ask that all resuscitative measures be used after delivery.

In the past 20 years, Chervenak, an obstetrician-gynecologist, and McCullough, an ethicist, have written extensively on the approach to maternal-fetal conflicts. They start with the concept of the fetus as a patient. They do not argue that the fetus is a person with the rights of personhood but argue that the fetus is a patient who should be managed according to beneficence principles. In an often-cited paper from 1985, they defined the ethical obligations of the parties involved in ethical conflict as the maternal autonomy-based obligations of the physician, the maternal beneficence-based obligations of the physician, the fetal beneficence-based obligations of the mother, and the fetal beneficence-based obligations of the physician. When maternal autonomy and fetal beneficence came into conflict, they recommended persuasion of the pregnant woman to undergo treatment to benefit the fetus and stated that coercion or court intervention may sometimes be justifiable on a moral basis (17). In 1993 they published "An Ethical Justification for Emergency, Coerced Cesarean Delivery," which allowed coerced delivery by cesarean section if the procedure was likely to prevent morbidity or mortality to the infant, there was no physical resistance from the woman, and there was no time to obtain a court order (18).

In 1990, the American Medical Association suggested guidelines for consideration of justifiable court-ordered interventions for pregnant women, including stipulations that the intervention must pose minimal risk to the woman's health, involve minimal invasion of her bodily integrity, and have a high probability of preventing substantial, irreversible fetal harm (19).

The American College of Obstetricians and Gynecologists (ACOG) has published several statements on the matter of coerced or court-ordered intervention during pregnancy. In 2004, ACOG published an ethics handbook that stated that in cases of maternal refusal of treatment, intervention by courts against the pregnant woman's wishes is "rarely if ever acceptable." The paper recommended examining the barriers to health-promoting behavior, addressing the social and cultural contexts of the woman's decisions, and recognizing the fallibility of medical knowledge (20).

In 2005 ACOG published a committee opinion, "Maternal Decision Making, Ethics, and the Law." In the opinion, the Committee on Ethics strongly opposes coercive and punitive legal approaches to pregnant women. The committee argued that (a) coercive and punitive actions violate the entitlement of competent adults to informed consent, (b) court orders for intervention neglect the fact that there are limitations to medical knowledge and prediction of outcomes, (c) coercive and punitive policies have a detrimental effect on prenatal care and the physician-patient relationship, (d) "coercive and punitive policies unjustly single out the most vulnerable women," and (e) these policies create the potential to criminalize otherwise legal behavior by pregnant women. The committee recommended that "in the absence of extraordinary circumstances . . . judicial authority should

not be used to implement treatment regimens . . . for such actions violate
the pregnant woman's autonomy" (21).

Lisa Harris, in an essay in *Obstetrics and Gynecology*, proposed new methods for framing and solving maternal-fetal conflicts. Framing maternal-fetal conflict as the "conflict between clinicians' moral obligations, not maternal and fetal rights," has worked best in the obstetrics literature, and Harris defined the ethical dilemmas in this way. She argued that the limitations of using principles to frame these dilemmas are that the principles are "difficult to use when negotiating moral dilemmas between intimates"; that life particularities, such as social class, race, politics, and religion, must also be considered when judging ethical dilemmas; and that principle-based ethics "neglects the broad social and political arrangements in which clinical care occurs," citing difficulties with the hierarchy of power that exists between physician and patient, particularly in cases of sex, race, and class inequality. Finally, she suggested that an alternative model for addressing perinatal ethical dilemmas would include attention to understanding the pregnant woman within the context of her social network and community, addressing the clinicians' standpoint and ethical judgment, and recognizing that the generation of a diversity of opinions may help to deal with issues of race and sex inequalities (22).

Brain Death in Pregnant Women with Periviable Fetuses

Although brain death in pregnant women with periviable fetuses has been and continues to be of interest to the media (and some ethicists), it is of little ethical value in illuminating decisions about premature infants. The pregnant woman who is now dead has no "interests" (other than perhaps the respectful disposition of her body, although the principle of "respect for the dead" is grounded in the moral obligations of the living rather than a right of the once living who survives death), and thus, there is no conflict between the now-dead pregnant woman and the still living fetus. These cases usually reflect conflict within the family or confusion about "brain death" (as in the headline "Brain Dead Pregnant Woman Dies").

Veatch defined the two potential ways to view these cases as (a) the pregnant woman is alive but terminally ill; therefore, continued treatment would be appropriate; or (b) the pregnant woman is newly dead, in which case the legal and ethical justifications for continued support are more difficult; but with no argument among family members, the life of the brain dead pregnant woman might be maintained if the fetus is near viability. Decisions under these circumstances hinge on states' definition of death and any prior expressed wishes of the now dead pregnant woman and/or her surrogate decision makers (23).

In a review of 10 cases of extended somatic support for pregnant women who had suffered brain death, it was reported that all 10 infants survived. They were born between 26 and 33 weeks of gestation, and of the six infants for whom follow-up information was available, none was developmentally delayed. A review such as this is subject to publication bias, as no cases of adverse neonatal outcomes in this setting were reported in the literature. The authors briefly raise some ethical questions inherent in providing somatic support for pregnant women, including the question of when and if the fetus becomes a patient and who should be the surrogate decision maker(s) for the mother and the fetus (24).

Decision Making in Situations of Maternal Illness

There are no general obstetric guidelines regarding when preterm delivery is indicated. However, in specific instances of maternal illness, preterm delivery may be required to restore the mother's health. ACOG guidelines for the treatment of preeclampsia state that the diagnosis of severe preeclampsia "usually warrants delivery." Immediate delivery is also the standard of care for pregnant women who have developed HELLP syndrome (hemolysis, elevated liver enzymes, and low platelet count) or who have eclampsia (25).

Intrauterine Intervention and Maternal-Fetal Surgery

The development of fetal treatments, including surgery, has contributed to conflicts of maternal and fetal best interests by offering interventions that are intended to benefit the fetus while placing the pregnant woman at some degree of risk. Some authors have promoted calling these interventions "maternal-fetal surgery" to acknowledge the intervention to both the pregnant woman and the fetus (26). The importance of informed consent becomes paramount in the decision-making process prior to intervention. Given the need to place the pregnant woman at risk during a fetal intervention, the evidence for the effectiveness of the intervention must be compelling and the risk to the pregnant woman must be negligible to warrant an attempt to compel fetal treatment over maternal objections. To date, there have been no published empirical studies to examine the ethics of fetal surgery.

Professional Guidelines and Ethical Commentary on Fetal Intervention

The AAP Committee on Bioethics published "Fetal Therapy—Ethical Considerations" in 1999. This statement acknowledges the ethical issues inherent in fetal therapies as they relate to the best interests of both the fetus and the pregnant woman. The committee advises a multidisciplinary collaborative approach to directly communicate with the pregnant woman and her partner about all the risks and benefits of fetal therapies. It also emphasizes that procedures of unproven efficacy should be undertaken only as research, with appropriate voluntary informed consent. To consider opposing a woman's refusal of intervention, the following criteria must be met: "1) there is reasonable certainty that the fetus will suffer irrevocable and substantial harm without the intervention, 2) the intervention has been shown to be effective, and 3) the risk to the health and well-being of the pregnant woman is negligible" (27).

In an analysis of the ethical issues relevant to maternal-fetal surgery, a group of bioethicists and obstetricians reviewed current practices and made recommendations for the scientifically and ethically sound practice of maternal-fetal surgery. They raised the following ethical issues: the risks and benefits to the pregnant woman, problems obtaining informed consent (i.e. "therapeutic misconception"), concerns about the ethics of intervention for nonlethal conditions, withholding intervention for those not in a randomized trial, concerns about entrepreneurship, and prioritization for funding. The group's recommendations included: " 1) innovation in maternal-fetal surgery should be conducted and evaluated as research, 2) women must be considered research subjects . . . , 3) the informed consent process must ensure adequate comprehension and genuine voluntariness . . . , 6) centers of excellence should be established for conducting research and providing maternal-fetal surgery, [and] 7) funding for research on maternal-fetal surgery should be considered in the context of societal needs" (26).

Chervenak and McCullough have proposed an ethical framework for consideration of initiating research in fetal surgery. Their framework is based on the concept of the viable fetus as a patient and the nonviable fetus as a patient if it is conferred that status by the pregnant woman. Their criteria for preliminary investigation state that (a) the intervention must either be life saving or prevent serious and irreversible disease or handicap; (b) the intervention must minimize risk and morbidity to the fetus; and (c) the intervention must pose a low risk of death to the pregnant woman and a low or manageable risk of disease, injury, or handicap. They further state that investigators have an ethical obligation to protect potential subjects from "unreasonably risky research" and consider "beneficence-based, risk-benefit analyses." The authors also emphasize the importance of "rigorously nondirective" counseling and voluntariness in consent (28).

Infertility Treatments and Ethical Conflict

There has been increasing recognition of the tension between maternal autonomy (for example, transferring multiple embryos to achieve at least one viable pregnancy) and fetal interests (for example, the risks associated with multiple fetuses). Selective reduction has not been a solution, as often couples opting for assisted reproductive technologies (ART) are also opposed to termination, even if a reduction in the number of fetuses is in the collective interest of the remaining fetuses. There is some concern that even singleton infants conceived by the use of ART procedures may have worse perinatal outcomes. If one assumes that this is true, then the decision to use ART may be thought of as a moral decision, balancing the desire of the parents to have children and the risks to their potential children. No published empirical research to date has specifically examined the ethics of ART.

ACOG recently issued a committee opinion, "Perinatal Risks Associated with Assisted Reproductive Technology." The report acknowledges data that have shown poorer birth outcomes in all infants conceived by the use of ARTs, including higher rates of perinatal mortality and higher incidences of prematurity, low birth weight, and small-for-gestational-age status. They recognize that measurement of these outcomes may be confounded by the etiologies for the infertility itself. The authors also describe an overall 30-fold increase in multiple pregnancies, although the rate of high-order multiples declined between 1998 and 2001. Recommendations for decreasing the rate of high-order multiples include preconception counseling about the option of multifetal pregnancy reduction and limiting the number of embryos transferred (29).

Several studies have shown that more preterm or low birth weight (LBW) infants are born to parents who conceived by the use of ARTs than to those who conceived spontaneously, but one recent prospective study refuted those findings. As well, ARTs contributed 15.5 percent of twins and 43.8 percent of triplets or higher-order multiples in the United States in 2002 (30).

In a study that used Centers for Disease Control and Prevention data regarding infants conceived by the use of ART from 1996 to 2000, the proportion of singletons born preterm and of low birth weight did not change over this period. The percentage of infants born with VLBWs declined overall, although for thawed embryos there was a 42 percent increase in VLBW infants. Singletons conceived by the use of ARTs had an increased risk for all five perinatal outcomes (LBW, VLBW, preterm delivery, preterm delivery and LBW, term LBW), which persisted after adjustment for maternal age, race-ethnicity, and parity (the risk ratios for the outcomes were 1.39 to 1.79). The outcomes for infants conceived by the use of ARTs were compared with secular trends, as there was no control group in that study. The authors concluded that by 2000, the absolute risk for LBW in singletons conceived by the use of ARTs had decreased and that the risk for preterm birth and LBW remained stable (31).

In a case-control study of twins conceived spontaneously compared with those conceived by in vitro fertilization (IVF), it was shown that twins conceived by IVF have a significantly higher incidence of preterm birth and a lower gestational age than twins conceived spontaneously (32).

In a recent prospective multicenter study with a large cohort and concurrent controls, neither ovulation induction nor IVF was significantly associated with increased odds of fetal growth restriction, low birth weight, preterm labor, or premature rupture of membranes (33).

THRESHOLD OF FETAL VIABILITY

Given the substantial, but improving, confidence interval on prenatal estimates of gestational age and fetal weight, neonatologists generally reserve the final decision about delivery room resuscitation for a fetus at the threshold of viability until the infant has been delivered and can be assessed. The ethical justification of this practice has been the independent moral obligation of the clinician to act in the "best interests" of the infant. When the right decision is unclear, the wishes of the parents become determinative. Recently, two court decisions have supported the strategy of resuscitation decision making at the time of delivery, yet are open to misinterpretation in the direction of overtreatment. In addition, the significance of parental input and consent has been challenged by the court decisions. Some empirical data from the United States and abroad suggests variation of resuscitation practices at 24 weeks of gestation (23 completed weeks), but at less than 23 completed weeks, clinicians consider resuscitation to be of minimal benefit. Professional guidelines strongly advocate parental involvement in decisions made at the limit of viability.

Legal Cases Concerning Delivery Room Resuscitation

Miller v. HCA (Texas, 2003)

The 2003 decision of the Texas Supreme Court in the case of Sidney Miller, a 615-gram, 23-week-gestation preterm infant born in 1990 and resuscitated against the wishes of her parents, affirmed the privilege of the physician to overrule parental wishes in emergent circumstances. The court concluded that the decision of whether to resuscitate an extremely premature infant can be made only at birth, at which time a physician can examine the infant (13).

In a commentary on the *Miller* decision, Annas agreed that "an informed decision . . . can be made only by actually examining the infant at birth." His concern was that clinicians may use the rules in a way they were not intended to support uniform resuscitation of newborns born preterm. "More troubling, the court implies that life is always preferable to death . . . and thus could be interpreted in the future to support the neonatologist who always resuscitates newborns, no matter how prematurne. . . . [S]uch a neonatologist is not exercising any medical judgment or making a split-second decision. . . . [T]he decision . . . has been made at a time during which the court believes it cannot reasonably be made: before the birth" (34).

Montalvo v. Borkovec (Wisconsin, 2002)

Emanuel (Montalvo) Vila was born in Wisconsin in 1996 at 23 $^3/_7$ weeks and with a birth weight of 615 or 679 grams. He was resuscitated with what his parents report was inadequate information about the prognosis of an infant at his gestational age. In this case, consideration of the requirement of informed consent presumed that the parents had a right to decide not to resuscitate the newly born child or to withhold LSMT. This presumption was incorrect, because the Wisconsin Supreme Court (*In re Edna*, 1997) concluded that withholding or withdrawing LSMT was not in the best interest of any patient who is not in a persistent vegetative state (PVS). In Wisconsin, in the absence of PVS, the right of a parent to withhold LSMT from a child does not exist (35).

The Wisconsin court also applied the federal child abuse amendments (i.e., the "Baby Doe" regulations) to the *Montalvo* case, arguing that because Wisconsin fulfilled the obligations for federal funds, Child Abuse Protection and Treatments Act (CAPTA; 1984) regulations were applicable in the case. CAPTA prevents "withholding of medically indicated treatment" defined as "failure to respond to the [disabled] infant's life-threatening conditions by providing treatment . . . which, in the treating physician's . . . reasonable medical judgment, will be . . . effective in . . . correcting all such conditions." The option of withholding resuscitation, argued by the plaintiffs, was exactly what CAPTA prohibited, regardless of gestational age or birth weight. Emanuel's parents did not have the right to withhold or withdraw immediate postnatal care because he was neither dying nor comatose. Because there was no alternative to treatment, the informed consent process was unnecessary. In Wisconsin, the informed consent statute states that it is unnecessary to disclose "information in emergencies where failure to [treat] would be more harmful to the patient than treatment." "In the exigent circumstances confronting the treating physician here . . . failure to treat was tantamount to a death sentence. Under the pleaded circumstances, informed consent was not required" (35).

Recent Legislation Defining Personhood

In 2002, the 107th U.S. Congress passed the Born-Alive Infants Protection Act of 2001. This law established personhood for all infants who are born "at any stage of development" who breathe, have a heartbeat, or "definite movement of voluntary muscles," regardless of whether the birth was due to labor or induced abortion (36). In the House Judiciary Committee's accompanying report, it was stated that the infant is "a person under the law—regardless of whether the child's development is believed to be, or is in fact, sufficient to permit long-term survival." The report goes on to acknowledge the uncertainty of whether infants below certain birth weights should be treated and states that "the standard of medical care applicable in a given situation involving a premature infant is not determined by asking whether that infant is a person. . . . HR 2175 would not affect the applicable standard of care" (37). In a brief commentary on the law, the Neonatal Resuscitation Program Steering Committee of AAP maintained that the act should not affect the current approach to treating the extremely premature infant and that comfort care was still an option for infants for whom resuscitation or continuation of life support is deemed inappropriate (38).

Empirical Data Concerning Limits of Viability in Current Practice in the United States and Abroad

The emerging professional standard of care in the United States and most Western nations appears to be full resuscitation for premature infants born at greater than 24 weeks gestational age and no resuscitation for premature infants born at less than 23 weeks gestational age. Parental wishes appear to have a role for infants born at between 23 and 24 weeks gestation but have a limited impact outside of that range.

In a survey of practicing neonatologists in Massachusetts conducted in 2002, differences in the perceived limits of viability were seen (41 percent of physicians saw treatment at >24 weeks gestation as clearly beneficial, and 84 percent saw treatment at >25 weeks gestation as clearly beneficial). At 23 weeks gestation or less, 93 percent of physicians considered resuscitation to be of no benefit. At 24 $^1/_7$ to 24 $^6/_7$ weeks gestation, physicians were split: 40 percent of physicians considered treatment to be beneficial and 60 percent considered the benefits to be uncertain. Thirty-three percent of physicians would resuscitate an infant upon parental request even if they considered the treatment to be of no benefit. When treatment benefits are uncertain, 100 percent of physicians would resuscitate the infant at parental request, 98 percent would resuscitate the infant if the parents were unsure, and 76 percent would withhold treatment at parental request. In addition to parental preferences, when the benefit of treatment was uncertain, factors that physicians thought were very important to consider were the medical condition of the infant at delivery (68 percent) and the likelihood of death (63 percent). Ninety-one percent of the respondents considered potential long-term suffering of the infant to be important or very important.

The authors concluded that most respondents would provide treatment that was beneficial, withhold treatment that was of no benefit, and defer to the parents' requests when the benefits were uncertain (39).

In a survey of neonatologists and neonatal nurses at Australian perinatal centers in 1997 and 1998, the majority of neonatologists (85 percent) and nurses (88 percent) would "always" or "almost always" resuscitate infants at 24 weeks gestation. More than half of respondents would occasionally resuscitate infants with birth weights of between 400 and 500 g. The most important factors influencing resuscitation decisions were parental wishes and the presence of congenital anomalies (40).

As part of the EURONIC project (a European questionnaire study examining the attitudes and practices of neonatal physicians and nurses), a case of extreme prematurity was presented and attitudes were assessed. At 24 weeks gestation, with a birth weight of 560 g, and with a 1-minute Apgar score of 1, 82 to 98 percent of physicians would resuscitate an infant in all countries studied except the Netherlands, where only 39 percent of the physicians surveyed would resuscitate the infant. The authors concluded that most physicians (except those in the Netherlands) considered this extremely preterm infant viable. Decision-making attitudes and practices after the infant's deterioration varied by country (41).

In an expert panel of North American neonatologists, pediatricians, and intensive care physicians, questions were asked regarding the initiation or withdrawal of treatment for several cases of ELBW infants. The principles that emerged from discussions of these cases were as follows: (a) that it is "difficult to make definite plans for treatment or non-treatment until the baby is born, and the neonatologist has a chance to assess size, maturity, and clinical status"; (b) that it is "essential to avoid misleadingly absolute predictions of viability or non-viability"; (c) that "shared and dynamic decision-making . . . ensures that decisions incorporate parental values, the infant's interests, and an optimal understanding of the facts and the inherent uncertainties in the child's clinical situation"; and (4) finally, that "in order for parents to choose to forgo life sustaining treatment on their child's behalf, survival does not have to be impossible or unprecedented—it only has to be very unlikely" (8).

In a questionnaire completed by 17 of 18 neonatologists in Alberta, gestational age was the most important factor involved in the decision to resuscitate or not resuscitate an infant. Parental requests, birth weight, and multiple anomalies also were important factors. Factors that were not important to the neonatologists included costs, medical-legal factors, and the religious beliefs of the physicians (42).

A longitudinal cohort study of live births at between 23 and 26 weeks gestation at the University of North Carolina in 1994 and 1995 found that 29 percent of infants were resuscitated at 23 weeks gestation, 67 percent were resuscitated at 24 weeks, 93 percent were resuscitated at 25 weeks, and 100 percent were resuscitated at 26 weeks. The likelihood of resuscitation was associated with increasing gestational age, higher birth weight, a better prognosis for survival and quality of life, and greater physician uncertainty about the accuracy of the prognosis. Withholding of resuscitation at delivery was associated with parental (not physician) preference for comfort care only. When physicians would have preferred comfort care only, resuscitation was provided in half of the live births. Physicians' prognoses for survival were relatively accurate. The authors concluded that physicians were more likely to resuscitate extremely preterm infants when the prognosis was uncertain or the parental wishes were unknown. When the parental wishes were known, parents usually determined the amount of resuscitation performed at delivery (43).

Professional Guidelines for Decision Making at the Limits of Viability

Professional guidelines advocate a model of joint decision making between parents and clinicians at the limits of viability, within the limits of appropriate medical care. However, the margins of viability at which parental discretion becomes a factor are increasingly limited (i.e., at between 23 and 24 weeks gestational age).

AAP provides guidelines for counseling and assisting families who face the delivery of an extremely preterm infant. The recommendations include (a) frequent reevaluation of the fetus or infant to assist in decision making and prognosis; (b) joint decision making with the family; (c) appropriately informing parents regarding "maternal risks associated with delivery options, potential for infant survival, and risks of adverse long-term outcomes"; (d) respect for parental choices in management within the limits of appropriate medical care; and (e) physician education about local and national outcomes associated with extremely preterm birth (44).

Despite all that is known about survival and outcomes at "periviable" gestational ages, the conclusions of a recent AAP workshop on the topic were primarily that major gaps in knowledge still exist and require study. Both obstetric and neonatal knowledge gaps exist, including the need for (a) improved gestational age and maturity assessments; (b) knowledge of the optimal mode of delivery; (c) studies on optimal delivery room management; as well as (d) evidence for appropriate management of nutrition, medications, infections, and other interventions in the postnatal period (45).

WITHHOLDING AND WITHDRAWING LIFE-SUSTAINING MEDICAL TREATMENT

The withholding and withdrawal of LSMT for infants are practiced in the United States and abroad. A significant number of preterm infants die with some limitation to their treatment. Most often, these are infants who are moribund and likely to die whether or not treatment is continued, but LSMT may also be withdrawn when long-term quality-of-life issues are the primary concern. Several authors speculate that the high rate of withholding or withdrawing life support is related to the sizeable number of extremely premature infants who are given initial trials of therapy. Over the last decade, the length of the initial trial appears to have increased dramatically. Ethicists and pediatricians have speculated that the Baby Doe regulations of the 1980s have affected clinicians' willingness to withhold or withdraw life support for newborns. Despite the Baby Doe regulations, AAP statements and guidelines continue to endorse the practice of limiting life support for critically ill infants with poor prognoses. Published data on end-of-life practices in parts of northern Europe have demonstrated that a minority of European physicians is willing to actively hasten death in critically ill neonates. Finally, familiarity with the use of pain management and palliative care is increasing.

Empirical Data Concerning Withholding and Withdrawing LSMT

Physicians have reported their experiences of withholding or withdrawing LSMT for infants in the medical literature since the 1970s. Several single-center studies have documented their practices of withholding or withdrawing LSMT. Prospective research is needed to accurately describe how these decisions are being made in modern clinical practice.

In 1973, Duff and Campbell at Yale published an early U.S. account of the limitation of medical treatment in the newborn period (primarily for term infants with congenital anomalies). In their retrospective review, 14 percent of deaths in the Yale nursery during a $2^1/_2$-year period were associated with the discontinuation of life-sustaining treatments. The authors concluded that families should be the primary decision makers, with guidance from society and health care professionals. The authors' discussion raised many questions about the ethics of withholding or withdrawing treatments, including issues around unclear prognosis, informed consent, and proxy decision making (46).

A similar case series from the 1980s at Hammersmith Hospital in London examined all cases in which withdrawal of treatment was discussed by the medical team over a 4-year period. Most of the infants in this series were born preterm or had acquired neurological damage. Of the 75 infants for whome withdrawal of treatment was discussed, 51 of their families were offered withdrawal by the medical team. In 47 cases, the families accepted the decision, and in 4 cases the families chose continued intensive treatment. The author concluded that withdrawal of treatment was the best course of action for infants who were certain to die or have "no meaningful life." He also concluded that effective communication and trust between physicians and families should preclude the need for involvement of the law or ethics committees (47).

A retrospective review of deaths in the NICU at the University of California at San Francisco (UCSF) between 1989 and 1992 documented the circumstances of the 165 infants who died during that period. One hundred eight died after the withdrawal of life-sustaining treatments, and another 13 died after additional treatments were withheld. A total of 73 percent of the deaths were attributable to the limitation of life-sustaining treatments. In the records of three-quarters of the infants whose treatments were withheld or withdrawn, the neonatologist documented the belief that continued treatment was futile and that death was imminent. In half of the infants' records, quality-of-life concerns were documented as a reason to limit treatment. For nearly one-quarter of the deaths, physicians cited quality-of-life concerns as the sole reason for the limitation of treatment. These findings were noted in the context of active delivery room resuscitation of 91 percent of live-born infants with birth weights of between 500 and 799 grams. In the cohort studied, the sequelae of extreme prematurity caused the highest proportion of deaths attributable to the withholding or withdrawal of therapies. The authors concluded that "the widespread application of neonatal intensive care has likely increased the proportion of infants for whom aggressive treatment is attempted but for whom it is subsequently determined to be ineffective or inappropriate." Conclusions from this study are limited by its retrospective design and an inability to abstract details of the decision making from the medical records (48).

In a case series of NICU deaths from Pittsburgh, Pennsylvania, 82 percent of deaths occurred after some limitation of treatment. In three-quarters of the deaths, the parents were involved in the decision to limit treatment, and disagreement between the parents and the care providers was rare. The authors concluded that decision making near the end of life for a critically ill neonate frequently results in limiting LSMT. They conclude, like the UCSF group, that "the rise in proportion of deaths after a decision of this nature may relate . . . to the increased number of extremely low birth weight infants who are given trials of aggressive therapy" (49).

A retrospective review of NICU deaths in 1988, 1993, and 1998 at the University of Chicago revealed local trends in withholding cardiopulmonary resuscitation (CPR) and withdrawal of LSMT. In 1993 and 1998, nearly 70 percent of nonsurvivors died without receiving CPR, which was a significant increase from the 16 percent in 1988. In 1993 and 1998, ~40 percent of all nonsurvivors died after withdrawal of mechanical ventilation, and ~40 percent of those infants for whom mechanical ventilation was withdrawn were hemodynamically stable. The vast majority of infants whose ventilation was withdrawn were full-term infants with congenital anomalies or asphyxia. Only rarely was ventilation withdrawn from ELBW infants with severe neurological injuries (<5 percent in all 3 years studied). Interestingly, the median and the average day of death did not differ significantly between the 78 nonsurvivors whose interventions were limited and the 100 nonsurvivors who received full intervention. The authors conclude that in their NICU, there has been a welcome increase in the number of infants who die in the arms of their parents, after removal of endotracheal tubes and without receiving CPR. They also suggest that a more nuanced examination of withholding and withdrawing therapies in the context of both physiologically stable and moribund infants is necessary to better understand the circumstances of end-of-life decision making (50).

Whether aggressive treatment of an ELBW infant is futile in terms of long-term survival is difficult to determine, as accurate predictors of survival have remained elusive. Researchers at the University of Chicago have raised the concern that a by-product of improved care and survival of ELBW infants is that the length of stay (LOS) for nonsurvivors has significantly increased. In a retrospective examination of ELBW (birth weight of <1,000 grams) infant survival at the University of Chicago during the 1990s, the median LOS for nonsurvivors rose steadily from 2 days in 1991 to 10 days in 2001. The authors concluded that the NICU "trial of therapy" for ELBW infants now takes much longer than it has in the past, and asking parents to "hold their breath" for 2 or 3 days to await improved prognostic estimates is no longer feasible (51).

Impact of the Baby Doe Regulations of the 1980s

The so-called Baby Doe regulations are often interpreted in a way that challenges physicians' authority to withdraw or withhold LSMTs from ELBW infants. In fact, in the *Montalvo* decision (2002) the Wisconsin court explicitly cited the regulations in arguing against a parental right to withhold resuscitation. However, these rules were not originally intended to apply to premature infants; rather, they were intended to apply to disabled full-term infants (35).

The original Baby Doe regulations (1984) were based on Section 504 of the Rehabilitation Act of 1973 and were struck down by the U.S. Supreme Court in 1986. The regulations held that nontreatment was discriminatory and violated an infant's civil rights.

The second set of Baby Doe regulations was enacted in 1984 and went into effect in 1985. They are amendments to CAPTA, which require the continuation of medical treatment unless an infant is "chronically and irreversibly comatose"; "the provision of such treatment would merely prolong dying, not be effective in ameliorating or correcting all of the infant's life-threatening conditions"; or "the provision of such treatment would be virtually futile in terms of the survival of the infant and the treatment itself under such circumstances would be inhumane." Adherence to these rules is required for states to receive federal child abuse funds. The existing rules have remained untested in the Supreme Court (52).

Interpretation of the Baby Doe regulations has been laden with pitfalls. The diagnosis of coma in the newborn period is impossible, and the concept of futility is too vague and subjective to be useful in decision making.

The Baby Doe regulations have affected the care of infants, including ELBW infants, as reflected in the attitudes of neonatologists. A questionnaire sent to members of the AAP Perinatal Section 1 year after the Baby Doe regulations went into effect asked physicians to consider several difficult neonatal cases and assessed their attitudes regarding the impact of the Baby Doe regulations. The results revealed that 30 percent of neonatologists thought that the Baby Doe regulations required the continuation of mechanical ventilation in a 550-gram preterm infant with seizures and a large intracerebral hemorrhage. Twenty-three percent of physicians stated that their approach to this case had changed as a result of the Baby Doe regulations. Eighty-one percent of those who responded did not think that the regulations would result in improved care for infants. Three-quarters did not believe that the regulations were needed to protect handicapped infants' rights. Kopelman et al., the study's authors, concluded that the regulations were not necessary and that they minimized the role of parents in decision making. The conclusions are limited by the survey methods of the study and the 49 percent response rate. The author also discussed additional concerns about the regulations, including concerns about the poor use of resources, difficulties with determining unconsciousness in the newborn period, changes in medical standards of care, and undermining of the best-interests standard in caring for ill neonates (53).

Kopelman, in commentaries 20 years after the enactment of the Baby Doe regulations, argued that AAP has interpreted the Baby Doe regulations incorrectly. She remains concerned that the regulations do not allow individualized decision making and use of the best-interests standard that AAP promotes. She disputes the benign interpretations of the terms of the regulations as understood by the AAP leadership and the Committee on Bioethics. She also argues that the rules are mistaken, as they do not allow for clinician discretion and do not treat infants in a way that adults would wish to be treated with regard to the relief of suffering. She raises concern that the Baby Doe rules have recently been applied in the *Montalvo* case in Wisconsin, where the appeals court decided that the parents had no right to decline treatment, as their 23-week-gestation infant was neither comatose nor dying (11, 54–56).

Professional Guidelines for Limitation of LSMT in the United States

There have been efforts over the past 15 years to develop a professional consensus on the limitation or withdrawal of LSMT from ELBW infants. Various committees within AAP have published guidelines for limiting life-sustaining treatments for newborns.

A group of prominent North American neonatologists, pediatricians, and intensive care physicians convened to review questions regarding the withdrawal of treatment for ELBW infants. The results of their discussions were published in 1994. The consensus of the group included the statement that "in order for parents to choose to forgo life sustaining treatment on their child's behalf, survival does not have to be impossible or unprecedented—it only has to be very unlikely." They acknowledge the uncertainties of prognosis, while emphasizing the importance of shared decision making between families and medical professionals. The group also discussed end-of-life decisions for chronically ill infants and concluded that a shared approach to decision making, with consideration of the child's suffering, the effects on the family, and the long-term prognosis, is the best course of action (8).

In 1994, the AAP Committee on Bioethics published *Guidelines on Forgoing Life-Sustaining Medical Treatment*. The general principles recommended were as follows: a presumption in favor of treatment, the patient or surrogate's right to decide and be informed, the patient or surrogate's right to refuse treatment, the fact that decisions to forgo treatment are limited to the specific treatment in question (not necessarily to all treatments), the preservation of respect for the patient, physicians' obligations to arrange for the care of their patient if they do not wish to participate in limiting LSMT, and the presumption against judicial involvement unless there are irresolvable disputes. The committee advocates the best-interests standard as a guideline for decision making for neonates. The document also emphasizes the importance of physician documentation in cases of limitation of LSMT (57).

A year later, the AAP Committee on Fetus and Newborn published "The Initiation or Withdrawal of Treatment for High-Risk Newborns." That document recommended the approach of the individualized prognostic strategy: providing care at an appropriate level at the time of initiation of care with constant reevaluation of the infant and dynamic decision making. Parents are to be informed and involved in decision making that could affect the infant's outcome. One physician should act as the spokesperson for the medical team. Treatments should be discontinued when "the condition is incompatible with life or when the treatment is judged to be futile" (9).

In 1996, the AAP Committee on Bioethics published *Ethics and the*

Care of Critically Ill Infants and Children. The committee expressed concerns that the Baby Doe regulations had caused physicians to overuse LSMT. However, the committee suggested that the language used in the regulations "may permit more physician discretion than some realize." The committee recommended parental involvement in decision making with physicians, using the principles of informed parental permission, and opposed clinical decision making on the basis of resource limitation (58).

End-of-Life Practices Abroad

European end-of-life practices vary by country, but there is great concern about the practice of active euthanasia in the Netherlands, France, and Belgium. A recent publication suggested a protocol designed to allow and regulate euthanasia of newborns in the Netherlands (59). In addition, infants at the border of viability (those born at less than 26 weeks gestation) are resuscitated much less frequently in the Netherlands than in other European countries and the United States. However, physicians in several European countries are uncomfortable with the practice of withholding or withdrawing life-sustaining treatments, according to the current literature.

EURONIC Data

The EURONIC research project has been carried out primarily in eight European countries and has amassed data via anonymous questionnaires on end-of-life practices and attitudes in neonatal intensive care self-administered to physicians and nurses.

In all countries, between 61 and 96 percent of the neonatologists reported that they had ever decided to limit intensive treatment. Between countries, a wide range of proportions of physicians withdrew ventilation, from a low of 23 percent in Italy to a high of 93 percent in the Netherlands. In that study, 86 percent of physicians in France and 45 percent of physicians in the Netherlands reported that they had given medications with the purpose of ending life. They conclude that variations in practice are culture and country dependent (60).

In a report that measured physicians' attitudes regarding quality of life versus absolute value of life, the country of origin remained the strongest predictor of physician response. Attitude scores were higher (i.e., indicating a greater concern for quality of life) in the Netherlands, the United Kingdom, and Sweden and lower (indicating a greater concern for life in general) in Hungary, Estonia, Lithuania, and Italy. The group concluded that increased concern for quality of life was associated with physicians' likelihood of reporting that they had ever set limits to intensive interventions. After controlling for potential confounders such as age, gender, years of experience, and religion, there were still important differences between countries, "suggesting an effect of cultural and social factors" (61).

Other European Empirical Data on End-of-Life Care

A questionnaire given to physicians caring for neonates in the Netherlands showed that during a 3-month period in 1995, 37 percent of neonatal deaths occurred following the administration of potentially life-shortening drugs. In 22 percent of cases, hastening of death was partially intended, and in 26 percent of cases, hastening of death was explicitly intended. In the vast majority of these cases (88 percent), the decision had been discussed with the infant's parents. The authors concluded that it is difficult to make the distinction between giving adequate palliative therapy for pain and discomfort and intentionally hastening death (62).

In a Belgian study, anonymous questionnaires regarding end-of-life decisions were sent to the attending physicians of infants who died over a 1-year period (in 1999 and 2000). Of the 194 nonsudden deaths during that year, 44 percent were preceded by a decision to withhold or withdraw treatment, 21 percent of infants were given opioids at doses that could be potentially life shortening, and 9 percent of patients received lethal doses or lethal drugs. Of the 143 deaths preceded by end-of-life decision making, half of the deaths occurred with the physician's explicit intention to hasten death. Lethal drugs were used five times more often for early neonatal deaths than for later deaths; and they were mainly used for preterm infants with intracerebral hemorrhage, infants with severe congenital malformations, and preterm infants with congenital malformations. In the attitude study, 79 percent of physicians thought that it was sometimes the physician's duty to prevent suffering by hastening death. The authors concluded that in the early neonatal period the severity of disorders is more apparent and that decisions based on estimates of survival are more easily made. They also concluded that the widespread willingness of physicians to participate in life termination is related to physicians' acceptance of best-interest standards and recognition of quality-of-life considerations (63).

In another study comparing end-of-life decisions in the Netherlands in 1995 and 2001, it was concluded that practices had changed little. Physicians completed questionnaires after the deaths of their patients. End-of-life decisions were made for 62 and 68 percent of all deaths in 1995 and 2001, respectively. Possible life-shortening drugs were used in 23 and 29 percent of patients who died after withholding or withdrawal of life-sustaining treatments. In 8 percent of deaths (in both years) following the withholding or withdrawal of life-sustaining treatments, drugs were given with the intention of hastening death. In 2001, more than 70 percent of end-of-life decisions were made because the infants had no chance of survival, and 23 percent were made because of a poor prognosis for later life. The authors concluded that despite liberal regulations around active ending of life in the Netherlands, the frequency of the practice had not increased (64).

Pain Management and Palliative Care at the End of Life

Despite concerns about respiratory depression and active ending of life, the use of opioids for pain management and analgesia is widespread after the withdrawal of life-sustaining therapies. There is also evidence, albeit sparse, that familiarity with and the use of palliative care in neonatology is increasing.

In a retrospective review of NICU deaths in a single center in the United States (from 1989 to 1992), 84 percent of infants received opioid analgesia when life support was withdrawn or withheld. The majority (64 percent) received doses in the usual pharmacologic range, whereas 36 percent received higher doses. (Ninety-four percent of those receiving suprapharmacologic doses had been receiving opioid analgesia previously and were likely to have developed tolerance.) The median time of death was 18 minutes for infants receiving pharmacologic doses of morphine and 20 minutes for infants receiving higher doses. All infants who died of necrotizing enterocolitis received opioids. The authors suggested that morphine was considered necessary treatment for abdominal pain in infants dying of necrotizing enterocolitis. Because of the methods used in the study, it was difficult to conclude anything about the physicians' intentions in administering analgesia (65).

A prospective study in the pediatric ICU literature showed that 89 percent of patients who were withdrawn from ventilatory support received sedation and analgesia. In patients who received analgesia or sedation as the ventilator was being withdrawn, the reasons for administering these medications that the physician and nurse stated were important were to decrease pain (83 percent), decrease anxiety (77 percent), and decrease air hunger (74 percent). Only 2 percent of physicians believed that it was important to give sedation and analgesia to hasten death (66).

At Children's Hospital of Wisconsin, a retrospective chart review evaluated the use of palliative care services in patients less than 1 year of age who died in the hospital over a 4-year period. Thirteen percent of infants who died had received a palliative care consultation, and the percentage had increased from 5 percent in 1994 to 38 percent in 1997 (the study was limited by the small number of patients). Those infants who had a palliative care consultation had fewer interventions, including blood product administration, blood draws, central lines, feeding tubes (including surgically placed tubes), endotracheal tubes, radiographs, and paralytic agent administration. There was also an increased rate of provision of supportive services, such as social work and pastoral services, for the palliative care patients. The authors concluded that palliative care services still are underutilized, but for patients who have consultations, the numbers of invasive and uncomfortable interventions are decreased. The study is limited by its small sample size and the exclusion of a significant number of patients who died at home after palliative care consultation (67).

The Concept of Futility in the Care of Extremely Ill Infants

Although much has been written about the concept of futility, there is a lack of agreement on its definition and of its utility as a concept. Within the realm of neonatal care, the concept has been invoked in cases both of extreme prematurity and of severe congenital anomalies that are incompatible with survival.

Futility arguments have been invoked when the health care team disagrees with parents regarding the provision of life-sustaining treatments to critically ill or severely neurologically impaired infants. Futility has been conceptualized in several ways, including physiological, or quantitative, futility; qualitative futility; resource-centered futility; professional integrity-based futility; and patient-centered, or goal-driven, futility (68). All but (probably) the concept of physiological futility are determined by the beliefs and values of the individuals involved in decision making. In a review article on decision making in extreme prematurity, Campbell and Fleischman assert that "although the concept of physiological futility provides a nearly value-free understanding of futility, it is not helpful in providing guidance about treatment decisions for infants for whom the level of benefit of the treatment and the overall prognosis is uncertain (69).

Bioethicists Veatch and Spicer contend that care is labeled futile "either because the care produces no demonstrable effect at a chosen level of probability, or because, even though it produces an effect, that effect is believed by the speaker to be of no net benefit" (70). Some authors have suggested that the concept of futility should be considered only in relation to specific treatment goals (68).

The paradigm case for futility conflicts for infants was the case of Baby K, an anencephalic infant born in Virginia in 1992. Although she was not a preterm infant, court rulings in her case could potentially be applied to decisions regarding the resuscitation of infants at the margins of viability or the continuation of life-sustaining treatment for neurologically devastated infants.

Although mechanical ventilation was not the standard of care for anencephalic infants, Baby K's mother insisted that she be ventilated after birth. Over the ensuing 2 years, the infant intermittently received mechanical ventilation for subsequent episodes of respiratory distress. The treating hospital went to court to have a guardian appointed and to obtain a declaratory motion to allow the provision of palliative care for the infant. The district court ruled that the hospital was required to continue to provide emergency treatment for respiratory distress under the Emergency Medical Treatment and Labor Act (EMTALA). In an appeal, the hospital argued that ventilating an anencephalic infant was not within normal standards of care, but the appeals court ruled that the hospital was required to provide care because the emergency condition was not anencephaly but respiratory distress. The court did, however, acknowledge that the EMTALA laws were not designed for application to this type of case. Court records document that the infant's mother objected to the limitation of treatment on religious grounds (71, 72). At least one author argues that parental religious beliefs should be respected in treatment decisions. Post is concerned that religious freedom and the free exercise clause of the First Amendment are at stake when religious concerns are ignored or trivialized during decision making (72).

Veatch and Spicer consider the physician's role limited in determining what treatments are futile. They define the problematic cases as ones in which the treatment has an effect, but it is an effect that clinicians believe has no benefit. They argue that in such cases, it is incorrect to refer to futility on medical grounds. The authors also maintain that in cases in which futility is considered, if the patient is competent or has clearly expressed wishes to have the treatment in question, he or she should receive the treatment, on the basis that the beliefs and the values of the patient or surrogate should take precedence. If the patient is incompetent and the treatment produces harm or pain for the patient, the clinician should seek to override the surrogate decision maker. If the patient is incompetent and the treatment is not injurious, there is no moral reason to override the surrogate. The only exceptions are in the case of compromising the clinician's professional integrity or unjustly using society's resources. The authors believe that the values of the patient or surrogate should take precedence, because clinicians' expertise is limited to medical knowledge and skills, not value judgments (70).

Whether aggressive treatment of an ELBW infant is futile has remained difficult to determine, as accurate predictors of survival have remained elusive. Some researchers have raised the concern that a by-product of improved care and survival of ELBW infants is that the LOS for nonsurvivors has significantly increased. In a retrospective examination of ELBW (birth weight of <1,000 grams) infant survival at the University of Chicago during the 1990s, the median LOS for nonsurvivors rose steadily from 2 days in 1991 to 10 days in 2001. The authors conclude that the NICU "trial of therapy" for ELBW infants now takes much longer than it has in the past, and asking parents to "hold their breath" for 2 to 3 days to await better prognostic news is no longer feasible (51).

SOCIETAL IMPLICATIONS OF PRETERM BIRTH

In the United States, where health care costs account for 15 percent of the gross domestic product, the costs of caring for premature infants have been the subject of some inquiry. The American public implicitly appears to be willing to accept the costs of preterm birth, in return for the improved survival of high-risk infants. It remains difficult to assess comprehensively the true costs of prematurity because of the fragmentation of the American health care system. There is a dearth of empirical literature examining the ethical concerns regarding the costs associated with preterm birth.

Several studies from the United States and abroad have examined predictors of the increased financial costs of caring for cohorts of premature infants during the neonatal period and beyond. Recent publications from Australia have evaluated the effectiveness and the efficiency of NICU care over the past 2 decades. In light of questions about the futility of expensive life-sustaining therapies, the costs of caring for nonsurvivors also have been examined and have been found to be small in proportion to the overall costs of caring for premature infants. One author explored whether ethically sound birth weight cutoffs would result in substantial savings to the health care system.

The long-term costs to society of supporting disabled individuals who were born premature have long been a subject of controversy. As a whole, American society has been willing to provide basic social services to support individuals who were born premature infants and seems unlikely to consider limiting health care spending on the basis of the prognosis for the infants' future quality of life. This is in contrast to the model of several northern European countries, in which infants born at less than 26 weeks of gestational age are typically not resuscitated, primarily because of quality-of-life concerns.

Access to perinatal care has improved in recent years, as more and more women with high-risk pregnancies are receiving care in perinatal centers. Some empirical data have confirmed that premature and LBW infants fare better at higher-level perinatal centers. There are differences in perinatal outcomes by race, ethnicity, and maternal age; but studies relating ethical concerns to those differences are few and far between.

Empirical Data on the Financial Costs of Prematurity

Multiple studies have shown an inverse relationship between gestational age or birth weight and hospital charges during the neonatal period. Preterm or LBW infants are more likely to consume community health services and special education services than term or normal birth weight infants. Families incur substantial long-term costs. It is difficult to measure the true costs (including direct and indirect costs) to patients, their families, and society. Cost-benefit studies are difficult to evaluate (73). In addition, one study empirically examined whether an ethically sound birth weight-specific cutoff for resuscitation would result in substantial savings in the cost of NICU treatment (74).

By using data from large national surveys of health behaviors and medical expenditures, it was estimated that LBW infants incurred more than one-third of all infant health care costs in the first year of life in 1988 ($4 billion of the $11.4 billion spent for all infants). The costs for an individual infant increased as gestational age decreased (75). Similarly, in a single-center retrospective study of preterm infants and hospital charges, gestational age, LOS, and survival were all independently related to cost (76).

In a single-center retrospective review and questionnaire study from an academic medical center in Finland, it was found that ELBW infants incurred significantly increased costs in the first year of life, including hospitalization costs, rehabilitation costs, loss of earnings for care givers, and travel costs. The study was limited by parental recall and participation bias, but the authors concluded that the total costs for ELBW infants, even those who were normally developed, were higher than those for normal-birth-weight infants (77).

The costs of caring for nonsurvivors are less than 10 percent of the overall costs of inpatient care for premature infants. Relative to the total cost of prematurity, the costs associated with NICU "trials of therapy" are small.

In a retrospective look at all ELBW infants born at the University of Chicago between 1991 and 2001, it was found that although the median LOS for nonsurvivors had increased significantly, the NICU bed-days occupied by nonsurvivors remained low (~7 percent) because of the overall improvement in survival (51).

In the retrospective study from Finland, the costs attributed to nonsurvivors constituted 9 percent of overall costs for ELBW infants. The authors concluded that the reason for the low proportion of costs attributable to nonsurvivors was their short life span (77).

A population-based cohort study of ELBW infants born in Victoria, Australia, determined that although the effectiveness of neonatal care had increased from 1979 to 1997 (as demonstrated by threefold increases in survival rates and quality-adjusted survival rates), efficiency (as measured by cost-effectiveness and cost-utility ratios) had remained relatively unchanged in nearly two decades (78, 79).

Cost and Resuscitation of ELBW Infants

Stolz and McCormick evaluated whether restricting access to neonatal care on the basis of reasonable birth weight cutoffs would result in substantial cost savings for NICU care. They found that infants born weighing <600 grams accounted for 3.2 percent of NICU charges and infants born at less than 25 weeks of gestation accounted for 5.4 percent of NICU charges. When the number of survivors was assessed at each birth weight cutoff, it was noted, for example, that a cutoff of 700 grams for resuscitation would save 10 percent in NICU costs but that in the United States ~2,700 potential survivors per year would not have been resuscitated. At a 600-gram cutoff, 3.2 percent of NICU charges would be saved, but 575 survivors would not have been resuscitated. In this study, nonsurvivors accounted for 8 percent of resource use by VLBW infants. The study was limited by its short-term assessment of costs, the biases incurred by studying the high-risk population of an academic metropolitan medical center, and a time period that spanned the introduction of surfactant. The authors conclude that ethically sound (i.e., extremely low) birth weight cutoffs for resuscitation would not result in substantial savings in the cost of NICU treatment (74).

Tyson et al., using Neonatal Research Network data, examined survival rates and LOSs for infants born weighing between 501 and 800 grams. That group estimated LOS at 127 hospital days per survivor and 148 days per survivor without severe brain injury. If mechanical ventilation had been used for all infants, the authors estimated a significant increase in resource use for eight additional survivors per 100 infants in this birth weight category (80).

A population-based study compared infants born at 23 to 26 weeks of gestation in the 1980s in New Jersey and the Netherlands, where treatment and resuscitation strategies were (and still are) quite divergent. The investigators found that the aggressive treatment strategies in New Jersey were associated with 24 additional survivors per 100 live births and 1,372 additional ventilator days per 100 live births. The prevalence of disabling cerebral palsy was also significantly increased among the survivors in the New Jersey cohort. The authors acknowledge the moral dilemmas inherent in strategies of either universally or selectively initiating intensive care (81).

Educational and Social Costs of Prematurity

The increases in long-term costs for individuals who were born premature are due to medical costs as well as educational and social costs. These individuals often require rehospitalization, specialized medical care, and special education or early intervention services. There are additional costs to their families, including transportation costs and the loss of wages if one parent leaves the workforce to care for the child.

In a population-based study conducted in the United Kingdom, it was shown that the total duration of hospital admissions during the first 5 years of life for individuals born at <31 gestational weeks was almost eight times that for individuals born at term. The largest component of the cost was the initial birth admission, but the cost differences persisted through the subsequent 4 years of life. Gestational age at birth was the strongest predictor of total costs during the first 5 years of life. The authors concluded that prematurity was a major predictor of the cost of medical services during the first 5 years of life (82).

Petrou et al. performed a meta-analysis of studies of the long-term costs of preterm birth and LBW. In their analysis, the authors used evidence from 20 studies to conclude that (a) "preterm or low birth weight infants are significantly more likely to be rehospitalized" than term or normal-birthweight infants; (b) "the increased use and cost of health care services consumed by preterm or low birth weight infants persists into childhood," with major neurologic abnormalities increasing the families' use of hospital and outpatient services in the longer term; (c) survivors have high rates of school failure and learning problems, requiring special education services; and (d) families have increased out-of-pocket expenses related to the consequences of prematurity and often have substantial reductions in family income (83).

In population-based surveys assessing medical expenditures and family health, it was noted that children born with LBWs were 50 percent more likely than normal-birth-weight children to require special education services and were slightly more likely to repeat a grade of school (75).

Access to Perinatal Care

In the 1980s and 1990s, perinatal care was regionalized in an attempt to improve maternal and neonatal outcomes. Women with complicated pregnancies were referred to higher-level perinatal centers for specialized care and neonatal therapies. It now appears that deregionalization is occurring, as the need for neonatal intensive care continues to grow (84). Community hospitals have begun offering intensive therapies, such as high-frequency ventilation and nitric oxide, raising concerns about quality of care. The ethical concerns that have arisen as a result of this deregionalization include the following: (a) parents who are less savvy or less informed may not be aware that their premature infant is not being treated at a perinatal center of the correct level, and (b) clinicians may be inadequately trained to use intensive therapies. As shown by the data that follow, premature infants delivered at hospitals without the proper level of neonatal care may have worse prognoses. One retrospective study looking at the outcomes for infants with necrotizing enterocolitis and mortality showed no difference in outcomes whether or not there was immediate access to surgical care. The study's conclusions are limited by its methodology.

Empirical Data Concerning Access to Perinatal Care

In a population-based cohort study done in South Carolina (from 1993 to 1995), total birth weight-adjusted mortality rates were significantly higher in Level I and II perinatal centers than in Level III centers (as many as 267 deaths per 1,000 births in Level I centers down to 146 deaths per 1,000 births in Level III centers [$p < 0.05$]). There was a trend toward lower mortality rates among VLBW infants born in Level III centers, although the numbers for some subgroups were too small for the trend to reach statistical significance (85).

In a population-based cohort study in Georgia (from 1994 to 1996), it was determined that 77 percent of VLBW infants were born at Level III or IV centers, 9.8 percent were born at Level II+ hospitals, and 13.1 percent were born at centers with other levels. The neonatal mortality rate, after adjustment for birth weight, correlated with the level of the perinatal center, with the lowest rate found for infants born at Level III centers (127.8/1,000 births) and the highest rate found for infants born at Level II centers (276.2/1,000 births). (Mortality rates were higher for infants born at Level IV hospitals [181.8/1,000 births] than at Level III centers because of the nature of the patient population.) The authors concluded that the highest mortality rates were at the centers with the lowest levels of care, even after consideration of the differences in the populations delivering at hospitals with various levels of care (86).

In a Swedish population-based cohort study, infants born at between 24 and 27 weeks (from 1992 to 1998) had increased mortality rates at general hospitals (32 percent) compared with those at university hospitals (23 percent). There was no difference in mortality rates for infants born at between 28 and 31 weeks gestation when the rates were compared by hospital type. The authors concluded that extremely preterm infants born at general hospitals suffered a substantially increased mortality rate. They question whether additional centralization may improve survival (87).

In a retrospective Australian review of outcomes for infants with necrotizing enterocolitis, infants cared for in centers with neonatal surgical facilities had neither improved survival nor improved outcomes such as LOS, resection for strictures, days on total parenteral nutrition (TPN), or mortality compared with the survival rates and outcomes for infants who were cared for in centers without neonatal surgical facilities. The study was confounded by factors that included the differential administration of antenatal steroids to the two groups. The authors concluded that the management of infants with necrotizing enterocolitis in centers without surgical capabilities was not associated with increases in morbidity or mortality (88).

One study conducted in the 1980s examined differences in the incidence of LBW or perinatal mortality between populations residing in metropolitan and nonmetropolitan areas in the United States. By using data from the National Linked Birth Death Data Set obtained between 1985 and 1987, it was found that at the national level, residence in a nonmetropolitan area was not associated with a higher risk of LBW or neonatal mortality, although the risks of postneonatal mortality and the late onset of prenatal care were slightly higher. The authors concluded that "non-metropolitan residence is not a strong risk factor for low birth weight outcome and neonatal mortality in the United States." The study was limited by its inability to assess other morbidities and by the fact that the data were collected in the mid-1980s, after which time major changes in clinical practice and mortality have occurred (89).

Race and Ethnicity and Access to Medical Care

Insidious racism or ethnic prejudice on the part of obstetricians or neonatologists may affect access to proper treatments. In a population-based retrospective cohort of women delivering singletons in the United States between 1989 and 2000, it appeared that preterm birth rates were declining among African American women (18.5 percent in 1989 versus 16.2 percent in 2000), although they were still substantially higher than the preterm birth rates among white women (9.4 percent in 2000). The numbers of medically indicated preterm births rose among both African American and white women, although they rose to a much higher degree among white women (an increase of 32 percent for African American women and an increase of 55 percent for white women). The authors concluded that the increase in preterm birth rates among white women was largely due to an increase in medically indicated preterm birth, whereas in African American women the preterm birth rate declined because of decreased rates of preterm rupture of membranes and spontaneous preterm birth. The authors raised concerns about the racial differences in obstetric interventions (90).

Distributive Justice and the Care of Preterm Infants

Ethical concerns about the distributive justice of caring for premature infants in light of the incidence of prematurity in high-risk populations of low socioeconomic status may be overstated, as the epidemiology of prematurity is changing. Rates of premature birth remain excessive in African American women, adolescents, and women of low socioeconomic status. Thus, there remain differences in perinatal outcomes between women of high and low socioeconomic status, and in particular, there are significantly poorer perinatal outcomes for African American women in the United States. However, preterm birth rates may be increasing among women of high socioeconomic status as they delay childbearing and use ARTs to conceive. As a result, the proportion of premature infants born to mothers of higher socioeconomic status may be rising. Some data have raised the concern that infants conceived by the use of ART are more likely to be born premature or of low birth weight. Achieving access to high-quality prenatal and obstetric care for all women, regardless of socioeconomic status, race, or ethnicity, would help the realization of justice for pregnant women and neonates.

In a population-based study of birth outcomes in North Carolina (1993 to 1997), it was found that Hispanic and white women had similar rates of infant mortality, low birth weight, and prematurity but that African American women had significantly higher rates of all adverse outcomes. In that study, Hispanic women had less education than African American women but had prenatal care patterns similar to those of African American women. Hispanic women also had significantly lower rates of daily tobacco use than white or African American women. The authors could not explain why, despite similar rates of use of prenatal care use, Hispanic women had significantly better birth outcomes than African American women. They did suggest that health behaviors such as smoking may be an important difference with respect to birth outcomes (91).

In an observational study from Arizona, adolescents had a greater incidence of delivering LBW infants, with 2 percent of their deliveries being VLBW, whereas the rate was 1.1 percent among women at least 19 years old ($p = 0.002$) (92).

In a large population-based study in New Zealand spanning the years from 1980 to 1999, it was found that the overall rates of premature births rose from 4.3 to 5.9 percent; however, the largest increase was among families living in the least-deprived areas (a 71.9 percent increase, from 3.2 to 5.5 percent). The authors concluded that preterm births were still on the rise, potentially because of changes in ultrasound dating techniques, changes in the definition of viability, decreased numbers of stillbirths, and increased rates of assisted conception. They also concluded that the social gradient in preterm birth had disappeared, with possible reasons including changes in maternal age and parity and women's participation in the workforce (93).

ETHICAL ISSUES IN PERINATAL AND NEONATAL RESEARCH

The ethical conduct of clinical research involving children was recently reviewed by the Institute of Medicine in a report published in 2004 (94). Overall, the regulations (referred to as Subpart D) and the associated ethical framework are appropriate for research involving premature infants.

Although the topic is not unique to neonatology, several themes have been the subject of investigation and commentary in the context of neonatal research. These include (a) the prospect of direct benefit to an infant from being included in the research, apart from any direct benefit from the re-search intervention (95, 96); (b) the documented prevalence of the "off-label" use of medications and the need for evidence-based medicine (97, 98); and (c) the need for alternative approaches to the retrieval of informed consent for neonatal research (16, 99–101). These topics are not reviewed in this appendix. Specific questions arise, however, in two main areas: (a) the applicability of Subpart B at the threshold for viability and (b) the abil-ity of adolescent pregnant women to consent to research. These two areas are discussed in more detail below.

Applicability of Subpart B: Additional Protections for Pregnant Women, Human Fetuses, and Neonates Involved in Research

Subpart B "applies to all research involving pregnant women, human fetuses, neonates of uncertain viability, or nonviable neonates" (102).

Definitions

"Nonviable neonate means a neonate after delivery that, although liv-ing, is not viable."

"Viable, as it pertains to the neonate, means being able, after delivery, to survive (given the benefit of available medical therapy) to the point of independently maintaining heartbeat and respiration" (102).

Research Involving Pregnant Women and Neonates

Pregnant women or fetuses may be involved in research if all of the conditions that are listed in §46.204 are met. Consistent with the research protections found in Subpart A and applicable to all human research sub-jects, there should be sufficient preclinical and clinical data to assess "po-tential risks to pregnant women and fetuses." Absent the prospect of direct benefit for either the pregnant woman or the fetus, the risk to the fetus must be minimal and the knowledge to be obtained must be important and unob-tainable by any other means.

The definition of minimal risk is found in Subpart A: "Minimal risk means that the probability and magnitude of harm or discomfort antici-pated in the research are not greater in and of themselves than those ordi-narily encountered in daily life or during the performance of routine physi-cal or psychological examinations or tests."

"If the research holds out the prospect of direct benefit solely to the fetus then the consent of the pregnant woman and the father is obtained in accord with the informed consent provisions of subpart A of this part, ex-cept that the father's consent need not be obtained if he is unable to consent because of unavailability, incompetence, or temporary incapacity or the pregnancy resulted from rape or incest." Otherwise, the consent of the pregnant woman is sufficient. "For children as defined in §46.402(a) who are pregnant, assent and permission are obtained in accord with the provisions of subpart D of this part."

Children are defined as "persons who have not attained the legal age for consent to treatments or procedures involved in the research, under the applicable law of the jurisdiction in which the research will be conducted." There must be an independent assessment of the viability of the neonate. In addition, "individuals engaged in the research will have no part in any decisions as to the timing, method, or procedures used to terminate a pregnancy."

Neonates of uncertain viability and nonviable neonates may be involved in research (§46.205) if the following conditions are met: Neonates of uncertain viability may not be involved in research unless the research holds out the prospect of enhancing the probability of survival of the neonate to the point of viability, and any risk is the least possible for achieving that objective, or the purpose of the research is the development of important biomedical knowledge which cannot be obtained by other means and there will be no added risk to the neonate resulting from the research. If neither parent is able to consent because of unavailability, incompetence, or temporary incapacity, the legally effective informed consent of either parent's legally authorized representative can be obtained.

After delivery a nonviable neonate may not be involved in research covered by this subpart unless all of the following additional conditions are met: (a) vital functions of the neonate will not be artificially maintained; (b) the research will not terminate the heartbeat or respiration of the neonate; (c) there will be no added risk to the neonate resulting from the research; (d) the purpose of the research is the development of important biomedical knowledge that cannot be obtained by other means; and (e) the legally effective informed consent of both parents of the neonate is obtained (unless either parent is unable to consent because of unavailability, incompetence, or temporary incapacity, or the consent of the father need not be obtained if the pregnancy resulted from rape or incest). The consent of a legally authorized representative of either or both of the parents of a nonviable neonate will not suffice.

A neonate, after delivery, that has been determined to be viable may be included in research only to the extent permitted by and in accord with the requirements of subparts A and D of this part.

Research Involving Pregnant Adolescents

Although the National Commission intended that the state consent laws for the treatment of minors apply in the research setting, this has been a point of contention and debate. For example, in adopting Subpart D, the

Food and Drug Administration specifically did not adopt the waiver of parental permission found in 45 CFR 46.408(c) (103). "Section 46.408(c) of DHHS [U.S. Department of Health and Human Services] subpart D allows an IRB [institutional review board] to determine that a research protocol is designed for conditions or for a subject population for which the permission of parents or guardians is not a reasonable requirement to protect the subjects." This section has often been used by institutional review boards to waive the requirement for parental permission for research involving adolescents, provided that the research involved procedures that the adolescent could consent to under applicable state law.

Although most states include marriage as a condition that results in the emancipation of an adolescent from parental control, only two states (New Jersey and Wisconsin) mention pregnancy or previous birth. The ability to independently consent for research participation as an "expanded" view of emancipation may be reasonable, but this has not been addressed explicitly in state laws (104).

State laws usually contain provisions for a minor to consent to health care (so-called mature minor statutes), with pregnancy often included as a qualifying condition. In addition, states allow a minor to consent to treatments for specific disorders or conditions such as sexually transmitted diseases, family planning, and alcohol or drug abuse. However, the applicability of these statutes to the research setting is far from clear (104).

REFERENCES

1. McHaffie HE, Lyon AJ, Hume R. Deciding on treatment limitation for neonates: the parents' perspective. European Journal of Pediatrics 2001;160:339–344.
2. Partridge JC, Martinez AM, Nishida H, et al. International comparison of care for very low birth weight infants: parents' perceptions of counseling and decision-making. Pediatrics 2005;116(2):e263–e271.
3. Brinchmann B. What matters to the parents? A qualitative study of parents' experiences with life-and-death decisions concerning their premature infants. Nursing Ethics 2002;9(4):388–404.
4. McHaffie HE, Laing IA, Parker M, McMillan J. Deciding for imperilled newborns: medical authority or parental autonomy? Journal of Medical Ethics 2001;27:104–109.
5. Bastek TK, Richardson DK, Zupancic JAF, Burns JP. Prenatal consultation practices at the border of viability: a regional survey. Pediatrics 2005;116(2):407–413.
6. Streiner DL, Saigal S, Burrows E, Stoskopf B, Rosenbaum P. Attitudes of parents and health care professionals toward active treatment of extremely premature infants. Pediatrics 2001;108(1):152–157.
7. Orfali K. Parental role in medical decision-making: fact or fiction? A comparative study of ethical dilemmas in French and American neonatal intensive care units. Social Science & Medicine 2004;58(10):2009–2022.
8. Lantos JD, Tyson JE, Allen A, et al. Withholding and withdrawing life sustaining treatment in neonatal intensive care: issues for the 1990s. Archives of Disease in Childhood: Fetal and Neonatal Edition 1994;71(3):F218–F223.

9. American Academy of Pediatrics. The initiation or withdrawal of treatment for high-risk newborns. Pediatrics 1995;96(2):362–363.

10. Leuthner S. Decisions regarding resuscitation of the extremely premature infant and models of best interest. Journal of Perinatology 2001;21(3):193–198.

11. Kopelman LM. Rejecting the Baby Doe rules and defending a "negative" analysis of the best interests standard. Journal of Medicine and Philosophy 2005;30(4):331–352.

12. *State v. Messenger.* In: Clerk of the Circuit Court: Circuit Court, County of Ingham, Michigan; 1994.

13. *Miller v. HCA, Inc.* SW 3rd 2003;118(75).

14. Blanco F, Suresh G, Howard D, Soll RF. Ensuring accurate knowledge of prematurity outcomes for prenatal counseling. Pediatrics 2005;115(4):e478–e487.

15. Haywood JL, Goldenberg RL, Bronstein J, Nelson KG, Carlo WA. Comparison of perceived and actual rates of survival and freedom from handicap in premature infants. American Journal of Obstetrics & Gynecology 1994;171(2):432–439.

16. Ballard HO, Shook LA, Desai NS, Anand KJ. Neonatal research and the validity of informed consent obtained in the perinatal period. Journal of Perinatology 2004;24(7):409–415.

17. Chervenak FA, McCullough LB. Perinatal ethics: a practical method of analysis of obligations to mother and fetus. Obstetrics & Gynecology 1985;66:442–446.

18. Chervenak FA, McCullough LB, Skupski DW. An ethical justification for emergency, coerced cesarean delivery. Obstetrics & Gynecology 1993;82:1029–1035.

19. Board of Trustees, American Medical Association. Legal interventions during pregnancy: court-ordered medical treatments for pregnant women. JAMA 1990;264:371–373.

20. American College of Obstetricians and Gynecologists (ACOG). Patient choice in the maternal-fetal relationship. In: Ethics in Obstetrics and Gynecology, 2nd ed. Washington, DC: ACOG; 2004:34–36.

21. American College of Obstetricians and Gynecologists. Committee Opinion No. 321: maternal decision making, ethics, and the law. Obstetrics & Gynecology 2005;106:1127–1137.

22. Harris LH. Rethinking maternal-fetal conflict: gender and equality in perinatal ethics. Obstetrics & Gynecology 2000;96(5):786–791.

23. Veatch RM. Maternal brain death: an ethicist's thoughts. JAMA 1982;248:1102–1103.

24. Powner DJ, Bernstein IM. Extended somatic support for pregnant women after brain death. Critical Care Medicine 2003;31(4):1241–1249.

25. American Academy of Pediatrics/American College of Obstetricians and Gynecologists. Guidelines for perinatal care. AAP and ACOG; 2002 October.

26. Lyerly AD, Gates EA, Cefalo RC, Sugarman J. Toward the ethical evaluation and use of maternal-fetal surgery. Obstetrics & Gynecology 2001;98(4):689–697.

27. American Academy of Pediatrics, Committee on Bioethics. Fetal therapy—ethical considerations. Pediatrics 1999;103(5 Pt 1):1061–1063.

28. Chervenak FA, McCullough LB. A comprehensive ethical framework for fetal research and its application to fetal surgery for spina bifida. American Journal of Obstetrics & Gynecology 2002;187(1):10–14.

29. American College of Obstetricians and Gynecologists. Committee Opinion No. 324: perinatal risks associated with assisted reproductive technology. Obstetrics & Gynecology 2005:1143–1146.

30. Wright VC, Schieve LA, Reynolds MA, Jeng G. Assisted reproductive technology surveillance—United States, 2002. Morbidity and Mortality Weekly Report 2005;54(SS-2):1–24.

31. Schieve LA, Ferre C, Peterson HB, Macaluso M, Reynolds MA, Wright VC. Perinatal outcome among singleton infants conceived through assisted reproductive technology in the United States. Obstetrics & Gynecology 2004;103(6):1144–1153.

32. Nassar AH, Usta IM, Rechdan JB, Harb TS, Adra AM, Abu-Musa AA. Pregnancy outcome in spontaneous twins versus twins who were conceived through in vitro fertilization. American Journal of Obstetrics & Gynecology 2003;189(2):513–518.

33. Shevell T, Malone FD, Vidaver J, et al. Assisted reproductive technology and pregnancy outcome. Obstetrics & Gynecology 2005;106(5):1039–1045.

34. Annas GJ. Extremely preterm birth and parental authority to refuse treatment—the case of Sidney Miller. New England Journal of Medicine 2004;351(20):2118–2123.

35. *Montalvo v. Borkovec.* In: WI App 147: 256 Wis. 2d 472; 2002.

36. U.S. Congress. An act to protect infants who are born alive. HR 2175, 107 ed. 107th Congress. Washington, DC: U.S. Congress; 2001.

37. Sensenbrenner FJ, Judiciary Committee. Report from the Committee on the Judiciary: Born-Alive Infants Protection Act of 2001. Washington, DC: U.S. Congress; July 26, 2001.

38. Boyle D, Carlo WA, Goldsmith J, et al. Born-Alive Infants Protection Act of 2001, Public Law No. 107-207. Pediatrics 2003;111(3):680–681.

39. Peerzada JM, Richardson DK, Burns JP. Delivery room decision-making at the threshold of viability. Journal of Pediatrics 2004;145:492–498.

40. Oei J, Askie LM, Tobiansky R, Lui K. Attitudes of neonatal clinicians towards resuscitation of the extremely premature infant: an exploratory survey. Journal of Paediatric and Child Health 2000;36:357–362.

41. De Leeuw R, Cuttini M, Nadai M, et al. Treatment choices for extremely preterm infants: an international perspective. Journal of Pediatrics 2000;137(5):608–616.

42. Byrne PJ, Tyebkhan JM, Laing LM. Ethical decision-making and neonatal resuscitation. Seminars in Perinatology 1994;18(1):36–41.

43. Doron MW, Veness-Meehan KA, Margolis LH, Holoman EM, Stiles AD. Delivery room resuscitation decisions for extremely premature infants. Pediatrics 1998;102(3):574–582.

44. MacDonald H, American Academy of Pediatrics, Committee on Fetus and Newborn. Perinatal care at the threshold of viability. Pediatrics 2002;110(5):1024–1027.

45. Higgins RD, Delivoria-Papadopoulos M, Raju TNK. Executive summary of the Workshop on the Border of Viability. Pediatrics 2005;115(5):1392–1396.

46. Duff RS, Campbell AGM. Moral and ethical dilemmas in the special-care nursery. New England Journal of Medicine 1973;289(17):890–894.

47. Whitelaw A. Death as an option in neonatal intensive care. Lancet 1986;8502(2):328–331.

48. Wall SN, Partridge JC. Death in the ICN: physician practice of withdrawing and withholding life support. Pediatrics 1997;99(1):64–70.

49. Cook LA, Watchko JF. Decision making for the critically ill neonate near the end of life. Journal of Perinatology 1996;16(2):133–136.

50. Singh J, Lantos J, Meadow W. End-of-life after birth: death and dying in a neonatal intensive care unit. Pediatrics 2004;114(6):1620–1626.

51. Meadow W, Lee G, Lin K, Lantos J. Changes in mortality for extremely low birth weight infants in the 1990s: implications for treatment decisions and resource use. Pediatrics 2004;113(5):1223–1229.

52. U.S. Department of Health and Human Services. US Child Abuse Prevention and Treatment Act; 1985;Public Law No. 42.

53. Kopelman LM, Irons TG, Kopelman AE. Neonatologists judge the "Baby Doe" regulations. New England Journal of Medicine 1988;318(11):677–683.

54. Kopelman LM. Are the 21-year-old Baby Doe rules misunderstood or mistaken? Pediatrics 2005;115(3):797–802.
55. Clark FI. Baby Doe rules have been interpreted and applied by an appellate court (letter). Pediatrics 2005;115(2):513–514.
56. Kopelman LM. Baby Doe rules have been interpreted and applied by an appellate court: in reply (letter). Pediatrics 2005;116(2):514–515.
57. American Academy of Pediatrics (AAP). Guidelines on forgoing life-sustaining medical treatment. Washington, DC: AAP; 1994:532–536.
58. American Academy of Pediatrics (AAP), Committee on Bioethics. Ethics and the care of critically ill infants and children. Washington, DC: AAP; 1996:149–152.
59. Verhagen AAE, Sauer PJJ. End-of-life decisions in newborns: an approach from the Netherlands. Pediatrics 2005;116(3):736–739.
60. Cuttini M, Nadai M, Kaminski M, et al. End-of-life decisions in neonatal intensive care: physicians' self-reported practices in seven European countries. EURONIC Study Group. Lancet 2000;355(9221):2112–2118.
61. Rebagliato M, Cuttini M, Broggin L, et al. Neonatal end-of-life decision making: physicians' attitudes and relationship with self-reported practices in 10 European countries. JAMA 2000;284(19):2451–2459.
62. van der Heide A, van der Maas PJ, van der Wal G, Kollee LA, de Leeuw R. Using potentially life-shortening drugs in neonates and infants. Critical Care Medicine 2000; 28(7):2595–2599.
63. Provoost V, Cools F, Mortier F, et al. Medical end-of-life decisions in neonates and infants in Flanders. Lancet 2005;365(9467):1315–1320.
64. Vrakking AM, van der Heide A, Onwuteaka-Philipsen BD, Keij-Deerenberg IM, van der Maas PJ, van der Wal G. Medical end-of-life decisions made for neonates and infants in the Netherlands, 1995–2001. Lancet 2005;365(9467):1329–1331.
65. Partridge JC, Wall SN. Analgesia for dying infants whose life support is withdrawn or withheld. Pediatrics 1997;99(1):76–79.
66. Burns JP, Mitchell C, Outwater KM, et al. End-of-life care in the pediatric intensive care unit after the forgoing of life-sustaining treatment. Critical Care Medicine 2000;28(8): 3060–3066.
67. Pierucci RL, Kirby RS, Leuthner SR. End-of-life care for neonates and infants: the experience and effects of a palliative care consultation service. Pediatrics 2001;108:653–660.
68. Moseley KL, Silveira MJ, Goold SD. Futility in evolution. Clinics in Geriatric Medicine 2005;21:211–222.
69. Campbell DE, Fleischman AR. Limits of viability: dilemmas, decisions, and decision makers. American Journal of Perinatology 2001;18(3):117–128.
70. Veatch RM, Spicer CM. Medically futile care: the role of the physician in setting limits. American Journal of Law and Medicine 1992;18(1–2):15–36.
71. Romesberg TL. Futile care and the neonate. Advances in Neonatal Care 2003;3(5): 213–219.
72. Post SG. Baby K: medical futility and the free exercise of religion. Journal of Law, Medicine, and Ethics 1995;23:20–26.
73. Petrou S. Economic consequences of preterm birth and low birthweight. British Journal of Obstetrics and Gynecology 2003;110(Suppl. 20):17–23.
74. Stolz JW, McCormick MC. Restricting access to neonatal intensive care: effect on mortality and economic savings. Pediatrics 1998;101(3):344–348.
75. Lewit EM, Baker LS, Corman H, Shiono PH. The direct cost of low birth weight. The Future of Children 1995;5(1):35–56.

76. St John EB, Nelson KG, Cliver SP, Bishnoi RR, Goldenberg RL. Cost of neonatal care according to gestational age at birth and survival status. American Journal of Obstetrics & Gynecology 2000;182(1):170–175.

77. Tommiska V, Tuominen R, Fellman V. Economic costs of care in extremely low birthweight infants during the first 2 years of life. Pediatric Critical Care Medicine 2003;4(2):256–257.

78. Doyle LW, Victorian Infant Collaborative Study Group. Evaluation of neonatal intensive care for extremely low birth weight infants in Victoria over two decades. II. Efficiency. Pediatrics 2004;113(3):510–514.

79. Doyle LW, Victorian Infant Collaborative Study Group. Evaluation of neonatal intensive care for extremely low birth weight infants in Victoria over two decades. I. Effectiveness. Pediatrics 2004;113(3):505–509.

80. Tyson JE, Younes N, Verter J, Wright LL. Viability, morbidity, and resource use among newborns of 501- to 800-g birth weight. National Institute of Child Health and Human Development Neonatal Research Network. JAMA 1996;276(20):1645–1651.

81. Lorenz JM, Paneth N, Jetton JR, den Ouden L, Tyson JE. Comparison of management strategies for extreme prematurity in New Jersey and the Netherlands: outcomes and resource expenditure. Pediatrics 2001;108(6):1269–1274.

82. Petrou S, Mehta Z, Hockley C, Cook-Mozaffari P, Henderson J, Goldacre M. The impact of preterm birth on hospital inpatient admissions and costs during the first 5 years of life. Pediatrics 2003;112(6):1290–1297.

83. Petrou S, Sach T, Davidson L. The long-term costs of preterm birth and low birth weight: results of a systematic review. Child: Care, Health, and Development 2001;27(2): 97–115.

84. McCormick MC, Richardson DK. Access to neonatal intensive care. The Future of Children 1995;5(1):162–175.

85. Menard MK, Liu Q, Holgren EA, Sappenfield WM. Neonatal mortality for very low birth weight deliveries in South Carolina by level of hospital perinatal service. American Journal of Obstetrics & Gynecology 1998;179(2):374–381.

86. Samuelson JL, Buehler JW, Norris D, Sadek R. Maternal characteristics associated with place of delivery and neonatal mortality rates among very-low-birthweight infants, Georgia. Paediatric and Perinatal Epidemiology 2002;16:305–313.

87. Johansson S, Montgomery SM, Ekbom A, et al. Preterm delivery, level of care, and infant death in Sweden: a population-based study. Pediatrics 2004;113(5):1230–1235.

88. Loh M, Osborn DA, Lui K, group NSW Neonatal Intensive Care Unit Study Group. Outcome of very premature infants with necrotising enterocolitis cared for in centres with or without on site surgical facilities. Archives of Disease in Childhood: Fetal and Neonatal Edition 2001;85:F114–F118.

89. Larson EH, Hart LG, Rosenblatt RA. Is non-metropolitan residence a risk factor for poor birth outcome in the U.S.? Social Science and Medicine 1997;45(2):171–188.

90. Ananth CV, Joseph KS, Oyelese Y, Demissie K, Vintzileos AM. Trends in preterm birth and perinatal mortality among singletons: United States, 1989 through 2000. Obstetrics & Gynecology 2005;105(5 Pt 1):1084–1091.

91. Leslie JC, Galvin SL, Diehl SJ, Bennett TA, Buescher PA. Infant mortality, low birth weight, and prematurity among Hispanic, white, and African American women in North Carolina. American Journal of Obstetrics & Gynecology 2003;188(5):1238–1240.

92. Miller H, Lesser K, Reed K. Adolescence and very low birth weight infants: a disproportionate association. Obstetrics & Gynecology 1996;87(1):83–88.

93. Craig ED, Thompson JM, Mitchell EA. Socioeconomic status and preterm birth: New Zealand trends, 1980 to 1999. Archives of Disease in Childhood: Fetal and Neonatal Edition 2002;86(3):F142–F146.

94. Field MJ, Behrman RE, eds. Ethical Conduct of Clinical Research Involving Children. Washington, DC: The National Academies Press; 2004.

95. Lantos JD. The "inclusion benefit" in clinical trials. Journal of Pediatrics 1999; 134(2):130–131.

96. Silverman WA. Disclosing the "inclusion benefit." Journal of Perinatology 2002; 22(4):261–262.

97. Choonara I, Conroy S. Unlicensed and off-label drug use in children: implications for safety. Drug Safety 2002;25(1):1–5.

98. Turner S, Nunn AJ, Fielding K, Choonara I. Adverse drug reactions to unlicensed and off-label drugs on paediatric wards: a prospective study. Acta Paediatrica 1999; 88(9):965–968.

99. Tyson JE, Knudson PL. Views of neonatologists and parents on consent for clinical trials. Lancet 2000;356(9247):2026–2067.

100. Manning DJ. Presumed consent in emergency neonatal research. Journal of Medical Ethics 2000;26(4):249–253.

101. Rogers CG, Tyson JE, Kennedy KA, Broyles RS, Hickman JF. Conventional consent with opting in versus simplified consent with opting out: an exploratory trial for studies that do not increase patient risk. Journal of Pediatrics 1998;132(4):606–611.

102. U.S. Department of Health and Human Services. 45 CFR Part 46: Protection of Human Subjects. Federal Register 2001;66(219):56775–56780.

103. Food and Drug Administration. Additional safeguards for children in clinical investigations of FDA-regulated products. Federal Register 2001;66(79):20589–20600.

104. Campbell AT. State regulation of medical research with children and adolescents: an overview and analysis. In: Field MJ, Behrman RE, eds. Ethical Conduct of Clinical Research Involving Children. Washington, DC: National Academies Press; 2004:320–387.

D

A Systematic Review of Costs Associated with Preterm Birth

John A. F. Zupancic[1]

The costs of prematurity have been the subject of close scrutiny for more than 2 decades. During that time, there have been dramatic advances in therapeutic interventions, improvements in mortality, and significant inflation in medical care costs. Although the neonatal intensive care phase is most prominent in discussions of these costs, the sequelae of prematurity constitute a chronic disease with significant long-term implications. This appendix has two parts: the first examines the literature on costs associated with the initial hospitalization for prematurity, whereas the second examines longer-term economic factors.

To evaluate the quality and applicability of cost-of-illness studies, it is important to have agreed-upon definitions of certain technical terms. There are, for example, several different categories of cost that might be important to stakeholders. Direct medical costs arise from resources directly consumed by patients. In the context of this review of costs of initial hospitalization, these include costs for the hospital bed and support services ("accommodation"), ancillary services (pharmacy, radiology, laboratory, and respiratory care services), and professional fees. In contrast to these direct costs, overhead costs are those expenses that are incurred in running the institution but that are not directly attributable to a particular patient.

---

[1]John A. F. Zupancic MD, ScD, Department of Pediatrics, Harvard Medical School, Boston, Massachusetts.

These include overhead expenditures for housekeeping, administration, and the physical plant. Costs to patients include nonmedical direct costs (such as the cost of transportation to the hospital, meals, and child care for other siblings). Finally, there are costs related to lost productivity, also referred to as indirect costs. In the short run, these are the lost contributions of labor by the parents; in the long run, they also include reduced work alternatives for the patient.

The particular choice of which costs to include is dependent on the perspective of the stakeholder who will be using the information. For example, hospital administrators will be most interested in the direct medical costs that affect hospital financial operations and less interested in wage losses by parents. However, in valuing the financial burden of prematurity to society, it is vitally important to understand the full extent of costs, regardless of the individuals to whom they accrue. In the absence of such information, policy makers may make decisions that appear to be fiscally desirable but in fact simply shift costs to another, unmeasured facet of care.

Studies that measure costs on their own without reference to the effectiveness of an intervention are known as "cost-of-illness studies." When costs are combined into a single metric with a measure of effectiveness, such as life years saved, the study is referred to as a "cost-effectiveness analysis." When patient preferences for particular outcomes are used as the measure of effectiveness, as they are in quality-adjusted life years, the study is a known as a "cost-utility analysis." Both cost-effectiveness and cost-utility analyses express costs and effects as a ratio measure. In contrast, cost-benefit analyses measure effects in monetary terms and subtract this value from the cost of the intervention to determine value for money.

METHODS

Population Description

Although much attention has been focused on infants at the borderline of viability, the large volume of children at higher gestational ages may drive the overall financial impact of prematurity. Therefore, broad inclusion criteria were maintained for the review and encompass children in the following categories: (a) premature, defined as birth at less than 37 weeks of gestational age, and (b) low birth weight, defined as a birth weight of less than 2,500 grams.

Although the assessment of efficiency is a critical component of technology assessment, the focus of this appendix is on the absolute financial burden of prematurity and low birth weight rather than on the value for money of treatment modalities. Therefore, only costing studies are included and cost-effectiveness, cost-utility, and cost-benefit studies are excluded, except when the population measurement of pertinent costs was a central component. In some cases cost descriptions of cohorts alongside trials of efficacy of therapeutic interventions are included, but these are restricted to control groups to optimize external validity.

Two factors have significant impacts on the generalizability of the findings from economic studies. First, the therapies offered in the field of neonatal intensive care and their resulting outcomes have changed substantially in the past 2 decades. In the late 1980s, there was a dramatic decrease in the rate of mortality because of prematurity with the introduction of surfactant replacement therapy, a therapy subsequently shown repeatedly to have important cost implications. Because the underlying structure of care has changed, this problem is difficult to overcome. For the review of short-run costs, therefore only studies reporting on cohorts after 1990 are included to optimize the external validity of the results and avoid bias against lower birth weight in incremental cost comparisons. Since follow-up care of infants following discharge has changed to a lesser degree, reports of long-run costs are included if the cohort was born after 1980. In a few cases, cohorts were assembled with patients from before and after 1980; these studies are included if >50 percent of the cohort met the inclusion date criterion.

Similarly, substantial effort has been made to assess the costs of neonatal intensive care in other countries. In some cases, as in the United Kingdom, Europe, and Canada, health care delivery and financing may have certain similarities that allow extrapolation of the results to the U.S. population. However, studies from middle-income and developing countries were excluded on the grounds that both outcomes and health care delivery cost structures are too different to interpret the applicability of the results in the U.S. context.

Data Sources and Search Strategies

The following databases were searched for candidate articles: Medline (1990 to 2005), electronic abstracts from the annual meetings of the Society for Pediatric Research (1998 to 2005), Econlit (1990 to 2005), and the Proquest dissertation and theses full-text index (1990 to 2005). The Science citation index was searched for articles citing any of the first authors of included studies. The bibliographies of other systematic or informal reviews were scanned (1–7). The websites of organizations known to be involved in similar research were also scanned; these included the websites of the March of Dimes, the Alan Guttmacher Institute, and the Centers for Disease Control and Prevention. The search strategies were intentionally broad to ensure optimal sensitivity. The intersection of the exploded MeSH headings "infant, newborn" and "costs and cost analysis" was used for Medline searches. For other databases, the keywords "econom*" OR "cost*" AND "infant" were used. The titles and abstracts of the articles retrieved with these strategies were manually screened to determine whether they met the inclusion criteria described above.

Cost Projections

Cost estimates were inflated to 2005 constant dollars by using both the medical component of the consumer price index (8) and the hospital producer price index (9). Currencies were converted to U.S. dollars by using purchasing power parities (10). Per-patient estimates of cost were projected to the U.S. birth cohort by multiplying by the number of infants in a given gestational age or birth weight category, according to the 2002 natality file of the National Center for Vital Statistics (11). State-level population cost estimates were projected to the U.S. birth cohort by dividing by the ratio of the state's birth cohort to the total number of births nationally for 2002 (the most recent year for which such statistics were available).

YIELD OF SEARCH STRATEGY

The manual screening of titles and abstracts from the initial literature searches yielded 170 articles. Of these, the majority were eliminated because they were review articles or economic evaluations of interventional studies, were based on data from middle-income or developing countries, were studies at the neonatal intensive care unit level not stratified by birth weight or gestational age, or had cohort dates prior to 1990 for short-run cost reports or 1980 for long-run cost reports. Descriptions and methodological assessment of the short-run (12–27) and the long-run (15, 27–41) cost studies retrieved are shown in Tables D-1 and D-2, respectively.

METHODOLOGICAL LIMITATIONS OF STUDIES RETRIEVED

Studies of Initial Hospitalization

The methodological quality of the short-run cost studies since 1990 was variable. Only five of the reports involved the collection of data alongside prospective research projects (12, 16, 23, 24, 27), whereas the remainder were retrospective analyses of administrative and clinical data collected for other purposes. In some cases, particularly those analyses involving state-level data in California, there was a preexisting process for checking the integrity of data through reabstraction (18, 25). However, the accuracy of the smaller secondary data sets was not reported in the publications.

TABLE D-1A Studies of Costs During Initial Hospitalization

Paper	Date of Cohort	Location of Cohort	Type of Cohort	Sample Size	Currency	Currency Date
Adams (13)	1996	US	Convenience sample	Total: 12,125 Normal preterm: 456 Extreme preterm: 513 Normal full term: 9,179	USD	Not specified
Brazier (14)	Not specified	UK	Hospital-specific	38	UK pounds	Not specified
Chollet (15)	1989-1991	US	Convenience sample	Total: 58,904 Normal preterm: 946 Extreme preterm: 986 Normal full term: 44,041	USD	Not specified
Doyle (16)	1997	Australia	Geographic (state)	233	Australian dollar	1997
Giacoia (17)	1983-1984	US	Hospital-specific	167	USD	Not specified
Gilbert (18)	1996	California	Geographic (state)	25-38 weeks: 147,224 500-3000 grams: 458,366	USD	Not specified
Kilpatrick (19)	1990-1994	California	Hospital-specific	138	USD	Not specified

Luke (20)	1991-1992	Illinois	Hospital-specific	Twins: 111 Singletons: 106	USD	Not specified
Marbella (21)	1989-1994	Wisconsin	Geographic (state)	Premature: 26,668 Full term: 368,955	USD	Not specified
McLoughlin (22)	Not specified	UK	Hospital-specific	109	UK pounds	Not specified
Rogowski (23)	1993-1994	US	25 self-selected hospitals	3,288	USD	1994
Rogowski (24)	1997-1998	US	29 hospitals in QI collaborative	6,797	USD	1998
Schmitt (25)	2000	California	Geographic (state)	518,697	USD	2003
St John (26)	1989-1992	Alabama	Hospital-specific	958	USD	Not specified
Tommiska (27)	1996-1997	Finland	Geographic (regional hospital)	<1000 g: 105	Euro	1997
Victorian Infant Collaborative Study Group (12)	1991-1992	Australia	Geographic (state)	429	Australian dollar	1992

TABLE D-1B Studies of Costs During Initial Hospitalization

Paper	Gestational Age	Birth Weight	Costs Included	Cost vs Charges	Data Sources	Uncertainty
Adams (13)	Not specified (premature and extreme preterm defined by ICD9)	Not specified	Hospital; professional	Paid claims	Claims database	Not specified
Brazier (14)	Not specified	Not Specified	Travel	Costs	Parent interview	Not specified
Chollet (15)	All	All	Hospital; professional	Billed charges	Claims database	Not specified
Doyle (16)	Not specified	500-999 grams	Hospital	Cost (ventilator and non-ventilator days, inflated from 1987 values)	Prospective research database	Sensitivity analysis
Giacoia (17)	Not specified	All	Travel	Costs	Parent interview	Statistical
Gilbert (18)	25-38weeks	500-3000 grams	Hospital	CCR (hospital-specific)	State-level linked vital statistics and discharge records	Not specified
Kilpatrick (19)	24-26 weeks	Not specified	Hospital	CCR (hospital-specific)	Hospital chart review and billing database	Not specified
Luke (20)	All	All	Hospital	Not specified	Hospital bills; hospital chart	Statistical

Study						
Marbella (21)	Not specified (premature defined as all prematurity-related DRG)	All	Hospital	Charges	State-level linked vital statistics and discharge records	Not specified
McLoughlin (22)	22-37	<2500 g	Travel	Costs	Parent interview	Not specified
Rogowski (23)	Not specified	501-1,500 grams	Hospital	CCR (department-specific)	Hospital financial data	Not specified
Rogowski (24)	Not specified	501-1,500	Hospital	CCR (department-specific)	Hospital financial data	Not specified
Schmitt (25)	All	All	Hospital	CCR (hospital-specific)	State-level linked vital statistics and discharge records	Statistical
St John (26)	24-32 vs 33-42	Not specified	Hospital; professionl	CCR (hospital-specific)	Hospital chart review and billing database	Not specified
Tommiska (27)	≥22 weeks	<1000 grams	Hospital; nonmedical direct; productivity losses	Cost (derivation not specified)	Hospital cost database and national ELBW registry; family questionnaire at 2 years	Statistical and sensitivity analysis
Victorian Infant Collaborative Study Group (12)	Not specified	500-999 grams	Hospital	Cost (ventilator and nonventilator days, inflated from 1987 values)	Prospective research database	Sensitivity analysis

TABLE D-2A Studies of Costs Following Discharge from Initial Hospitalization

Paper	Date of Cohort	Location of Cohort	Type of Cohort	Sample Size	Currency	Currency Date
Broyles (28)	1988-1996	Texas	Hospital-specific	388 (control group of RCT)	USD	1997
Chaikand (29)	1987-1988	US	National	6,788	USD	1989-1990
Chollet (15)	1989-1991	US	Convenience sample	Total: 58,904 Normal preterm: 946 Extreme preterm: 986 Normal full term: 44,041	USD	Not specified
Gennaro (30)	1990-1994	US	Hospital-specific	224	USD	Not specified
Lewit (31)	1988	US	National	35,000	USD	1988
McCormick (32)	1983-1984	Pennsylvania	Hospital-specific	VLBW: 32 Controls: 34	USD	Not specified
Medstat (41)	2001	US	Convenience sample	Total: 28,958 All preterm: 3,214 Normal full term: 15,795	USD	2004
Petrou (33)	1970-1993	UK	Geographic (regional)	>37 weeks: 226,120 32-36 weeks: 11,728 28-31 weeks: 1,346 <28 weeks: 500	UK Pounds	1998-1999

Study	Period	Location	Basis	Data	Currency	Year
Petrou (34)	1978-1988	UK	Geographic (regional)	>37 weeks: 90,236 32-36 weeks: 4,485 28-31 weeks: 596 <28 weeks: 241	UK Pounds	1998-1999
Pharaoh (35)	1979-1981	UK	Geographic (regional)	109	UK Pounds	1984
Rogowski (36)	1986-1987	California	Geographic (state)	Inception: 887 Survived: 591	USD	1987
Rolnick (37)	1993, 1995	Minnesota	Hospital-specific (single health plan)	2500-4499: 1203 =1500-2499: 38	USD	Not specified
Roth (38)	1990-1991	Florida	Geographic (state)	120,533	USD	2001
Stevenson (39)	1980-1981	UK	Geographic (regional)	Total: 641 <1,000: 20 1,000-1,500: 153 1,501-2,000: 468	UK Pounds	1979
Stevenson (40)	1980-1981	UK	Geographic (regional)	Total: 52 <1,000: 9 1,000-1,500: 25 1,501-2,000: 18	UK Pounds	1979
Tommiska (27)	1996-1997	Finland	Geographic (regional hospital)	<1000 g: 105 >36 weeks: 75	Euro	1997

TABLE D-2B Studies of Costs Following Discharge from Initial Hospitalization

Paper	Gestational Age	Birth Weight	Costs Included	Cost vs Charges	Data Sources	Uncertainty	Discounting
Broyles (28)	Not specified	<1000 or <1,500 and ventilated except drugs	Hospital; outpatient	CCR (department-specific)	Prospective research database	Statistical	3%
Chaikand (29)	Not specified	<2,500	Education	Costs	NCHS Child Health Supplement to National Health Interview Survey	Statistical	2%
Chollet (15)	All	All	Hospital; professional	Billed charges	Claims database	Not specified	Not specified
Gennaro (30)	Not specified	<2,500	Wages; transportation; unreimbursed med	Costs	Interviews	Statistical	Not specified
Lewit (31)	All	All	Hospital; education	Charges	National Medical Expenditure Survey	Not specified	Not specified
McCormick (32)	Not specified	<1,500	Hospital; outpatient MD; transportation; childcare	Charges	Diary; interviews	Statistical	Not specified

Medstat (41)	Not specified	All	Hospital; outpatient medical; drugs	Paid claims	Marketscan proprietary database of 100 payers	Not specified	Not specified
Petrou (33)	All	Not Specified	Hospital	Costs	Linked vital statistics and National Health Service records; NHS financial returns	Statistical	Not specified
Petrou (34)	All	Not Specified	Hospital	Costs	Linked vital statistics and National Health Service records; NHS financial returns	Statistical	Not specified
Pharaoh (35)	Not specified	<1,500	Hospital; outpatient medical	Costs	Prospective research database	Not specified	5%
Rogowski (36)	Not specified	<1,500	Hospital; outpatient MD except drugs	Inpatient: CCR (department-specific) Outpatient: charges	Medicaid claims data	Not specified	Not specified

continued

TABLE D-2B Continued

Paper	Gestational Age	Birth Weight	Costs Included	Cost vs Charges	Data Sources	Uncertainty	Discounting
Rolnick (37)	Not specified	>1,500	Hospital; Outpatient MD except drugs	Charges	Claims database	Statistical	Not specified
Roth (38)	Not specified	All	Education	Costs	Linked birth and school records	Statistical	Not specified
Stevenson (39)	Not specified	<2,000	Hospital; outpatient MD; drugs	Costs	Medical records; MD interview	Not specified	6%
Stevenson (40)	Not specified	<2,000	Hospital; outpatient MD; drugs	Costs	Medical records; MD interview; department of education	Not specified	6%
Tommiska (27)	≥22 weeks	<1000 grams	Hospital; nonmedical direct; productivity losses	Cost (derivation not specified)	Hospital cost database and national ELBW registry; family questionnaire at 2 years	Statistical and sensitivity analysis	Not specified

The inconsistent level of regionalization in neonatal care delivery makes the nature of the cohort critically important for cost analyses of prematurity. Six of the reports (12, 16, 18, 21, 25, 27) involved cohorts that were geographically based at the state or regional level. Others used claims data from nationally representative insurance organizations (13, 15) or data from a large number of self-selected hospitals in a neonatal quality improvement network (23, 24). Although the latter data do not guarantee freedom from selection bias, the large number of patients and hospitals involved makes such bias less likely than the likelihood of selection bias with the two small single-center studies (20, 26). In most cases, the inclusion criteria were adequately described; however, three studies defined gestational-age exclusively by diagnosis-related group (DRG) codes (13, 15, 21) rather than by direct observation of patient information. Because there is some discretion in the use of some DRG codes (specifically, "normal preterm" and "preterm with problems"), generalization of the findings to a larger population is more difficult.

Because of the very low incidence of extreme prematurity and the marked variability and skew of cost data, it is also important that studies have adequate sample sizes. As these studies were targeted toward the estimation of costs rather than inference, it is difficult to define an appropriate sample size a priori. The U.S. state-level geographic studies (18, 21, 25), insurance-claims studies (13, 15), and neonatal-network studies (23, 24) all based cost estimates on at least 1,000 premature infants. In contrast, the hospital-specific studies (19, 20, 26) and non-U.S. studies (12, 16, 27) examined as few as 105 premature infants, a sample size that is unlikely to yield useful confidence intervals, especially when the data are projected to national levels.

Earlier cost-of-illness studies in neonatalogy often relied on hospital charges, as these were easily available in administrative databases. However, the use of charges as a measure of economic cost may distort cost estimates because charges reflect a hospital's decisions regarding markups and internal cost transfers. Information on actual costs may be derived from proprietary cost accounting systems or from conversion factors known as cost-to-charge ratios, which are mandated for the reporting of cost information to federal agencies. Two studies in the current review relied only on billed charges (15, 21), one relied on paid insurance claims (13), two relied on older costing studies corrected for inflation (12, 16), and two referred to costs but did not specify the means of derivation (20, 27). The remaining six studies used Medicare cost to charge ratios and are likely to be more comparable to each other.

Given the issues of variance in cost data and the number of comparisons made between groups of infants in the costing studies, it is particularly surprising that they relied almost entirely on point estimates without any quantification of statistical or parameter uncertainty. Statistical uncertainty was reported in only three studies (20, 25, 27), and sensitivity analyses were performed in three studies (12, 16, 27).

Because almost any medical care involves a net expenditure of resources, it is important that the costs of prematurity be viewed as incremental on the medical costs for neonatal care had the premature infant been delivered later in gestation. Five of the studies did not include a cohort of infants delivered at full term (12, 16, 19, 23, 24).

In regionalized systems of neonatal care, infants are often transferred to other hospitals for higher levels of care or to less intensive care settings for a period of further maturation following the resolution of acute cardiorespiratory instability. Failure to include posttransfer costs would lead to underestimates of the cost of care, whereas failure to include transferred infants would affect the external validity of the estimates and possibly overestimate treatment costs, as retrotransferred infants are more stable. Three studies explicitly noted that transferred infants were excluded (19–21), two explicitly included them (15, 25), and the remainder did not specify the inclusion or exclusion of transferred infants.

Several authors also excluded nonsurviving infants from cost estimates (18, 21). One article that did measure the costs for nonsurviving infants observed that they represented 9 percent of total costs (27). Because nonsurviving infants have shorter lengths of stay, they are likely to be less costly (24, 26), even with increased per diem resource utilization due to their higher illness acuity. Including only the costs accruing to survivors will yield underestimate, as resources must also be invested in nonsurvivors to yield a surviving infant.

The currency date was not provided in seven of the articles; when this information was necessary for calculations, the most recent year of the cohort was assumed.

Studies of Costs Following Discharge from the Initial Hospitalization

The longer-run costing studies were similarly methodologically variable. Several of these limitations overlapped with those of the short-run studies.

Most of the studies were secondary analyses of data collected for other purposes. One study was a randomized trial with prospective data collection (28), six used linked governmental vital statistics and administrative or survey databases (27, 29, 31, 33, 34, 38), four used commercial or governmental claims databases (15, 36, 37, 41), three used clinical data (35, 39, 40), and two collected primary data through patient interviews (27, 30, 32). For preexisting data sets, validation was generally not described.

The majority of long-run studies were from broadly representative cohorts. These geographically based cohorts were at the regional (27, 33–35, 39, 40), state (36, 38), and national (29, 31) levels. Only six smaller studies used convenience or hospital-specific samples (15, 28, 30, 32, 37, 41).

There were, however, other problems with generalizability. Six of the 16 long-run studies were from countries other than the United States (27, 33–35, 39, 40). Of note, these were all geographical cohorts and represented the only studies in the review with assessment of direct medical costs beyond 2 years of age. Generalizability was also compromised by the broad time range of the studies. As noted above, the literature search was restricted only to studies conducted after 1980, given that postdischarge care is not as technologically sophisticated and therefore not as rapidly changing. This decision also allowed the inclusion of longer periods of follow-up. The cohort dates of these studies, however, ranged from 1980 to 2001; and the degree of comparability or applicability of earlier studies to the current context is unclear. Most studies did specify the birth weight and gestational age inclusion criteria for the samples, which allowed projection of the results for health policy. Studies that relied on claims databases used DRG designations, which must be applied with a degree of discretion, thus limiting external validity (15, 41).

In contrast to the studies of initial neonatal hospitalization, the sample sizes of most of these studies were adequate, possibly because of the greater reliance on administrative data. Four of the 16 studies had sample sizes of >20,000 infants (15, 31, 33, 34). Although these were heavily weighted toward full-term controls, the sizes of the subsamples of infants born preterm still comprised several hundred to several thousand infants. Only five studies had sample sizes of <150 infants (27, 30, 32, 35, 40). Although the confidence intervals around the cost estimates are consequently broad, most of these studies involved direct patient interviews or questionnaires and yielded unique information that would otherwise not have been obtainable.

Ten of the studies stated that they used costs derived from cost-to-charge ratios or other cost-accounting systems. None of the authors conducted primary costing research, and direct validation of preexisting cost-accounting systems was not presented; however, in at least some of the studies, these appear to be well-established and accepted systems (33, 34). The validity of patient-reported costs is equally difficult to ascertain. None of the studies presenting data from patient interviews, diaries, or questionnaires provided validation of these sources (27, 30, 32).

Uncertainty was again assessed inconsistently. Seven of the studies presented no information on sampling or parameter uncertainty, either through descriptive statistics or sensitivity analysis (15, 31, 35, 36, 39–41).

The assessment of costs for premature infants over the longer term is a more complex exercise, requiring the assembly of data from multiple sources. In some studies, this led to a large number of assumptions regarding the applicability of data, the choice of unit costs, and natural history (29, 31). Although these assumptions were well explained, it is very difficult to know the extent to which they are valid.

Unlike the assessment of initial hospital costs, the study of postdischarge resource utilization ideally tracks costs over several years. Most individuals have a positive rate of time preference; that is, they prefer to receive benefits sooner rather than later and to defer negative factors such as costs. To take account of this preference, economists apply a discount rate to reduce the weight of future investments in a stream of costs over time. This is variably set at 0 to 5 percent, with a 3 percent rate generally being considered reasonable for application in the base case. Only 5 of the 16 studies in the present review applied a discount rate (28, 29, 35, 39, 40).

CONTENT LIMITATIONS OF RETRIEVED STUDIES

Studies of Initial Hospitalization

Cost Categories

Cost categories in the studies of initial hospitalization costs for prematurity were variable. Only one study included both direct nonmedical costs and productivity losses (27). Only three studies included professional fees as a component of direct medical costs (13, 15, 26). The inclusion of overhead costs could be inferred in most cases but was usually not specified.

Only one author disaggregated costs into their component parts, in two studies. Rogowski showed that for infants with birth weights of <1,500 grams, accommodation costs represented most of the total cost of care (72 percent). Of the remaining ancillary costs, 22 percent was for respiratory therapy, 24 percent was for laboratory work, 7 percent was for radiology, and 16 percent for pharmacy (24).

Maternal Costs

This review was not specifically targeted to maternal costs, but these were measured in several of the studies reviewed (13, 15, 18, 20, 21). This is an important potential confounder, as the marginal contribution of maternal care may introduce bias in the comparison of costs for various gestational ages. For example, for infants born at from 25 to 29 weeks gestation, maternal costs were approximately 8 percent of the neonatal costs, for infants born at from 30 to 34 weeks gestation they were 32 percent, for infants born at from 37 to 38 weeks gestation they were 192 percent (18).

Corresponding U.S. population projections were as follows: for infants born at 25 to 29 weeks gestation, $100 million; for infants born at 30 to 34 weeks gestation, $429.5 million; and for infants born at 37 to 38 weeks gestation $1.94 billion. Adams et al., found that maternal costs were $7,451 for those with full-term infants, $10,626 for those with healthy preterm infants, and $11,508 for those with extreme preterm infants (13). Chollet et al. found that maternal costs were $7,850 for the full-term DRG, $13,017 for the healthy preterm DRG, and $14,815 for the extreme preterm DRG (15). Thus, maternal costs vary inversely with birth weight, in parallel with neonatal costs, but to a lesser degree.

The articles that do include maternal costs list only the cost for the delivery admission; other costs are often associated with premature delivery (closer monitoring, repeat admissions, etc.) that may not be captured and would inflate the costs of the delivery itself. In an exception to this pattern, Schmitt et al. showed that, for pregnancies that resulted in births of infants less than 1,500 grams, prenatal hospitalizations accounted for $6.4 million of a total of $49.6 million of maternal hospital expenditures in California (25). Infertility treatments were also not captured in the studies reviewed.

Birth Weight and Gestational Age Cohorts

The majority of studies reported only on very low birth weight infants (in some cases with full-term controls). Although the per-infant cost is significantly lower for moderately preterm infants, the much higher incidence of moderate prematurity results in significant population costs. Schmitt et al. showed that infants with birth weights of 1,500 to 2,500 grams had total projected costs of $2.46 billion nationally (25). St John et al. projected that the costs for infants born at 30 to 34 weeks of gestation were $2.29 billion (26).

No studies determined the incremental contribution of low birth weight after controlling for gestational age.

Financial Burden on Minorities

Although certain ethnic and racial groups experience an increased burden of prematurity, the cost studies reviewed here did not specifically examine the issue of which populations are associated with the initial hospitalization costs.

Financial Burden on Payers

The studies reviewed did not provide specific disaggregations of the sources of payment for care for prematurity. Two of the studies relied on claims databases from large third-party payers. Chollet et al. calculated that prematurity accounts for $4.7 billion to employer-sponsored health insurance plans, beyond the costs for normal-term deliveries (15). Older studies suggested that the newborn period is a major source of uncompensated care (42), accounting for as much as 19 percent of the direct delivery and uncompensated care dollars allocated to maternity and neonatal care (43). The March of Dimes estimates that 11 percent of newborns covered by employer health plans are born premature and that $7.4 billion (in 2002 dollars) in hospital charges was billed to private insurers (44).

Studies of Costs Following Discharge from the Birth Hospitalization

Cost Categories

Thirteen of 16 studies included direct medical costs (15, 27, 28, 31–37, 39–41). However, three of these included only rehospitalization costs and omitted the costs of outpatient physician visits or pharmaceuticals (31, 33, 34). Several of the studies failed to disaggregate the costs of rehospitalization from outpatient care (35, 37) or the costs of initial hospitalization from those of postdischarge care (31).

Educational costs were assessed in only four studies (27, 29, 31, 38). Two of these dealt with preschool costs (27, 31), one dealt with kindergarten costs (38), and two dealt with educational costs beyond kindergarten (29, 31). None followed an incidence cohort of infants longitudinally through school or assessed costs throughout the school spectrum by a consistent methodology.

Parental out-of-pocket expenditures were assessed in five studies (14, 17, 22, 27, 30). All of these included travel costs. Only one, non-U.S. study examined parental wage losses (27). None of the studies retrieved examined the lost productivity of the child.

Only one study attempted to ascertain costs in the direct medical, educational, and parental out-of-pocket expense categories (27).

Time Horizon

Only four of the studies tracked costs beyond 5 years of age. Despite the availability of cohorts reporting clinical follow-up to young adulthood (45, 46), there is almost no information on the cost implications of prematurity beyond early childhood.

Birth Weight and Gestational Age Cohorts

In contrast to the studies of initial hospitalization, most studies of longer-term costs included infants across the birth weight and gestational age spectra.

Comorbid and Resulting Conditions

The studies retrieved did not make any attempt to attribute postdischarge costs to particular neonatal or postnatal conditions other than birth weight or gestational age. Thus, limited information is available on the proportion of rehospitalization or outpatient costs that are associated with chronic lung disease, retinopathy of prematurity, or cerebral palsy. There are, however, estimates of the costs of certain of these (47–52) conditions separately, without the prematurity denominator afforded by the studies reviewed here. Studies of premature infants with chronic lung disease, for example, show that the costs for infants with admissions for respiratory syncytial virus infection are significantly higher; however, the proportion of costs for the entire birth cohort cannot be derived directly (51, 52). Similarly, although costs are available for cerebral palsy, most children with this condition were not born prematurely; the extent to which the costs for cerebral palsy drive the longer-term costs for premature infants is not known.

CHARACTERIZATION AND ESTIMATES OF COSTS OF INITIAL HOSPITALIZATION

Direct Medical Costs

Despite the heterogeneity of methods, designs, and sources, estimates of the per-patient cost are moderately consistent. The second column of Table D-3 shows the per-patient costs derived from the studies, expressed in 2005 U.S. dollars. For infants with birth weights of 500 to 999 grams, cost estimates ranged from $67,027 to $221,450, with four of six estimates in the range $84,847 to $126,380 per infant.

There are several potential sources of variability in cost estimates. First, the studies were performed with cohorts spanning a 15-year period. The characteristics of the adjusters for differences over time are therefore significant. The results are reported with both the medical component of the consumer price index (CPI), which relies on charges and may therefore overestimate charges, and the hospital producer price index (PPI), which used the actual net costs of resources, purchased by both public and private sources. As shown in Table D-3, use of these indices had a minimal effect on the results, suggesting that the source of variation lies elsewhere. A second potential source of variability in estimates is in the geographic diversity of the cohorts. International comparisons are facilitated to some extent by

TABLE D-3 Direct Medical Costs During Initial Hospitalization

Study	Per Patient Cost	Per Patient Cost - 2005 Dollars Using Medical CPI	Per Patient Cost - 2005 Dollars Using Hospital PPI
Adams (13)	Normal preterm: 10,416 Extreme preterm: 49,933 Normal full-term: 1,139	Normal preterm: 14,634 Extreme preterm: 70,151 Normal full-term: 1,600	Normal preterm: 13,506 Extreme preterm: 64,744 Normal full-term: 1,477
Chollet (15)	Normal preterm: 15,363 Extreme preterm: 55,424 Normal full-term: 2,376	Normal preterm: 27,827 Extreme preterm: 100,389 Normal full-term: 4,303	Normal preterm: 22,430 Extreme preterm: 80,919 Normal full-term: 3,469
Doyle (16)	500-999: 81,956 Aust dollars per live birth	500-999: 73,920	500-999: 68,801
Gilbert (18)	25 week survivor: 202,700 30 week survivor: 46,400 38 week survivor: 1,100	25 week survivor: 284,775 30 week survivor: 65,188 38 week survivor: 1,545	25 week survivor: 262,825 30 week survivor: 60,163 38 week survivor: 1,426
Kilpatrick (19)	24 week survivor: 294,749 25 week survivor: 181,062 26 week survivor: 166,215	24 week survivor: 447,851 25 week survivor: 275,111 26 week survivor: 252,552	24 week survivor: 405,210 25 week survivor: 248,918 26 week survivor: 228,506
Luke (20)	25-27 weeks: 195,254 28-30weeks: 91,343 31-34 weeks: 18,367 39-42 weeks: 2,230	25-27 weeks: 329,292 28-30weeks: 154,048 31-34 weeks: 30,976 39-42 weeks: 3,761	25-27 weeks: 285,070 28-30weeks: 133,361 31-34 weeks: 26,816 39-42 weeks: 3,256
Marbella (21)	"premature survivor": 16,973 3000-4500 gram: 1,300	"premature survivor": 25,789 3000-4500 gram: 1,975	"premature survivor": 23,334 3000-4500 gram: 1,787
Rogowski (23)	501-1500 grams: 49,457 501-1000 grams: 83,176 24-26 weeks: 95,560 27-29 weeks: 61,724 30-32 weeks: 35,106	501-1500 grams: 75,147 501-1000 grams: 126,380	501-1500 grams: 67,992 501-1000 grams: 114,347
Rogowski (24)	501-1500 grams: 53,316 501-1000 grams: 90,015 24-26 weeks: 101,638 27-29 weeks: 62,960 30-32 weeks: 34,258	501-1500 grams: 70,633 501-1000 grams: 119,251	501-1500 grams: 68,043 501-1000 grams: 114,879

Population st Projection - 05 Dollars ing Medical CPI	US Population Cost Projection - 2005 Dollars Using Hospital PPI	Per-Patient LOS	Per-Patient Ventilator Days	Per-Patient Maternal Costs
7 weeks: 7.04 billion 8 weeks: 2.06 billion 41 weeks: 5.17 billion	<37 weeks: 6.50 billion <28 weeks: 1.90 billion 37-41 weeks: 4.77 billion	Normal preterm: 6.1 Extreme preterm: 19.9 Normal full-term: 1.9	N/A	Normal preterm: 10,626 Extreme preterm: 11,508 Normal full-term: 7,452
7 weeks: 13.38 billion 8 weeks: 2.95 billion 41 weeks: 13.9 billion	<37 weeks: 10.78 billion <28 weeks: 2.38 billion 37-41 weeks: 11.20 billion	N/A	N/A	Normal preterm: 13,017 Extreme preterm: 14,815 Normal full-term: 7,850
)-999 grams: 4 billion	500-999 grams: 1.81 billion	500-999: 82.1 per live birth	500-999: 34.4 per live birth	N/A
7 weeks: 4.62 billion 34 weeks: 1.87 billion)-1499 grams: 2.82 billion)-2499 grams: 3.50 billion	<37 weeks: 4.26 billion 30-34 weeks: 1.73 billion 500-1499 grams: 2.60 billion 500-2499 grams: 3.23 billion	25 week survivor: 92 30 week survivor: 30.4 38 week survivor: 1.8	N/A	25 week survivor: 7,500 30 week survivor: 7,200 38 week survivor: 2,500
week survivor: 1.79 billion week survivor: 1.28 billion week survivor: 1.36 billion	24 week survivor: 1.62 billion 25 week survivor: 1.16 billion 26 week survivor: 1.23 billion	24 week survivor: 120 25 week survivor: 86 26 week survivor: 80	24 week survivor: 76 25 week survivor: 58 26 week survivor: 45	N/A
27 weeks: 5.25 billion 30weeks: 4.76 billion 34 weeks: 4.35 billion 42 weeks: 8.7 billion	25-27 weeks: 4.55 billion 28-30weeks: 4.12 billion 31-34 weeks: 3.77 billion 39-42 weeks: 7.54 billion	25-27 weeks: 71.2 28-30weeks: 39.0 31-34 weeks: 11.8 39-42 weeks: 3.1	N/A	25-27 weeks: 84,892 28-30weeks: 81,971 31-34 weeks: 23,759 39-42 weeks: 7,573
weeks: $8.16 billion 00-4500 grams: $5.85 billion	<37 weeks: 7.38 billion 3000-4500 grams: 5.29 billion	"premature survivor": 14.1 N/A 3000-4500 gram: 1.7	N/A	N/A
-1500 grams: 3.93 billion -1000 grams: 2.89 billion	501-1500 grams: 3.56 billion 501-1000 grams: 2.61 billion	501-1500 grams: 49 501-1000 grams: 75 24-26 weeks: 82 27-29 weeks: 58 30-32 weeks: 39	N/A	N/A
-1500 grams: 3.69 billion -1000 grams: 2.72 billion	501-1500 grams: 3.55 billion 501-1000 grams: 2.62 billion	501-1500 grams: 47 501-1000 grams: 73 24-26 weeks: 79 27-29 weeks: 55 30-32 weeks: 36	N/A	N/A

continued

TABLE D-3 Continued

Study	Per Patient Cost	Per Patient Cost - 2005 Dollars Using Medical CPI	Per Patient Cost - 2005 Dollars Using Hospital PPI
Schmitt (25)	500-999 grams: 205,218 500-1499 grams: 136,456 >2,500 grams: 1,647	500-999 grams: 221,450 500-1499 grams: 147,249 >2,500 grams: 1,777	500-999 grams: 222,104 500-1499 grams: 147,684 >2,500 grams: 1,783
St John (26)	24 week survivor:145,892 30 week survivor: 37,569 40 week survivor: 1,127	24 wk survivor: 246,044 30 week survivor: 63,359 40 week survivor: 1,900	24 wk survivor: 213,002 30 week survivor: 54,851 40 week survivor: 1,645
Tommiska (27)	<1000 gram survivor: 70,290 Euro Full term: 515 Euro	<1000 gram survivor: 105,662 Full term: 774	<1000 gram survivor: 90,338 Full term: 662
Victorian Infant Collaborative Study Group (12)	500-999 grams: 53,655 Aust dollars per live birth	500-999 grams: 67,865	500-999 grams: 58,752

Weighted averages calculated from data in articles to correspond to weight categories above.

the Organisation for Economic Co-operation and Development purchasing power parity, although this accounts only for differences in price and not differences in practice style. Within the United States, neonatal care is fairly homogeneous, so it is likely that price differences will outweigh geographic practice style differences. An adjustment for geographic differences was not made because of the difficulty in defining the location of care for most of the cohorts, which were often either at the state level or at institutions in several states. Finally, variability arises because of the authors' choices of which types of costs to include. Unfortunately, most authors did not disaggregate costs into components, thus making an assessment of the contributions of these choices to the cost estimates difficult to quantify. Table D-3 presents neonatal costs separately from maternal costs, showing a greater degree of variability for the former.

Because it is difficult to fully address variability in prices, an attempt was also made to describe resource utilization independent of its price. Table D-3 shows the length of stay (LOS) and the number of days of assisted ventilation for the studies reviewed. Although not all studies reported these measures, the variability in the direct markers of resource utilization appears to be somewhat less than that for cost. The LOSs for infants with birth weights of 500 to 999 grams ranged from 64 to 106 days in six studies, with four studies showing LOSs in the narrow range of 73 to 82 days.

S Population ost Projection -)05 Dollars sing Medical CPI	US Population Cost Projection - 2005 Dollars Using Hospital PPI	Per-Patient LOS	Per-Patient Ventilator Days	Per-Patient Maternal Costs
)0-999 grams: 7.70 billion)0-1499 grams: 5.06 billion ,500 grams: 6.58 billion	500-999 grams: 7.70 billion 501-1499 grams: 5.06 billion >2,500 grams: 6.58 billion	500-999 grams: 64.4 500-1499 grams: 47.9 >2,500 grams: 2.3	N/A	500-999 grams: 11,609 500-1499 grams: 12,183 >2,500 grams: 3,378
37 weeks: 9.92 billion -34 weeks: 3.86 billion 7-42 weeks: 7.34 billion	< 37 weeks: 8.59 billion 30-34 weeks: 3.34 billion 37-42 weeks: 6.35 billion	N/A	N/A	N/A
)0-999 grams: 2.41 billion 7-41 weeks: 2.50 billion	500-999 grams: 2.06 billion 37-41 weeks: 2.14 billion	<1000 gram survivor: 106 Full term: N/A	N/A	N/A
0-999 grams: 1.55 billion	500-999 grams: 1.34 billion	500-999 grams: 77 per live birth	500-999 grams: 23 per live birth	500-999 grams: N/A

Studies that reported both birth weight- and gestational age–specific costs show that these are consistent. Gilbert et al. give a per-patient cost of $202,700 for a survivor born at 25 weeks gestation and a per-patient cost of $224,400 for a survivor born with a birth weight of 500 to 750 grams (18). For survivors born at 30 weeks gestation, the per-patient cost is $46,400, whereas for a survivor with a birth weight of 1,250 to 1,499 grams, the per-patient cost is $51,900. These authors excluded infants whose birth weights and gestational ages did not match; the birth weight-specific costs may therefore be less biased, as the gestational age on vital statistics records is more often likely to be inaccurate. Across all studies, under the assumption that DRG Code 387 for extreme prematurity corresponds to gestational ages of <28 weeks, costs ranged from $70,451 to $100,389, similar to those for the corresponding birth weight range of 500 to 999 grams.

When the costs were projected to the U.S. population, the range for infants born at <37 weeks gestation was $4.62 billion to $13.38 billion, with the latter estimate derived from a study based on charges (15). For infants with birth weights of 500 to 999 grams, the costs ranged from $1.53 billion to $5.06 billion, with the range for the U.S. population being $2.72 billion to $5.06 billion.

Full-term controls had per-patient costs of $734 to $4,303. If the studies that used charges or failed to specify this were excluded, the range for the U.S. population was $1,545 to $1,900. Corresponding population projections were $2.37 billion to $6.58 billion.

The previously noted inverse relationship between costs and gestational age or birth weight was observed in all studies. The marked right skew of the cost data was also noted in those studies that reported means and medians (23–25, 27).

Direct Nonmedical Costs and Lost Productivity

Table D-4 describes studies that assessed parental out-of-pocket expenditures and lost productivity. In the single study that examined both nonmedical direct costs and productivity losses, parental mean costs before discharge for extremely low birth weight infant were €2,755, or 4 percent of total costs (27). These were composed of 64 percent travel costs, 30 percent lost earnings, and 6 percent accommodation. An earlier interview study of travel costs for mothers of 109 low-birth-weight infants in Britain showed that 36 percent of families traveled more than 21 miles, that 88 percent of families visited the infants daily, and that the median total expenditure was between £101 and £200 (in 1990 United Kingdom pounds sterling), with a maximal expenditure of £1,000 (22). More recently, Gennaro observed the families of 224 infants born at less than 37 weeks of gestational age discharged from a single center between 1990 and 1994 (30). That study did not detail the productivity losses during the initial hospitalization. The average mother in that study used 4 weeks of maternity leave during the initial hospitalization. Out-of-pocket expenses averaged $433, with the largest category being transportation.

CHARACTERIZATION AND ESTIMATES OF COSTS FOLLOWING DISCHARGE FROM THE BIRTH HOSPITALIZATION

Direct Medical Costs

Estimates of direct medical resource utilization and costs following discharge from the birth hospitalization are given in Table D-5. There was a greater degree of heterogeneity compared with that in the studies of initial hospitalization, in large degree because of the various time horizons and costs included. For this reason, it is problematic to provide a single estimate or range of estimates for these costs. As for short-run costs, costs and resource utilization were inversely related to gestational age. In addition, in studies with longer follow-ups, the majority of the costs accrued in the first year of life. In studies that measured both outpatient and rehospitalization costs, the latter accounted for the majority of costs in the first year of life,

TABLE D-4 Parental Out of Pocket Expenses and Lost Productivity During Initial Hospitalization

Paper	Parental Wages	Lost Productivity of Child	Child Care	Other	Travel
Brazier (14)	N/A	N/A	N/A	N/A	Per visit: 3-17 Per week: 27.98
Gennaro (30)	N/A	N/A	N/A	Total initial hosp <2,500: 433	<2,500: 271
Giacoia (17)	N/A	N/A	N/A	N/A	Total: 250 Per visit: 25
McLoughlin (22)	N/A	N/A	N/A	N/A	Median: Approx 100 (from figure)
Tommiska (27)	<1000: 827[a]	N/A	N/A	Accomodation <1,000: 165[a] Total initial hospital <1,000: 2,755	<1,000: 1763[a]

[a]Calculated from data in article.

TABLE D-5 Direct Medical Expenses Following Discharge from the
Initial Hospitalization

Paper	Time Horizon	Rehospitalization (cost)	Outpatient MD, Drug and Other (cost)
Broyles (28)	1 year adjusted age	<1,500: 6,982	<1,500: 2,931
Chollet (15)[a]	2 years (1 year detail)	Not separated from initial hospitalization	Normal preterm: 4,463 Extreme preterm: 6,329 Normal full-term: 2,243 Other preterm: 4,195
Lewit (31)	15 years of age	<1,500 <1 year (not separated from initial hospitalization) 3-5 years: 290 6-10 years: 470	N/A
McCormick (32)	1 year of age	<1,500: 8,250 Term: 900	MD visits <1,500: 564 Term: 232 Other Outpatient: <1,500: 1,311 Term: 63
Medstat (41)	1 year of age	Preterm: 35,034 Normal full-term: 1,210	Preterm: 6,576 Normal full-term: 1,620
Petrou (33)	5 years of age	Year 1: >37 weeks: 297 32-36 weeks: 2,016 28-31 weeks: 7,272 <28 weeks: 10,630 Total (inc birth hosp): >37 weeks: 1,333 32-36 weeks: 4,378 28-31 weeks: 14,059 <28 weeks: 13,639	N/A
Petrou (34)	10 years of age	Including birth hosp: >37 weeks: 1,659 32-36 weeks:7,394 28-31 weeks:17,751 <28 weeks: 17,820	N/A

Post-Discharge Total	Rehospitalization (mean or median)	Rehospitalization (mean total days)	Rehospitalization (LOS)	Outpatient Visits (Clinic, MD, ER)
1,500: 9,913	<1,500: 0.7	<1,500: 7.6	N/A	<1,500: Clinic: 6.4 ER: 1.9 Total: 8.2
Not separated from initial hospitalization	N/A	N/A	N/A	N/A
1,500 1 year (not separated from initial hospitalization) 5 years: 290 10 years: 470	N/A	N/A	N/A	N/A
1,500: 10,139 Term: 1,179	N/A	N/A	N/A	<1,500: 18.5 Term: 9.3
Preterm: 41,611 Normal full-term: 831	Preterm: 1.3 Normal full-term: 1.1	N/A	Preterm: 16.8 Normal full-term: 2.3	Preterm: 8.9 Normal full-term: 5.9
Year 1: 37 weeks: 297 32-36 weeks: 2,016 28-31 weeks: 7,272 28 weeks: 10,630 Total (inc birth hosp): 37 weeks: 1,333 32-36 weeks: 4,378 28-31 weeks: 14,059 28 weeks: 13,639	>37 weeks: 2 32-36 weeks: 2 28-31 weeks: 1 <28 weeks: 1	>37 weeks: 6.3 32-36 weeks: 16.2 28-31 weeks: 48.7 <28 weeks: 49	N/A	N/A
Excluding birth hosp: 37 weeks: 1,659 32-36 weeks:7,394 28-31 weeks:17,751 28 weeks: 17,820	>37 weeks: 0.75 32-36 weeks: 1.48 28-31 weeks: 2.54 <28 weeks: 1.9	Including birth hosp: N/A >37 weeks: 6.2 32-36 weeks:18 28-31 weeks:58.2 <28 weeks: 59.2		N/A

continued

TABLE D-5 Continued

Paper	Time Horizon	Rehospitalization (cost)	Outpatient MD, Drug and Other (cost)
Pharaoh (35)	4 years of age	N/A	N/A
Rogowski (36)	1 year of age	<1,000: 12,800 <1,500: 5,290	<1,500: 870
Rolnick (37)	1 year postdischarge	N/A	N/A
Stevenson (39)[c]	8-9 years of age	<1,000: 421 1,001-1,500: 433 1,501-2,000: 270	<1,000: 876 1,001-1,500: 793 1,501-2,000: 430
Stevenson (40)[d]	8-9 years of age	<1,000: 1,861 1,001-1,500: 1,439 1,501-2,000: 570	<1,000: 1,617 1,001-1,500: 1,447 1,501-2,000: 1,149
Tommiska (27)[e]	2 years of age	Year 1: <1,000: 12,185 control: 225 Year 2: <1,000: 2,575 control: 195	Year 1: <1,000: 1,995 control: 295 Year 2: <1,000: 1,420 control: 315

[a]Mothers and infants combined
[b]Calculated from data in article
[c]Per infant with no disability
[d]Per infant with disability
[e]Total cost includes nonmedical (See Tables D-5 and D-6)

with a range of 54 to 60 percent of the costs in the non-U.S. studies and 70 to 86 percent of the costs in the U.S. cohorts.

Petrou examined factors associated with higher rehospitalization costs (33). These included maternal conditions, such as hospitalization, age >35 or <20 years, or smoking; perinatal factors, such as instrumental delivery or delivery complications; demographic factors, such as lower socioeconomic status; and prematurity.

Postdischarge Total	Rehospitalization (mean or median)	Rehospitalization (mean total days)	Rehospitalization (LOS)	Outpatient Visits (Clinic, MD, ER)
<1,500: 2,620[b]	N/A	N/A	N/A	N/A
<1,500: 6,160	<1,000: 1.8 1,000-1,249: 1.9 1,250-1,499: 2.1	<1,500: 5.5	<1,000: 13.6 1,000-1,249: 9.6 1,250-1,499: 9.8	N/A
2,500-4,499: 2,919 1,500-2,500: 5,938	N/A	N/A	N/A	N/A
<1,000: 1,297 1,001-1,500: 1,226 1,501-2,000: 699	N/A	N/A	N/A	N/A
<1,000: 3,475 1,001-1,500: 2,886 1,501-2,000: 1,719	N/A	N/A	N/A	N/A
Year 1: 1,000: 20,390 control: 1,415 Year 2: 1,000: 13,955 control: 1,205	Year 1: <1,000: 1.8 control: 0.1 Year 2: <1,000:1.0 control: 0.1	Year 1: <1,000: 8.4 control: 0.3 Year 2: <1,000: 4.2 control: 0.4	N/A	Year 1: <1,000: 7.1 control: 2.9 Year 2: <1,000: 6.5 control: 3.8

Educational Costs

Details of studies assessing educational costs are given in Table D-6. As noted above, the assessment of educational costs was inconsistent with respect to both the study methodology and the age at the time of the assessment. After controlling for medical, economic, and social factors, Chaikind and Corman found a 49 percent relative risk for special education placement in low-birth-weight infants (29). This translated to a net present value

TABLE D-6 Educational Expenditures Following Discharge from Initial Hospitalization

Paper	Pre-School Age	School Age
Chaikand (29)	N/A	<2500 Age 6-15: 1,240 (370.8 million total/yr)
Lewit (31)	<1500 Preschool: 290	<1500 Age 6-10: Special Ed 150 Age 6-15: Grade Rep 45
Pharaoh (35)	N/A	<1,500: 4,211
Roth (38)	N/A	Kindergarten <1,000: 6979 1,000-1,499: 5,740 1,500-2,499: 4,870 >2,500: 4,375

Tommiska (27)	"Special Day Care"
	Year 1:
	  <1,000: 0
	  control: 0
	Year 2:
	  <1,000: 1,285
	  control: 0
		N/A

Clements	Early intervention (0-3 years cumulative) <28 weeks: 7,182 28-30 weeks: 5254 31-33 weeks: 2,654 34-36 weeks: 1,321 37-39 weeks: 770 >40 weeks: 613	N/A

of $1,240 (in 1988 U.S. dollars) per low birth weight infant, or $370 million per year for special education costs alone. Roth et al. found that infants with birth weights of <1,000 grams had kindergarten costs 60 percent higher than those for normal birth weight controls (38). However, the authors noted that low levels of maternal education and poverty accounted for more than three quarters of the total excess costs of kindergarten, whereas low birth weight accounted for only 1 percent of the total excess costs because of the relative numbers of children with these predisposing conditions.

Early intervention costs may also be significant. A recent study of state-level data in Massachusetts assessed costs from birth to age 3 years for early intervention services by gestational age. Infants born at less than 28 weeks of gestation had early intervention costs of $7,182 (in 2003 U.S. dollars), whereas the early intervention costs were $613 for those delivered at 40 weeks of gestation or more (53).

Direct Nonmedical Costs and Lost Productivity

Table D-7 shows the costs associated with postdischarge parental out-of-pocket expenses and lost productivity. Tommiska et al. documented first-year parental wage losses of €5,990 for infants with birth weights of <1,000 grams, whereas the loss was €880 for controls. These costs increased to €8,175 in the second year for the parents of children born with low birth weights (27). Similar data are not available for the United States.

SUMMARY OF COST STUDIES FOR PREMATURITY

Several themes emerged from this systematic review of cost-of-illness studies:

1. Most studies had significant methodological limitations. These included a reliance on administrative data sets without adequate checks on data validity, small sample sizes and possible selection bias, a lack of quantification of uncertainty through the use of descriptive statistics or sensitivity analysis, the use of charges or inadequately described costing, the lack of a control group, and a failure to discount appropriately for longer studies.

2. All cost estimates in the literature omitted at least some potentially important components of costs and are therefore likely to underestimate true resource use. These omissions included professional fees, hospital costs for transferred infants, costs for nonsurviving infants, and out-of-pocket costs for parents. There is almost no information on the lost earnings of parents and no information on the productivity losses of the infants themselves. Maternal costs for the delivery hospitalization and the costs of antenatal admissions were omitted by most studies. The analysis of infants and mothers separately risks both an underestimation of the costs of prematurity and the possibility of missed shifting of costs between the two groups. Very few studies have addressed educational costs, and these do not provide adequate information across the spectrum of school age and disability.

3. Most authors did not disaggregate costs into their components, making it problematic to target the sources and predictors of high costs.

4. Studies confirmed the previously noted inverse relationship of maternal, neonatal, and postdischarge costs with birth weight and gestational age.

TABLE D-7 Out-of-Pocket Expenses and Lost Productivity Following Discharge from Initial Hospitalization

Paper	Parental Wages	Lost Productivity of Child	Child Care	Other	Travel
Tommiska (27)	Year 1: <1,000: 5,990 control: 880 Year 2: <1,000: 8,175 control: 595	N/A	N/A	"Home Aid" Year 1: <1,000: 0 control: 0 Year 2: <1,000: 255 control: 85	Year 1: <1,000: 75 control: 15 Year 2: <1,000: 85 control: 15
McCormick (32)	N/A	N/A	<1,500: 563 Term: 1,082	N/A	<1,500: 180 Term: 23
Gennaro (30)	N/A	N/A	N/A	Non-reimbursed Health <2,500: 69 Total Out of Pocket <2,500: 445	N/A

5. Although the per-patient cost for moderately preterm infants is lower than that for extremely preterm infants, the larger numbers of these infants results in population costs of similar magnitudes in both groups. This has important implications for the setting of policy, as interventions that ameliorate moderate prematurity may be as cost-effective as the more difficult interventions that would eliminate extreme prematurity.

6. The time horizon for economic follow-up is inadequate. Very few studies have followed infants beyond 5 years, and none have documented the implications of prematurity in young adulthood, despite the availability of appropriate cohorts.

7. Most of the studies with longer time horizons or more comprehensive methods of cost ascertainment have been from countries other than the United States. The appropriateness of generalizing these cost estimates to the United States is uncertain.

RECOMMENDATIONS FOR POLICY AND FURTHER RESEARCH

The findings summarized above have direct implications for policy and research:

1. Because policy makers are likely to accept the dollar estimates of the costs of illness without adequately assessing the quality of the underlying studies, it is important that the peer review process identify the more significant methodological limitations, such as the use of unadjusted charges or the lack of assessment of uncertainty.

2. In light of the prominence of the economic implications on health policy decision making for this population, it is essential that a U.S. study with a societal perspective be performed. This should include a comprehensive assessment of productivity losses and parental out-of-pocket expenditures in the U.S. context.

3. Studies with longer time horizons should be undertaken and should preferably use an incidence approach rather than a prevalence approach to costing. At a minimum, these should extend well into school age. The implications of prematurity as young adults enter the work force should be examined, as should lifetime labor force implications.

4. Because of the interactions between socioeconomic status and outcome, costing studies should include specific analyses of the increased burden on particular racial and ethnic populations.

5. The focus of short-run costing studies should be shifted toward a perinatal perspective, in which the unit of analysis is the maternal-infant dyad. This is now feasible with improved data linkage.

6. Attention should be directed toward the economic implications of moderate prematurity, in addition to extreme prematurity.

7. A longitudinal analysis of the economic implications of prematurity to the educational system should be undertaken.
8. A comprehensive longitudinal study of the long-term economic implications of prematurity should be undertaken.

REFERENCES

1. Mugford M. The cost of neonatal care: reviewing the evidence. Soz Praventivmed. 1995;40(6):361–368.
2. Petrou S. Economic consequences of preterm birth and low birthweight. Br J Obstet Gynaecol. 2003 Apr;110(Suppl 20):17–23.
3. Petrou S, Davidson LL. Economic issues in the follow-up of neonates. Semin Neonatol. 2000 May;5(2):159–169.
4. Petrou S, Sach T, Davidson L. The long-term costs of preterm birth and low birth weight: results of a systematic review. Child Care Health Dev. 2001 Mar;27(2):97–115.
5. Richardson DK, Zupancic JA, Escobar GJ, Ogino M, Pursley DM, Mugford M. A critical review of cost reduction in neonatal intensive care. I. The structure of costs. J Perinatol. 2001 Mar;21(2):107–115.
6. Richardson DK, Zupancic JA, Escobar GJ, Ogino M, Pursley DM, Mugford M. A critical review of cost reduction in neonatal intensive care. II. Strategies for reduction. J Perinatol. 2001 Mar;21(2):121–127.
7. Zupancic JA, Richardson DK, Lee K, McCormick MC. Economics of prematurity in the era of managed care. Clin Perinatol. 2000 Jun;27(2):483–497.
8. U.S. Bureau of Labor Statistics. Consumer Price Index—All Urban Consumers—Medical Care (Series ID CUUR0000SAM). [Online]. Available: www.bls.gov/data [accessed August 1, 2005].
9. United States Bureau of Labor Statistics. Producer Price Index Industry Data—Hospitals (ID PCU622). 2005 [Online]. Available: www.bls.gov/data [accessed September 20, 2005].
10. Organization for Economic Cooperation and Development. Purchasing Power Parities for OECD Countries since 1980. 2005 [Online]. Available: www.oecd.org [accessed August 1, 2005].
11. Martin JA, Hamilton BE, Sutton PD, Ventura SJ, Menacker F, ML M. Births: Final Data for 2002. National Vital Stat Rep. 2003;52(10): 1-113.
12. The Victorian Infant Collaborative Study Group. Economic outcome for intensive care of infants of birthweight 500-999 g born in Victoria in the post surfactant era. J Paediatr Child Health. 1997 Jun;33(3):202–208.
13. Adams EK, Nishimura B, Merritt RK, Melvin C. Costs of poor birth outcomes among privately insured. J Health Care Finance. 2003 Spring;29(3):11–27.
14. Brazier L, Harper K, Marrington S. Hospital visiting costs. An exploratory study into travelling expenses incurred by parents with babies in a regional neonatal unit. J Neonat Nurs. 1995;1(2):29–31.
15. Chollet DJ, Newman JF Jr, Sumner AT. The cost of poor birth outcomes in employer-sponsored health plans. Med Care. 1996 Dec;34(12):1219–1234.
16. Doyle LW. Evaluation of neonatal intensive care for extremely low birth weight infants in Victoria over two decades. II. Efficiency. Pediatrics. 2004 Mar;113(3 Pt 1):510–514.
17. Giacoia GP, Rutledge D, West K. Factors affecting visitation of sick newborns. Clin Pediatr (Phila). 1985 May;24(5):259–262.
18. Gilbert WM, Nesbitt TS, Danielsen B. The cost of prematurity: quantification by gestational age and birth weight. Obstet Gynecol. 2003 Sep;102(3):488–492.

19. Kilpatrick SJ, Schlueter MA, Piecuch R, Leonard CH, Rogido M, Sola A. Outcome of infants born at 24-26 weeks' gestation. I. Survival and cost. Obstet Gynecol. 1997 Nov;90(5):803–808.

20. Luke B, Bigger HR, Leurgans S, Sietsema D. The cost of prematurity: a case-control study of twins vs singletons. Am J Public Health. 1996 Jun;86(6):809–814.

21. Marbella AM, Chetty VK, Layde PM. Neonatal hospital lengths of stay, readmissions, and charges. Pediatrics. 1998 Jan;101(1 Pt 1):32–36.

22. McLoughlin A, Hillier VF, Robinson MJ. Parental costs of neonatal visiting. Arch Dis Child. 1993 May;68(5 Spec No):597–599.

23. Rogowski J. Measuring the cost of neonatal and perinatal care. Pediatrics. 1999 Jan;103(1 Suppl E):329–335.

24. Rogowski J. Using economic information in a quality improvement collaborative. Pediatrics 2003 Apr;111(4 Pt 2):e411–e418.

25. Schmitt SK, Sneed L, Phibbs CS. The costs of newborn care in California: a population-based study. Pediatrics. 2006;117:154–160.

26. St John EB, Nelson KG, Cliver SP, Bishnoi RR, Goldenberg RL. Cost of neonatal care according to gestational age at birth and survival status. Am J Obstet Gynecol. 2000 Jan;182(1 Pt 1):170–175.

27. Tommiska V, Tuominen R, Fellman V. Economic costs of care in extremely low birthweight infants during the first 2 years of life. Pediatr Crit Care Med. 2003 Apr;4(2):157–163.

28. Broyles RS, Tyson JE, Heyne ET, Heyne RJ, Hickman JF, Swint M, et al. Comprehensive follow-up care and life-threatening illnesses among high-risk infants: a randomized controlled trial. JAMA 2000 Oct 25;284(16):2070–2076.

29. Chaikand S, Corman H. The impact of low birthweight on special education costs. J Health Econ. 1991 Oct;10(3):291–311.

30. Gennaro S. Leave and employment in families of preterm low birthweight infants. Image J Nurs Sch. 1996 Fall;28(3):193–198.

31. Lewit EM, Baker LS, Corman H, Shiono PH. The direct cost of low birth weight. Future Child. 1995 Spring;5(1):35–56.

32. McCormick MC, Bernbaum JC, Eisenberg JM, Kustra SL, Finnegan E. Costs incurred by parents of very low birth weight infants after the initial neonatal hospitalization. Pediatrics. 1991 Sep;88(3):533–541.

33. Petrou S. The economic consequences of preterm birth during the first 10 years of life. Br J Obstet Gynaecol. 2005 Mar;112 Suppl 1:10–15.

34. Petrou S, Mehta Z, Hockley C, Cook-Mozaffari P, Henderson J, Goldacre M. The impact of preterm birth on hospital inpatient admissions and costs during the first 5 years of life. Pediatrics. 2003 Dec;112(6 Pt 1):1290–1297.

35. Pharoah PO, Stevenson RC, Cooke RW, Sandu B. Costs and benefits of neonatal intensive care. Arch Dis Child. 1988 Jul;63(7 Spec No):715–718.

36. Rogowski J. Cost-effectiveness of care for very low birth weight infants. Pediatrics. 1998 Jul;102(1 Pt 1):35–43.

37. Rolnick SJ, Jackson JM, O'Connor P, DeFor T. Impact of birthweight on healthcare charges within a managed care organization. Am J Manag Care. 2000 Dec;6(12):1289–1296.

38. Roth J, Figlio DN, Chen Y, Ariet M, Carter RL, Resnick MB, et al. Maternal and infant factors associated with excess kindergarten costs. Pediatrics. 2004 Sep;114(3):720–728.

39. Stevenson RC, McCabe CJ, Pharoah PO, Cooke RW. Cost of care for a geographically determined population of low birthweight infants to age 8-9 years. I. Children without disability. Arch Dis Child Fetal Neonat Ed. 1996 Mar;74(2):F114–F117.

40. Stevenson RC, Pharoah PO, Stevenson CJ, McCabe CJ, Cooke RW. Cost of care for a geographically determined population of low birthweight infants to age 8-9 years. II. Children with disability. Arch Dis Child Fetal Neonat Ed. 1996 Mar;74(2):F118–F121.

41. Thomson Medstat. The Cost of Prematurity to U.S. Employers. http://www.marchofdimes.com/prematurity/15341_15349.asp : March of Dimes; 2004.

42. Imershein AW, Turner C, Wells JG, Pearman A. Covering the costs of care in neonatal intensive care units. Pediatrics. 1992 Jan;89(1):56–61.

43. Long SH, Marquis MS, Harrison ER. The costs and financing of perinatal care in the United States. Am J Public Health. 1994 Sep;84(9):1473–1478.

44. March of Dimes. Impact on Business. http://www.marchofdimes.com/prematurity/15341_15349.asp : March of Dimes; 2005.

45. Hack M, Youngstrom EA, Cartar L, Schluchter M, Taylor HG, Flannery D, et al. Behavioral outcomes and evidence of psychopathology among very low birth weight infants at age 20 years. Pediatrics. 2004 Oct;114(4):932–940.

46. Saigal S, Pinelli J, Hoult L, Kim MM, Boyle M. Psychopathology and social competencies of adolescents who were extremely low birth weight. Pediatrics. 2003 May;111(5 Pt 1):969–975.

47. Darmstadt GL, Bhutta ZA, Cousens S, Adam T, Walker N, de Bernis L. Evidence-based, cost-effective interventions: how many newborn babies can we save? Lancet. 2005 Mar 12-18;365(9463):977–988.

48. Leader S, Yang H, DeVincenzo J, Jacobson P, Marcin JP, Murray DL. Time and out-of-pocket costs associated with respiratory syncytial virus hospitalization of infants. Value Health. 2003 Mar-Apr;6(2):100–106.

49. Stang P, Brandenburg N, Carter B. The economic burden of respiratory syncytial virus-associated bronchiolitis hospitalizations. Arch Pediatr Adolesc Med. 2001 Jan;155(1): 95–96.

50. Waitzman NJ, Romano PS, Scheffler RM. Estimates of the economic costs of birth defects. Inquiry. 1994 Summer;31(2):188–205.

51. Greenough A, Alexander J, Burgess S, Bytham J, Chetcuti PA, Hagan J, et al. Health care utilisation of prematurely born, preschool children related to hospitalisation for RSV infection. Arch Dis Child. 2004 Jul;89(7):673–678.

52. Greenough A, Cox S, Alexander J, Lenney W, Turnbull F, Burgess S, et al. Health care utilisation of infants with chronic lung disease, related to hospitalisation for RSV infection. Arch Dis Child. 2001 Dec;85(6):463–468.

53. Clemens K, Avadi F, Wilber N, Barfield WD. The cost of prematurity: birth to age three early intervention costs [abstract]. Pediatr Res., in press.

E

Selected Programs Funding
Preterm Birth Research

On August 10, 2005, the Institute of Medicine Committee on Understanding Premature Birth and Assuring Healthy Outcomes hosted a workshop on barriers to research on preterm birth (see Chapter 13 for discussion). Presenters at that workshop provided information on the funding of research on premature birth and preterm infants, the primary sources of which are the National Institutes of Health (NIH), the Centers for Disease Control and Prevention (CDC), and nonprofit voluntary health or philanthropic organizations, including the March of Dimes (MOD) and the Burroughs Wellcome Fund (BWF). The information that these agencies and organizations provided at the workshop are described below.

NATIONAL INSTITUTES OF HEALTH

An overview of the funding dollars that are being provided through the NIH, the National Institute of Child Health and Development (NICHD), and the Pregnancy and Perinatology Branch (PPB) of NICHD provides a snapshot of its grant portfolio in fiscal year (FY) 2004 for nonnetwork and network grants as well as some background about its FY 2004 R01 (grants for health-related research and development) grantees and trainees. Pinpointing how much NIH spends specifically on preterm birth research is difficult because it is codified under a broad general category called prenatal birth-preterm low birth weight that encompasses research concerned with normal and preterm labor, intrauterine growth retardation, and fetal and infant physiology and nutrition. Separating funding for preterm birth and its consequences from the general category is not possible with the information currently available from NIH.

Between FYs 2000 and 2004, funding in the category prenatal birth–preterm low birth weight increased from $306.5 million to $393 million in grants, contracts, and intramural research. Approximately 80 percent ($311.7 million) of these dollars came from the National Institute of Allergies and Infectious Diseases, NICHD, and the National Institute on Drug Abuse. PPB's share of the NICHD contribution was about $70 million. The remainder of the NICHD funds is primarily allocated to research conducted in components of NICHD's intramural research programs (Division of Epidemiology, Statistics, and Prevention Research).

The PPB portfolio of grants relevant to preterm birth is divided between two areas. One area is parturition, in which basic research on the events leading to labor and delivery, which is fundamental to understanding preterm birth, is conducted. The other area is preterm birth, in which research directly related to preterm birth is conducted. In addition, two PPB networks are substantially involved in research on premature birth and its sequelae: the Maternal-Fetal Medicine Unit (MFMU) Network and the Neonatal Research Network (NRN). Both of these networks conduct clinical trials, as well as observational and mechanistic studies. The budget for MFMU in FY 2004 was about $10 million per year, approximately 75 percent of which goes to research on premature birth. The NRN FY 2004 research budget was approximately $8.5 million, with 75 percent going to research on infants born preterm ($6.4 million).

In FY 2004, PPB supported 264 grants, which included new and ongoing grants; 41 (15.6 percent of the total PPB funding) were related to research on parturition or spontaneous premature birth. Twenty of these grants (7.6 percent of the total) were for research on parturition, and 21 of these grants (8 percent of the total) were for research on premature birth. PPB also supported 30 network grants (11.4 percent of the total dollars) that dealt with research on premature birth or premature infants. These were all U10 grants, which are cooperative programs between sponsoring institutions and participating principal investigators. The preterm birth–related grants can also be divided into two categories: nonnetwork preterm birth grants (a total of $8.4 million) and grants into the MFMU for preterm birth research (a total of $7.5 million). About $11 million, representing about 10.3 percent of the total for research on infants born preterm, was expended. Nonnetwork grants for research on infants born preterm totaled $4.6 million, and funds going to NRN for research on infants born preterm were $6.4 million.

The portfolio of research on parturition was allocated into three general research areas: the uterus, which involves research on contractility and relaxation; fetal membranes, which involves research on fetal membrane rupture and amniotic fluid regulation; and the cervix, which involves research on cervical ripening. For the first category, the PPB funded 15 grants, including 1 F32 grant for postdoctoral research training, 2 K08 mentored career development awards, 3 R03 small research grants, 8 R01 grants, and 1 R01 supplemental grant. In the area of fetal membrane research, PPB funded three R01 grants; in the area of research on the cervix, PPB funded two grants, one F32 grant and one R01 grant. The spontaneous premature birth research portfolio can be broken down into seven areas: interventions, premature rupture of membranes, infection and inflammation/cytokines, epidemiology, transgenic mouse models, proteomics, and bioinformatics. The numbers and types of grants funded in each of these areas were as follows: interventions, two U01 grants; premature rupture of membranes, two R01 grants; infection and inflammation/cytokines, eight R01 grants; epidemiology, six R01 grants and one R01 supplemental grant; transgenic mouse models, one R03 grant; proteomics, one R01 grant; and bioinformatics, one K08 grant. The paylines, or funding levels, for these grants were the 14th percentile for R01 grants and the 20th percentile for R03 grants.

In the intramural research program, NICHD conducts epidemiological, clinical. and laboratory research on those maternal and fetal diseases responsible for excessive infant mortality in the United States. The Perinatology Research Branch of the Division of Intramural Research focuses on the study of the mechanisms of disease responsible for premature labor and delivery, with particular emphasis on the role of subclinical intrauterine infection. The prenatal diagnosis of congenital anomalies is another major area of interest. NICHD also recently awarded a major contract and lease for continued support of the Perinatology Research Branch, located in Michigan. The new campus offers access to a patient population with a high rate of pregnancy complications and brings to bear the academic resources of three major universities: Wayne State University, the University of Michigan, and Michigan State University. These clinical and laboratory facilities opened in the spring of 2005.

MFMU Network

Some notable studies on preterm birth by the MFMU network have included the preterm premature rupture of the membranes (pPROM) trial, which demonstrated that broad-spectrum antibiotic therapy for pPROM prolongs latency and improves neonatal outcome; the bacterial vaginosis (BV) trial, which demonstrated that antibiotic treatment of asymptomatic BV does not reduce the rate of preterm delivery; and a progesterone trial, which indicated that weekly injections of 17-hydroxyprogesterone caproate reduced the incidence of recurrent preterm birth and improved the neonatal outcome for pregnancies at risk because of a previous preterm delivery.

Neonatal Research Network Studies

In the area of research on infants born preterm, notable studies included a surfactant trial that showed that lung surfactant prevents respiratory distress syndrome and an ongoing follow-up study of extremely-low-birth-weight infants. The latter study involved a long-term assessment of developmental and cognitive functions. In addition, NRN conducted a trial that demonstrated that nitric oxide administered by inhalation was of no benefit to extremely-low-birth-weight infants.

R01 Grantees in FY 2004

A total of 28 R01 grantees and 2 U01 (R01 equivalent) grantees were supported in the areas of parturition or preterm birth research. Twelve were in the area of parturition and 18 were in the area of premature birth. In the area of parturition, the typical grantee was a Ph.D. and a full professor in a basic science department who received NIH-supported training or did postdoctoral research and conducted animal research. In the area of preterm birth, the typical grantee was an M.D. or Ph.D. associate or full professor in a department of obstetrics and gynecology, did postdoctoral training, and conducted human research.

Trainee Grants for FY 2004

In 2004, 24 individual training and career development awards, which included new or ongoing awards, were supported. These included 3 F31 grants, which are for predoctoral fellowships; 2 F32 grants, which are for postdoctoral fellowships; 10 K08 grants, which are mentored, nonclinical research grants; and 9 mentored clinical research grants known as K23 grants. In the area of parturition, PPB funded four grants: one K31 grant, one F32 grant, and two K08 grants. In the area of premature birth, PPB funded only one K08 grant.

NICHD also awarded one new institutional training (T32) grant in FY 2004. These grants provide support for basic or clinical pre- or postdoctoral training. PPB currently supports five of these T32 grants. Three are in the area of perinatal medicine or biology, one is in the area of perinatal epidemiology, and one is in the area of developmental neonatal biology. In total, this provides funding for about 19 postdoctoral trainees (M.D.'s or Ph.D.'s) per year. NICHD also supports a mentored clinical research development program for clinicians.

In 2005, PPB supported two P01 grants relevant to research on preterm birth. One is entitled Initiation of Human Labor: Prevention of Prematurity. This grant focuses on investigation of the physiological and molecular bases for the initiation of human parturition and the causes of preterm birth. It involves studies of fetal adrenal activity, fetal signaling to the myometrium, fetal lung surfactant, and cervical remodeling and competency. The other P01 grant is entitled Overall Gene-Environmental Interaction to Human Parturition. Its overall goal is to identify the genetic and environmental risk factors that contribute in a multifactorial manner to preterm birth and to model the gene, environment, and maternal-fetal interactions that may contribute to the risk of prematurity. This research involves the analysis of the allelic frequencies of numerous polymorphisms in 16 candidate genes implicated in parturition.

A new initiative that will be funded in 2006 is the genomic and proteomic network for premature birth research, which aims to accelerate the pace of research on premature birth by focusing on genomic and proteomic strategies in the human and providing for the scientific community a web-based database for data mining and the deposition of genomic and proteomic data.

CENTERS FOR DISEASE CONTROL AND PREVENTION

The CDC Division of Reproductive Health, Extramural, has funded several grants relevant to preterm research. The project Preterm Birth among Inner City Women: Bacterial Vaginosis, Stressors and Race was funded by multiple awards made through cooperative agreements with the CDC's intramural program. The project investigates the hypothesis that there is a disproportionate risk of BV and preterm birth in selected populations, mostly the African-American population, which could be an expression of susceptibility resulting from immunosuppression and that immunosuppression may be exacerbated by the health-eroding effects of chronic stressful experiences.

Functional Genomics and Proteomic Markers of Preterm Delivery and Their Variation by Race is a 5-year collaborative project investigating four pathways to preterm birth: infection, decidual hemorrhage, premature activation of normal parturition by maternal or fetal stress, and myometrial stretching.

As part of the Pregnancy Outcomes in Community Health (POUCH) Study, CDC is funding a case-cohort investigation of the relationship between preterm delivery and selected immune system-related gene polymorphisms in a multiethnic community. The second goal of the project is to develop prediction models for preterm delivery.

Another project is investigating whether providing 17-hydroxyprogesterone caproate to women with a history of spontaneous preterm birth seen in the context of routine prenatal care will result in a significant reduction in the rate of preterm birth.

MARCH OF DIMES

MOD receives between 800 and 900 letters of intent for requests for research funding. Of these, approximately 550 potential applicants are invited to apply for funding, and of those applications, 15 to 20 percent are funded (depending on the annual budget). The letters of intent are screened and selected by a committee.

Applications are reviewed in the traditional peer review system by study sections. All applications are for investigator-initiated grants. The applicants are approximately 40 percent M.D.'s and 60 percent Ph.D.'s. The proposals span a range of subjects, all of which must be relevant to birth defects and reproductive health. This translates into the support of research on genetics, developmental biology, and neurobiology. However, research of a more clinically directed nature that addresses, in particular, the problems of neonates and problems related to pregnancy is also supported. Among these are studies that relate to premature birth, including both its potential causes and its consequences. These grants are awarded for 3 years and may be renewed three times, based on reapplications that compete with other renewals and new proposals.

Research in social and behavioral sciences relating to the mission of MOD is also supported. Among these grants are included those that address such issues as the development of speech, hearing, vision, and intelligence, as well as social influences on health. These are also awarded for 3 years.

The Basil O'Connor grants are directed toward support of newly independent investigators who are just emerging from their training but who have a faculty appointment on a tenure line, or its equivalent. These awards currently have a fixed budget of $75,000 per year for 2 years.

The average annual award in 2005 for all grants comprising 410 projects, except the Basil O'Connor grants, was $83,000. In 1999, a special group of grants that considered the causes of prematurity was awarded. Those research studies needed to address external conditions but had to have biological plausibility, and they have been completed. Two of these generated successful research. A new initiative began in 2004 and offered six grants for research on causes of prematurity.

BURROUGHS WELLCOME FUND

The mission of BWF is to advance the medical sciences through the support of research and education by providing grants totaling $25 million to $35 million per year. Its major strategy is to invest in people, particularly young scientists working in undervalued or underfunded areas of research. BWF currently funds four competitive programs that rely on institutions to nominate their best young scientists. Two of these programs are bridging awards: they provide support for 2 years at the postdoctoral level and then continue for 3 years into the assistant professorship level. This funding is viewed as risk capital that young scientists can use to innovate and gather some preliminary data that help them to be more successful in obtaining subsequent NIH grants. Another of the four programs provides support to clinical investigators at the late assistant and early associate professor level who are engaged in translational research that spans the gap between the bench and the bedside. The fourth program supports assistant professors studying infectious diseases.

In addition to these national programs, BWF provides support for science education within the state of North Carolina. The centerpiece of this effort is a competitive program for student science enrichment at the secondary school level. About 85 percent of the BWF funding goes to its competitive awards, and 15 percent of the funding goes to other catalytic efforts to improve the environment for BWF researchers. Within its national programs, BWF actively encourages the support of reproductive science as a broad category, but these grants are not specified for research in subcategories, such as prematurity.

F

Committee and Staff Biographies

COMMITTEE BIOGRAPHIES

Richard E. Behrman (*Chair*) is the executive of the Federation of Pediatric Organizations (FOPO) and chair of FOPO's Pediatric Education Steering Committee. Until July 1, 2002, he held the position of Senior Vice President for Medical Affairs at the Lucile Packard Foundation for Children's Health and Senior Advisor for Health Affairs at the David and Lucile Packard Foundation. Dr. Behrman is also clinical professor of pediatrics at Stanford University; the University of California, San Francisco; and George Washington University, Washington, D.C. He recently served as chair of the Institute of Medicine Committee on Clinical Research Involving Children. Dr. Behrman's areas of special interest include perinatal medicine, intensive and emergency care of children, the provision and organization of children's health and social services, and related issues of public policy and ethics. Dr. Behrman has published extensively in critically reviewed scientific journals and is editor-in-chief of the *Nelson Textbook of Pediatrics* and the journal *The Future of Children*. He is a member of the Institute of Medicine of the National Academy of Sciences.

Eli Y. Adashi is currently dean of medicine and biological sciences at Brown University. Dr. Adashi has until recently served as chair of the Department of Obstetrics and Gynecology at the University of Utah Health Sciences Center. Dr. Adashi has authored or coauthored more than 250 peer-reviewed publications and more than 120 book chapters or reviews, as well as coedited or edited 13 books focusing on intraovarian regulation, reproductive medicine, and novel gene discovery. A member of the Institute of Medicine of the National Academy of Sciences, a member of the Association of American Physicians, and a fellow of the American Association for the Advancement of Science, Dr. Adashi has been the recipient of several academic honors and awards. A past recipient of a Research Career Development Award from the National Institute of Child Health and Development, Dr. Adashi has been continuously funded by the National Institutes of Health since 1985, most recently in the area of ovarian genomics and gene-targeting technology. Dr. Adashi is former president of the Society for Reproductive Endocrinologists, the Society for Gynecologic Investigation, and the American Gynecological and Obstetrical Society. Dr. Adashi is a founding member, treasurer, and most recently, chair, on the advisory committee of the Geneva, Switzerland-based Bertarelli Foundation, which is dedicated to promoting the welfare of infertile couples and to addressing the "epidemic" of infertility therapy-associated high-order multiple gestations.

Marilee C. Allen is a professor of pediatrics and associate director of neonatalolology at The Johns Hopkins School of Medicine. She is board certified in both neonatology and neurodevelopmental disabilities. She is an active clinician in the neonatal intensive care unit (NICU) at Johns Hopkins and is codirector of the NICU Developmental Clinic at the Kennedy Krieger Institute. Dr. Allen is an international expert on neonatal intensive care follow-up, the neurodevelopmental outcomes of high-risk infants, and early intervention strategies. She has authored or coauthored nearly 50 scientific papers. She has served on the Neonatal-Perinatal Sub-Board of the American Board of Pediatrics. Dr. Allen is also a member of the Society for Pediatric Research, the American Pediatric Society, the American Academy of Cerebral Palsy and Developmental Medicine, and the American Academy of Pediatrics.

Rita Loch Caruso, is a professor of environmental health sciences at the University of Michigan School of Public Health. Dr. Caruso received a Ph.D. in toxicology from the University of Cincinnati in 1984. She was assistant professor of pediatrics and human development at Michigan State University before joining the Toxicology Program at the University of Michigan. She has served on several National Institutes of Health study sections and is a member of the City of Ann Arbor Environmental Commission. She has been elected to university, regional, and national offices by her professional peers. Her research focus is female reproductive toxicology. Continuously funded by competitive external grants since 1984, her research emphasizes the mechanisms of toxicity related to pregnancy at the molecular, biochemical, and cellular levels and the integration of this knowledge at the tissue and whole-animal levels. She has a particular emphasis on environmentally persistent chemicals, such as polychlorinated biphenyls, lindane, and dichlorodiphenyltrichloroethane (DDT). Major projects involve the development of models for reproductive toxicity study, the mechanisms of disruption of uterine muscle gap junctions, toxicant-induced alteration of myometrial intracellular signaling (phosphorylation, calcium, phospholipids), and endocrine-mediated modulation of uterine contractions. She is a participating faculty member in the Environmental Toxicology, Reproductive Sciences, Pharmacological Sciences, and Cellular and Molecular Basis of Systems and Integrative Biology graduate and post-doctoral training programs.

Jennifer Culhane is an associate professor of obstetrics and gynecology at the Drexel University College of Medicine and of biostatistics and epidemiology at the Drexel University School of Public Health. Dr. Culhane's work focuses on the social determinants of adverse reproductive outcomes and the contribution that these social exposures play in racial and ethnic differences in the rates of preterm birth and low birth weight. In addition, Dr. Culhane explores the physiological mechanisms that underpin these associations. Her current funded research explores the efficacy of interpregnancy interventions on the reduction of repeat preterm birth. Specifically, nonpregnant women with a recent history of early preterm birth are assessed for a wide range of risk factors, including urogenital tract and periodontal infections, depression, body mass index, housing instability, smoking, and low levels of literacy. After randomization, women in the intervention group are provided treatment for all identified risk factors. Both the timing of the intervention (prepregnancy) and the simultaneous treatment of numerous risk factors are novel aspects of this work. Other studies employ multilevel modeling techniques to examine the association between various socioenvironmental influences—including measures of area-level poverty, crime, homelessness, housing abandonment, and sexually transmitted diseases—on the risk of preterm birth after adjustment for individual characteristics and behaviors.

Christine Dunkel Schetter is a professor in the Department of Psychology at the University of California, Los Angeles, and is director of the Health Psychology Program there. She has conducted research on pregnancy and birth from an multidisciplinary perspective since 1983, including several prospective studies of ethnically diverse and low income populations in California. Her research has focused broadly on the role of stress in preterm delivery, especially identifying the components of stress and emotion that predict preterm birth, the biological and behavioral pathways involved, ethnic disparities and cultural factors in pregnancy, and the roles of other psychosocial factors such as social support and resilience resources in birth outcomes. She has collaborated with Dr. Calvin Hobel, Dr. Curt Sandman, Dr. Susan Scrimshaw, Dr. Ruth Zambrana, and others in this research. In 2004 she received the Distinguished Senior Research Award in Health Psychology (Division 38) from the American Psychological Association. She has served in many editorial and professional capacities pertaining to psychology and health. She is part of a National Institute of Child Health and Human Development–funded network project on community and child health using a community partnership model and investigating, among other issues, the role of stress and allostatic load in preterm birth.

Michael G. Gravett is professor and vice-chairman of Obstetrics & Gynecology and director of Maternal-Fetal Medicine at the University of Washington School of Medicine. Dr. Gravett is active in obstetrical research related to prematurity. He has authored numerous scientific papers and chapters and is internationally recognized for his research on infectious causes and consequences of preterm birth. His work has been cited by other investigators nearly 1,000 times and he has received many national and international awards. He is active in several national and international societies, including the Infectious Disease Society for Obstetrics and Gynecology, the Society for Gynecologic Investigation, and the Society for Maternal-Fetal Medicine. He is listed in *The Best Doctors in America.*

Jay D. Iams holds the Frederick P. Zuspan Endowed Chair at Ohio State University in Columbus where he is professor and vice chair of the Department of Obstetrics & Gynecology. He has conducted clinical research in prematurity since 1982, including trials of risk scoring and patient education, outpatient uterine contraction monitoring, and antibiotics to prevent preterm birth. Dr. Iams has been the principal investigator at Ohio State in the National Institute of Child Health and Human Development Maternal Fetal Medicine Network since 1992, with publications on prematurity and cervical sonography, fetal fibronectin, uterine contraction frequency, antibiotics, and supplemental progesterone. He is an associate editor of *The American Journal of Obstetrics and Gynecology* and was president of the Society for Maternal Fetal Medicine in 2002–2003. He is a member of the American Gynecological and Obstetrical Society and the March of Dimes National Strategic Advisory Committee on Prematurity and sits on the American Board of Obstetrics and Gynecology's Division of Maternal Fetal Medicine.

Michael C. Lu is an assistant professor of Obstetrics & Gynecology at the University of California, Los Angeles (UCLA) School of Medicine. He holds a joint faculty appointment in the Department of Community Health Sciences at the UCLA School of Public Health. Dr. Lu's research examines racial-ethnic disparities in birth outcomes, with a focus on preterm birth. He is a co-principal investigator on a National Institutes of Health grant to plan and conduct a multisite, academic-community partnership study on child health disparities. He is also a co-principal investigator for the Los Angeles Best Babies Collaborative, a countywide collaborative funded by Proposition 10 to develop a plan for improving birth outcomes in Los Angeles. He is currently working with the California Maternal Child Health (MCH) Branch on developing a framework for quality monitoring and improvement of maternal health care in California. He is the associate director of the Maternal Child Health Bureau–funded leadership training program at the UCLA School of Public Health (through the Center for Healthier Children, Families, and Communities). He recently received the 2003 National MCH Epidemiology Young Professional Achievement Award, and the 2004 American Public Health Association MCH Section Young Professional Award.

Marie McCormick is the Sumner & Esther Feldberg Professor of Maternal & Child Health in the Department of Society, Human Development, and Health at the Harvard School of Public Health and a professor of pediatrics at the Harvard Medical School. In 1987, she joined the faculty of the Department of Pediatrics at Harvard Medical School in the Joint Program in Neonatology as the director of its Infant Follow-up Program and chief of the section of neonatal epidemiology and health policy. In 1991, she became professor and chair of the Department of Maternal and Child Health at the Harvard School of Public Health and a professor of pediatrics. Her research has focused on the effectiveness of perinatal and neonatal health services on the health of women and children, with a particular concern in the outcomes of very premature infants. Recent awards include election to the Johns Hopkins Society of Scholars (1995), the Ambulatory Pediatric Association Research Award (1996), and election to membership to the Institute of Medicine. She has served on several advisory and study panels at the Institute of Medicine, for which she has been recognized as a National Associate of the National Academies in recognition for exceptional pro bono service. She has just completed a 3-year term as the chair of the Institute's Committee on Immunization Safety, for which she was awarded the David Rall Medal at the annual meeting.

Laura E. Riley is the medical director of labor and delivery at Massachusetts General Hospital, with a focus on high-risk pregnancy and an emphasis on infectious disease complications of obstetrics. She has provided clinical service for more than 10 years, working initially at Boston City Hospital with indigent, high-risk pregnant women and with an emphasis on HIV disease in pregnancy. Dr. Riley has participated in multiple research initiatives, including the Women and Infants Transmission Study, which is a study of the natural history of HIV in pregnancy. Her current National Institutes of Health–sponsored research project investigates the causes of epidural-related fever in women randomized to receive an epidural for labor analgesia compared with that in women using a doula for labor support. Nationally, she continues to be interested in projects related to infectious disease complications of pregnancy, serving as a consultant to the Centers for Disease Control and Prevention on perinatal HIV testing and the recent guidelines on the prevention of group B streptococcus infection. She is in year 3 as the chair of the Obstetric Practice Committee at the American College of Obstetricians and Gynecologists, a committee that drafts guidelines for obstetric care.

Jeannette A. Rogowski is a university professor in the Department of Health Systems and Policy at the University of Medicine and Dentistry of New Jersey School of Public Health. She is the director of the Center for Health Economics and Health Policy. Dr. Rogowski is a research associate of the National Bureau of Economic Research. She is an internationally recognized authority in the economics of preterm birth. Dr. Rogowski has written extensively on the cost and quality of neonatal intensive care. Her research has examined the costs of care for high-risk infants and the economic implications of collaborative quality improvement efforts. Related research has focused on the measurement of the quality of neonatal intensive care and on studying the determinants of high-quality care.

Saroj Saigal is a neonatologist and professor of pediatrics at McMaster University in Hamilton, Ontario, Canada. She is also a senior career scientist of the Canadian Institutes of Health Research (CIHR). Dr. Saigal has been involved in outcome studies for the last 25 years. She and her collaborators have followed a population-based cohort of extremely low birth weight survivors (those with birth weights of <1,000 grams) from infancy to adulthood. The outcomes on a broad range of measures for this cohort in comparison with that of their normal birth weight peers have been reported in several waves at age 3, 5, and 8 years and adolescence. In the most recent investigative period (funded jointly by CIHR and the National Institute of Child Health and Human Development), the sociological (educational attainment, social and emotional functional limitations, and quality of life) and health (chronic illness, growth trajectories, physical activity, body composition, and economic burden of health care) outcomes were examined at young adulthood (age 24 years). Dr. Saigal is involved in several academic and policy meetings on issues related to prematurity. She was awarded the Distinguished Neonatologist Award (2005) by the Canadian Pediatric Society for her contributions to the field.

David Savitz is a professor in the Department of Community and Preventive Medicine of the Mount Siani School of Medicine, New York, N.Y. Dr. Savitz's primary research activities and interests are in reproductive, environmental, and cancer epidemiology. He is developing and applying epidemiological methods in reproductive studies of pregnancy outcomes, specifically the roles of social factors, infection, nutrition, tobacco, illicit drug use, and stress in birth weight and preterm birth. His other research addresses the causes of pregnancy loss, child development, and a range of environmental and occupational exposures. He has served as editor of the *American Journal of Epidemiology* and as a member of the Epidemiology and Disease Control—1 Study Section of the National Institutes of Health and is currently an editor for the journal *Epidemiology*. He was president of the Society for Epidemiologic Research, was North American Regional Councilor for the International Epidemiological Association, and is president of the Society for Pediatric and Perinatal Epidemiologic Research.

Hyagriv Simhan serves as medical director of the Center for Prematurity at the University of Pittsburgh. Dr. Simhan engages in both clinical and basic research exploring the role of infection and inflammation in early preterm birth. He is currently involved in single-center and multicenter international clinical cohort studies that explore the interactive contribution of genetics and the environment to the risk of preterm birth. He is also actively investigating anti-inflammatory and immunomodulatory agents among women with preterm premature rupture of membranes for reduction of neonatal morbidity. His laboratory focus is on the response of uterine decidual cells to infectious and inflammatory stimuli and the ability of anti-inflammatory cytokines and antimicrobials to attenuate that response.

Norman J. Waitzman is an associate professor in the Department of Economics at the University of Utah. He is a health economist with research concentrations in the areas of the societal burden of illness and the socioeconomic determinants of health. In the former area, he was the primary author of the most comprehensive study to date on the societal cost of birth defects. He has authored or coauthored several articles evaluating screening programs and other public health interventions, including the proposed U.S. Food and Drug Administration rule to supplement grains with folate in the late 1990s to prevent birth defects. Part of this research has also been devoted to the methodological problems encountered in estimates of the societal burden of illness and in the evaluation of interventions to reduce that burden. In his area of expertise on the socioeconomic determinants of health, Dr. Waitzman has written several articles on the effects of socioeconomic characteristics of areas, independent of individual sociodemographic characteristics, on individual health and mortality.

Xiaobin Wang is an attending pediatrician, the Mary Ann and J. Milburn Smith Research Professor, and director of the Mary Ann and J. Milburn Smith Child Health Research Program at the Children's Memorial Medical Center and Northwestern University Feinberg School of Medicine. In the past 10 years, Dr. Wang's research has focused on the molecular epidemiology of complex human diseases, in particular, adverse pregnancy outcomes. At present, Dr. Wang is the principal investigator of three National Institutes of Health–funded projects and one March of Dimes Birth Defect Foundation–funded molecular epidemiological project related to pregnancy outcomes. She leads a multidisciplinary research team that consists of a representative(s) from each of the areas of clinical medicine, epidemiology, molecular biology, population genetics, biostatistics/bioinformatics, and environmental health sciences. The current research focus of her team is investigation of the environmental and genetic factors and gene-environment interactions in determining the risk of adverse pregnancy outcomes and the integration of epidemiological, clinical, and laboratory methods to better understand the pathogenic pathways and biological mechanisms of adverse pregnancy outcomes. Dr. Wang has served as scientific grant reviewer for National Institutes of Health Study Sections and a scientific journal article reviewer for 18 scientific journals.

IOM STAFF BIOGRAPHIES

Andrew Pope is director of the Board on Health Sciences Policy in the Institute of Medicine (IOM). With a Ph.D. in physiology and biochemistry, his primary interests are in science policy, biomedical ethics, and the environmental and occupational influences on human health. During his tenure at the National Academies and since 1989 at the Institute of Medicine, Dr. Pope has directed numerous studies on topics that range from injury control, disability prevention, and biological markers to the protection of human subjects of research, National Institutes of Health priority-setting processes, organ procurement and transplantation policy, and the role of science and technology in countering terrorism. Dr. Pope is the recipient of the National Academy of Sciences' President's Special Achievement Award and the Institute of Medicine's Cecil Award.

Adrienne Stith Butler is a senior program officer in the Board on Health Sciences Policy of the Institute of Medicine (IOM). Previously, Dr. Stith

Butler served as study director for the IOM report, *Preparing for the Psychological Consequences of Terrorism: A Public Health Strategy*, conducted within the Board on Neuroscience and Behavioral Health. She has also served as a staff officer for IOM reports, *In the Nation's Compelling Interest: Ensuring Diversity in the Health-Care Workforce* and *Unequal Treatment: Confronting Racial and Ethnic Disparities in Health Care*, conducted within the Board on Health Sciences Policy. Prior to working at IOM, Dr. Butler served as the James Marshall Public Policy Scholar, a fellowship cosponsored by the Society for the Psychological Study of Social Issues and the American Psychological Association (APA). In this position, based at APA in Washington, D.C., she engaged in policy analysis and monitored legislative issues related to ethnic disparities in health care and health research, racial profiling, and mental health counseling provisions in the reauthorization of the Elementary and Secondary Education Act. Dr. Butler, a clinical psychologist, received a doctorate in 1997 from the University of Vermont. She completed postdoctoral fellowships in adolescent medicine and pediatric psychology at the University of Rochester Medical Center in Rochester, New York.

Eileen J. Santa is a research associate with the Board on Health Sciences Policy at the Institute of Medicine (IOM). Prior to working at IOM, Ms. Santa worked with the American Psychological Association's public policy office, analyzing policy, monitoring legislation, and advocating for increased access to language services for in hospital settings for patients whose dominant language is not English and increased services for women and ethnic minority veterans. Ms. Santa is also a doctoral candidate in clinical psychology at the University of Massachusetts, Boston, where she conducted research on the postpartum mental health of Latinas. She has also coauthored a chapter on clinical issues in working with immigrant Latinas.

Thelma L. Cox is a senior program assistant in the Board on Health Sciences Policy. During her years at the Institute of Medicine (IOM), she has also provided assistance to the Division of Health Care Services and the Division of Biobehavioral Sciences and Mental Disorders. Ms. Cox has worked on several IOM reports, including *In the Nation's Compelling Interest: Ensuring Diversity in the Health-Care Workforce; Unequal Treatment: Confronting Racial and Ethnic Disparities in Health Care;* and *Ethical Issues Relating to the Inclusion of Women in Clinical Studies*. She has received the National Research Council Recognition Award and two IOM Staff Achievement Awards.

Index

A

Academic/school problems, 350, 357, 363-366, 374
Access to care, 9, 19, 34, 138, 673, 676-678
Acidosis, 200, 330, 331
Actin, 175, 182, 291
Adenyl cyclase, 291
Adenylate cyclase, 173
Administration for Children and Families, 447
Adolescents, 44, 120, 125-126, 265, 349, 364, 377, 381, 382, 448, 449, 463, 628-629, 678, 679, 681-682
Adrenocorticotropic hormone (ACTH), 172, 173, 179, 188
Advisory Committee on Infant Mortality, 452, 464
African Americans
  alcohol use, 27
  birth certificate data, 81
  birth weights, 25, 77, 105, 112, 113, 114, 121, 130, 138, 139, 140, 154, 209
  BMI (maternal), 151, 152
  depression, 109
  douching practices, 100
  drug abuse, 27
  educational attainment, 114, 130
  environmental toxicant exposure, 251
  estimates of gestational age in, 67-68
  fetal maturation rate, 78
  foreign-born vs. U.S.-born, 26, 129
  growth outcomes, 382
  income and net worth, 146
  infant mortality rates, 50-51, 77, 112, 130, 315-316, 630
  infections, 27, 100, 132
  infertility, 158
  interpregnancy interval, 153, 154
  low-income, 106-107, 112, 113, 120-121, 125
  marital status–related risks, 125, 127, 128
  maternal age–related risks, 126, 128
  neighborhood environment, 137, 138-139, 140, 142, 143
  personal resources, 119
  PPROM, 211-212
  prenatal care, 64, 131
  prepregnancy health, 125
  rates of preterm birth, 5, 12, 26, 48-49, 76, 112, 130, 133, 222, 250, 315, 614, 616, 620-621, 678, 679
  risk of preterm birth, 106-107, 109, 120-121, 126, 149, 151, 152, 209, 233, 265, 271, 628-629
  stressors, 105, 106-107, 109, 112, 113, 114, 132, 142
  survival advantage of preterm infants, 77, 315, 630

tobacco use, 27, 92, 131
unintended pregnancy, 120-121
Age. *See also* Maternal age
    perinatal terminology, 61
Agency for Healthcare Research and
    Quality, 17, 158, 447
Agent Orange, 243, 250
Agricultural chemicals, 231, 237-241, 251,
    252
Air pollution exposures
    carbon monoxide, 234, 236
    exposure assessment, 232-233
    gestation stage and, 235-236
    location of residence and, 138, 232, 235,
        250
    nitrous oxides, 234-235, 236
    ozone, 234, 235, 236-237
    particulates, 22-23, 231, 234, 235-236,
        237, 252
    PCBs, 242
    sulfur dioxide, 22-23, 231, 233-234,
        235-236, 237, 252
Alabama, 450, 651, 693
Alan Guttmacher Institute, 690
Albuterol, 291
Alcohol use, 27, 92, 120, 131, 134, 142,
    371
Aldrin, 239
Alkaline phosphatase, 270, 272
α-Amino-3-hydroxy-5-methyl-4-isoxazole
    propionate (AMPA), 199
α-Fetoprotein, 270, 272
Altitude, and birth weight, 70
Aluminum sulfate, 249
American Academy of Pediatrics, 35, 57,
    320-321, 647, 649, 655, 660, 663,
    666, 667-668
American Association of Gynecology and
    Obstetrics Foundation, 437
American Board of Obstetric and
    Gynecology, 437
American Board of Pediatrics, 439
American College of Obstetricians and
    Gynecologists, 18, 33, 64, 258, 278,
    292, 448
    ethics handbook, 653, 655
    sample antepartum record, 302-307
    workforce data, 441
American Indians/Alaska Natives
    birth weights, 77
    educational attainment, 130

marital status, 128
    maternal age, 128
    preterm birth rates, 5, 49, 128
American Medical Association, 653
American Society for Reproductive
    Medicine (ASRM), 17, 18, 33, 165-
    166, 168, 258
Amniocentesis, 66
Amnionitis, 70, 184, 185-186, 191, 195,
    200, 220
Ampicillin, 295, 296
Amplitude-integrated EEG, 68, 69
Anemia, 94-95, 163, 266, 327-328
Anencephaly, 671-672
Aneuploidy, 163, 269
Angelman syndrome, 164
Angiotensin II, 179
Animal models
    intrauterine infections, 22, 181, 184,
        185, 186, 195-196, 199-200
    neonatal sequelae, 196-200, 202, 203,
        206
    parturition pathways, 22, 181, 184, 185,
        186, 187, 192-196, 199-200, 251,
        254
    prenatal stress, 102, 180
    PWMD, 196-197, 199-200
    relevance to humans, 192, 193
    species comparison of reproductive
        characteristics, 194-195
Antenatal counseling, 646
Antenatal maternal treatments, 12, 77, 74,
    287, 289, 291, 295-300, 318, 651
Antibiotics. *See also individual antibiotics*
    efficacy for prevention of preterm birth,
        22, 132, 151, 186, 274, 275, 276-
        280, 296, 727
    gestational age and, 278
    maternal infection, 132, 151, 186, 196,
        276-280
    neonatal side effects, 319, 322
    for PPROM, 278, 296, 727
    preconceptional use, 278-279
    for preterm labor, 273, 295-296
Anticonvulsant drugs, 199
Anxiety, 24, 103, 104, 107-108, 111-112,
    180, 371
Apnea, 318, 321
Apoptosis, 175, 188, 191, 199, 200, 325
Appendicitis, 279
Arab Americans, 158

Arachidonic acid, 174, 191, 205, 251, 293
Arginine, 294
Arizona, 679
Aroclor 1254, 251
Arsenic, 248-249, 252
Artificial insemination, 16, 45, 157
Asians/Pacific Islanders
    birth weights, 140
    educational attainment, 130
    marital status, 128
    maternal age, 128
    neighborhood environment, 140
    preterm birth rates, 5, 26, 48, 49-50, 76,
        128, 133, 222
Asphyxia, 328, 664
Assisted reproductive technologies (ART).
    See also specific procedures
    accreditation of embryo laboratories,
        165
    ASRM practice guidelines, 17, 165-166,
        168, 258
    birth defects, 163-164
    definition, 16, 155
    delivery method, 163
    estimated date of confinement, 61
    ethical issues, 656-658
    fetal reduction, 166, 657
    incidence of pregnancies, 155-157, 167-
        168
    infant mortality rates, 17, 162, 657
    international comparisons, 166-167
    live birth trends, 46-47, 157, 164, 165
    low birth weights, 46, 162, 657, 679
    maternal age and, 16, 45, 46-47, 159,
        166, 167
    maternal and child health risks, 162-164
    multiple gestations, 16-17, 45-47, 135,
        154, 157, 159-160, 161, 163-165,
        258, 266, 424, 606, 631
    number of embryos transferred, 159,
        165-168, 258, 656-658
    oversight/regulation, 164-165, 258
    parturition pathways, 177
    preterm birth trends and risks, 16, 17,
        37, 45-47, 161, 265, 266-267, 631,
        657, 678, 679
    procedures, 155-157
    reporting of outcomes, 16, 18, 45, 155,
        157
    singletons, 17, 46, 159, 162-163, 168,
        266-267, 657

success rate, 166
    utilization rate, 156, 157, 159
Association of American Medical Colleges,
    438, 442
Association of Pediatric Department Chairs,
    437
Asthma, 14, 32, 149
Atherosclerosis, 152
Atosiban, 293, 294, 295
Atrazine, 240
Attention deficit hyperactivity disorder, 14,
    32, 348, 370, 371, 374, 463
Australia, 42, 43, 209, 369, 646, 661, 674,
    677, 692, 693
Autism, 371, 422
Autoimmune diseases, 82
Avon Premature Infant Project, 394-395

B

Baby Doe regulations, 659, 665-666
Bacterial vaginosis (BV), 27, 100, 102, 110,
    132, 135, 151, 185, 186, 217, 269,
    270, 271, 272, 274, 276, 277, 278,
    279, 727, 729
Bacteriuria, asymptomatic, 110, 132, 133,
    184, 276
Bacteroides, 269
Ballard Score, 67, 68, 71, 78, 612, 613
Bangladesh, 248-249
Bayley Scale of Infant Development, 357,
    392
Bax protein, 191
Bcl2 protein, 191
BEAM Trial, 300
Bechwith-Wiedermann syndrome, 164
Behavioral influences. *See also* Nutrition,
    maternal; Physical activity; Tobacco
    use
    alcohol use, 27, 92, 120, 131, 134, 142
    clustering of, 90-91
    cultural context, 142
    douching, 99-100, 121, 131
    employment-related, 26, 36, 97-99, 110,
        121, 133, 134-135, 149, 265
    illicit drug use, 24, 26, 27, 36, 63, 89,
        92-93, 121, 130-131, 133, 134, 180,
        626
    infections, 94
    interventions, 471-472
    methodological issues, 23-24, 90-91, 93

racial/ethnic disparities and, 26, 27, 36, 92, 100, 129-131, 133
sexual activity, 99
socioeconomic disparities, 90, 93, 133, 134-135
stress and, 180-181
Behavioral and socio-emotional outcomes, 14, 32, 47, 349, 350, 370-372, 375, 376-377, 381, 394, 396
Belgium, 167, 168, 470, 668, 669
Berendes, H., 605
β-adrenergic receptor agonists, 290-291, 295
β_2-adrenergic receptor, 212, 215
β-hexachlorocyclohexane, 239
Beta-mimetic drugs, 291-292, 293, 294
Betamethasone, 297, 298, 299, 334
Biological mechanisms. *See also* Parturition process; Preterm premature rupture of membranes
in environmental toxicant exposures, 251-252
prenatal stress, 101, 110, 143-144, 179-180, 626
proteomic modifications, 219-221
RDS, 66, 202
Biophysical profile, 66
Biotin, 219
Birth certificates, 9, 60, 78, 79, 80, 81, 209
Birth defects, 150-151, 162, 163-164, 263, 315, 415, 422
Birth weight. *See also* Low birth weight; Very low birth weight
categories, 57-59
and costs of medical care, 705, 706-707
depression and, 109
gender differences, 63, 70, 77
geographic differences, 70
and gestational age, 8-9, 10, 59, 79, 242
and infant mortality, 21, 446
infections and, 186, 278
interpregnancy interval and, 152, 153-154
and length of hospital stay, 407, 408, 710
methodological issues, 56-59, 62, 347, 386
misclassification, 79
neighborhood conditions and, 137-142
neurodevelopmental disabilities by, 356, 357, 358-363, 364, 365, 366, 367, 368, 420-421

nutrition and, 95, 96, 134
personal resources and, 119
population differences, 25, 63, 70
prenatal stress and, 104, 180
program eligibility based on, 461
as proxy for maturity, 4, 5, 8, 25, 31, 34, 36, 56-59, 62, 347, 386, 606
racial/ethnic disparities, 25, 63, 70, 76, 77, 105, 112, 113, 114, 121, 130, 138-139, 140, 154, 209
reporting, 9
smoking and, 90, 217, 283
social support and, 116, 143
socioeconomic disparities, 139-140
unintended pregnancy and, 120, 121
violence and, 110, 138
Blacks. *See* African Americans
Blood pressure, 102. *See also* Hypertension, maternal
Body mass index, 80, 94, 95, 134, 151, 152
Born-Alive Infant Protection Act of 2001, 659-660
Botulinum Toxicum injections, 353
Bradycardia, 321, 327
Brazillian cohort, 239
Breast cancer, 163, 338
Breastfeeding, 338, 343
Bromodichloromethane, 244
Bronchodilators, 319
Bronchopulmonary dysplasia (BPD), 202, 297, 298, 317, 318, 319-321, 324, 327, 331, 336, 343, 378-379, 390, 707
Budin, Pierre, 57
Building Interdisciplinary Careers in Women's Health Program, 437
Burroughs Wellcome Fund, 33, 438, 446, 731

C

C-CPEP Trial, 274
C-reactive protein, 270
Cadmium, 248
Caffeine, 321
Calcium
channel blockers, 291, 292-293
mobilization, 171, 174, 175, 182, 251, 293
supplementation, 95
Calgranulins, 220

California, 234, 236, 403, 406, 407, 408, 417, 428, 646, 691, 692, 693, 697, 705
Calmodulin, 171, 175, 182
Canada, 26, 42, 43, 133, 233, 234, 240, 365-366, 384, 385, 647-648, 661, 690
Cancer, 163, 243, 338
Candida, 325
CAP gene, 173, 181
Carbon monoxide, 234, 236
CARDIA study, 113
Cardiometabolic disease, 388-389
Cardiovascular development, 326
Cardiovascular disease
    adulthood risk, 386, 388, 389
    maternal, 149, 150, 152
Cardiovascular function, 101, 114, 321
Career development in clinical research. *See also* Training clinical researchers
    board certification, 439
    faculty vitality, 442-443, 453
    liability concerns and, 438-439, 440, 441
    mentors, 436, 439, 453
    need for change, 7-8, 439-440
    ob/gyn physician researchers, 7, 32, 438, 440-446
    women, 439-442
Caspase, 191
Catalase, 199
Catecholamines, 110, 179, 205
Cefetamet-pivoxil, 276
Centers for Disease Control and Prevention (CDC), 16, 33, 35, 165, 258, 415, 425, 657, 690
    funding for preterm research, 17, 446, 447, 729-730
    perinatal data collection, 10, 45, 79, 84
Centers for Medicare and Medicaid Services, 447
Central nervous system complications. *See also* Cerebral palsy; Cognitive impairment; Neurodevelopmental disabilities; Neurodevelopmental support; Periventricular white matter disease
    delivery method and, 332
    diagnosis, 333, 379
    germinal matrix injury, 333, 334
    IPH, 333, 334, 379
    IVH, 295, 296, 297, 298, 300, 326, 331, 33-334, 336, 366, 379, 385

    neuroimaging, 379
    neuroprotective medications, 336
    treatment, 333-334, 336
Cerebral atrophy, 334, 335, 336, 379
Cerebral palsy (CP), 14, 32, 196, 199-200, 300, 320, 325, 335-336, 348, 350-353, 371, 372, 374, 378, 399, 403, 415-421, 424, 425, 675, 707
Cervical
    cerclage, 273, 274, 275, 281-282
    examination, 12, 268-269
    inflammation, 272
    injury or abnormality, 189, 266
    length, 189, 268, 270, 271, 272, 275, 281-282, 283, 286
    ripening, 170, 172, 174-175, 181
    scores, 268
Cesarean delivery, 43-44, 163, 181, 234, 332, 622, 623, 651-652, 653
Charge to committee, 3-4, 33, 52
Child abuse and neglect, 143, 463, 659
Child Abuse Protection and Treatments Act, 659, 665-666
Child Health and Developmental Studies of the San Francisco Bay Area, 238
Children's Hospital of Wisconsin, 670
China, 42, 50, 233, 234, 237, 248
Chlamydia trachomatis, 135, 270
Chlorination disinfection by-products, 244-245
3-Chloro-4-(dichloromethyl)-5-hydroxy-2(*5H*)-furanone, 244
Chloroform, 244, 245
Chorioamnionitis, 82, 184, 185-186, 200, 205, 296, 335
Choriocarcinoma, 219
Chromosomal disorders, 69, 80, 162
Chronic lung disease (CLD). *See* Bronchopulmonary dysplasia
Chronological age, 61
Citrulline, 294
Classifications of preterm birth, 607-608
Clindamycin, 276, 277, 278
Clinical research on preterm birth. *See also* Career development in clinical research; Funding for clinical research and training; Training clinical researchers
    adolescent subjects, 448, 449, 681-682
    barriers to, 7, 32, 34, 435-436, 438-439
    ethical issues, 447-451, 679-682

federal activities, 446-447
informed consent, 448, 449, 680-681
institutional review boards, 448, 449
leadership challenges and needs, 8, 452-454
liability issues, 450-452
minimal risk vs no added risk, 448, 450-451, 680
multidisciplinary approach, 32, 452-453, 473-474
ob/gyn physician researcher workforce, 7, 32, 438-439, 440-446, 453-454
protections for subjects of, 448-451, 680-681
reimbursement for clinical services, 451-452, 453
Clinical Risk Index for Babies, 67
Co-amoxicillin-clavulanic acid treatment, 295, 296
Cocaine use, 24, 93-94, 134, 180, 191, 471, 631. See also Drug abuse
Cochrane database, 292, 342
Cognitive impairment
academic problems, 350, 357, 363-366, 374
attention deficits, 14, 32, 348, 363, 370
auditory processing and discrimination, 369
Bayley Scale of Infant Development, 357
birth weight and, 356, 357, 358-363, 364, 365
cystic PVL and, 335
development quotient, 355, 357
doxapram and, 321
economic costs of, 399, 403, 415-421, 424, 425
executive function disorder, 370
fetal brain sparing and, 71
gestational age at birth and, 356, 357, 358-363, 365, 372, 374
infections and, 325, 378
IQ scores, 71, 349, 354-363, 370, 371, 394, 425
language disorders, 14, 32, 328, 348, 363, 369-370, 374, 394
learning disabilities, 14, 32, 348, 363, 364-365, 369, 371, 374
memory, 363, 365, 369, 370
mental retardation, 14, 32, 47, 348, 353, 355-356, 374, 376, 399, 403, 415-421, 424, 425

spatial skills, 363, 394
and special education, 11, 47, 363, 364, 423-424, 717-719
steroid therapy and, 320
visual processing and perceptual deficits, 362-363, 365, 368-369, 394
Cohabitation, 127, 129
Collaborative Perinatal Project, 349
Colombia statistics and studies, 240, 343
Colony stimulating factors, 213
Colorado, 70
Community factors. See also Neighborhood conditions
ethical issues, 654
methodological issues, 136, 144-146
modeling, 136, 139-140, 144-146
quality index, 145
racial/ethnic disparities, 136, 137, 138-139, 140
research needs, 141
social class disparities, 136, 139-141, 142, 233
stressful, 137, 142, 143-144
Complications. See Neonatal complications of preterm birth
Computerized tomography, 333
Conduct disorders, 371
Conferences on preterm birth, 605
Congenital anomalies, 63, 64, 69, 163, 327, 328, 661, 663, 664, 669, 671-672
Congestive heart failure, 152
Connective tissue disorders, 189
Connexins
CX-26, 181
CX-43, 171, 172, 174, 181
Contraction-associated proteins (CAPs), 171, 173, 174
Contractions. See Preterm labor; Uterine
Coronary artery disease, 386
Corrected age, 61
Corticotropin-releasing hormone (CRH), 102, 110, 170, 172-173, 174, 176, 179, 180, 187, 215, 269, 270
Cortisol, 102, 110, 172, 174, 179, 185, 192, 194, 297, 340
Costs of preterm birth. See Medical care costs of preterm birth; Societal costs of preterm birth
Croatia, 233
CRYO Trial, 384
Cuban statistics and studies, 42, 49

Cultural factors. *See also* Racial/ethnic
    disparities
  neighborhood characteristics, 142
  in risk behaviors, 142
  and stress, 26, 36, 111-112, 142
Cyclic adenosine monophosphate (cAMP),
    171, 173, 174, 291
Cyclic guanosine monophosphate, 171, 294
Cyclooxygenase inhibitors, 293
Cyclooxygenase-2 (COX-2), 174, 187
Cystine, 199
Cytochrome P450, 216, 243
Cytokines, proinflammatory, 102, 132, 173,
    174, 177, 179, 180, 184, 186, 187,
    195, 205, 222, 252, 335
Cytomegalovirus, 82, 325, 329
Czech Republic statistics and studies, 233,
    234, 235

D

Data collection
  cause of death, 82
  gene-environment interactions, 227
  fetal deaths, 81, 82
  perinatal, 9-10, 45, 79, 84
  recommendations, 6, 8-10, 73, 84-85,
    480-482
  vital records, 9, 43, 60, 78, 79-81, 209
Data reporting
  ART-related outcomes, 16, 18, 45, 155,
    157
  artifacts of, 78, 635-636
  birth weight, 9
  infant outcomes, 15-16, 18, 45, 73-74,
    155, 157
  international differences, 43, 636-637
  LMP, 80
  quality of vital records, 79-81
  resuscitation at delivery, 73
  standards, 79
  vital statistics, 9-10, 60, 78, 79-83
DDT, 231, 237-239, 241, 251, 252
Decidual
  hemorrhage, 17, 182-183, 269
  membrane activation, 170, 172, 174,
    175
Defensins, 220, 269, 272
Definitions of preterm birth, 4, 8, 31, 36,
    56, 57-59, 72, 224, 230, 606-609

Delayed childbearing, 154. *See also*
    Maternal age
Delinquency, 371, 394
Delivery method, 43-44. *See also* Cesarean
    delivery
Denmark, statistics and studies, 42, 96, 103,
    104, 112, 155, 371, 385
Depression
  maternal, 14, 103, 104, 107, 109, 111-
    112, 120, 380, 390
  premature children, 371
Developmental disabilities. *See*
    Neurodevelopmental disabilities
Dexamethasone, 297, 298, 299, 320
DHEA-S, 172, 173-174, 179
Diabetes mellitus
  fetal origins hypothesis, 387, 388
  maternal, 44, 71, 80, 82, 148, 149, 150,
    163, 263, 617, 622, 630-631
Diagnosis
  CNS complications, 333, 379
  preterm labor, 12, 220, 268, 273, 284-
    287, 289-290; *see also* Prediction/
    predictors of preterm birth
Dichloroacetic acid, 244
Dichlorobromomethane, 244
Dieldrin, 239, 241
Diet. *See* Nutrition, maternal
Dioxin, 243-244, 250
Dipalmitoylphosphatidylcholine, 202
District of Columbia, 168
Diuretics, 219, 333-334
DNA methylation, 164, 218
Domestic/personal violence, 110, 120, 135,
    143
Douching, 99-100, 121, 131
Doxapram, 321
Drug abuse, 24, 26, 27, 36, 63, 89, 92-93,
    121, 130-131, 133, 134, 180, 371,
    471-472, 626
Dubowitz score, 67, 68, 71, 78, 612, 613
Due date, 60-61
Dysmorphic syndrome, 69

E

Ear infections, 14, 370
Early intervention programs, 11, 15, 82,
    202, 353, 380, 393-396, 399, 400,
    402, 422-423, 469-470, 718-719

Early and Periodic Screening Diagnosis and Treatment (EPSDT) program, 459
Earned Income Tax Credits, 471
Earthquakes, 106, 111
Eclampsia, 655
Economic costs. *See* Medical care costs of preterm birth; Societal costs of preterm birth
Education
  costs of preterm birth, 11, 47, 400, 423-424, 460, 706, 717-719
  early intervention services, 393-395, 458, 460, 469, 472
Education for All Handicapped Children Act, 373
Educational attainment, 114, 130, 390, 622, 628-629
Ehlers-Danlos syndrome, 209
Electroencephalography (EEG), 68
Electroretinography, 68
Embryonic chorionic gonadotropin, 187
Emergency Medical Treatment and Labor Act, 672
Emotional and affective states. *See also* Anxiety; Depression; Prenatal stress, maternal
  intrusive thought, 112
  linkages to preterm birth, 24, 102, 103, 104, 107-109, 110, 111
Employment
  occupational exposures to toxins, 231, 237, 240-241, 242, 246, 248, 249-250
  physical demands of, 26, 36, 97-99, 110, 121, 133, 134-135, 136, 149, 265, 471
  stress related to, 47, 97, 109-110, 135, 391
Endocrine pathways, 144, 179, 215
Endometrial cancer, 163
Endorphins, 340
Endotoxin, 200
Enterovirus, 82
Environmental Genome Project, 211
Environmental Protection Agency, 33
Environmental toxicants. *See also* Air pollution exposures
  agricultural chemicals, 231, 237-241, 251, 252
  animal studies, 251
  biological mechanisms, 251-252

chlorination disinfection by-products, 244-245
co-exposures, 231
cumulative exposures, 231-232
dioxin, 243-244, 250
environmental tobacco smoke, 22, 231, 245-247, 252, 321
exposure assessment, 231-232, 237, 244, 253
gene interactions, 226
and gestational age at birth, 237
maternal age and, 246
metals and metalloids, 22, 230, 231, 232, 247-249, 252
occupational exposures, 231, 237, 240-241, 242, 246, 248, 249-250
paternal exposures, 240, 243, 249-250
PCBs, 241-243, 251
phthalates, 252, 253
racial/ethnic disparities, 138, 233, 235, 240, 250-251
research needs, 253-254
residence as exposure proxy, 231, 232, 233, 235, 236, 250
socioeconomic disparities, 232-233, 240, 250
Epigenetics, 218-219
Epilepsy, 353
Erythromycin, 151, 275, 276, 277, 278, 296
Escherichia coli, 200
Estonia, 668
Estrogen receptor-alpha, 238
Estrogens, 172, 173-174, 175, 179, 187, 215
Ethical issues
  access to perinatal care, 673, 676-678
  adolescents, 448, 449, 678, 681-682
  Baby Doe regulations, 659, 665-666
  brain death in pregnant women with periviable fetuses, 654-655
  in decision making, 287, 645-652, 655
  delivery room resuscitation, 658-659, 674-675
  distributive justice of care, 678-679
  end-of-life and LSMT practices, 645-652, 658-672
  financial costs, 673-675
  infertility treatments, 656-658
  informed consent, 448, 449, 649-652, 653, 655, 656, 658, 659, 663, 668, 681

intrauterine interventions, 448, 655-656
legal precedents, 649-651, 658-659
maternal-fetal conflicts, 287, 652-658
maternal illness, 655
paternal rights, 448, 680-681
personhood, 653, 659-660
professional guidelines, 655-656, 662, 667-668
racism or ethnic prejudice, 678
in research, 447-448, 679-682
social and community context, 654
societal costs of preterm birth, 673-679
termination of pregnancy, 448, 681
viability threshold, 314, 448, 450-451, 647, 658-662, 681
Etiologies of preterm birth. *See also* Behavioral influences; Community factors; Gene-environment interactions; Genetic susceptibility; Medical and pregnancy conditions; Psychosocial factors
animal models, 22
biological pathways, 21, 22, 37, 89, 143-144
environmental pollutants and, 22-23, 37
life course perspective, 37
modeling complex interactions, 25-26, 37, 141-142, 143, 144-147, 256-257, 272, 273
racial/ethnic disparities, 37, 77
research recommendations, 6, 21-23, 122-123, 255-256, 488-489
EURONIC project, 661, 668-669
European Society of Human Reproduction and Embryology, 166
Expression proteomics, 220
Extracorporeal membrane oxygenation, 198
Extremely low birth weight, 59, 314, 448, 450-451, 647, 648, 650, 651, 658-662
Eye. *See* Ophthalmic impairment; Visual processing and perceptual deficits

F

Factor V, 82, 212
Family
costs of preterm birth, 3, 47, 371, 391, 402, 426-427, 459, 675, 676, 706, 712
early intervention services, 393-395, 458, 460, 469

history of preterm birth, 12, 22, 152, 209
impacts of premature infants on, 14, 47, 389-393
parental leave policies, 638
participation in medical decision making, 72, 287, 645-652, 655, 659, 660, 664, 665, 666, 667, 668
public policies affecting, 471
Faroe Islands, 96
Fas-caspase apoptosis pathway, 191
Fatty acids, long-chain, 24, 94, 96-97
Feeding intolerance, 322, 337
Fenoterol, 291
Fentanyl, 340
Ferritin, 270
Fertility Clinic Success Rate and Certification Act of 1992, 165
Fetal
adrenal androgen, 172, 185
brain sparing, 69, 71
congenital abnormalities, 64, 163, 327, 328
cortisol, 172, 185
death, 73, 74, 79, 81, 82, 152, 162, 186, 209, 279
developmental milestones, 317-318, 322, 326, 327, 328, 331-332
effects of tocolytics, 293
fibronectin, 267, 270, 271, 272, 275, 277, 285, 286
glucocorticoid effects, 297
growth, 58, 59, 95, 96, 109, 263, 298; *see also* Intrauterine growth restriction
HPA axis, 171-172, 179, 185, 188, 269
immune interactions with maternal system, 150, 324
intrauterine interventions, 448, 655-656
lung development, 66, 70-71, 201-202, 317-318
membrane activation, 175
movement, 332
neurological development, 298, 331-332, 338-339
origins of adult disease, 386-389
red cell alloimmunization, 150
stress, 287
twin-to-twin transfusion sequence, 150
Fetomaternal hemorrhage, 82, 327

Fibronectins, 175, 267, 270, 271, 272, 275, 277, 285, 286
Filipino women, 49-50
Finland, 26, 42, 129, 133, 693, 697
First And Second Trimester Evaluation of Risk trial, 162
Fish and fish oil, 96-97, 242
Flame retardants, 252
Florida, 450, 465, 697
Fluconazole, 325
Fluorescent polarization, 66
Folate, 24, 95, 219
Food and Drug Administration, 291, 447, 682
Foster care, 28
France, 42, 470, 605, 648, 668
Free radicals, 198-199, 204, 205, 333, 335
Functional Genomics and Proteomic Markers of Preterm Delivery and Their Variation by Race project, 729
Functional maturity, 68-69
Functional proteomics, 220
Funding for clinical research and training
  Burroughs Wellcome Fund, 438, 446, 731
  CDC, 17, 446, 447, 729-730
  clinical revenues and, 451-452, 453
  March of Dimes, 20, 33, 446, 730
  NICHD, 437, 447, 725, 726, 727
  NIH, 227, 436, 437, 438, 446, 447, 452, 453-454, 725-729
  by professional associations, 437
  recommendations, 8, 32, 255
  by subject area, 725-731
Fungal infections, 325

G

G proteins, 173, 182
Gamete intrafallopial transfer (GIFT), 155, 156, 162. *See also* Assisted reproductive technologies
Gamma-interferon (IFN-γ), 132, 213, 214, 222
Gap junctions, 171, 173, 174, 175, 177, 181, 293
Gardnerella vaginalis, 269
Gastroesophageal reflux, 321, 323-324
Gelatinase B, 175
Gender differences
  behavioral outcomes, 371
  birth weight, 63, 70, 77

growth outcomes, 382
infant mortality rate, 77
pulmonary morbidity, 77
Gene-environment interactions
  epigenetic approaches, 218-219
  goals of studies, 211, 216-217
  infection/inflammation, 187, 211, 213-214, 217
  methodological issues, 223-228
  and parturition, 177, 187
  racial/ethnic disparities and, 132-133, 223
  smoking, 217
  toxic agents, 226
General Health Questionnaire, 107
Genetic susceptibility
  analytical challenges, 224-228
  candidate genes, 210, 212-216, 225
  data management and integration, 227
  disease-associated, 222-223
  evidence of, 22, 209-216
  family history of preterm birth, 12, 22, 152, 209
  gene-gene interactions, 224
  genetic association studies, 209-211, 226
  haplotype analysis, 224
  inflammation pathway, 212, 213-214
  international comparisons, 209
  maternal history of preterm labor/birth, 107, 149, 209
  maternal vs. fetal genes, 226
  microarray analysis, 216, 219
  phenotype definition, 224
  population admixture, 223, 225-226
  positional cloning, 210
  PPROM, 211-212, 223
  and racial/ethnic disparities, 26, 27, 130, 132, 152, 209, 211-212, 221-223
  reporting and replication of results, 228
  sample size and power, 227
  single-gene candidates, 209, 211-212
  twin studies, 209
  uteroplacental pathway, 214-215
  whole-genome scanning, 210
Genital tract infections. *See* Infection and inflammation, maternal
Geographic differences. *See also* International comparisons; *individual states and countries*
  comparisons, 636-638
  infant mortality rate, 627, 631, 634, 638
  malpractice insurance, 450

in preterm birth, 40-41, 617, 618
racial/ethnic disparities, 638-639
Geographic information systems, 144
Geonomic and Proteomic Network for
 Premature Birth Research, 221
Georgia, 41, 316-317, 677
Germany, 42
Gestational age
 fetal growth curves by, 58, 59, 63, 69-70
 measurement, 9, 10, 38, 43, 59-65, 67-
  68, 70, 72, 78, 80, 83, 337, 609-614;
  see also Measurement of maturity
 and stress effects, 104
Gestational age at birth. *See also* Large for
 gestational age; Small for gestational
 age
 antibiotic therapy and, 278
 ART and, 61
 and birth defect–related preterm birth,
  150
 and birth weight, 8-9, 10, 59, 79, 242
 categories, 58-59, 75, 79, 608
 and cesarean delivery, 43-44
 and cognitive impairment, 356, 357,
  358-363, 365, 372, 374
 and complications of preterm birth, 3,
  13-14, 76, 201-202, 314, 349
 data collection, 9-10, 79
 defining preterm birth, 4, 8, 31, 36, 56,
  57-59, 72, 606-609
 environmental exposures, 237
 interpregnancy interval, 153
 and intrauterine infections, 184
 and length of hospital stay, 407, 408
 and lung development, 76, 201-202,
  318, 319, 336
 and management of care, 74, 76
 maternal hypertension and, 617, 622
 and medical costs, 401, 410-414, 428,
  673, 674, 689, 694-695, 698-700,
  704-705, 706-707, 711
 misclassification, 79, 80
 and mortality, 3, 13, 31, 40, 72-74, 79,
  287, 288, 314-315, 406, 412, 627,
  630, 632-635
 multiple gestations and, 75, 161-162, 622
 and neurodevelopmental disabilities, 14,
  349, 350-351, 352, 353, 366, 367,
  372, 416, 419
 and ophthalmic impairment, 366
 and outcomes, 347-348

as proxy for prematurity, 56-57, 59-65,
 337, 609-614
serum eicosapentanoic acid levels and,
 96
tobacco use and, 622
trends, 2-3, 31, 38-39, 614, 615, 616,
 619, 623
and survival, 32, 74, 288, 289, 290
use of data, 79, 609-610
viability threshold, 65, 314, 448, 450-
 451, 647, 658-662, 681
Glaucoma, 331, 368
Glucocorticoids, 172, 179-180, 203, 287,
 297
Glucose metabolism, 99, 386, 387
Glutamate, 199, 212, 335
Glutamic acid, 212
Glutathione, 199
Glutathione peroxidase, 199
Glycoprotein, 271
Granulocyte colony stimulating factor (G-
 CSF), 270, 272
Greece, 153
Growth
 fetal, 58, 59, 95, 96, 109, 263, 298; *see
  also* Intrauterine growth restriction
 premature infants, 3, 32, 320, 321, 381-
  382
Gsα regulatory proteins, 173
Guatemala, 42

H

Haloacetic acids, 244
Hammersmith hospital, 663
Haplotypes, 210
Harris, Lisa, 654
Hawaiian women, 49-50
Health insurance
 ART coverage, 158, 165, 167
 burden on private payers, 705-706
 interconception care, 466
 managed care reimbursement policies,
  467
 Medicaid and Medicare, 19, 20, 28, 404,
  406, 417, 456-460, 462-463, 464-
  465, 466
 reimbursement for clinical services in
  research, 451-452
 SCHIP, 19, 457, 458, 465
 and utilization of services, 638

Health Resources and Services
    Administration, 33, 447
Health Status Classification System for
    Preschool Children 383-384
Healthcare Cost and Utilization Project, 417
Hearing impairment, 14, 47, 328-329, 348,
    367, 369-370, 371, 372, 376, 399,
    403, 415-421, 424, 425
Hearing screening for newborns, 328-329,
    370
HEDIS (Health Plan Employer Data and
    Information Set), 18-19, 467
HELLP syndrome, 655
Heparin-binding epidermal growth factor,
    187
Heptachlor, 239, 241
Heterogeneity of preterm population, 55,
    68-76
    fetal maturation, 70-71
    IUGR, 69-71
    late-term or near-term infants, 75-76
    perinatal mortality at limit of viability,
       72-74
    small for gestational age, 69-70
Hexachlorobenzene, 239, 241
Hexoprenaline, 291
High blood pressure, 163, 330. *See also*
    Hypertension, maternal
High-risk pregnancy, 97, 108, 117
Hispanics/Latinos
    birth certificate data, 81
    birth weights, 77, 679
    BMI (maternal), 151
    educational attainment, 130
    environmental exposures, 240
    infant mortality rate, 51
    infertility, 158
    inter- and intra-group variations, 129
    interpregnancy interval, 153
    marital status, 128
    maternal age, 128
    neighborhood conditions, 140, 143
    prenatal care, 64
    rates of preterm birth, 5, 26, 49, 76,
       105, 128, 129, 315, 679
    risk of preterm birth, 151
    social supports, 143
    stress, 105, 108, 112
Histone deacetylases, 218
History of preterm labor or birth, 12, 22,
    107, 149, 152, 209, 226, 265, 266,
    271, 272, 274, 276, 277, 278-279

Homelessness, 105, 106
Hopkins Symptom Checklist, 107
Human Genome Epidemiology workshop,
    228
Human immunodeficiency virus, 325
Human Proteomics Organization, 221
Hungary, 668
Hurricane Katrina, 111
Hydatiform moles, 219
Hydrocephalus, 334, 353, 379
Hydrocortisone, 320, 327, 336
Hydrogen peroxide, 199, 204
17-Hydroxylase, 173
Hyperbilirubinemia, 328
Hyperglycemia, 389
Hyperoxia, 203, 329
Hypertension, maternal
    chronic, 70, 71, 148, 149, 150
    gestational, 82, 102, 149
    and gestational age at birth, 617, 622
    and indicated preterm birth, 149, 630-
       631
    and IUGR, 70, 71
    maternal age and, 44
Hypertension, neonatal, 333
Hyperthyroidism, 149
Hypocarbia, 198
Hypoglycemia, 76, 200, 336
Hypoplastic left heart syndrome, 198
Hypotension, 198, 200, 293, 299, 323, 326,
    327, 333
Hypothalamic pituitary axis (HPA), 101,
    111, 170, 171-172, 177, 179, 180,
    185, 188, 269
Hypoxia, 203, 329
Hypoxia-ischemia, 198-199, 333

                              I

Ibuprofen, 293, 326
Illinois, 693
Immigrants, 458
Immune and inflammatory processes. *See
    also* Infection and inflammation,
    maternal
    environmental toxicants and, 251, 252
    gene-environment interactions, 187
    genetic factors, 212, 213-214
    mechanical ventilation and, 205
    stress and, 101, 110, 144, 179-180
Immunomodulators, 22, 196

Implantation, 187-188, 220
Imprisonment, 105
In vitro fertilization (IVF), 16, 17, 155, 156, 159, 160, 162, 163, 165, 166, 167. *See also* Assisted reproductive technologies
India, 42, 239, 388
Indian Health Service, 447
Indicated preterm birth
    alcohol use and, 93
    defined, 36, 149
    fetal conditions and, 150
    history of, 149
    hypertension and, 90, 149
    maternal age and, 45
    racial/ethnic disparities, 77-78
    rates, 608
    risk factors, 149, 150, 262, 609
Individuals with Disabilities Educational Act, 395 n.1, 460
Indomethacin, 293, 295, 326, 334, 336
Induction of labor, 43
Infant Health and Development Program, 393-394
Infant mortality rate. *See also* Neonatal mortality rates; Perinatal mortality rates
    ART and, 17, 162
    birth defects and, 150, 315
    birth weight and, 21, 446
    data collection, 79
    early intervention and, 82, 202
    fungal infections, 325
    gender differences, 77
    geographic variations, 627, 631, 634, 638
    gestational age at birth and, 3, 13, 31, 40, 72-74, 79, 287, 314-315, 406, 412, 627, 630, 632-635
    intranational and international comparisons, 315-316
    leading causes, 315
    neuroprotective substances and, 336
    prenatal care and, 465
    racial/ethnic disparities, 76, 77, 78, 112, 113, 130, 315-316, 630, 638-639
    regionalization and NICU access and, 21, 315, 468
    smoking and, 90
    trends, 31, 39-40, 77, 315, 351, 604, 605, 627, 630, 632-655
    unintended pregnancy and, 120

Infant Toddler Quality of Life Questionnaire, 383
Infection and inflammation, maternal. *See also individual agents and diseases*
    animal models, 22, 181, 184, 185, 186, 195-196, 199-200
    antibiotic treatment, 132, 151, 186, 196, 276-280, 625
    biomarkers of preterm birth risk, 269, 271
    and birth weight, 186, 278
    endometrial, 185, 188
    and fetal death, 186
    genetic factors, 187, 211, 213-214, 217, 220
    group B streptococcus, 185, 191, 263, 276
    immunomodulators, 196
    and implantation errors, 188
    intracervical inflammation, 282
    intrauterine, 22, 82, 181, 184-186, 189, 191, 195-196, 199-200, 625-626
    lifestyle factors and, 94
    lower genital tract, 185-186, 187; *see also* Bacterial vaginosis
    and neonatal lung injury, 203, 205, 319, 325, 326, 336
    neurodevelopmental effects, 325, 333, 378
    nosocomial, 343
    nutrition and, 95
    and parturition process, 21, 22, 36, 135, 176, 179-180, 184-187, 195-196, 199-200, 213-214, 251, 252, 265, 325
    periodontal, 110, 184, 186, 187, 265, 279-280
    and PPROM, 189, 190-191
    and preeclampsia, 186
    and preterm labor, 211, 295
    prevalence, 184
    and PWMD, 199-200, 317, 326, 335
    racial/ethnic disparities and, 26, 36, 50-51, 100, 130, 132, 133, 278
    sexual activity and, 99
    sexually transmitted, 27, 110, 132, 133, 135, 325
    socioeconomic disparities, 26-27, 135
    systemic, 186, 187, 279
    in underweight women, 151
Infertility and subfecundity
    causes, 158
    defined, 154

endometrial cancer and, 163
racial/ethnic disparities in, 158
and risk of preterm birth, 16, 154, 163
Infertility treatments. *See also* Assisted
  reproductive technologies
  data collection, 10, 157
  delay in seeking, 158
  economic barriers, 158, 168
  insurance coverage, 158, 165, 167, 168
  live births, 158
  maternal age and, 154
  and multiple gestations, 154, 159-168
  racial/ethnic disparities in, 158
  and risk of preterm birth, 155
  socioeconomic disparities, 158
  and spontaneous abortions, 158
  utilization rates, 154
Informed consent, 448, 449, 649-652, 653,
  655, 656, 658, 659, 663, 668, 681
Institute of Medicine, Roundtable on
  Environmental Health Sciences,
  Research, and Medicine, 32
Insulin growth factor binding protein-1, 220
Interagency Coordinating Council on Low
  Birth Weight and Preterm Birth, 446
Interleukin (IL)
  IL-1, 174, 179, 184, 187-188, 191, 200,
    213, 222
  IL-1α, 188, 212, 213, 222
  IL-1β, 185, 211, 212, 213
  IL-2, 212, 213, 222
  IL-6, 132, 179, 185, 200, 211, 212, 213,
    222, 270, 271
  IL-8, 174, 175, 181, 183, 185, 213, 271,
    282
  IL-10, 213, 222
Intermountain Healthcare (IHC) Health
  Plans cohort, 404-410, 426
International comparisons
  ART-related multiple gestations, 166-
    167
  data reporting, 43, 637-638
  genetic susceptibility, 209
  infant mortality rate, 315-316
  interpregnancy interval, 153
  life-sustaining medical treatment, 646,
    647, 648, 661, 668-670, 673
  low birth weight, 637
  preterm birth rates, 26, 42-43
International HapMap Project, 208
Interpregnancy interval, 152-154, 466

Interstitial collagenase, 175
Interventions for premature infants. *See*
  Neonatal lung disease/injury;
  Neurodevelopmental support; Post-
  NICU discharge interventions
  for cerebral palsy, 353
  early intervention programs, 11, 15, 82,
    202, 353, 380, 393-396, 399, 400,
    402, 422-423, 469-470, 718-719
  economic costs, 11, 399, 400, 402, 422-
    423
  educational, 393-395
  effectiveness, 15, 353, 380, 393-396,
    606, 690
  intrauterine, 448, 655-656
Intracytoplasmic sperm injection (ICSI),
  155, 156, 160, 164. *See also* Assisted
  reproductive technologies
Intraparenchyal hemorrhage (IPH), 333,
  334, 379
Intrauterine growth restriction (IUGR), 45,
  163, 606
  causes, 63, 69, 70, 148
  community environment and, 138
  and fetal death, 82
  maternal illness and, 148, 150
  and maturation rate, 70-71, 80, 217
  multiple gestations and, 63
  and preterm birth, 262
  smoking and, 217
  socioeconomic disparities and, 60
  stress and, 104, 107, 111, 138
  unintended pregnancy and, 120
Intrauterine insemination, 16, 45, 157, 160
Intraventricular hemorrhage (IVH),
  neonatal, 295, 296, 297, 298, 300,
  326, 331, 333-334, 336, 366, 379,
  385
IQ scores, 71, 349, 354-363, 370, 371, 394,
  425
Ireland, 42
Iron deficiency anemia, 94-95
Iron supplementation, 24, 94, 328
Israel, 239
Italy, 126, 243, 668

J

Japan, 42, 60
Jaundice, 76
Juvenile justice system, 28

K

Kaiser Permanente Medical Care System, 406, 407
Kessel, H., 605
Kopelman, Loretta, 649, 666
Krieger's measures of racism, 113

L

Labor. *See* Parturition process; Preterm labor
Lamellar body count, 66
Language disorders, 14, 32, 328, 348, 363, 369-370, 374, 394
Large for gestational age, 9, 58
Last menstrual period (LMP) for pregnancy dating, 60-62, 80
Lead exposure, 22, 141, 230, 231, 232, 247-248, 249, 252
Leapfrog Group, 468
Learning disabilities, 14, 32, 348, 363, 364-365, 369, 371, 374
Lecithin, 202
Lecithin/sphingomyelin (L/S) ratio, 66, 70
Leiomyomas, 158
Leukemia-inhibiting factor, 187
Liability issues, 34, 285, 438-439
Life-sustaining medical treatment. *See also* Mechanical ventilation; Neonatal intensive care units
  accuracy of physician prognoses, 651-652, 662
  attitudes of neonatologists, 666, 668
  Baby Doe regulations, 659, 663, 665-666, 668
  "best interests" standard, 645, 646, 648-649, 658, 666, 667, 669
  counseling for parents, 646, 651, 662
  delivery-room resuscitation, 72, 73, 74, 82, 647, 649, 650-651, 658-659, 660-662, 673-675
  EURONIC project, 661, 668-669
  euthanasia, 668, 669, 670
  futility-of-care concept, 664, 665-666, 671-672
  informed consent, 649-652, 659, 668
  international attitudes and practices, 646, 647, 648, 661, 668-670, 673
  legal precedents, 649-651, 658-659, 666
  pain management and palliative care, 660, 662, 663, 669, 670-671, 672

  parental wishes and rights, 649-652, 659, 660, 664, 665, 666, 667, 668
  personhood legislation and, 659-660
  professional guidelines, 662, 663, 667-668
  proxy decision making, 645-648, 663
  quality-of-life issues vs. value of life, 663, 664, 668, 669, 673
  religious beliefs and, 661, 672
  standard of care, 660-662
  at viability threshold, 314, 448, 450-451, 647, 658-662
  withholding and withdrawal, 662-672
Lindane, 239, 241
Lipopolysaccharide, 190, 196
Lithuania, 235, 668
Live births
  data reporting, 9, 60, 78, 79, 80, 81-82, 157
  defined, 73, 74
  infertility treatments and, 46-47, 157, 158, 159, 164, 165
Long-term care, 417, 418, 422, 459
Low birth weight, 120, 121, 137-142, 152, 153-154, 186, 278. *See also* Birth weight
  and adult disease risk, 386-389
  antenatal maternal steroids and, 299, 651
  ART and, 46, 162, 657
  defined, 57, 79
  family history, 22
  international comparisons, 42-43, 315
  IUGR and, 606
  preterm births, 606-607
  prior reports on, 34
  trends, 604
Lung. *See also* Asthma; Bronchopulmonary dysplasia; Fetal; Neonatal lung disease/injury; Respiratory distress syndrome; Restrictive lung disease, maternal
  phospholipid profile, 66
  surfactant production, 202
Lymphotoxin-alpha (LTA), 212, 213

M

Macrosomia, 181
Magnesium sulfate, 291, 293, 294, 300, 652
Magnetic resonance imaging, 333

Malaria, 325
Malaysia, 42
Malpractice insurance, 438-439, 441, 450-452
March of Dimes, 20, 33, 446, 467, 690, 706
    Basil O'Connor grants, 730
    Prematurity Campaign, 34-35, 605-606
Marijuana use, 93, 134
Marital status and preterm birth risk, 127-129, 135, 622, 628-629
Maryland, 168
Massachusetts, 168, 402, 422, 423, 660, 718
Maternal age
    and ART, 16, 45, 46-47, 159, 166, 167
    and cesarean delivery, 44
    and environmental toxicants, 246
    and indicated preterm deliveries, 45, 149
    and infertility treatments, 154
    and multiple gestations, 16, 45, 47, 159, 166
    protective effect of marriage, 127, 128
    and rehospitalization, 716
    and risk of preterm birth, 125-127, 135, 149, 265, 627, 628-629
    and tobacco use, 92
    and trends in preterm birth, 44-45, 125-127, 606
    and unintended pregnancy, 120
    weathering hypothesis, 126
Maternal and Child Health Bureau, 447, 462-463
    block grants, 19, 465
Maternal depression, 14, 47
Maternal-Fetal Medicine Units (MFMU) Network Study, 271-272, 298, 726
Maternal stature, 80
Maternal weight. *See also* Body mass index
    duration of gestation and, 94
    gain during pregnancy, 94, 151, 283
    interpregnancy interval and, 154
    obesity, 94, 148, 151-152
    prepregnancy, 93
    and spontaneous preterm birth, 151-152, 188, 265
    underweight, 109, 148, 151, 154, 188, 265, 276, 283
Matrix metalloproteinases (MMPs), 174, 177, 178, 182-183, 185, 195, 271
    MMP-1, 175, 183, 190, 191, 211, 215

MMP-2, 190, 215
MMP-3, 183, 191, 215
MMP-8, 175, 190, 211, 215
MMP-9, 175, 183, 187-188, 190, 191, 211, 215
    tissue inhibitors of (TIMP), 190, 191
Maturity/maturation. *See also* Gestational age; Measurement of maturity
    adaptations to adverse intrauterine conditions, 70-71, 80, 188
    defined, 8, 56
    and morbidity and mortality, 8, 56
    neurological, 67, 340-342
    racial/ethnic disparity in rate, 78
    signaling mechanisms for labor, 171-172, 179, 188
McHaffie, Hazel, 646, 648
Measurement of maturity
    ART and, 61
    biophysical profile, 66, 297
    birth weight as, 8, 25, 31, 34, 56-59, 62, 347
    comparability of methods, 613-614, 635-636
    definition of preterm birth and, 55, 57-59
    fetal growth curves, 58, 59, 63, 69-70
    functional, 68-69
    gestational age as proxy, 56-57, 59-65, 337, 609-614
    heterogeneity of preterm population, 69-76
    LMP, 60-62, 63, 78, 80, 610, 611, 612, 613, 614
    lungs, 66
    and management of care, 8, 72-76, 83, 337
    methods, 62, 85, 609-614
    obstetric, 610, 611, 612
    neurological, 67, 68-69
    physiological severity, 66-67
    postnatal, 62, 67-68, 78, 80, 81, 611-613
    public health implications, 79-81, 609-610
    quality of vital records, 79-81
    racial and ethnic disparities, 67-68, 76-78, 80, 612
    research implications, 10, 76-83, 612-614
    standards of practice, 80

ultrasound, 9, 10, 59, 62-65, 68-69, 78, 80, 81, 83, 85, 610-611, 612
validity and reliability, 610, 613
Mechanical ventilation, 202, 203-204, 205, 334, 340, 341, 342, 343, 403, 664-665, 666, 671-672, 710. *See also* Life-sustaining medical treatment
Medicaid, 19, 20, 28, 404, 406, 417, 456-460, 462, 464-465, 466
Medical care costs of preterm birth, 47, 604-605
   assistive devices, 418
   birth to early childhood, 47, 399, 400, 403-415
   birth weight or gestational age and, 401, 410-414, 428, 673, 674, 689, 694-695, 698-700, 704-705, 706-707, 711
   burden on minorities, 705
   burden on payers, 705-706
   categories of costs, 702, 704, 706
   characterization and estimates, 707-719
   co-morbid and resulting conditions, 11, 415, 707
   content limitations of studies, 704-707
   direct costs, 402, 415, 688, 707-717
   disability-specific beyond early childhood, 415-422
   ethical issues, 673-675
   geographic adjustment, 409-410, 426, 710
   initial hospitalization, 10-11, 406-409, 428, 688, 691-695, 701-702, 704-706, 707-712
   inpatient, 410-411, 412, 414, 417, 418
   lengths of stay, 406-409, 709, 710, 711
   long-term care, 417, 418, 422, 459
   maternal, 11, 47, 399, 400, 401, 402, 403, 426, 704-705, 709, 711
   national, 412, 421-422, 428
   nonsurvivors, 673, 674, 702
   outpatient, 411-412, 413, 414, 417, 422, 715, 717
   physician visits, 417, 418
   post-discharge, 167, 696-700, 702-704, 706-707, 712-719
   prescription medications, 418, 714
   public burden, 456-457
   readmissions, 408, 706, 707, 714-717
   therapy and rehabilitation, 418
   time horizon of studies, 706
   total, 411, 414

Medical and pregnancy conditions. *See also* Genetic susceptibility; Infection and inflammation, maternal; Infertility treatments; Maternal weight; *individual conditions*
   fetal, 150-151
   interpregnancy interval, 152-154
   and IUGR, 148, 150
   maternal, 148-150, 151-154
Medicare, 406, 417
Medline, 690-691
Meningitis, 325
Menstrual cycle, 60
Mental retardation, 14, 32, 47, 348, 353, 355-356, 374, 376, 399, 403, 415-421, 424, 425
Metabolic pathways, 215-216
Metabolomic technologies, 272
Metals and metalloids, 22, 230, 231, 232, 247-249, 252. *See also individual metals*
Metaproterenol, 291
Methodological issues
   aggregation bias, 130
   analytical challenges, 136, 224-228
   behavioral measures, 23-24, 90-91, 93
   birth weight as measure of prematurity, 56-59, 62, 347, 386
   community factors, 136, 144-146
   confounders, 24, 90, 93, 94, 97, 99, 101, 106, 121, 133, 136, 151, 180, 224-225, 226, 233, 235, 239, 242, 635
   cost studies, 691-707
   data management and integration, 78, 227
   diagnostic criteria, 14, 349, 701
   ecological-level effects, 145, 231, 233, 253
   exposure assessment, 231-232, 235, 239, 244, 245, 253
   follow-up studies, 14, 349
   generalizability of findings, 690, 702
   genetic studies, 223-228
   infant mortality rates, 315
   international comparisons, 42, 43, 112, 612, 637-638
   intervention research, 115, 116-118, 142
   maternal vs. fetal genes, 226
   measurement error, 130, 145, 231
   misclassification error, 130, 245
   modeling social context, 136, 139-140, 141-142, 144-146

multilevel studies, 141-142, 143, 144-147
multiple-gene testing, 225
nested data structures, 139
observational studies, 91, 95, 101-102,
    115-116, 136
outcome measures, 14, 25, 36, 59, 349
phenotype for preterm birth, 224
population admixture, 223, 225-226
psychosocial "exposure" assessments,
    97, 99, 101, 107, 109, 112, 114, 115
quality standards, 228
quasiexperimental designs, 107
recall/self-report, 90, 93, 114, 231, 245
reporting and replication of results, 228
sample selection criteria, 14, 118, 349,
    377, 701
sample size and power, 101, 227, 342,
    701
social exposure assessments, 144
terminological/linguistic, 4-5, 8, 36, 56,
    99, 112
Methyl-binding domain proteins, 218
Methylxanthines, 321, 341
Metronidazole, 151, 275, 276, 277, 278,
    279, 280
Metropolitan Atlanta Developmental
    Disability Surveillance Program, 403
Mexican women, 49, 105, 129, 133
Mexico, 42
MFM Units Network Preterm Prediction
    study, 152
Michigan, 242, 650, 727
Michigan State University, 727
Miller, Nikolaus T., 57
Minnesota, 697
Missouri, 467-468
Mitogen-activated protein kinase (MAPK)
    system, 181, 251
Mobiluncus, 269
Morphine, 340
Mortality rates. *See also* Infant mortality
    rate; Perinatal mortality
    clarifying, 81-83
    intra- and international comparisons,
        315-316
Moscow Foundling Hospital, 57
Müllerian duct abnormality, 149
Multiple gestations
    ART-related, 16-17, 45-47, 135, 154,
        157, 159-160, 161, 163-165, 424,
        606

and delivery method, 163
and gestational age at birth, 75, 161-
    162, 622
and IUGR, 63, 71
live birth rates, 45, 46, 164-165
maternal age and, 44, 45, 47, 159
maternal and child risks, 163-164
measurement of maturity, 80
mycotoxin exposure and, 241
and neuromaturation, 71
ovulation promotion and, 16, 17, 45,
    160-161
and PPROM, 189, 191
protective nutrients, 97
and rate of preterm birth, 45-46
reducing rates of, 164-168
reporting requirements, 45, 160
and risk of preterm birth, 12, 46, 47, 97,
    159-168, 265, 266, 270, 627, 630-
    631
socioeconomic differences and, 135, 158
spontaneous, 160, 161
twin-to-twin transfusion sequence, 150
ultrasound detection, 64
and uterine overdistension, 181
Mycoplasma hominis, 99
Mycoplasma species, 269
Mycotoxins, 241
Myosin, 175, 182, 290, 291
Myosin light-chain kinase (MLCK), 171,
    174, 175, 182, 291, 292
Myotonic dystrophy, 209

N

Narcotic abstinence syndrome, 341
National Center for Birth Defects and
    Developmental Disabilities, 447
National Center for Chronic Disease
    Prevention and Health Promotion,
    447
National Center for Complementary and
    Alternative Medicine, 447
National Center for Health Statistics, 9, 10,
    48, 79, 80, 84, 126, 127, 131, 401,
    447, 614
National Center on Minority Health and
    Health Disparities, 447
National Center on Quality Assurance, 18-
    19, 467

National Center for Vital Statistics, 691
National Early Intervention Longitudinal
    Study, 395-396
National Health Interview Survey, 417
    Disability Supplement, 415, 417
National Health and Nutrition Examination
    Survey (NHANES), 253, 375
National Human Genome Research
    Institute, 208
National Human Research Protection
    Advisory Committee, 448
National Institute on Alcohol Abuse and
    Alcoholism, 447
National Institute of Allergy and Infectious
    Disease, 447, 726
National Institute of Child Health and
    Human Development, 32-33, 35,
    152, 221, 279
    career development funding, 437, 447,
        727, 728
    Consensus Conference Panel, 298
    MFMU Network Study, 271-272, 298,
        300, 726
National Institute on Deafness and Other
    Communication Disorders, 447
National Institute of Dental and
    Craniofacial Research, 447
National Institute of Diabetes and Digestive
    and Kidney Diseases, 447
National Institute on Drug Abuse, 447, 726
National Institute of Environmental Health
    Sciences, 210-211, 447
National Institute of Mental Health, 447
National Institute of Neurological and
    Communicative Disorders and
    Stroke, 35, 300, 349
National Institute of Nursing Research, 447
National Institute of Occupational Safety
    and Health, 249
National Institutes of Health (NIH), 446,
    447
    Consensus Conference, 297
    F grants, 727, 728
    funding for preterm birth research, 227,
        452-453, 725-729
    K grants, 437, 727, 728
    Medical Scientist Training Program, 440
    MFMU network, 726, 727-728
    Neonatal Research Network studies, 728
    Office of Research on Women's Health,
        33, 158

P grants, 729
R grants, 436, 437, 438, 453-454, 727,
    728, 731
recommendations for, 7-8, 15, 17
Roadmap initiative, 7
trainee grants, 437, 727, 728-729
U grants, 436, 453, 727, 728
National Linked Birth Death Data Set, 678
National Medical Expenditure Survey, 417
National Survey of Family Growth, 158
National Vital Statistics System, 79
Necrotizing enterocolitis, 295, 296, 297,
    298, 317, 322-323, 326, 670, 677
Neighborhood conditions
    adverse, 24-25, 37, 136, 137-142, 471
    aggregations, 140
    and birth weight, 137-142
    environmental toxicants, 233, 250
    fixed effects models, 140
    index of disadvantage, 141
    individual-level interactions, 136, 140,
        142-143, 147
    physical, 138-139, 471
    random effects models, 140
    service, 137-138
    social and cultural characteristics, 137,
        142-143, 250
    socioeconomic context, 139-141, 142
Neonatal complications of preterm birth.
    See also Central nervous system
    complications; Neurodevelopmental
    disabilities; *individual conditions*
    animal models, 196-200, 202, 203, 206
    auditory, 328-329
    breastfeeding and, 338, 343
    cardiovascular, 198, 293, 295, 296, 297,
        298, 299, 300, 317, 320, 321, 323,
        326-327, 331, 333
    CNS, *see* Central nervous system
        complications
    gastrointestinal, 76, 295, 296, 297, 298,
        317, 320, 321, 322-324, 326, 327
    gestational age and, 3, 13-14, 76, 201-
        202, 314, 349
    hematologic, 87, 327-328
    iatrogenic, 349
    infections and immune system, 76, 322-
        323, 324-326, 331, 334, 343, 422
    jaundice, 336-337
    late-onset problems, 331
    management practices and, 343-344

near-term or late-preterm infants, 4, 14, 76, 336-337
ophthalmic, 67, 317, 326, 329-331
parenteral nutrition, 323
rehospitalization, 14, 202, 320, 380-381
respiratory, *see* Neonatal lung disease/injury
severity measures, 66-67
side effects of treatment, 300, 320, 322, 326, 328, 331, 334-335, 336
skin, 324
thermoregulation, 76, 336, 343
transfusions, 327-328
variations in rates, 56, 343-344
viability limit and, 324
Neonatal Individualized Developmental Care and Assessment Program (NIDCAP), 338, 342
Neonatal intensive care units (NICU). *See also* Life-sustaining medical treatment
access, 315, 317
costs of care, 403, 406, 429; *see also* Medical care costs of preterm birth
environment, 337-338
family-centered care, 338, 339
length of stay, 407, 408, 674
neurodevelopmental support, 337-343
nursing care, 468-469
organizational and management structures, 468-469
outcomes, 19, 349, 351, 468, 673, 674
quality of care, 18, 19, 20, 67, 408, 409, 466, 469-469
regionalization, 20, 21, 315, 316-317, 467, 468, 469, 701, 702
"trials of therapy," 672, 674
utilization rate, 406
volume and level of care, 468
Neonatal lung disease/injury. *See also* Respiratory distress syndrome
alveolarization disruption, 202-203
animal models, 202, 203, 206
apnea, 318, 321, 327
and asthma, 14, 321
BPD/CLD, 202, 297, 298, 317, 318, 319-321, 324, 327, 331, 336, 343, 378-379, 390
corticosterid treatment, 203, 299, 320
gastrointestinal reflux and, 323-324
gestational age at birth and, 201-202, 319

infection/inflammation and, 203, 205, 319, 325, 326, 336
long-term effects, 320, 321
mechanical ventilation and, 202, 203-204, 205, 299, 320, 328, 343
medications, 319-320, 321
and neurodevelopmental outcomes, 318, 319, 320, 321, 378-379
oxidative stress and, 204-205
pneumonia, 295, 319, 323, 325
positive end-expiratory pressure and oscillatory ventilation, 204, 319
pulmonary hypoplasia, 318
and reactive airway disease, 14, 32, 319, 323-324, 422
RSV infections, 320-321, 707
and SIDS, 321
surfactant deficiency, 66, 202, 204, 299, 318, 320
viral bronchiolitis, 320
Neonatal mortality rates, 73, 76, 77, 78, 79, 184, 292, 295, 314, 412, 677. *See also* Infant mortality rate; Perinatal mortality
Neonatal Research Network, 675, 726
NEOPAIN trial, 652
Netherlands, 163, 364, 383, 661, 668, 669, 670, 675
Neural tube defects, 269
Neurodevelopmental disabilities. *See also* Central nervous system complications; Cognitive impairment
antenatal maternal treatments, 299-300
assessment, 68-69
behavioral and socio-emotional problems, 14, 32, 349, 350, 370-372, 375, 376-377
birth weight and, 356, 357, 358-363, 364, 365, 366, 367, 368, 420-421
coordination disorders, 349-350, 353-354
early intervention, 15, 380, 393-396
economic costs of, 399, 403, 415-421
factors influencing outcomes, 318, 319, 320, 321, 378-380
functional outcomes, 349, 369, 374-377
gestational age and, 14, 349, 350-351, 352, 353, 366, 367, 372, 416, 419
hearing impairment, 14, 47, 328-329, 348, 367, 369-370, 371, 372, 376, 399, 403, 415-421, 424, 425
in late preterm or near-term infants, 4, 14, 374

lung disease/injury and, 318, 319, 320, 321
motor impairment, 14, 32, 47, 334, 335-336, 348-349, 350-354, 374, 375; *see also* Cerebral palsy
physical therapy and medical interventions, 353
predictors, 349, 379
prevalence, 349, 415, 416, 417, 419, 420-421
PWMD and, 335-336
risks of, 3, 14, 32, 325, 327
sensorimotor integration problems, 354
severity of, 14-15, 372-374
special education costs, 47
treatment-related risks, 334-335
visual impairment, 14, 47, 329-331, 348, 353, 354, 366-369, 371, 372, 375, 376, 399, 403, 415-421, 424, 425
Neurodevelopmental support
breastfeeding, 338
clustered care, 339
kangaroo care, 338, 343
NIDCAP, 338, 342
pain and discomfort, 339, 340
positioning and handling, 337-338, 340-342
sensory input in NICU environment, 338-339
and weight gain, 339, 343
Neuroendocrine processes, stress-related, 179
Neurofibromatosis, 209
Neurological morbidity. *See* Central nervous system complications; Neurodevelopmental disabilities
Neurotrophins, 214
Neutrophil collagenase, 175
Neutrophil elastase, 175
Nevada, 41
New Freedom Initiative, 463
New Jersey, 168, 423, 450, 675, 682
New York, 239, 242
New Zealand, 679
Niacin, 219
Nifedipine, 292-293
Nitrates, 240, 241, 252
Nitric oxide, 676
donors, 291, 294-295
and parturition process, 171, 173, 175, 213
synthase, 294

6-Nitro-7-sulfamoylbenzo(f)quinoxaline-2,3-dione, 199
L-Nitro-arginine methylester, 175
Nitroglycerin, 294-295
Nitrous oxides, 234-235, 236
North Carolina, 104, 679, 731
Norway, 42, 240-241, 248, 249, 265, 647
Nutrition, maternal. *See also* Maternal weight
access issues, 138
and birth weight, 95, 96, 134
cultural context, 142
dietary composition, 24, 94-95, 134
education, 472
and epigenetic modifications, 219
fish and fish oil, 96-97, 242
measurement of diet, 94
multivitamin supplements, 94
and PPROM, 189
prepregnancy weight, 93
and risk of preterm birth, 265, 273
socioeconomic disparities, 26, 133, 134
starvation, 194
vitamins and minerals, 24, 94, 95-97, 121, 189, 219, 247, 274
Nutrition, neonatal, 203, 338, 343
Nylidrin, 291

O

Obesity, 94, 134, 151-152
Office of Behavioral and Social Sciences Research, 158
Oligohydramnios, 293
Olive oil, 96-97
Operation Ranch Hand, 250
Ophthalmic impairment
amblyopia, 331, 366, 368
birth weight and, 366, 367, 368
cataracts, 331, 368
cortical visual impairments, 331, 368
CP-related impairment, 353
gestational age and, 366
glaucoma, 331, 368
lens anterior vascular capsule, 67, 329
optic nerve atrophy, 331, 368
plus disease, 330
refractive disorders, 331, 366, 368, 376
retinal detachment, 331, 368
ROP, 317, 326, 329-331, 366, 368, 375, 378, 384, 707
strabismus, 14, 331, 366

Oral contraceptive use, 60
Orciprenaline, 291
Organisation for Economic Co-operation and Development, 710
Organophosphate pesticides, 239-240, 241
Otitis media, 328
Outcomes for premature infants. *See also* Cognitive impairment; Neurodevelopmental disabilities
    accuracy of professional estimates of, 651-652
    antibiotic therapy and, 22, 132, 151, 186, 274, 275, 276-280
    ART and, 17, 46, 162, 657
    behavioral and socio-emotional problems, 14, 32, 47, 349, 350, 370-372, 375, 376-377, 381, 394, 396
    early intervention and, 15, 82, 202, 353, 380, 393-396, 469-470
    educational achievement, 365-366, 376, 377, 381, 394
    family impacts, 389-393, 395-396
    fetal-origins hypothesis, 386-389
    functional, 349, 369, 374-377, 384, 392, 396
    gestational age at birth and, 347-348
    growth, 3, 32, 320, 321, 381-382, 387, 388
    health, 3, 14, 32, 202, 320, 380-381, 386-389
    intact survival, 373-374
    maternal mental health and, 378, 380, 390
    measures, 14, 25, 36, 59, 349
    methodological issues, 14, 25, 36, 59, 347, 349, 377, 386-387, 396-397
    multiple disabilities, 371-372
    neonatal factors, 318, 319, 320, 321, 378-379
    prenatal and intrapartum predictors, 378
    quality of care and, 409, 465, 631, 633, 677-678
    quality of life, 383-386
    reporting, 15-16, 18, 45, 73-74, 155, 157
    research recommendations, 13-16, 349, 378, 392-393, 430-431, 484-485
    severity of disability and, 372-374, 390
    social support and, 390
    socioeconomic conditions and, 379-380, 396
    treatment interventions, 12, 288-301

Ovarian cancer, 163, 338
Ovulation hyperstimulation syndrome, 163
Ovulation promotion, 16, 17, 18, 45, 157, 160, 162, 163, 167, 168, 258
Oxidative stress, 197, 204-205
Oxytocin
    and parturition process, 170, 171, 172, 175, 178, 179, 215
    receptor antagonists, 291, 293-294
    receptors, 174, 177, 181, 215, 294
Ozone, 234, 235, 236-237

P

p53 protein, 191
Pancuronium, 334
Papiernik, Émile, 605
Parathyroid hormone-related peptide, 171
Parity, and risk of preterm birth, 628-629
Parturition process
    animal models, 22, 181, 184, 185, 186, 187, 192-196, 199-200, 251, 254
    ART and, 177
    behavioral response, 180-181
    Braxton-Hicks contractions, 171
    cervical ripening, 170, 172, 174-175, 181
    CRH and, 170, 172-173, 174, 176, 179, 180, 187, 215
    decidual and fetal membrane activation, 170, 172, 174, 175
    decidual hemorrhage and, 17, 182-183
    environmental toxicants and 251-252, 254
    estrogens and, 172, 173-174, 175, 179, 187, 215
    gene-environment interactions and, 177, 187
    implantation errors and, 187-188
    infection and inflammation and, 21, 22, 36, 135, 176, 179-180, 184-187, 195-196, 199-200, 213-214, 251, 252, 265, 325
    intrauterine vascular lesions and, 176-177
    involution, 170, 175
    maternal health risk, 13
    myometrial activation, 170, 171-172, 263
    myometrial stimulation, 170, 171, 172-175

NIH research portfolio, 726-727
normal pathways, 170-176
obesity and, 94
oxytocin and, 170, 171, 172, 174, 175, 177, 178, 179, 181, 215, 293
placental clock, 111, 172-173, 176, 177-181, 188
preterm pathogenesis, 12, 111, 176-189
progesterone and, 171, 172, 173, 174, 179, 181, 187, 215
prostaglandins and, 96, 170, 171, 172, 173, 174-175, 177, 178, 184, 185, 195, 215, 251, 293
quiescence, 170, 171, 173, 292
research needs, 189
signaling mechanisms for labor, 68, 110, 171-173, 179, 185, 251
stress and, 111, 177-181
uterine contractility, 170, 171, 172, 174, 175, 182, 185, 215, 251
uterine overdistension and, 181
uteroplacental thrombosis and, 182-183, 214-215
Parvovirus infection, 82
Patent ductus arteriosus, 198, 293, 297, 326-327
Paternal
exposure to environmental toxicants, 240, 243, 249-250
perceptions of impacts, 391
rights, 448, 680-681
Pennsylvania, 234, 450, 664, 696
Perhydroxyl, 204
Perinatal care. *See also* Neonatal intensive care units
access to, 673, 676-678
evidence-based selective referral, 20-21, 468
quality of, 19, 20, 31-32, 133, 469, 631, 633, 676
regionalization, 20, 316-317, 676
Perinatal mortality
antenatal maternal treatment and, 297, 298, 300
ART and, 657
data reporting, 10, 82
defined, 73-74, 82
gestational age and, 288
regionalization and NICU access and, 289, 292, 677-678
viability limit and, 73-74, 82, 630

Periodontal infections, 110, 184, 186, 187, 265, 279-280
Peritonitis, 323
Periventricular white matter disease (PWMD)
animal models, 196-197, 199-200
antenatal corticosteroid therapy and, 297
cerebral atrophy, 334, 335, 336, 379
cerebral white matter lesions, 196, 197, 199-200
cerebrovascular regulatory impairment and, 198, 333, 335
hypoperfusion and, 197
incidence, 196
infection or inflammation and, 199-200, 317, 326, 335
and neurodevelopmental diabilities, 335-336
periventricular leukomalacia, 196-197, 199-200, 297, 298, 333, 335, 336, 366, 379
pre-OL vulnerability, 198-199, 335
and strabismus, 366
in ventilated premature infants, 198
Peroxisome proliferator-activated receptors, 252
Personal resources, 118-120, 127
Personal Responsibility Work Opportunity and Reconciliation Act, 462
Personhood, 653, 659-660
PGDH, 174
PGE, 181
PGE2, 174, 191
PGF2α, 174
PGHS, 174
PGHS-2, 181
Pharmacogenetics Research Network and Knowledge Base (PharmGKB), 227
Phenobarbital, 300, 334
Philippines, 153
Phosphatidylglycerol, 66
Phospholipase A$_2$, 191, 251
Phospholipase C, 182
Phthalates, 252, 253
Phthisis, 331
Physical activity
leisure, 24, 99
neonatal, 341
occupational demands, 26, 36, 97-99, 110, 121, 133, 134-135, 136, 149, 265, 471

protective effects, 99, 341
    reduction, 273, 282, 283
Physiological severity measures, 66-67
Placenta previa, 163, 262, 265
Placental
    abruption, 45, 70, 90, 150, 162-163,
        182, 183, 189, 265
    clock, 172-173, 177-181
    infarction, 70
    separation, 175
Plasmin, 175
Platelet-activating factor, 205
Pneumonia, neonatal, 295, 325
Pneumothorax, 202, 334
Poland, 248
Polybrominated diphenyl ethers, 252
Polychlorinated biphenyls, 241-243, 251
Polyhydramnios, 181, 191, 209, 610
Porencephaly, 379
Post-NICU discharge interventions
    Avon Premature Infant Project, 394-395
    early infant and childhood, 393-394
    National Early Intervention Longitudinal
        Study, 395-396
Post-term infants, 80
Post-traumatic stress disorder, 112
Postdate pregnancy, 263
Postmenstrual age, 61, 69
Postpartum endometritis, 185
Prediction/predictors of preterm birth
    biological, 220, 269-271
    biophysical, 267-269, 270, 272
    Bishop scores, 267
    cervical examination, 267, 268-269
    clinical, 265-267
    fetal fibronectin, 267, 270, 271, 272
    lower genital tract markers, 269, 270,
        271, 272
    multiple-marker approach, 271-273
    rationale for, 264-265, 272
    research needs, 272-273
    sensitivity, 3, 270
    serum biomarkers, 269, 270
    uterine contractions, 267-268
Preeclampsia, 45, 70, 82, 148, 150, 162,
    163, 186, 188, 219, 220, 221, 262,
    263, 655
Pregnancy Outcomes in Community Health
    Study, 729
Pregnancy Risk Assessment Monitoring
    System, 105, 120

Premature rupture of membranes (PROM).
    See also Preterm premature rupture
    of membranes
    corticosteroid therapy, 297
    defined, 182
    emotional and affective factors, 111
    lead exposure and, 247
    mechanisms, 183, 220
    nutrition and, 95
    occupational fatigue and, 98
    prolonged, 70
    smoking and, 90
Prenatal care. See also Neonatal intensive
    care units; Perinatal care
    access to, 9, 19, 26-27, 34, 36, 64, 133,
        143, 273, 282, 316
    data reporting on, 79, 81
    focus of, 263
    Medicaid eligibility, 19, 465
    and preterm birth rate, 131, 139, 143,
        265, 465, 633
    prior reports on, 34
    racial/ethnic disparities and, 26-27, 36,
        64, 131, 133, 679
    socioeconomic conditions and, 133, 135,
        143
    stress and, 181
    time of initiation, 79, 81, 606
    ultrasound standard, 9, 64, 83
Prenatal counseling, 651
Prenatal education, 101
Prenatal stress, maternal
    animal models, 102, 180
    behavioral response, 180-181
    biological responses, 101, 110, 144,
        179-180, 626
    and birth weight, 104, 180
    catastrophic events, 24, 27, 105-106,
        107, 111, 121, 180
    chronic exposures, 24, 27, 105, 106-
        107, 110, 111, 121, 135, 137, 142,
        180, 626
    community context, 137, 142, 143-144
    coping strategies, 137, 180
    cultural considerations, 26, 36, 111-112,
        142
    defined, 177
    developmental effects, 102
    domestic/personal violence, 24, 110, 135
    emotional components, 24, 102, 103,
        104, 107-109, 110, 111, 121-122

fetal response, 71, 102, 104
gestational age and, 104
household strain, 110
immune and inflammatory processes, 101, 110, 144, 179-180
intervention trials, 101
life events, 24, 103, 104-105, 108, 112, 121, 132, 135, 181, 625
linking mechanisms, 110-111
measuring, 146
methodological issues, 101, 103-104, 146, 180
and neurobehavioral indices, 102
neuroendocrine processes, 144, 179
observational studies, 101
occupational/work, 47, 97, 109-110, 135
physiologic reactivity, 111
and placental clock, 177-181
and racial/ethnic disparities, 105, 106-107, 109, 112, 113-114, 130, 132, 133
racism and discrimination and, 24, 113-114, 123, 132, 136
reduction, 273, 282
research recommendations, 122-123
and risk of preterm birth, 265
socioeconomic conditions and, 27, 97, 106-107, 112, 113, 135, 142
unintended pregnancy and, 120, 135
vulnerable time during pregnancy, 108
Preterm Birth Among Inner City Women: Bacterial Vaginosis, Stressors and Race project, 729
Preterm labor, 608-609. *See also* Parturition process
antibiotic therapy, 273, 295-296
anxiety and, 108, 111
bed rest, 275
clinical evidence, 263
contraction monitoring, 274, 275, 276
diagnosis, 12, 220, 268, 273, 284-287, 289-290
efficacy of interventions, 289
ethical issues, 287
genetic markers, 223
history of, 107, 274, 275
infections/inflammation and, 211, 295
racial/ethnic disparities, 77
and risk of preterm birth, 267-268, 286-287, 608

sexual activity and, 99
symptoms, 284
tocolytic agents and, 184, 273, 275, 276, 280, 285, 289, 290-295
twins, 275
Preterm Prediction Study, 93, 94, 271-272
Preterm premature rupture of membranes (PPROM), 608. *See also* Premature rupture of membranes
antibiotic therapy and, 278, 296, 727
genetic susceptibility, 211-212, 223
potential mechanisms, 183, 190-191, 211
previous, 189
racial/ethnic disparities, 77-78, 211-212
risk factors, 189-190, 608-609
uteroplacental thrombosis and, 182-183
Prevention of preterm birth. *See also* Treatment interventions
antibiotic therapy, 22, 132, 274, 275, 276-280
cerclage, 273, 274, 281-282
early detection and suppression of labor, 264, 273, 275-276
economic evaluation, 427-428
efficacy of interventions, 12, 264, 272-283, 633
focus of efforts, 3, 264
medical interventions, 273-280
neighborhood interventions, 143
nonmedical interventions, 273, 274, 282-283
preconception care, 264, 278-279
progesterone supplements, 272, 273, 274, 280-281
research needs, 4
surgical interventions, 273, 281-282
Prevotella, 269
Progesterone
antagonist, 194
and parturition process, 171, 172, 173, 174, 179, 181, 187, 192
receptor, 173, 215
supplements, 272, 273, 274, 280-281, 727-728, 729-730
Project on Human Development in Chicago Neighborhoods, 143
Prolactin, 214
Prostacyclin (PGI2), 171
Prostaglandins
H2 synthase, 173

and parturition process, 96, 170, 171,
    172, 173, 174-175, 177, 178, 184,
    185, 186, 191, 195, 251
  receptors, 174, 215
Protease-activated receptors, 182
Proteinuria, 149
Proteoaminoglycans, 174-175
Proteomics, 219-221, 272
Psychosocial factors. *See also* Prenatal
    stress, maternal
  emotional response and affective states,
    110-111, 121-122
  individual-level perspective, 37, 89, 123
  intendedness of pregnancy, 24, 118,
    120-121, 123
  personal resources, 118-120, 123
  research recommendations, 122-123
  social support, 115-118, 122, 136
  violence, 24
Public health databases, 79-81
Public policies and programs. *See also*
    individual programs
  coordination of, 469-470
  early intervention, 28, 469-470
  economic burdens of preterm birth, 28,
    456-472
  education, 28, 456, 460
  expenditures, 456-463
  financing health care, 28, 456-460, 462-
    63, 464-466, 470
  foster care, 456, 458, 463
  income supports, 28, 456, 457, 459,
    460-462, 470
  juvenile justice, 458, 463
  options for improving outcomes, 464-472
  pro-family, 471
  quality-of-care initiatives, 466-469
  research recommendations, 6-7, 28-29,
    474-475, 479, 491-492
  social reforms, 470-472
Puerto Rican women, 49, 129
Pyelonephritis, 279

                              Q

Quality of care
  managed care and, 467
  measures of, 467
  NICU, 18, 20, 466
  perinatal, 466-469
  prenatal, 18-19, 20

  racial/ethnic disparities, 77
  regionalization and, 20, 467-469, 676
Quality of life, 383-386, 428, 663, 668, 669

                              R

Racial/ethnic disparities, 638-639. *See also*
    individual racial or ethnic groups
  access to care, 315, 678
  behavioral and social factors, 26, 27, 36,
    92, 100, 129-131, 133
  birth weight, 25, 63, 70, 76, 77, 105,
    112, 113, 114, 121, 130, 138-139,
    140, 154, 209
  classification of racial and ethnic groups,
    48, 221
  community context, 136, 137, 138-139,
    140
  educational attainments and, 130
  etiology of preterm birth, 77-78
  exposure to environmental toxicants,
    138, 233, 235, 240, 250-251
  fetal maturation rate, 78
  gene-environment interactions, 132-133,
    223
  genetic influences, 26, 27, 130, 132,
    152, 209, 211-212, 221-223
  gestational age distributions at birth,
    619
  gestational age estimates, 67-68, 76-78,
    80, 612
  geographic differences, 638-639
  infant mortality rates, 26, 36, 50-51, 76,
    77, 78, 112, 113, 130, 315-316, 630,
    638-639
  infections, 26, 27, 36, 50-51, 100, 130,
    132, 133, 278
  infertility problems, 158
  interpregnancy interval, 153
  intra- and inter-group variations, 129,
    146
  life-course perspective, 37
  marital status-related risks, 125, 127,
    128
  maternal-age-related risks, 126, 127, 128
  measuring risk, 138
  nativity and duration of residence and,
    26, 129, 133, 140, 146, 628-629
  prenatal care, 9, 26-27, 36, 64, 131, 133
  prenatal stress, 26, 27, 36, 111-112,
    130, 132, 133

psychosocial factors and, 105, 106-107, 109, 112, 113, 114, 119, 132
quality of care, 77
rates of preterm birth, 4, 5, 12, 26-27, 36, 48-49, 76, 105, 106-107, 109, 112, 113, 120-121, 126, 130, 133, 465, 631
research recommendations, 6, 26-27, 48, 147, 158, 257, 490-491
risk of preterm birth, 106-107, 109, 120-121, 126, 129-135, 149, 151, 152, 209, 233, 265, 271, 628-629
sociodemographic risk factors, 125, 126, 129-133
socioeconomic disparities, 26, 51, 106-107, 112, 113, 114, 120-121, 125, 129, 130, 133-135, 147, 250
vital record reporting, 617
Racism and discrimination, 24, 36, 113-114, 132, 471, 678
RAND Corporation, 465
Reactive airway disease, 14, 32, 319, 323-324, 422
Reactive oxygen species, 191, 205
Recombinant human erythropoietin, 329, 336
Recommendations. *See* Research recommendations
Rehabilitation Act of 1973, 665
Rehabilitation services, 459
Relaxin, 171, 215, 270
Renal disorders, maternal, 149
Reporting. *See* Data reporting on preterm birth
Reproductive research. *See* Clinical research on preterm birth
Reproductive Scientist Development Program, 437
Research recommendations. *See also* Clinical research on preterm birth; Funding for clinical research and training
behavioral and psychosocial risk factors, 23-26, 122-123
causes of preterm birth, 255-258
clinical and health services research, 6, 12-21, 473-474, 482-488
data collection, 6, 8-10, 84-85, 480-482
delivery of health care, 19-21, 474, 488
diagnosis and treatment, 12-13, 308-309, 483-484

economic consequences, 6, 10-12, 431, 482
etiology of preterm birth, 6, 21-23, 188, 255-256, 488-489
evaluation of public programs and policies, 6-7, 28-29, 474-475, 479, 491-492
infertility treatments, 16-18, 257-258, 485-487
multidisciplinary research centers, 6, 7-8, 473-474, 479-480
multiple gestations, 16-18, 258, 485-487
multiple risk factors, 256-257, 489-490
outcomes of preterm birth, 13-16, 349, 430-431, 484-485
priorities, 6, 8-27, 478-479, 480-491
quality of care, 18-19, 474, 487
racial/ethnic and socioeconomic disparities, 6, 26-27, 48, 257, 490-491
Respiratory distress syndrome
antenatal maternal steroids and, 77, 296, 297, 298, 299-300, 318
biological mechanisms, 66, 202
gestational age at birth and, 76, 318, 336
incidence, 318, 336
inflammation and, 205
management practices and, 343
mortality rate, 202, 318
racial/ethnic disparities, 77, 318
respiratory support, 204, 296, 318-319, 403
surfactant therapy, 202, 204, 296, 299-300, 318, 690, 728
thyrotropin releasing hormone and, 300
Respiratory syncytial virus (RSV), 320-321, 707
Restrictive lung disease, maternal, 149
Resuscitation at delivery, 72, 73, 74, 82, 647, 649, 650-651, 658-659, 673-675
Retinoblastoma, 164
Retinopathy of prematurity (ROP), 317, 326, 329-331, 366, 368, 375, 378, 384, 707
Retroplacental hematomas, 183
Rhode island, 168
Risk factors for preterm birth. *See also* Prediction/predictors of preterm birth
behavioral and psychosocial, 625-626
demographic, 625
efficacy of interventions by, 274-275

for indicated preterm birth, 149, 150, 262

medical, 624, 625

multifactoral nature of, 5, 37, 626

mutable, 626

sensitivity of biomarkers, 270

strongest factors, 12, 265-267

trends in preterm birth by, 624-627, 628-631, 632

Risk factors for rehospitalization, 716

Ritodrine, 291-292, 294-295

Robert Wood Johnson Foundation, 467

RU-486, 194

Rubella, 263, 325

Russian Federation, 42, 243

S

Salbutamol, 291

Saturated phosphatidylcholine, 66

Scoring for Neonatal Acute Physiology, 67

Scotland, 26, 133, 646, 647

Sepsis, neonatal, 76, 295, 296, 298, 323, 325, 330, 331, 334

Sexual activity, 99, 377

Sexually transmitted infections, 27, 110, 132, 133, 135, 325

Shake test, 66

Sickle cell disease, 222

Single mothers, 127, 129, 135, 606, 617, 628-629

Single-nucleotide polymorphisms (SNPs), 210, 211, 216, 224

Small for gestational age, 4, 36, 58-59, 69-70, 79, 97-98, 212, 315, 386, 387, 606, 607, 609, 637, 657

Smith-Lemli-Opitz syndrome, 209

SNP Consortium Ltd., 209

Social Security Administration, 461

Social support

and birth weight or fetal growth, 116, 143

conceptualizations, 115

defining and measuring, 115

emotional support, 115

information, 115

instrumental aid, 115

intervention research, 101, 115, 116-118

marital status and, 127

neighborhood environment and, 137, 143

observational studies, 115-116

and outcomes, 390

Societal costs of preterm birth. *See also* Medical care costs of preterm birth

aggregate annual, 31, 47, 399

caregiver, 402, 426-427

cognitive impairment, 399, 403, 415-421, 424, 425

cost-effectiveness and cost-utility analyses, 689-690

cost-of-illness methodology, 402-403, 688, 689

data sources and search strategies, 690-691

definitions, 688-689

direct costs, 402, 415, 688, 707-717

early intervention services, 11, 399, 400, 402, 422-423, 675

economic evaluation of preventive measures, 427-428

education, 11, 47, 399, 400, 401, 402, 403, 415, 417, 423-424, 456, 457, 675, 706, 717-719

ethical issues, 673-679

family, 3, 47, 371, 402, 426-427, 459, 675, 676, 706, 712

indirect (household and labor market productivity), 11, 47, 399, 400, 402, 403, 415, 417, 425, 712, 713, 719, 720

international comparisons, 690, 692-699, 707, 710

methods, 689-691

per patient, 399, 691, 705, 707, 708, 710, 711-712

policy and research recommendations, 6, 10-12, 431, 482, 721-722

population description, 689-690

projections, 691

public programs, 28, 456-463

studies of, 691, 692-700

Society for Assisted Reproductive Technology, 165

Society for Maternal-Fetal Medicine, 33, 437

Society for Pediatric Research, 690

Sociodemographic risk factors. *See also* Geographic differences; Maternal age; Racial/ethnic disparities; Socioeconomic conditions

birth defects, 151

and impacts of preterm birth, 14-15
marital or cohabitation status, 127-129,
  135, 628-629
Socioeconomic conditions
  and behavioral factors, 90, 93, 133, 134-
    135
  and birth weight, 139-140
  clustering of disadvantages, 138
  community context, 139-141, 142, 233
  confounding in behavioral and
    psychosocial studies, 90, 93, 94, 97,
    98, 121, 133
  and costs of preterm birth, 718
  distributive justice issues, 678-679
  exposure to environmental toxicants,
    232-233, 240, 250
  infections, 26-27, 135
  international comparisons, 133
  mediators of preterm birth, 133-135
  and multiple gestations, 135, 158
  and nutrition, 94, 95, 133, 134
  and outcomes of preterm birth, 379-380,
    396
  and personal resources, 119
  prenatal care, 135
  and racial/ethnic disparities, 51, 129,
    130, 133-135, 147
  and risk of preterm birth, 4, 5, 24, 26,
    36, 51, 60, 98, 126, 133-135, 136,
    470-471, 628-629
  and stress, 27, 97, 106-107, 112, 135,
    142
Sodium nitroprusside, 175
Solvents, 249
South Africa, 42
South Carolina, 77, 677
Spain, 26, 42, 133, 239, 247-248
Special education, 11, 47, 363, 364, 399,
  400, 415, 417, 423-424, 458, 460,
  673, 717-718
Special Education Expenditure Project, 424
Spina bifida, 150
Spontaneous preterm birth, defined, 36. *See
  also* Parturition process
State Children's Health Insurance Program
  (SCHIP), 19, 457, 458, 465
Stem cells, 327
Strabismus, 14, 331, 366
Streptokinase, 333-334
Stress. *See also* Prenatal stress, maternal
  defined, 100-101
  on families, 47

neonatal, 340
oxidative, 204-205
Substance Abuse and Mental Health
  Services Administration, 447
Sudan, 42
Sudden infant death syndrome (SIDS), 321
Sulindac, 293
Sulfur dioxide, 22-23, 231, 233-234, 235-
  236, 237, 252
Superovulation therapies, 16, 17, 18, 45,
  157, 160, 258
Superoxide, 199, 204
Supplemental Security Income, 28, 457,
  458, 459, 460-462
Survey of Income and Program
  Participation, 417, 425
Sweden
  end-of-life practices, 668
  health care policies, 26, 166-167, 168,
    470, 677
  preterm birth studies and statistics, 42,
    110, 133, 209, 234, 248, 351, 353,
    369, 376, 677
Switzerland, 42
Sympathoadrenal-medullary (SAM) system,
  179
Syphilis, 325
Systemic lupus erythematosus, 148, 149,
  150

T

Taiwan, 244
Tay-Sachs disease, 222
Temporary Assistance to Needy Families,
  28, 458, 459, 462, 470, 471
Terbutalin, 291, 292
Termination of pregnancy
  induced, 64, 73, 657, 660, 681
  spontaneous abortion, 60, 81, 188
Terrorist attacks of 9/11, 105-106, 111
Tetracycline, 276, 278
Texas, 650, 696
Th1-type cytokine, 188
Th2-type cytokines, 188
Thailand, 97-98
Theophylline, 321
Thompson, Tommy, 446
Thrombin, 177, 182-183, 191
Thrombin-antithrombin III (TAT) complex,
  183, 269

Thrombin receptor agonist peptide type 14, 191
Thrombophilias, 82
Thromboxane B$_2$, 205
Thyroid disease, 82
Thyroxine, 336
Title V Maternal and Child Health programs, 28, 458, 462-469
Tobacco use
  and birth weight, 90, 217, 283
  confounding in environmental studies, 235
  cultural context, 142
  gene-smoking interaction, 217
  and gestational age at birth, 622
  and hypertension, 91
  interventions, 101
  and IUGR, 217
  maternal age and, 92
  as outcome of preterm birth, 371
  prenatal stress and, 181
  and preterm birth, 36, 90, 91-92, 130-131, 134, 136, 217, 266, 317, 622, 630-631
  prevalence, 217
  and PPROM, 189, 191
  racial/ethnic disparities and, 27, 36, 92, 131, 317, 679
  and rehospitalization risk, 716
  second-hand smoke, 22, 231, 245-247, 252, 321
  socioeconomic conditions and, 90, 133, 134
  unintended pregnancy and, 120
Tocolytic (labor-inhibiting) agents, 184, 273, 280, 290-295
Toll-like receptors, 187, 211, 214
Topiramate, 199
Toxics Release Inventory, 253
Toxoplasma, 325
Training clinical researchers
  costs, 438
  funding, 436, 437
  length of training, 438-439
Transforming growth factor, 214
Treatment interventions. *See also* Antibiotics; Life-sustaining medical treatment
  antenatal, to reduce neonatal morbidity, 12, 77, 74, 287, 289, 291, 295-300, 318
  CNI complications, 333-334, 336

  corticosteroids, 296-299, 334
  informed decision making, 287-288, 289
  maternal transfer, 12-13, 287, 289, 291, 292, 295, 300-301
  off-label medicine use, 447-448
  strategies and effectiveness, 12, 288-301
  tocolytic drugs, 184, 273, 275, 276, 290-295
Trends in preterm birth
  ART and, 45-47, 617
  data reporting issues, 635-636
  delivery method, 43-44, 622, 623
  extremely low risk mothers, 622, 624
  geographic differences, 40-41, 614-617, 618, 620-621, 630, 631
  by gestational age, 2-3, 31, 38-39, 614, 615, 616, 619, 623
  hypertensive or diabetic mother, 617, 622
  infant mortality rate, 39-40, 627, 630-631, 632-625
  international comparisons, 42-43
  marital status, 617
  maternal age, 44-45, 617, 632
  multiple births, 45-47, 617, 622, 623
  racial/ethnic disparities, 614, 616, 617, 619-622, 631
  rates, 2-3, 38, 406, 604, 614-617
  by risk factor, 624-627, 628-631, 632
  singleton, 39
  smokers, 617, 622
  socioeconomic status, 622-623
Trichloroacetic acid, 244
Trichomonas vaginalis, 99, 277, 279
Trihalomethanes, 244, 245
Tryptophan, 219
Tumor necrosis factor-alpha (TNF-α), 132, 174, 179, 185, 191, 200, 205, 211, 212, 213-214, 217, 269, 271

U

Ultrasound
  access to, 64, 611
  cervical evaluation, 268-269, 271, 281-282, 285
  costs and benefits, 64-65, 68
  cranial, 68
  gestational age measurement, 9, 10, 59, 62-65, 68-69, 78, 80, 81, 83, 85, 610-611, 612

neuroimaging, 333, 335
safety, 65
standards of practice, 9, 64, 83
timing of, 80
training of personnel, 83, 611
weight estimates by, 70
Underweight women, 109, 148, 151, 154, 188
Unintended pregnancy, 24, 120-121, 135
United Arab Emirates, 153
United Kingdom, 42, 385, 394-395, 409, 376, 668, 675-676, 690, 692, 693, 696, 697, 712
United Nations Children's Fund (UNICEF), 42
University of California at San Francisco, 664
University of Chicago, 665, 672, 674
University of Michigan, 727
University of North Carolina, 661
Urban Institute, 463
Ureaplasma urealyticum, 185, 270, 276
Urinary tract infections
maternal, 110, 132, 133, 184, 276
neonatal, 325
U.S. Collaborative Perinatal Project, 238
U.S. Department of Education, 15
Office of Special Education Programs, 395
U.S. Department of Health and Human Services, 446, 448
U.S. National Maternal and Infant Health Survey, 209
U.S. Office of Management and Budget, 48
Utah Birth Defects Prevention Network, 150
Uterine
abnormality, 266
artery resistance, 102
contractility/contractions, 170, 171, 172, 174, 175, 182, 185, 215, 251, 267-268, 291
overdistension, 181, 269
stretch, 170, 171, 181
tumors, 158
Uterine-derived catecholestrogen, 187
Uteroplacental
genetic pathways, 214-215
insufficiency, 63, 69, 611
thrombosis, 182-183

V

Vaginal bleeding, 12, 62, 183, 191, 265
Vaginal microflora, 100
Vaginosis. *See* Bacterial vaginosis
Vascular epithelial growth factor, 187
Ventricular peritoneal (VP) shunt, 333-334
Vermont, 651
Vermont Oxford Network, 404, 408, 409, 468, 469
Very low birth weight, 21, 47, 59, 79, 105, 113, 114, 196, 202-203, 325, 403-404, 409, 423, 468, 646, 657
Viability threshold, 65, 314, 448, 450-451, 647, 658-662, 681
Vietnam, 243, 250
Violence, 24, 110, 138
Virginia, 41, 671-672
Visual processing and perceptual deficits, 362-363, 365, 368-369, 394. *See also* Ophthalmic impairment
Vital records, 43
Vitamin A, 319
Vitamin C, 24, 95, 189, 274
Vitamin E, 274, 331, 334
Vitamin K, 300, 334

W

Wayne State University, 727
Weight. *See* Maternal weight
West Africa, 240
Whites (non-Hispanic)
alcohol use, 27
birth certificate data, 81
birth weights, 77, 130, 140, 209, 679
BMI (maternal), 151
douching practices, 100
educational attainment, 130
estimates of gestational age in, 67-68
illicit drug use, 27
income and net worth, 146
infant mortality rate, 51, 130, 630
infections/inflammation, 27, 100, 132, 222
infertility, 158
interpregnancy interval, 153
IUGR, 107
marital status, 128
maternal age, 128
multiple births, 617

neighborhood environment, 137, 138,
140, 143
prenatal care, 131
rate of preterm birth, 5, 26, 48, 76, 128,
130, 315, 614, 616, 617, 620-621,
622, 678, 679
risk of preterm birth, 209, 212, 265
stress, 107, 108, 132
tobacco use, 27, 92, 131, 617
WIC program, 470
Wisconsin, 242, 659, 665, 666, 682, 693
Women's Reproductive Health Research
program, 437
World Health Organization, 42, 57, 72, 383

Y

Yaffe, S., 605
Yeast infection, 277

Z

Zinc supplementation, 95
Zygote intrafallopian transfer (ZIFT), 155,
156. *See also* Assisted reproductive
technologies